Contents

Preface

The first edition of this book was a monograph written by the late H Brendan Devlin and was a landmark in the scientific analysis of surgery of the abdominal wall, which discarded many of the older out of date concepts. We are heavily indebted to Brendan not only for providing the basis for this text but also for the inspiration to follow along a line of inquiry for evidence based material to present to our readers. At the same time we have not neglected the important historical and economic aspects of hernia surgery and some of our own personal views. Andrew Kingsnorth assisted Brendan in writing the 2nd edition of this book and Karl Le Blanc now adds an entirely new perspective from North America with particular emphasis on the use of prosthetic materials and laparoscopic techniques.

We have thoroughly revised and added to all the chapters resulting in an increase in material of approximately 50% and the addition of hundreds more up to date references. We have also provided the reader with clear line drawings of operative techniques, photographs and several short video clips on CD-Rom which are referred to/referenced in the text by the icon (CD). This extra effort should allow the reader the ability to adopt and apply much of the information and operative techniques that are presented. The technological revolution that began a decade ago and still continues to evolve has therefore been fully recognised in this text which we believe will appeal to surgeons in training and those already experienced in managing abdominal wall hernias. It is hoped that this work will be an effective reference to all those that possess this book.

General introduction and history of hernia surgery

ANCIENT AND RENAISSANCE HERNIA SURGERY

The high prevalence of hernia, for which the lifetime risk is 27% for men and 3% for women[926] has resulted in this condition inheriting one of the longest traditions of surgical management. The Egyptians (1500 BC), the Phoenicians (900 BC) and the Ancient Greeks (Hippocrates, 400 BC) diagnosed hernia. During this period a number of devices and operative techniques were recorded. Attempted repair was usually accompanied by castration, and strangulation was usually a death sentence. The word 'hernia' is derived from the Greek (hernios), meaning a bud or shoot. The Hippocratic school differentiated between hernia and hydrocele – the former was reducible and the latter transilluminable.[946] The Egyptian tomb of Ankh-ma-Hor at Saqqara dated around 2500 BC includes an illustrated sculpture of an operator apparently performing a circumcision and possibly a reduction of an inguinal hernia[1096] (Figure 1.1). Egyptian pharaohs had a retinue of physicians whose duty was to preserve the health of the ruler. These doctors had a detailed knowledge of the anatomy of the body and had developed some advanced surgical techniques for other conditions and also for the cure of hernia. The mummy of the Pharaoh Meneptah (1215 BC) showed a complete absence of the scrotum, and the mummified body of Rameses 5th (1157 BC) suggested that he had had an inguinal hernia during life with an associated fecal fistula in the scrotum and signs of attempts at surgical relief.

Greek and Phoenician terracottas (Figures 1.2 and 1.3) illustrate general awareness of hernias at this time (900–600 BC) but the condition appeared to be a social stigma and other than bandaging, treatments are not recorded. The Greek physician Galen (129–201 AD) was a prolific writer and one of his treatises was a detailed description of the musculature of the lower abdominal wall in which he also describes the deficiency of inguinal hernia. He described the peritoneal sac and the concept of reducible contents of the sac.

Celsus (AD 40) was a prolific writer and although he had no medical training he documented in encyclopedic detail Roman

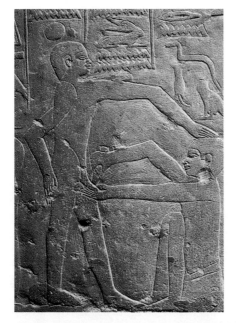

Figure 1.1 *Egyptian Tomb of Ankh-ma-Hor (Saqqara). The operator (bottom right) rubs in something with an instrument, and seems to perform a reduction of an inguinal hernia.*

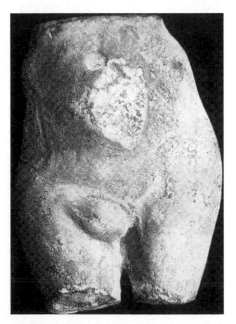

Figure 1.2 *Terracotta ex voto shows femoral hernia. (From Geschichte der Medizin, 1922.)*

surgical practice: taxis was employed for strangulation, trusses and bandages could control reducible hernia, and operation was only advised for pain and for small hernias in the young. The sac could be dissected through a scrotal incision, the wound then being allowed to granulate. Scar tissue was perceived as the optimum replacement for the stretched abdominal wall. A common method of treating hernia at this time was to reduce the contents of the sac and then attempt to obliterate it by a process of inflammation and gangrene by applying pressure to the walls of the sac through clamping the hemiscrotum between two blocks of wood. The last of the Graeco-Roman medical encyclopedists, Paul of Aegina (625–900 AD), distinguished complete scrotal from incomplete inguinal herniation or bubonocele. For scrotal hernia, he recommended ligation of the sac and the cord with sacrifice of the testicle. Paul was the last of the great surgeons who wrote several books, which gave detailed descriptions of operative procedures including inguinal hernia.

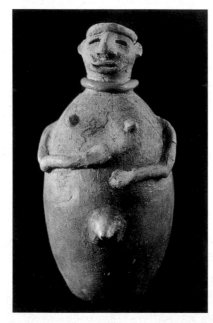

Figure 1.3 *Phoenician terracotta figure (female) shows umbilical hernia (5th–4th century BC). (From Museo Arquelogico, Barcelona, Spain.)*

During the dark time of the Middle Ages there was a decline of medicine in the civilized world and the use of the knife was largely abandoned. Few contributions were made to the art of surgery, which was now practised by itinerants and quacks. With the rise of the universities such as the appearance of the school of Salerno in the 13th century, there was some revival of surgical practice.[1096] At this time three important advances in herniology were made: Guy de Chauliac, in 1363, distinguished femoral from inguinal hernia. He developed taxis for incarceration, recommending the head-down, Trendelenburg position.[274] Guy was French and studied in Toulouse and Montpelier and later learned anatomy in Bologna from Nicole Bertuccio. Guy wrote extensively about hernia in his book Chirurgia (Figure 1.4), principally about diagnosis and methods of treatment. He described four surgical interventions one of

which was a herniotomy without castration, another consisting of cauterization of the hernia down to the os pubis and a third consisting of transfixion of the sac to a piece of wood by a strong ligature. His fourth method however was conservative treatment with bandaging and several weeks' bedrest accompanied by enemas, bloodletting and special diet. At the time he was the authorative expert on hernia.

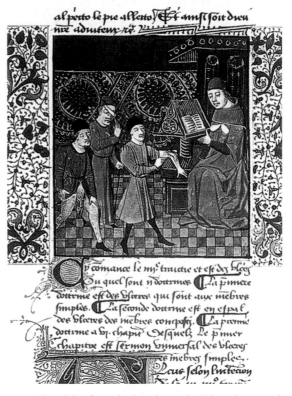

Figure 1.4 *The visit of surgical patients, in* Chirurgia. *Guy de Chauliac, 15th century manuscript. (From the Bibliothèque Nationale, Paris, France.)*

Franco's book Traites des Hernies (1561)[372] standardized the practice of hernia surgery at the time and diminished the influence of the itinerant practitioners (Figure 1.5). Franco popularized the punctum aurium and using this instrument made a small incision in the upper scrotum, isolated the hernia sac from the spermatic cord and then encircled it with a gold thread thus sparing the testis. He chose gold thread because this was considered to be the best non-reactive material. In spite of the known hazards and high mortality of operating on a strangulated hernia, Franco advised early intervention and rejected the conservative measures employed such as bloodletting and tobacco enemas. As a result he cured numerous patients with life-saving operations. He wrote many up as case reports illustrating his management and surgical techniques. He recommended reducing the contents and closing the defect with linen suture (Figure 1.6). His beautifully written manuscript was rediscovered and published again in 1925 by Walter van Brunn. As shown in the illustration the unusual feature of the book was the patients posing in their usual attire as if they were going about their everyday life.

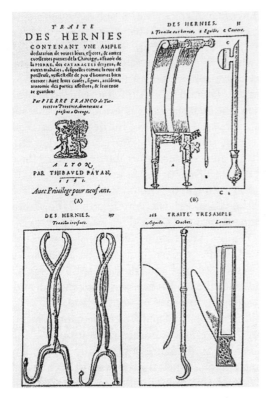

Figure 1.5 *Frontispiece and surgery instruments in* Traités des Hernies, *by Pierre Franco, Vincent, Lyon, 1561.*

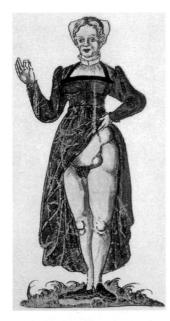

Figure 1.6 *Woman with femoral hernia. In* Die Handschrift des Schmitt-und Augenartztes. *Caspar Stromayr. By Walter von Brunn, 1925.*

In 1559 Stromayr, a German surgeon from Lindau, published a remarkable contribution to surgery. His book Practica Copiosa describes 16th-century hernia surgery in great detail and is comprehensively illustrated. Stromayr differentiated direct and indirect inguinal hernia and advised excision of the sac and of the cord and testicle in indirect hernia.[1103] Having differentiated and classified the two types of inguinal hernia,

Stromayr recommended a testis-sparing procedure for the direct type. His operation for high ligation of an indirect sac at the internal ring is illustrated in Figure 1.7. Stomayr also advanced the technology of trusses, which he designed to be adapted to the rigors of everyday life. The Renaissance brought burgeoning anatomic knowledge, now based on careful cadaver dissection. William Cheselden successfully operated on a strangulated right inguinal hernia on the Tuesday morning after Easter 1721. The intestines were easily reduced and adherent omentum was ligated and divided. The patient survived and went back to work[211] (Figure 1.8).

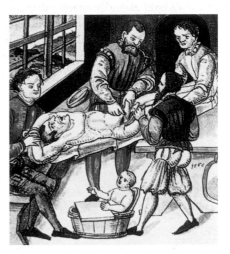

Figure 1.7 *The dissection of the sac and cord in an indirect hernia, carried to the level of the internal ring. In von Brunn, 1925.*

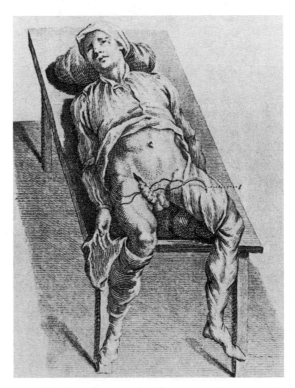

Figure 1.8 *Ligation of strangulated omentum in a strangulated right scrotal hernia. The wound then granulated. The patient survived and the hernia did not recur. Operation by Cheselden in 1721.[211]*

Without adequate interventional surgery some patients survived hernia strangulation when spontaneous, preternatural fistula occasionally followed infarction and sloughing of a strangulated hernia. Cheselden's Margaret White survived for many years 'voiding the excrements through the intestine at the navel' after simple local surgery for a strangulated umbilical hernia.[211] The closure of such a fistula in the absence of distal bowel pathology was described by Le Dran, who had noted that it was quite common for poor people with incarcerated hernias to mistake the tender painful groin lump for an abscess and incise it themselves. He found that these painful wounds with fecal fistulas required no more than cleaning and dressing. Often the wound would heal, nature preferring to send the feces along the natural route to the anus[673] (Figure 1.9).

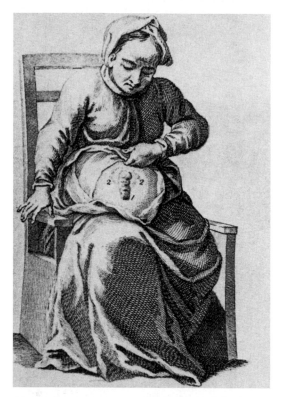

Figure 1.9 *Development of a preternatural colon fistula (colostomy) after strangulation of an umbilical hernia. The wound was trimmed. The patient survived many years 'voiding' the excrements at the umbilicus. Operation by Cheselden about 1721.[211]*

THE ANATOMICAL ERA

The great contribution of the surgical anatomists was between the years 1750–1865 and was called the age of dissection.[1096] The main contributors were Antonio Scarpa and Sir Astley Cooper and few major advances in our knowledge of the anatomy of the groin have been made since this time. The names of these great anatomists are Pieter, Camper, Antonio Scarpa, Percival Pott, Sir Astley Cooper, John Hunter, Thomas Morton, Germaine Cloquet, Franz Hesselbach, Friedrich Henle and Don Antonio Gimbernat.

The Dutchman Camper was a polymath who described a fascia, which is sandwiched in between the skin and deep fascia and can only be separated from this fascia below the inguinal ligament where the space between them accommodates lymph glands and cutaneous vessels of the groin. Below the external ring, Camper's fascia becomes the dartos muscle of the scrotum, which like the platysma is a muscle of the superficial fascia. Camper was the author of the definitive surgical text on hernia at the time. Antonio Scarpa was educated at the University of Padua (Figure 1.10) and he occupied the chairs of anatomy at the University of Modena and later Pavia. He was said to be arrogant and tyrannical and as a result despised by his colleagues. Sir Percival Pott described the pathophysiology of strangulation in 1757 and recommended surgical management (Figure 1.11): 'I am perfectly satisfied that the cause of strangulated hernia is most frequently … a piece of intestine (in other respects sound and free of disease) being so bound by the said tendon, as to have its peristaltic motion and the circulation through it impeded or stopped.'[922] Pott was trained at St Bartholomew's Hospital and wrote the manuscript 'A Treatise on Rupture'. This publication brought him into conflict with the Hunters who accused him of plagiarism for his description of congenital hernia, which they claimed to have described two years previously. He emphasized that the hernia sac was peritoneum continuous with the general peritoneal cavity and had not been in any way ruptured or broken, which until that time was the popular theory of causation of hernia.

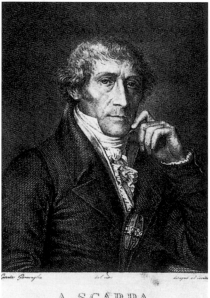

A. SCARPA

Figure 1.10 *Antonio Scarpa (1752–1832) Professor of Surgery and anatomy in Pavia, Italy.*

Fifty years later Astley Cooper (Figure 1.12) implicated venous obstruction as the first cascade in the circulatory failure of strangulation: 'By a stop being put to the return of blood through the veins which produces a great accumulation of this fluid and a change of its colour from the arterial to the venous hue.' Nevertheless ligature, the insertion of setons and castration remained the mainstays of treatment prior to the publication

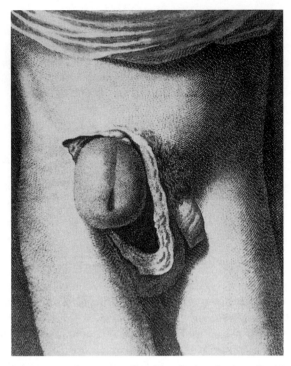

Figure 1.11 *Intestine strangulated by the 'tendon' so that the venous circulation through it is stopped, leading to gangrene. Described by Pott in 1757.*[922]

of Astley Cooper's monograph in 1804[238] (Figure 1.13). Sir Astley Cooper (1768–1841) trained at St Thomas's hospital, London, became a surgeon at Guy's Hospital and from 1813–1815 was Professor of Comparative Anatomy of the Royal College of Surgeons. Cooper published six magnificent books, two of which covered the subject of hernia, which were liberally illustrated by his own hand from dissections he had performed personally. Cooper was a charismatic lecturer and socialite and

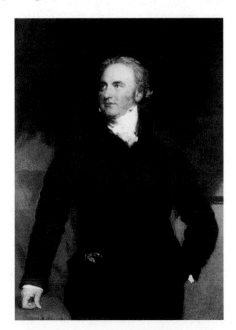

Figure 1.12 *Sir Astley Paston Cooper (1768–1841). Surgical anatomist, London, England.*

had an extensive surgical practice, which included being Sergeant Surgeon to King George IV. Cooper's recognition of the transversalis fascia positions him as one of the most important contributors to present day surgery which emphasizes this layer as being the first layer to be breached in groin hernias.

John Hunter (1728–1793) was born in Glasgow but became a pupil at St Bartholomew's Hospital to Percival Pott and later served as a surgeon at St George's Hospital where he established his well-known anatomy lessons and later the Hunterian museum which is now housed in the Royal College of Surgeons of England. Hunter's contribution was to define the role of the Gubernaculum testis that directed the descent of that organ with the spermatic vessels into the scrotum around the time of birth. Thomas Wharton (1813–1849), also a London surgeon working at the North London Hospital, in his short life wrote three anatomical texts, two of which were the subject of inguinal hernia and the groin. He first gave an accurate description of the conjoined tendon of the internal oblique and transversus muscles and their termination and attachment to the outer portion of the rectus sheath.

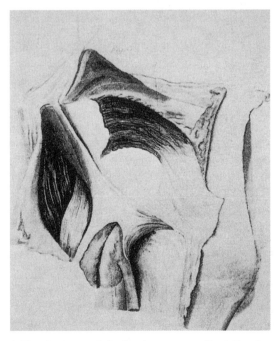

Figure 1.13 *Anatomy of the fascia transversalis. Astley Cooper (1804) demonstrated the fascia extending behind the inguinal ligament into the thigh to be the femoral sheath. He first recognized the fascia transversalis and its importance in groin herniation.*[238]

The first accurate description of the iliopubic tract, an important structure utilized in many sutured repairs for inguinal hernia, was made by Jules Cloquet (1790–1883).[225] Cloquet was Professor of Anatomy and Surgery in Paris and surgeon to the Emperor. Cloquet researched the pathological anatomy of the groin in numerous autopsy dissections and their reconstruction in wax models. He was the first to observe the frequency of patency of the processus vaginalis after birth and its role in the production of a hernia sac later in life. Franz Hesselbach was an anatomist at the University of Wurzburg who described the triangle now so important in laparoscopic surgery which originally defined the pathway of direct and external and supravesical hernias (Figure 1.14). The triangle as defined today is somewhat smaller. Friedrich Henle (1809–1885) was another German latterly working in the University of Gottingen. Henle described an important ligament running from the lateral edge of the rectus sheath and fusing with the pectineal ligament. This structure when present could be utilized to anchor sutures in herniorrhaphy. Finally Don Antonio Gimbernat (1742–1790) was a Spanish surgeon working in Barcelona and also surgeon to King Charles III and President of the College of Surgeons of Spain. Gimbernat not only defined the lacunar ligament as a distinct anatomical structure but also showed how its division in strangulated femoral hernia was usually the point of obstruction and allowed reduction of the contents of the sac.

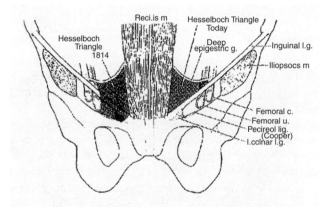

Figure 1.14 *The triangle of Hesselbach described in 1814, and as understood today. In* Hernias, *by JE Skandalakis, SW Gray, JS Rowe Jr, 1983.*

THE ERA OF ANTISEPSIS AND ASEPSIS

Before bacteria were recognized and with it the need for meticulous cleanliness in the environment of the operating theater, postoperative sepsis was virtually routine and mortality rates extremely high. Oliver Wendell Holmes in 1842 and Semmelweiss in 1849 emphasized the importance of handwashing before operating. However, identifying and understanding the problem of infection and the causal bacteria, had to await the discoveries of Louis Pasteur which were later put into practice by Joseph Lister (1827–1912). The application of Lister's principles of providing clean linen and special coats, special receptacles for antiseptic dressings, cleansing sponges soaked in carbolic acid and thymol, and the segregation of post-mortem examinations and operating theaters profoundly influenced British and European surgeons and decimated postoperative infection rates. Modern surgery commenced with Lister's discoveries.[700]

Other important innovations were acquired before operative surgery presented a minimal danger to the patient. Ernst

von Bergman invented the steam sterilizer in 1891 and introduced the word 'aseptic'. Halsted with the nurse Caroline Hampton introduced rubber gloves in 1896 and together with the introduction of a face-mask by von Miculicz the conversion from antiseptic to aseptic technique was finally set for the techniques of modern hernia surgery to develop.[295]

THE DAWN OF ANESTHESIA

The removal of pain during surgical operations not only eliminated the terror of the surgical operation from the patient but also enabled more careful anatomical dissection and reconstruction and the evolution of planned surgical procedures.[1096] An American dentist Horace Wells pioneered the use of nitrous oxide as an anesthetic but his first public attempt at demonstrating a painless dental extraction was a failure. It was left to his associate William Thomas Green Morton to demonstrate the first successful anesthetic using sulfuric ether in the theater of the Massachusetts General Hospital in Boston. The operation on Edward Gilbert Abbott was for removal of a tumor angioma in the neck. Following this demonstration on 16 October 1846 the practice spread widely into Europe and Lister in London used it for a thigh amputation on Frederick Churchill on 21 December 1846. With patients no longer fearing pain, the scene was set for the great technological advances of the second half of the 19th century.

THE TECHNOLOGICAL ERA

Initial surgical attempts at hernioplasty were based on static concepts of anatomic repair using natural or modified natural materials for reconstruction. Wood (1863)[1221] described subcutaneous division and suture of the sac and fascial separation of the groin from the scrotum. Czerny (1876), in Prague, pulled the sac of an inguinal hernia through the external ring, ligated it, amputated the redundant sac and allowed the neck to spring back to the deep ring.[262] MacEwen (1886), of Glasgow, bundled the sac up on itself and stuffed it back along the canal so that it would act as a cork or tampon and stop up the internal ring[724] (Figure 1.15). Kocher (1907), surgery's first Nobel Prize winner, invaginated the sac on itself and fixed it laterally through the external oblique[607] (Figure 1.16). Suffice to say, none of these operations has stood the test of time.

As so often in surgery a new concept was needed before further progress could be made in herniology. Two pioneers – the American Marcy and the Italian Bassini (1884) – vie for priority for the critical breakthrough[90–92,742] (Figures 1.17 and 1.18). Both appreciated the physiology of the inguinal canal and both correctly understood how each anatomic plane, transversalis fascia, transverse and oblique muscles, and the external oblique aponeurosis, contributed to the canal's stability. Read, having carefully surveyed all the evidence, agrees with Halsted[462] that Bassini got there first.[944]

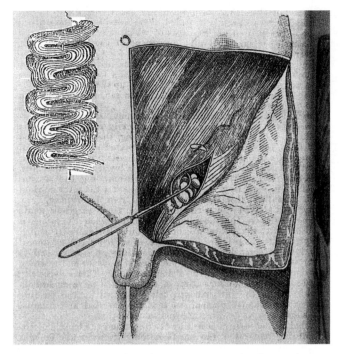

Figure 1.15 *The operation of McEwan 1886. The dissected indirect sac is bundled up and then used as an internal stopper or pad to prevent further herniation along the valved canal.*[724]

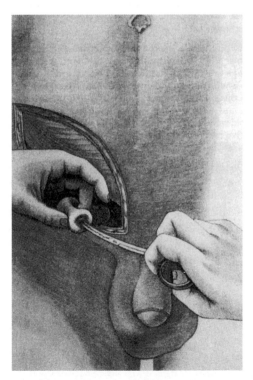

Figure 1.16 *Invagination of the sac which is fixed laterally by suturing its stump to the external oblique. No formal dissection or repair of the deep ring was made. Operation by Kocher in 1907.*[607]

Although both contributed to herniology, Bassini made another seminal advance when he subjected his technique to the scrutiny of the prospective follow-up. Bassini's 1890 paper is truly a quantum leap in surgery;[92] indeed, if it is read alongside

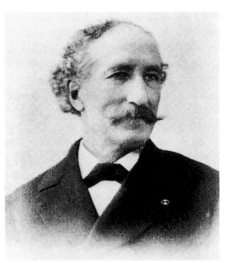

Figure 1.17 *Henry Orville Marcy (1837–1924); Boston surgeon, anatomist, and philanthropist. The first American student of Lister. (Courtesy of the New York Academy of Medicine Library.)*

the contribution of Haidenthaller, from Billroth's clinic – reporting a 30%, early recurrence rate – which appears in the same volume of Langenbeck's Archiv für Klinische Chirurgie, Bassini's stature is further enhanced.[457]

Marcy directed his attention to the deep ring in the fascia transversalis; his operation for indirect inguinal hernia entailed closure of the deep ring with fascia transversalis only, the object being the recreation of a stable and competent deep ring. In 1871 he reported two patients operated on during the previous year 'in which I closed the (deep) ring with the interrupted sutures of carbolized catgut followed by permanent cure'.[741]

Bassini had become interested in the management of inguinal hernia in about 1883, and from 1883 to 1889 he operated on 274 hernias. After trying the operations of Czerny and

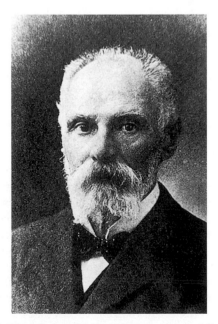

Figure 1.18 *Edoardo Bassini (1844–1924); invented first successful inguinal hernioplasty.*

Wood, he modified his approach and attempted a radical cure, so that the patient would not require a truss after surgery. He decided to open the inguinal canal and approach the posterior wall of the canal; gradually he was focusing onto the deep ring and fascia transversalis. Seven times he opened the canal, resected the sac and closed the peritoneum at the internal ring. He then constructed a tampon of the excess sac at the internal ring and sutured this sac stump, or tampon, to the deep surface of the external oblique. One of his seven patients died 3 months after the operation from an unrelated cause. Post-mortem examination showed the sutured portion of the neck, the 'stopper' or tampon, to be completely reabsorbed. Bassini deduced that although the risk of recurrent herniation was diminished by this technique it did not afford adequate tissue repair; and some external support – a truss – would still be needed to prevent recurrence. He now proceeded to complete anatomical reconstruction of the inguinal canal:

> … 'this might be achieved through reconstruction of the inguinal canal into the physiological condition, a canal with two openings one abdominal the other subcutaneous and with two walls, one anterior and one posterior through the middle of which the spermatic cord would pass. Through a study of the groin, and with the help of an anatomical knowledge of the inguinal canal and inguinal hernia, it was easy for me to find an operative method, which answered the above-described requirements, and made possible a radical cure without subsequent wearing of a truss. Using the method exclusively I have, during the year 1884, operated on 262 hernias of which 251 were either reducible or irreducible and 11 strangulated'.

His series included 206 men and 10 women; the non-strangulated cases were 115 right, 66 left and 35 bilateral inguinal hernias. The age range was 13 months to 69 years. The operations were performed under general narcosis and there were no operative deaths; however; three patients who each had strangulated hernias died postoperatively – one of sepsis, one of shock and one of a chest infection. Bassini's patients were carefully followed up, some to 4¾ years, and seven recurrences were recorded. There were, in fact, eight recurrences; Bassini failed to tabulate case 65, a 54-year-old university professor in Padua with a strangulated right direct inguinal hernia, with a recurrence at eight months. The wound infection rate was 11 in 206 operations and the time to healing averaged 14 days.[92] These statistics compare favorably with reports made up to the 1950s.

Bassini dissected the indirect sac and closed it off flush with the parietal peritoneum. He then isolated and lifted up the spermatic cord and dissected the posterior wall of the canal, dividing the fascia transversalis down to the pubic tubercle. He then sutured the dissected conjoint tendon consisting of the internal oblique, the transversus muscle and the 'vertical fascia of Cooper', the fascia transversalis, to the posterior rim of Poupart's ligament, including the lower lateral divided margin of the fascia transversalis. Bassini stresses that this suture line must be approximated without difficulty; hence the early dissection separating the external oblique from the internal oblique must be adequate and allow good development and mobilization of the conjoint tendon (Figure 1.19).

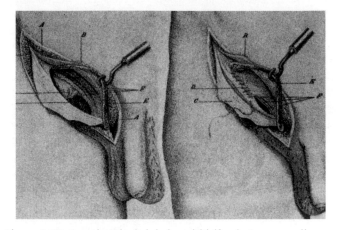

Figure 1.19 *Suturing the 'triple layer' (F) (fascia transversalis, transversus tendon and internal oblique) to the upturned edge of the inguinal ligament. An anatomical and physiological repair of the posterior wall of the inguinal canal preserving its obliquity and function. Operation by Bassini in 1890.[92]*

The Bassini legacy was popularized by Attilio Catterina, Bassini's assistant in Padua in 1887 who later became professor in Genoa in 1904. Catterina was entrusted by Bassini to teach the exact surgical technique. To do this he wrote an atlas of 'The Operation of Bassini'! This adds 16 life-sized color plates by the artist Orazio Gaicher of Cortina. This book was published in London, Berlin, Paris and Madrid in the 1930s and described in detail the uncorrupted Bassini technique, especially the division of the transversalis fascia, resection of the cremaster muscle and complete anatomical survey of all the relevant anatomy nowadays considered so essential.[195,196] This was a foretaste of the Shouldice operation.[1186] The illustrations show quite clearly that Bassini resected the Cremaster muscle and completed division of the posterior wall of the inguinal canal. The Shouldice and Bassini hernioplasties are therefore essentially the same.

By contrast, Haidenthaller; from Billroth's Clinic in Vienna, reported 195 operations for inguinal hernia, with 11 operative deaths and a short-term recurrence rate of 30.8%.[457] Although Halsted made important contributions to herniology, his general technical contributions of precise hemostasis, absolute asepsis and the crucial importance of avoiding tissue trauma are easily overlooked. Halsted was always concerned to achieve optimum wound healing, and he not only practiced surgery but he experimented and theorized. His observation on closing skin wounds is best repeated verbatim: 'The skin is united by interrupted stitches of very fine silk. These stitches do not penetrate the skin, and when tied they become buried. They are taken from the underside of the skin and made to include only its deeper layers – the layers which are not occupied by sebaceous follicles.[461–463] In today's world hematoma, sepsis and damaged tissue leading to delayed healing mean not only a poor surgical outcome but weigh heavily on the debit side of any economic evaluation. These Halstedian principles should be rigidly applied by any surgeon who undertakes hernia surgery.

Halsted must also be given priority for recognizing the value of an anterior relaxing incision, first described by Wolfler in 1892[1220] and subsequently popularized in the USA by Rienhoff[954] and in England by Tanner (1942).[1116] Apart from Halsted, countless other authors have corrupted or simplified the original Marcy–Bassini concept of a review of the posterior wall of the canal and the correction of any deficits in it, the reconstruction of the patulous deep ring for indirect herniation and the repair of the stretched fascia transversalis in cases of direct herniation. Bull and Coley independently sutured the internal oblique and the aponeurosis over the cord,[158,232] whereas Ferguson (1899) advised against any mobilization of the cord and, therefore, any review of the posterior wall of the canal.[352]

Imbrication, or overlapping, of layers was introduced by Wyllys Andrews in 1895 in Chicago.[35] Andrews confessed that his technique was an outgrowth of experience with MacEwan, Bassini, Halsted and similar operations. Andrews laid great stress on careful aseptic technique: 'Finally, I unite the skin itself with a buried suture which does not puncture any of its glands or ducts.' Andrews used cotyledon only as a dressing. Again the importance of careful surgical technique is emphasized. Andrews stressed the importance of the posterior wall of the canal: 'The posterior wall of the canal … is narrowed by suturing the conjoined tendon and transversalis fascia firmly to Poupart's ligament.' Andrews recommended the kangaroo tendon introduced by Marcy. Andrews then reinforced the posterior wall with the upper (medial) margin of the external oblique aponeurosis, which he drew down behind the cord and sutured to Poupart's ligament. Andrews' intention was to interlock or imbricate the layers. The lower (lateral) flap of the external oblique aponeurosis was then brought up anterior to the cord. Andrews concluded his article: 'Any successful method of radical cure must be a true plastic operation upon the musculoaponeurotic layers of the abdominal wall. Cicatricial tissue and peritoneal exudate are of no permanent value.' Andrews had visited Bassini in Padua on several occasions to acquaint himself with the revolutionary operation. However, in his future descriptions of the operation, Andrews failed to mention that Bassini had divided the posterior wall of the inguinal canal and these erroneous observations were passed on to a generation of European and American surgeons because Catterina's atlas was not published in Europe until the 1930s. Andrews' description of Bassini's operation was therefore the only definitive description and the classical Bassini operation became corrupted until it was reintroduced as the Shouldice operation in the 1950s.

Perhaps we should pause at about 1905 and summarize what empiricism had achieved thus far. First, all authors agree that division of the neck of the sac and flush closure of the peritoneum is imperative to success. Second, dissection of the deep ring with exploration of the extraperitoneal space to allow adequate closure of the fascia transversalis anterior to the peritoneum emerges as a cardinal feature. Marcy and Bassini stress the fascia transversalis repair, Halsted emphasized it, Andrews' diagram suggests it. Ferguson did not examine the entire posterior wall, but tightened the internal ring lateral to the emergent cord. All are agreed that the deep ring is patulous in indirect herniation and consequently the fascia transversalis must be repaired. In the English

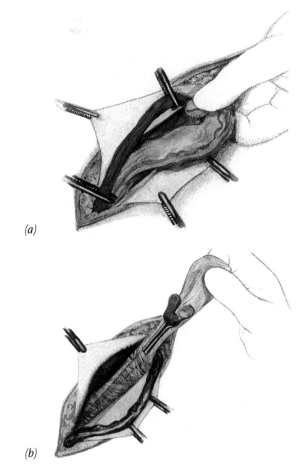

(a)

(b)

Figure 1.20 *(a) Bassini completely isolated and excised the cremaster muscle and its fascia from the cord. He thus ensured complete exposure of the deep ring and all the posterior wall of the inguinal canal, an essential pre-requisite to evaluate all the potential hernial sites. (b) Bassini stressed the complete exposure and incision of the fascia transversalis of the posterior wall of the inguinal canal. To complete the repair he sutured the divided fascia transversalis, together with the transversus muscle, and the internal oblique muscle, 'the threefold layer' to the upturned inner free margin of the inguinal ligament. (From Catterina, The Bassini Procedure, published by H.K. Lewis, 1934.)*

literature, Lockwood in 1893 clearly emphasized the fascia transversalis and Bassini's 'triple layer'. Lockwood obtained good results by repairing this important layer.[702,703] Third, preservation of the obliquity of the canal is suggested by Marcy and Bassini, and by the later Halsted and Bloodgood papers.

Fourth, double-breasting (imbrication) of aponeurosis gives improved results and is recommended by Andrews. Lastly, all the authors stress careful technique. Avoidance of tissue trauma, hematoma and infection leads to impressively better results. Sepsis is an important antecedent of recurrence.

After the 19th-century advances of Marcy and Bassini, and the important contribution to surgical technique by Halsted, little of major importance was contributed until the 1920s. Countless modifications of Marcy's and Bassini's operations were made and reported frequently. The Bassini operation re-emerged as the Shouldice repair in 1950s (Figure 1.20). Erle Shouldice

(1890–1965) also promulgated the benefits of early ambulation and opened the Shouldice clinic, a hospital dedicated to the repair of hernias to the abdominal wall. A huge experience accumulated with an annual throughput of 7000 herniorrhaphies per year, enabled the surgeons at the Shouldice clinic to study the pathology in primary and recurrent hernias and to emphasize adjuncts to successful outcomes. Continuous monofilament wire was used in preference to other suture materials and the hernioplasty incorporated repair of the internal ring, the posterior wall of the inguinal canal and the femoral region. The Cremaster muscle and fascia with vessels and genital branch of genitofemoral nerve were removed and the posterior wall after division was repaired by a four-layer imbrication method using the iliopubic tract as its main anchor point. The landmark publication with long-term follow-up was produced by Shearburn and Myers in 1969 and from this time until the introduction of mesh, the Shouldice operation became the gold-standard for inguinal hernia repair.[1042]

THE EXTRAPERITONEAL–PREPERITONEAL APPROACH TO THE GROIN

Alternatives to the anterior (inguinal) approach to the internal ring include the transabdominal (laparotomy)[634,1114] and the extraperitoneal (preperitoneal).[206] Marcy recognized the advantages of the transabdominal intraperitoneal approach to the ring in 1892:

> 'It may rarely happen to the operator who has opened the abdomen for some other purpose to find the complication of hernia. When the section has been made considerably large, as in the removal of a large tumour; the internal ring is within reach of the surgeon. Upon reflection, it would naturally occur to any operator that under these conditions it is better to close the internal ring, and reform the smooth internal parietal surface from within by means of suturing. My friend, Dr N. Bozeman of New York, easily did this at my suggestion in a case of ovariotomy more than 10 years ago'.

Marcy attributed the transabdominal technique to the French in 1749.[743] Lawson Tait recommended midline abdominal section for umbilical and groin hernia in 1891.[1114] LaRoque, in 1919, recommended transabdominal repair of inguinal hernias through a muscle-splitting incision about 1 inch (2.5 cm) above the ring. The peritoneum was opened, the sac dissected and then inverted into the peritoneal cavity by grasping its fundus and pulling it back into the peritoneal cavity. The sac was excised and a repair of the deep ring effected[634] (Figure 1.21). LaRoque believed that the transabdominal approach provided absolute assurance of high ligation of the hernia sac and wrote three papers with accumulative experience of almost 2000 inguinal hernia repairs.[993]

Battle, a surgeon at St Thomas' Hospital, London and the Royal Free Hospital, described his approach to repair of a femoral hernia in 1900. Battle pointed out the difficulties of diagnosing femoral hernia and the difficulties, principally the age, sex and comorbidity, of managing patients with femoral

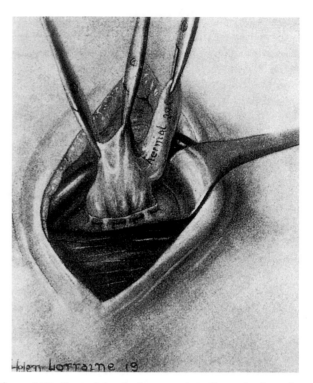

Figure 1.21 *Transabdominal approach to the groin through a muscle-splitting incision above the inguinal canal with subsequent closure of the peritoneal sac away from the canal.*[634]

hernia. He approached the hernia sac from above through an incision splitting the external oblique above the inguinal ligament. After dealing with the peritoneal sac, Battle repaired the femoral canal, constructing a 'shutter' of the aponeurosis of external oblique which he sutured to the pectineus fascia and the pectineal ligament across the abdominal opening of the femoral canal.[93,993] The Battle operation like many operations for groin hernia has now passed into oblivion.

The extraperitoneal–preperitoneal approach owes its origin to Cheatle (1920) who initially used a midline incision but subsequently (1921) changed to a Pfannenstiel incision.[206,207] Cheatle explored both sides, and inguinal and femoral protrusions were reduced and amputated. If needed, for strangulation or adhesions, the peritoneum could easily be opened. The fascia transversalis was visible and easily repaired. Cheatle advised against this approach for direct hernia because the direct region was usually obscured and distorted by the retraction of the rectus muscles. However, Cheatle's landmark contribution had a minimal impact at the time and remained little used for many years.[993]

A.K. Henry, a master anatomist, rediscovered and popularized the extraperitoneal approach in 1936.[494] At this time he was the Director of the Surgical Unit, Kasr-el-Aini Hospital and Professor of Clinical Surgery in the University of Cairo although he later returned to the Hammersmith Hospital and subsequently became Professor of Anatomy at the Royal College of Surgeons in Ireland. The full impact of the Cheatle/Henry operation was not recognized until after the Second World War, when McEvedy,[770] adopted a unilateral oblique incision retracting the rectus muscle medially to approach a femoral hernia. In the USA, Musgrove and McCready (1949) adopted the Henry approach to femoral hernia.[830] Mikkelsen and Berne (1954) reported inguinal and femoral hernias repaired by this technique and commended the excellent access obtained even in the obese. Furthermore femoral, inguinal and obturator hernias were all repairable through this 'extended suprapubic approach'.[788]

TWO EUROPEANS – LYTLE AND FRUCHAUD

In the immediate aftermath of the Second World War two European Surgeon Anatomists, Lytle and Fruchaud, are important contributors. Lytle was principally concerned with the anatomy and shutter mechanism of the deep inguinal ring. He dissected the deep ring and in a remarkable film demonstrated its prophylactic mechanism in indirect herniation. He was concerned to preserve the mechanism of the ring and at the same time to reinforce its patulous medial margin in indirect herniation. He emphasized that maneuvers which damaged the lateral 'pillars of the ring' inevitably compromised the physiological shutter mechanism. In a subsequent study he clearly described the embryological anatomy of the ring and how it could be repaired, in the fascia transversalis layer, without losing its function[720] (Figure 1.22).

A remarkable Frenchman, Henri Fruchaud published two books in Paris in 1956: L'Anatomie Chirurgicale de la Region de l'Aine (Surgical Anatomy of the Groin Region)[376] and Le Traitement Chirurgical des Hernies de l'Aine (Surgical Treatment of Groin Hernias).[377] Fruchaud combined traditional anatomical studies of the groin, the work of Cooper; Bogros and Madden, with his own extensive anatomical and surgical experience.

He invented an entirely new concept – 'the myopectineal orifice' – which combined the traditionally separate inguinal and femoral canals to form a unified highway from the abdomen to the thigh. The abdominocrural tunnel of fascia transversalis extended through this myopectineal orifice, through which all inguinal and femoral hernias pass, as do the iliofemoral vessels. Based on this anatomical concept Fruchaud recommended complete reconstruction of the endo-fascial wall (fascia transversalis) of the myopectineal orifice. This unifying concept forms the basis for all extraperitoneal mesh repairs, open or laparoscopic, of groin hernias (Figure 1.23). Fruchaud's two books were never

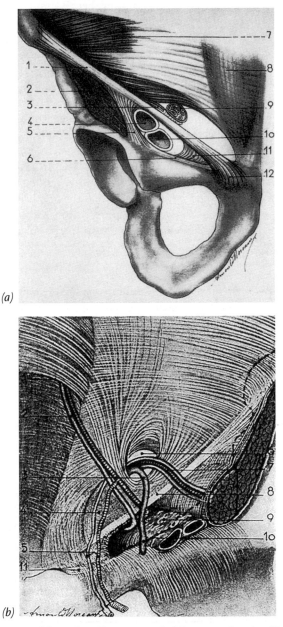

(a)

(b)

Figure 1.23 (a) Fruchaud's concept of the myopectineal orifice ('l'orifice crural classique') incorporating the inguinal and the femoral canals. An external view showing the two canals separated by the inguinal ligament and internal dissection (b) demonstrating how the muscles of the groin form a tunnel down to the myopectineal orifice.[376]

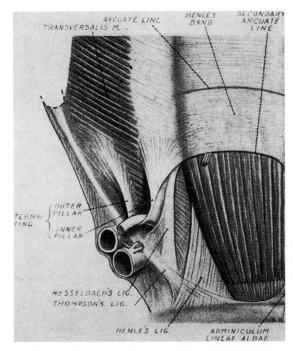

Figure 1.22 The 'shutter mechanism' of canal and the internal anatomy of the deep ring, demonstrating the sling of fascia transversalis which pulls the deep ring up and laterally when the muscles contract.[720]

published in English and therefore his findings remained relatively obscure and did not have the full impact and recognition until the laparoscopic era of hernia repair.[1096] The concept of Fruchaud has been expanded by Stoppa in France and Wantz in the USA into the 'giant reinforcement of the peritoneal sac' repairs of inguinal hernias.[1098,1185,1188]

TENSION-FREE HERNIA REPAIR

Irving Lichtenstein is the seminal thinker who introduced tension-free prosthetic repair of groin hernias into everyday, commonplace, outpatient practices. As well as being an office procedure under local anesthetic, Lichtenstein pioneered the idea that hernia surgery is special, that it must be performed by an experienced surgeon and cannot be relegated to the unsupervised trainee doing 'minor' surgery. The key feature of Lichtenstein's technique is the 'tensionless' operation. With his co-workers Shulman and Amid, he has developed a simple prosthetic operation, which can be performed on outpatients[25,694] (Figure 1.24). As a pioneer, Lichtenstein worked hard to promulgate his ideas but even so the first edition of his book 'Hernia Repair Without Disability' written in 1970 sold rather poorly and never went beyond the first printing.[990] Subsequent editions however, required numerous reprints to meet demand paralleling the increase in popularity and worldwide success of the mesh-patch repair devised by Lichtenstein.

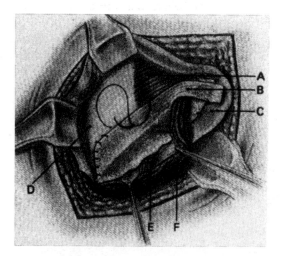

Figure 1.24 *The Lichtenstein's tension-free hernioplasty.*[691]

LAPAROSCOPIC REPAIR

Laparoscopic repair continues to develop its place in the surgical armamentarium of inguinal hernia. The use of the laparoscope has been extended to repair incisional, ventral, lumbar, and paracolostomy hernias. This latter technique is rapidly gaining in popularity.

The first attempt to treat an inguinal hernia with the laparoscope was made by P. Fletcher of the University of the West Indies in 1979.[398] He closed the neck of the hernia sac. The first report of the use of a clip (Michel) placed laparoscopically to close the neck of the sac was made by Ger in 1982, who reported a series of 13 patients: all the patients in this series were repaired through an open incision except the thirteenth patient who was repaired under laparoscopic guidance with a special stapling device. The three-year follow-up of that patient revealed him to be free of an identifiable recurrence. Ger continued his efforts to repair these hernias laparoscopically. He reported the closure of the neck of the hernia sac using a prototypical instrument called the 'Herniostat' in beagle dogs.[399] The results in these models appeared to be promising. In that same article, he reported the potential benefits of the laparoscopic approach to groin hernia repair as: (1) creation of puncture wounds rather than formal incisions; (2) need for minimal dissection; (3) less danger of spermatic cord injury and less risk of ischemic orchitis; (4) minimal risk of bladder injury; (5) decreased incidence of neuralgias; (6) possibility of an outpatient procedure; (7) ability to achieve the highest possible ligation of the hernial sac; (8) minimal postoperative discomfort and a faster recovery time; (9) ability to perform simultaneous diagnostic laparoscopy; and (10) ability to diagnose and treat bilateral inguinal hernias. These potential advantages and advances in the laparoscopic repair of hernias continue to be the recognized goals that each method is attempting to achieve.

Bogojavalensky, a gynecologist, presented the first known use of a prosthetic biomaterial in the laparoscopic repair of inguinal and femoral hernias in 1989.[133] He placed a roll of polypropylene mesh into indirect hernias of female patients. The neck of the internal inguinal ring was then closed with sutures. Popp repaired a coincidental direct hernia that was found at the time of a uterine myomectomy.[918] He recognized the need to provide coverage of a wider area than that of the defect itself. To accomplish this, he placed a 4 × 5 cm oval dehydrated dura mater patch over the defect. This was secured to the peritoneum with catgut sutures that were tied extracorporeally. Popp expressed concerns that the intra-abdominal repair of inguinal hernia could lead to adhesive complications and suggested that a preperitoneal approach might be preferable.

Schultz published the first patient series of laparoscopic herniorrhaphy in 1990.[1026] Rolls of polypropylene were stuffed into the hernial orifice, which was then covered by two or three flat sheets of polypropylene mesh (2.5 × 5 cm) over the defect. These rolls of mesh were not secured to either the fascia or peritoneum. To achieve access to the hernia defect he incised the peritoneum. Following the placement of the rolls he closed the peritoneum with clips. This probably represents the earliest attempt at a type of transabdominal preperitoneal (TAPP) repair that is commonly used today. Corbitt modified this technique by inverting the hernia sac and performing a high ligation with sutures or with an endoscopic stapling device.[245] Despite the initial success of these early reports, because of recurrence rates approaching 15–20% these techniques were abandoned.[244] The lack of extensive dissection with the above methods, however, remained appealing. A similar concept was applied in the intraperitoneal onlay patch (IPOM) technique. Salerno, Fitzgibbons and Filipi investigated this type of repair in the porcine model.[1009] They placed rectangular pieces of flat polypropylene mesh to cover the myopectineal orifice and secured it with a stapling device. The success of these repairs led them to apply this method in clinical trials.

At about the same time, Toy and Smoot reported upon their first ten patients that were repaired with the IPOM technique.[1135] They secured an expanded polytetrafluoroethylene patch (ePTFE) patch to the inguinal floor with staples that were introduced by a prototypical-stapling device of their own design, the 'Nanticoke Hernia Stapler'. They successfully used this fixation device in 20–30 patients without adverse results. A subsequent report of their first 75 patients was published in 1992.[1136] In this later series, the same prosthetic biomaterial (7.5 × 10 cm) was attached with the Endopath EMS® stapler. After a follow-up of up to 20 months, the recurrence rate was 2.4%. They noted a significant decrease in postoperative pain and an earlier return to normal activity as compared to the open repair of the hernia defect. Others reported similar results.[668,670,1080]

Fitzgibbons later abandoned the IPOM repair except for simple indirect inguinal hernias.[360] One patient developed a postoperative scrotal abscess that may or may not have been related to the placement of the mesh in that position. This patient was noted to have firm attachment of the appendix to the site of the polypropylene mesh. He also noted that, in follow-up of these patients, the patch material could be pulled into the hernial defect because it was affixed to the peritoneum alone rather than fascia. Because of these adverse events, he believed that the transabdominal preperitoneal (TAPP) approach, which had been reported by Arregui[48] for inguinal hernia repair, was more appropriate. In this repair, the peritoneum is incised and dissected away from the transversalis fascia to expose the inguinal floor. The mesh material is then secured to that fascia which was believed to ensure superior fixation and tissue ingrowth. Both the TAPP and IPOM techniques require the entry into the abdominal cavity.

In a continuing effort to prevent bowel contact to the prosthesis, Popp described a method to dissect the peritoneum away from the abdominal wall prior to the incision of the peritoneum in the TAPP repair in 1991.[919] Saline was inserted into the preperitoneal space with a percutaneous syringe. This 'aquadissection' was found to be helpful in the dissection of this area to create a space in which to operate within the preperitoneal space. This early concept probably led to the idea that the entire dissection could be accomplished from within the preperitoneal space, thereby eliminating the need to enter the abdominal cavity.

Additional variations that did not gain acceptance were the 'ring-plasty' and a preperitoneal iliopubic tract repair. The former method was simply a sutured repair that approximated the deep structures of the lateral iliopubic tract to the proximal arching musculotendinous fibers of the transversus abdominis muscle.[306,573] The latter technique was also a 'tissue' repair but secured the iliopubic tract to the transversus abdominis muscle.[393,394] This repair incorporated the use of an inlay of a prosthetic material but still had the disadvantage of being a repair under tension. These methods may have limited usage in rare circumstances.

In these earlier years, the predominant laparoscopic method of inguinal herniorrhaphy was the TAPP approach using either a polypropylene mesh or an expanded polytetrafluoroethylene material.[178,573,919] In 1992, Dulucq[318,319] was the first surgeon to perform 'retroperitoneoscopy' to effect a repair of an inguinal hernia without any direct entry into the abdominal cavity. In 1993, Phillips and Arregui separately described a technique that did not utilize a peritoneal incision in the repair of the inguinal floor.[50,908] The dissection of the preperitoneal space was accomplished under direct visualization of the area via a laparoscope placed into the abdominal cavity. The laparoscope was then moved into the newly dissected preperitoneal space to complete the repair. Ferzli and McKernan later popularized the technique of Dulucq preferring the term 'totally extraperitoneal'.[353,773] Using the 'open' entry into the preperitoneal space, the dissection of the space was carried out under direct visualization. This totally extraperitoneal (TEP) repair was identical to that of the TAPP but appeared to incur less risk of injury to the intra-abdominal organs.

Currently, the majority of laparoscopic inguinal hernia repairs are approached by either the TAPP or TEP method and utilize a polypropylene mesh biomaterial. The majority of the surgeons that perform the TEP repair utilize the commercially available dissection balloons to create the space within the preperitoneal area to perform the repair.

In a multicenter report, the recurrence rate of these repairs was 0.4% in 10 053 repairs with a median follow-up of 36 months.[350] The surgeons that continue to perform the laparoscopic herniorrhaphy believe that the goals that were anticipated by Ger have been realized.

The improvement in recovery in laparoscopic cholecystectomy patients and results that were seen in herniorrhaphy patients encouraged attempts to repair ventral and incisional hernias in 1991. The initial report by LeBlanc involved only five patients using an ePTFE patch biomaterial.[669] Although the overlap of the hernia defect by the prosthesis was only 1.5–2 cm, these patients were free of recurrence after seven years of follow-up. The fixation used was that of the 'box-type' of hernia stapler without the use of sutures. Sutures were used only to aid in the positioning of the patch. These sutures were removed from the prosthesis at the completion of the stapling of the patch. With further patients and follow-up, no recurrences were noted.[664,667] Barie proposed the use of a polyester material covered on the visceral side with a mesh of absorbable polyglactin.[77]

Park modified the technique for the repair of large ventral hernias by utilizing the transfascial fixation of the ePTFE or Prolene® mesh with transabdominally placed Prolene® sutures passed through a Keith needle.[887] In their series of 30 cases, only one recurrence was noted. This repair used a fascial overlap of 2 cm. Holzman placed a Marlex® prosthesis with a 4 cm overlap onto normal fascial edges and secured them with an endoscopic stapler.[511] He found this technique to be safe and effective. In separate investigations, Holzman, Park and others compared the open versus laparoscopic methods and found that the laparoscopic repair was associated with fewer postoperative complications, a shorter hospital stay and lower recurrence rates than open prosthetic repair.[184,282,511,886,939] The largest study published to date confirms that the laparoscopic repair of incisional and ventral hernias can be accomplished with reproducibility and with excellent results.[492] Additionally, the long-term follow-up of LeBlanc's patients has proven that this is a durable procedure when the tenets that are noted below are applied:

1 a minimum prosthetic overlap of 3 cm;
2 helical tacks placed at 1–1.5 cm intervals; and
3 transfascial sutures are placed at 5 cm intervals.[655,663]

Others, however, do not share this view. Some surgeons, notably in Spain, prefer the use of the 'double crown' technique.[185,804] In this technique no sutures are used. Instead, two concentric rows of helical tacks are placed. The first at the periphery of the biomaterial as in the sutured technique and the second, inside of this one, near the hernia defect itself. The initial reports seem to have similar results as that of the authors using the transfascial sutures but only a longer interval of follow-up will prove or disprove if either one or both of these approaches is best.

CHRONOLOGY OF HERNIA SURGERY

Ancient

1500 BC	Inguinal hernia described in an Egyptian papyrus. An inguinal hernia is depicted on a Greek statuette from this period.[946]
900 BC	Tightly fitting bandages are used to treat an inguinal hernia by physicians in Alexandria. A Phoenician statue depicts this.[946]
400 BC	Hippocrates distinguished hernia and hydrocele by transillumination.[946]
AD 40	Celsus described the older Greek operations for hernia.[197]
AD 200	Galen introduced the concept of 'rupture' of the peritoneum allowed by failure of the belly wall tissues.[946]
AD 700	Paul of Aegina distinguished complete and incomplete hernia. He recommended amputation of the testicle in repair.[946]

Medieval

1363	Guy de Chauliac distinguished inguinal and femoral hernia.[274]
1556	Franco recommended dividing the constriction at the neck of a strangulated hernial sac.[372]
1559	Stromayr published Practica Copiosa, differentiating direct and indirect hernia and advocating excision of the sac in indirect hernia.[989]

Renaissance

1700	Littre reported a Meckel's diverticulum in a hernial sac.[701]
1724	Heister distinguished direct and indirect hernia.[490]
1731	De Carengeot described the appendix in a hernial sac.[276]
1756	Cheselden described successful operation for an inguinal hernia.[211]
1757	Pott described the anatomy of hernia and of strangulation.[922]
1785	Richter described a partial enterocele.[956]
1790	John Hunter speculated about the congenital nature of complete indirect inguinal hernia.[524]
1793	De Gimbernat described his ligament and advocated medial rather than upward division of the constriction in strangulated femoral hernia. This avoided damage to the inguinal ligament and the serious bleeding, which sometimes followed.[277]
1804	Cooper published his three-part book on hernia – The plates are a tour de force; they are almost life-sized and depict anatomy as never before. Cooper defined the fascia transversalis; he distinguished this layer from the peritoneum and demonstrated that it was the main barrier to herniation. He carefully delineated the extension of the fascia transversalis behind the inguinal ligament into the thigh as the femoral sheath and the pectineal part of the inguinal ligament – Cooper's ligament.[196–198]
1811	Colles, who had worked as a dissector for Cooper, described the reflected inguinal ligament.[233]
1816	Hesselbach described the anatomy of his triangle.[502]
1816	Cloquet described the processus vaginalis and observed it was rarely closed at birth. He also described his 'gland', so important in the differential diagnosis of lumps in the groin.[225] Anesthesia discovered.[745]
1870	Lister introduced antiseptic surgery and carbolized catgut.[700]
1871	Marcy, who had been a pupil of Lister, described his operation.[742]
1874	Steele described a radical operation for hernia.[1084]
1875	Annandale successfully used an extraperitoneal groin approach to treat a direct and an indirect inguinal and a femoral hernia on the same side in a 46-year-old man. Annandale plugged the femoral canal with the redundant inguinal hernial sacs.[37]
1876	Czerny pulled the sac down through the external ring, ligated it at its neck, excised it and allowed it to retract back into the canal.[262]
1881	Lucas-Championniere opened the canal and reconstructed it by imbrication of its anterior wall.[713]
1886	MacEwan operated through the external ring; he rolled up the sac and used it to plug the canal.[724]
1887	Bassini published the first description of his operation.[91]
1889	Halsted I operation described.[461]

1890 Coley's operation – placing the internal oblique anterior to the cord which emerged at the pubic end of the repair. This was the most pernicious and least effective corruption of Bassini's operation.[232]

1891 Tait advocated median abdominal section for hernia.[1114]

1892 Wolfler designed the anterior relaxing incision in the rectus sheath to relieve tension on the pubic end repair and prevent recurrence at that site.[1220]

1893 Lockwood emphasized the importance of adequate repair of the fascia transversalis.[702]

1895 W.J. Mayo – a radical cure for umbilical hernia.[761]

1895 Andrews introduced imbrication or 'double-breasting' of the layers.[35]

1898 Lotheissen used Cooper's ligament in repair of femoral hernia.[711]

1898 Brenner described 'reinforcing' the repair by suturing the cremaster between the internal oblique arch and the inguinal ligament. The fascia transversalis is not inspected. A serious corruption of the Marcy-Bassini strategy.[142]

1899 Ferguson advised leaving the cord undisturbed – a more serious corruption of Bassini.[352]

1901 McArthur darned his inguinal repair with a pedicled strip of external oblique aponeurosis.[764]

1902 Berger turned down a rectus flap to repair inguinal hernia.[115]

Modern aseptic

1903 Halsted II operation. Halsted abandoned cord skeletonization to avoid hydrocele and testicular atrophy, and adopted Andrews' imbrication and the Wolfler–Berger technique of a relaxation incision and a rectus sheath flap.[462]

1906 Russell – the 'saccular theory' of hernias, postulating that all indirect inguinal hernias are congenital.[987]

1907 Kocher – revised operation for indirect hernia without opening the canal. The sac was dissected, invaginated and transposed laterally.[607]

1909 McGavin used silver filigree to repair inguinal hernias.[771]

1909 Nicol reported pediatric day-case inguinal herniotomy in Glasgow.[844]

1910 Kirschner used a free transplant of fascia lata from the thigh to reinforce the external oblique.[601]

1918 Handley reconstructed the canal using a darn/lattice technique.[470]

1919 LaRoque – transperitoneal repair of inguinal hernia through grid iron (muscle splitting) incision.[634]

1920 Cheatle – extraperitoneal approach to the groin through a midline incision.[206]

1921 Gallie used strips of autologous fascia lata to repair inguinal hernia.[381]

1923 Keith – classic review of the causation of inguinal hernia. He remarked that aponeurosis and fascia are living structures and speculated that a tissue defect could be responsible for the onset of hernias in middle age.[578]

1927 Keynes – surgeon to the London Truss Society – advocated elective operation using fascial graft techniques.[584]

1936 Henry – extraperitoneal approach to groin hernia.[494]

1940 Wakeley – a personal series of 2020 hernias.[1179]

1942 Tanner popularized rectus sheath 'slide'.[1116]

1945 Lytle reinterpreted the importance of the internal ring.[718]

1945 Mair introduced the technique of using buried skin to repair an inguinal hernia.[737]

1952 Douglas – first experimental studies of the dynamics of healing (aponeurosis) showed that aponeurotic strength was slow to recover and only reached an optimum at 120 days.[314]

1953 Shouldice – a series of 8317 hernia repairs with overall recurrence rate to 10 years of 0.8%. Emphasis on anatomic repair and early ambulation.[1046]

1955 Farquharson – an experience of 485 adults who had their hernias repaired as day cases.[344]

1956 Fruchaud – the concept of the myopectineal orifice and fascia transversalis tunnel for all groin hernias.[376]

1958 Marsden – a 3-year follow-up of inguinal hernioplasties. An important contribution to the evaluation of results.[749]

1958 Usher – the use of knitted polypropylene mesh in hernia repair.[1155]

1960 Anson and McVay – classic dissections and evaluation of musculoaponeurotic layers based on a study of 500 body halves.[39]

1962 Doran described the pitfalls of hernia follow-up and set out criteria for adequate evaluation.[312]

1970 Lichtenstein showed the interdependence of suture strength and absorption characteristics with wound healing. Demonstrated experimentally the critical role of non-absorbable or very slowly absorbable sutures in aponeurotic healing.[689]

1972 Doran – critical review of short-stay surgery for inguinal hernia in Birmingham.[313]

1973 Glassow reported 18 400 repairs of indirect hernia with a recurrence rate less than 1%.[423]

1979 Laparoscopic hernia repair first attempted.[398]

1981 Read demonstrated a tissue defect, metastatic emphysema, in smokers with direct herniation.[181]

1981 Chan described patients developing hernia while undergoing continuous ambulatory peritoneal dialysis.[202]

1983 Schurgers demonstrated an open processus vaginalis in a man 5 months after commencement on peritoneal dialysis.[1029]

1984 Gilbert described the umbrella plug for inguinal hernia repair.[406]

1985 Read postulated an etiological relationship between smoking, inguinal herniation and aortic aneurysm.[180]

1986 Lichtenstein described the tension-free repair of inguinal hernias.[690]

1989   Gullmo demonstrates the value of herniography in patients with obscure symptoms in the groin or pelvis and to exclude primary or recurrent hernia.[451]

1990   Robbins and Rutkow introduced the concept of a pre-formed mesh plug introduced into the hernia defect covered by a loose lying mesh patch.[960]

1990   Schultz first used a synthetic prosthetic biomaterial in the laparoscopic repair of an inguinal hernia.[1026]

1991   LeBlanc performs laparoscopic incisional hernia repair.[669]

1992   Dulucq repairs an inguinal hernia laparoscopically without direct entry into the abdominal cavity.[318]

1993   Environmental factors in hernia causation redefined.[186]

1994   Gilmore describes the surgical treatment of 1400 sportsmen with groin disruption detailing the patho-physiology and treatment.[415]

2

Essential anatomy of the abdominal wall

The anatomy of the abdominal wall is well-documented in several standard texts on anatomy, which contain accurate and detailed information that is readily available. The lined drawings in this chapter have been adapted from published reports for anatomists and surgeons with particular attention to applied surgical anatomy and anatomical variance of the normal. Pathological processes further disorganize the underlying anatomy and the surgeon who seeks to make a success of hernia repairs should fully understand these anatomical variations. Today the surgeon should individualize the operation for the anatomy encountered.

The shortcomings of the Bassini operation encouraged surgeons to re-examine the anatomy of the abdominal wall in order to generate practical advice for surgeons encountering pathological or anatomical variations from the standard descriptions.

Under normal circumstances the musculo-aponeurotic layers of the abdominal wall are designed to retain the contents of the peritoneal cavity. There are certain limited areas however where the underlying anatomical structure is deficient and where hernias develop. This deficiency is most notable in the groin area in relation to the inguinal and femoral canals but there are several other sites notably the umbilicus, epigastrium, lumbar triangle, obturator canal, sciatic foramina, perineum, pelvic sidewall and the spigelian line. The list is quite long and the clinician may or may not encounter one of the rarer types of abdominal wall hernias in a lifetime.

The work of Anson and McVay on the inguinal canal appeared in 1938, and since then they and their associate Zimmerman have published extensively. Other notable contributors include Askar, Condon, Fruchaud, Griffith, Harkins, Kark, Lytle, Madden, Mizrachy, Nyhus, Ruge, Skandalakis and Van Mameren.

EXTERNAL ANATOMY – THE SURFACE MARKINGS

The abdominal wall, bounded by the lower margin of the thorax above, and by the pubes, the iliac crests and the inguinal ligaments below, is easily recognized in the upright man. Vertically down the center of the abdomen the depression of the linea alba is obvious and is usually more apparent above the umbilicus. The umbilicus lies at the junction of the upper three-fifths and lower two-fifths of the linea alba. In the healthy young adult the rectus muscle is prominent on either side of the linea alba. The rectus muscle is particularly prominent inferolaterally to the

umbilicus: this infra-umbilical rectus mound is of surgical importance. With ageing and obesity the lower abdomen sags but the infra-umbilical rectus mound remains obvious and visible to the subject, even into old age.

The outer margin of each rectus is indicated by a convex vertically directed furrow, the semilunar line (linea semilunaris), which is most distinct in the upper abdomen where it commences at the tip of the ninth costal cartilage. At first it descends almost vertically, but inferior to the umbilicus it gently curves medially to terminate at the pubic tubercle. It is along this line that the internal oblique aponeurosis bands and splits to enclose the rectus muscle in the upper two-thirds of the abdomen. The broad furrow of the inferior semilunar line is also described as the Spigelian fascia and is the site of herniation (Chapter 21). In the lower abdomen the configuration varies, a wider pelvis and greater pubic prominence being important female characteristics (Figure 2.1).

The surgeon must be aware of the elastic and connective tissue lines in the skin (Langer's lines) if optimum healing is to be obtained. Incisions made at right angles to Langer's lines gape and tend to splay out when they heal. The longitudinal contraction of the healing wound, particularly when the wound crosses a skin delve or body crease, can make healing very unsightly with contracture and for these reasons vertical incisions over the groin should be avoided. However, rapid abdominal access requires adequate vertical incisions and they continue to remain in everyday general surgical and gynecological practice particularly in emergency surgery (Figure 2.2).

THE SUBCUTANEOUS LAYER

Beneath the skin there is the subcutaneous areolar tissue and fascia. Superiorly over the lower chest and epigastrium this layer is generally thin and less organized than in the lower abdomen where it becomes bilaminar – a superficial fatty stratum (Camper's fascia) and a deeper, stronger and more elastic layer (Scarpa's fascia). Scarpa's fascia is well developed in infancy, forming a distinct layer which must be separately incised when the superficial inguinal ring is approached in childhood herniotomy.

In the lower abdomen the deeper fascia (Scarpa's) is more membranous with much elastic tissue and almost devoid of

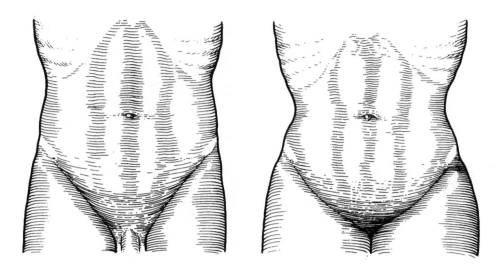

Figure 2.1 *Topographical anatomy of the abdomen – the distinctly different male and female characteristics are important in hernia surgery. The boundaries of the abdomen, the costal cartilages above and the crests of the iliac and pubic bones and the inguinal ligament inferiorly are illustrated. The umbilicus, the rectus muscle and the semilunar lines are important surface landmarks.*

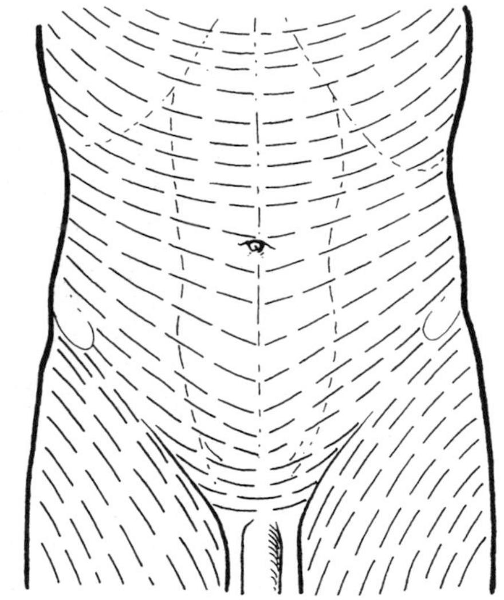

fatty in texture and is easily distorted by the dilatation of any of the structures in its neighborhood, a varicose saphenous vein, enlarged lymph nodes and lymphatics, and a femoral hernia. The cribriform fascia is the anterior boundary of the femoral canal at this site (Figure 2.4).

After deciding the site of an incision in the abdominal wall the surgeon will encounter a reasonably constant pattern of blood vessels. Superficially they anastomose to make a network in the subcutaneous tissue. The lower intercostal arteries, the musculophrenic and the right and left superior epigastric arteries (continuations of the internal thoracic from the subclavian) supply the abdominal wall cephalad to the umbilicus. Caudal to the umbilicus the superior epigastric vessels are continuous with the inferior epigastric vessels lying deep to the rectus muscle; the inferior epigastric artery arises from the external iliac artery just proximal to the inguinal ligament.

Figure 2.2 *Tension lines of the skin (Langer's lines). Incisions at right angles tend to splay and lead to unsightly scars. This adverse phenomenon is enhanced if the incision also crosses a joint crease. Vertical incisions in the groin for hernia repair are particularly unsightly.*

fat. This fascia does not pass down uninterrupted to the thigh and perineum as the superficial fatty fascia does; instead, the deep fascia is attached to the inner half of the inguinal ligament, to the anterior fascia lata of the thigh and to the iliac crest laterally. Medially it forms a distinct structure containing much elastic tissue and descends, almost as a band, from the pubis to envelop the penis as the suspensory ligament. Internally it can be traced as a thin layer over the penis and scrotum. Behind the scrotum it becomes continuous with the deep layer of the superficial fascia of the perineum (Colles' fascia) (Figure 2.3).

The superficial fascia in the upper medial thigh has important anatomic features for the hernia surgeon. It is interrupted by the passage, from superficial to deep, of the saphenous vein and other structures, at the saphenous opening or fossa ovalis. Attenuated connective tissue, the cribriform fascia, packs and 'closes' the saphenous opening. Although the cribriform fascia lies in the same plane as the deep fascia, it has many of the structural characteristics of the superficial fascia: it is loose and

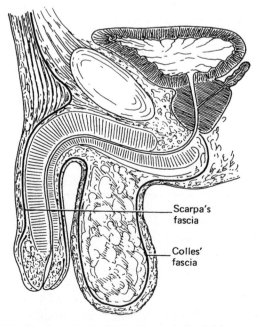

Scarpa's fascia

Colles' fascia

Figure 2.3 *The deep elastic fascia (Scarpa's fascia) is stronger over the lower abdomen where it forms a distinct layer that requires division in groin hernia operations.*

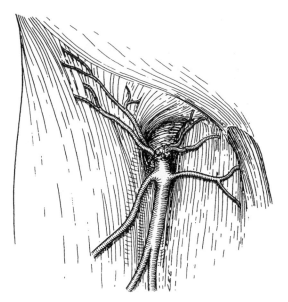

Figure 2.4 *In the upper thigh the long saphenous vein goes from superficial to deep to join the femoral vein which is contained in the femoral sheath, an extension of the abdominal fascia transversalis. The femoral sheath is deficient anteriorly where the saphenous vein penetrates it. This weak part of the femoral sheath is the sieve-like cribriform fascia.*

The inferior epigastric artery forms the lateral margin of Hesselbach's triangle;[502] the neck of an indirect inguinal hernia is lateral and a direct inguinal hernia medial to this artery.

In addition to the serially arranged vessels, there are three small superficial branches of the femoral artery in the upper thigh (and accompanying veins draining to the saphenous vein) which spread out from the groin over the lower abdomen. These vessels are the superficial circumflex iliac passing laterally and upwards over the inguinal canal, the superficial epigastric coursing upward and medially and the superficial external pudendal making its way medially to supply the skin of the penis and scrotum and, importantly, to anastomose with the spermatic cord vessels to the scrotal contents. All these arteries are encountered in inguinal and femoral hernioplasty; all anastomose adequately both with the serial intercostal and lumbar arteries and across the midline. In most instances they can be divided with impunity, but sometimes they are an important auxiliary blood supply to the testicle (Figure 2.5). The veins accompanying the arteries drain ultimately into the femoral vein at the saphenous opening from the lower abdomen and into the subclavian vein from the upper abdomen.

SUPERFICIAL NERVES

The cutaneous nerves are arranged segmentally, similarly to the intercostal nerves in the thorax. The lower five or six nerves sweep around obliquely to supply the abdominal parietes, giving a lateral cutaneous branch which passes between the digitations of the external oblique muscle; this branch divides into a small posterior nerve which extends back over the latissimus

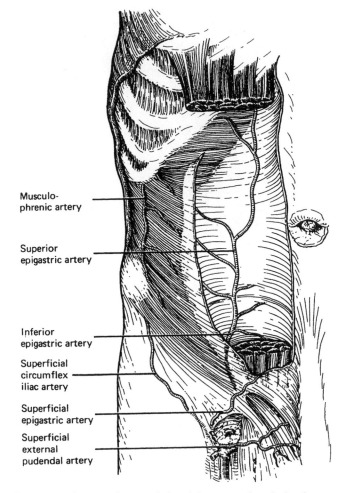

Musculo-
phrenic artery

Superior
epigastric artery

Inferior
epigastric artery

Superficial
circumflex
iliac artery

Superficial
epigastric artery

Superficial
external
pudendal artery

Figure 2.5 *The vasculature of the abdomen and groin is of particular interest to the surgeon. Fortunately the vessels all anastomose freely, so surgery does not need to be locked into vascular anatomy, except for the anastomosis of the pudendal with the cord vessels over the pubis. Care should be taken not to dissect the superficial tissues medial to the pubic tubercle to avoid threat to the pudendal anastomosis and the testicle.*

dorsi and a larger anterior nerve which supplies the external oblique and the overlying subcutaneous tissue and skin. The main stem of the intercostal nerve continues forwards and gains the surface by passing through the rectus muscle and emerging through the anterior rectus sheath a centimeter or so from the midline (Figure 2.6).

The most caudal of the abdominal wall nerves are derived from the first lumbar nerve; they are the iliohypogastric and ilio-inguinal nerves. The ilio-inguinal nerve is generally smaller than the iliohypogastric nerve – if one is large the other is smaller and vice versa. Occasionally the ilio-inguinal nerve is very small and may be absent. The anterior cutaneous branch of the iliohypogastric nerve emerges through the aponeurosis of the external oblique just above the superficial inguinal ring and innervates the skin in the suprapubic region. The ilio-inguinal nerve passes through the lower inguinal canal and becomes superficial by emerging from the superficial inguinal ring to supply the skin of the scrotum and a small area of the medial upper thigh (Figure 2.7).

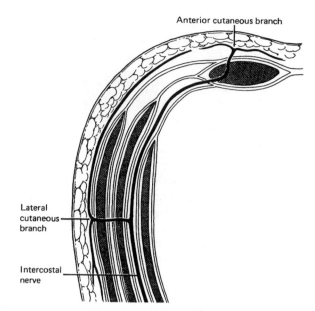

Figure 2.6 *The lower abdomen is segmentally supplied by the intercostal nerves. Each nerve has a lateral cutaneous branch which gives anterior and posterior divisions in the subcutaneous tissue. When a local anesthetic is administered it is important to block the anterior division of the lateral cutaneous branch of these nerves.*

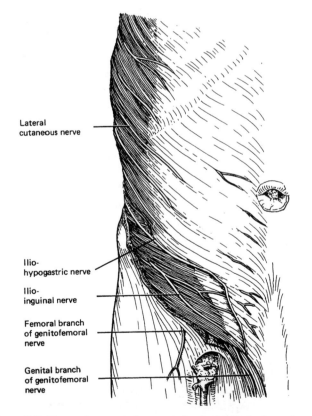

Figure 2.7 *The groin area is innervated principally by branches of the first lumbar nerve – the iliohypogastric and ilio-inguinal nerves. These nerves innervate the skin area over the iliac crest (the lateral branch of the iliohypogastric nerve), the suprapubic region (the anterior iliohypogastric nerve) and the side of the scrotum and upper medial thigh (the ilio-inguinal nerve after it emerges from the inguinal canal).*

The genitofemoral nerve arises from the first and second lumbar nerves and completes the innervation of the abdominal wall and groin areas. At first it passes obliquely forwards and downwards through the substance of the psoas major. It emerges from the muscle and crosses its anterior surface deep to the peritoneum, going behind, posterior to, the ureter. It divides a variable distance from the deep inguinal ring into a genital and a femoral branch.

The posterior two-thirds of the scrotum are supplied by S2 and S3 through the perineal and posterior femoral cutaneous nerves. The anterior scrotal cutaneous supply is frequently disrupted in inguinal hernioplasty (Figure 2.8).

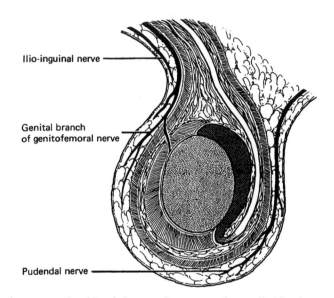

Figure 2.8 *The skin of the anterior scrotum is supplied by the ilio-inguinal nerve, L1, and the genital branch of the genitofemoral nerve, L1. These nerves are often disrupted in hernioplasty.*

The sensory nerve supply of the upper anterior thigh is from the lateral cutaneous nerve of the thigh, the femoral branch of the genitofemoral nerve, the ilio-inguinal nerve and the genital branch of the genitofemoral nerve (Figure 2.9). There is overlap between the territories of these nerves and their pathways also show considerable variation.

The lateral cutaneous nerve of the thigh arises from the dorsal branches of the ventral rami of the second and third lumbar nerves. It emerges from the lateral border of the psoas major and crosses the iliacus obliquely, running towards the anterior superior spine. It lies in the adipose tissue between the iliopsoas muscle fascia and the peritoneum.

Usually the lateral cutaneous nerve of the thigh forms one single trunk but it may divide into two branches a variable distance proximal to the inguinal ligament[986] (Figure 2.10). The nerve then penetrates the anterior surface of the body by passing deep to the lateral portion of the inguinal ligament; it may lie superficial to the sartorius muscle here or may pass through the sartorius before it becomes superficial to supply the skin of the lateral side of the thigh. The variability of the course of the

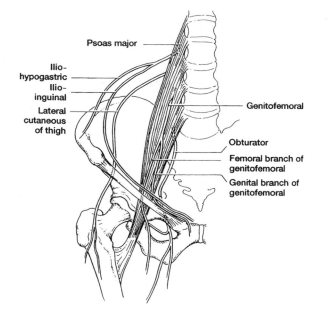

Figure 2.9 *The nerves of the lower abdomen, the groin and upper thigh. The lateral cutaneous nerve of the thigh and the femoral branch of the genitofemoral nerve are at special risk in extraperitoneal operations on groin hernia.*

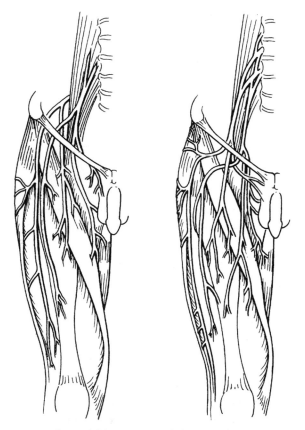

Figure 2.10 *The variable anatomy of the lateral cutaneous nerve of the thigh and the femoral branch of the genitofemoral nerve. Both these nerves are in close proximity to the inguinal ligament as they progress to the thigh. (After Ruge, 1908 – from Van Mameren and Go, 1995.)[986]*

nerve in the abdomen is considerable and the distance between nerve and the deep inguinal ring also variable.[515] The nerve may traverse the anterior abdominal wall cranial to the inguinal ligament or through the attachment of the ligament to the anterior superior iliac spine.

The genital branch, a mixed motor and sensory nerve, crosses the femoral vessels and enters the inguinal canal at or just medial to the deep ring. The nerve penetrates the fascia transversalis of the posterior wall of the inguinal ligament either through the deep ring or separately medially to the deep ring. The nerve traverses the inguinal canal lying between the spermatic cord above and the upturned edge of the inguinal ligament inferiorly; the nerve is vulnerable to surgical trauma as it progresses along the floor of the canal (the gutter produced by the upturned internal edge of the inguinal ligament). The genital nerve supplies the motor function to the cremaster muscle and the sensory function to the skin of the scrotum.

The femoral branch enters the femoral sheath lying lateral to the femoral artery and supplies the skin of the upper part of the femoral triangle (Figure 2.11).

The scrotal nerve supply is complex.[1227] The autonomic supply of the testis is from T10 to T12, via nerves which accompany the spermatic vessels. These autonomic nerves are motor to the vasculature and to the smooth muscle of the tunica albuginea. However, they also have free, sensory, endings in the interstitial spaces of the testis and convey noxious stimuli which give referred pain in the lower abdomen (T10–T12 segments). The autonomic supply of the vas and epididymis are distinct from those of the testis; pain from these structures is felt in the L1 segment, lower than testicular pain, in the distributions of the genitofemoral nerve.

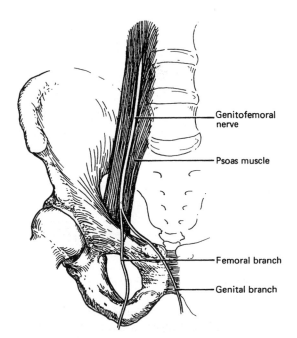

Figure 2.11 *The genitofemoral nerve, from L1 and L2, innervates the femoral sheath and the skin over it. It needs blocking when a femoral hernia is to be operated under local anesthetic.*

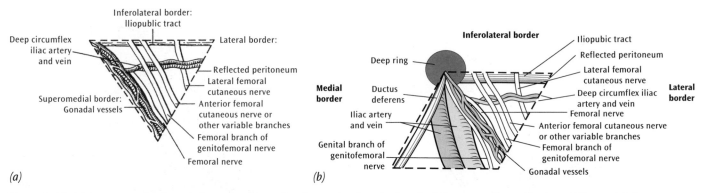

Figure 2.12 *(a) Laparoscopic view of the nerves immediately proximal to the inguinal ligament after reflection of the parietal peritoneum. These nerves lie in the adipose tissue just deep to the peritoneum and superficial to the iliopsoas muscle: the 'triangle of pain'. (b) Laparoscopic view of the deep inguinal ring and adjacent structures, the 'triangle of doom'. (After Skandalakis et al. 1996.)*

The somatic nerve supply is the genitofemoral nerve, L1 and L2, and the sacral nerve, S2 and S3. The genital branch of the genitofemoral nerve supplies the cord, the cremaster, the tunica vaginalis and, along with the L1 component of the ilio-inguinal nerve, the anterior third of the scrotal skin.

The area lateral to the cord vessels and above the inguinal ligament where the femoral branch of genitofemoral nerve and lateral cutaneous nerve of the thigh lie has been dubbed the 'triangle of pain' by laparoscopic surgeons because of the hazard of nerve injury by entrapment with staples. In this area thick globular adipose tissue can surround and conceal the nerves. On a deeper plane the femoral nerve crosses this triangle with the genitofemoral and lateral cutaneous nerve superficial to it (Figure 2.12). This entire area is considered to be the 'quadrangle of doom'. All of the nerves that can be injured during the laparoscopic inguinal hernia repair are located in this anatomic region.

THE EXTERNAL OBLIQUE MUSCLE

The external oblique muscle arises by eight digitations from the external surfaces of the lower eight ribs; the upper three digitations alternate with the origins of the serratus anterior and the lower four with those of the latissimus dorsi muscle. The fibers pass downwards and forwards from their origins; the posterior fibers are nearly vertical and are inserted into the anterior external lip of the iliac crest: in contrast, the uppermost fibers run almost horizontally towards the contralateral side. The intervening fibers pursue an intermediate oblique course. All the superior and intermediate fibers end in the strong external oblique aponeurosis.

Superiorly the aponeurosis is relatively thin and passes medially to be attached to the xiphoid process. Inferiorly the aponeurosis is very strong. Along its lower margin the aponeurosis forms the inguinal ligament, which is attached superolaterally to the anterior superior iliac spine and inferomedially to the pubic tubercle. The aponeurosis of the muscle forms the anterior rectus sheath and is inserted, along with its fellow of the opposite side, into the linea alba and the front of the pubis.

The aponeurosis is broadest inferiorly, narrowest at the umbilicus and broad again in the epigastrium.

The aponeurosis of the external oblique muscle fuses with the aponeurosis of the internal oblique in the anterior rectus sheath. This line of fusion is considerably medial to the semilunar line – the fusion line is oblique and somewhat semilunar, being more lateral above and more medial below. In fact, the external oblique aponeurosis contributes very little to the lower portion of the anterior rectus sheath. This latter point is of considerable importance in inguinal hernioplasty[776] (Figure 2.13).

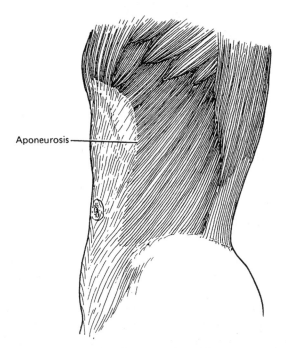

Figure 2.13 *The external oblique muscle and its aponeurosis invests the abdomen. The aponeurosis of this muscle forms the anterior rectus sheath by fusion to the underlying aponeurosis of the internal oblique. However, this line of fusion, in the lower abdomen especially, is considerably medial to the semilunar line, a point of great importance in inguinal hernioplasty, allowing a 'slide operation' on the internal oblique without compromising the anterior rectus sheath (see page 31).*

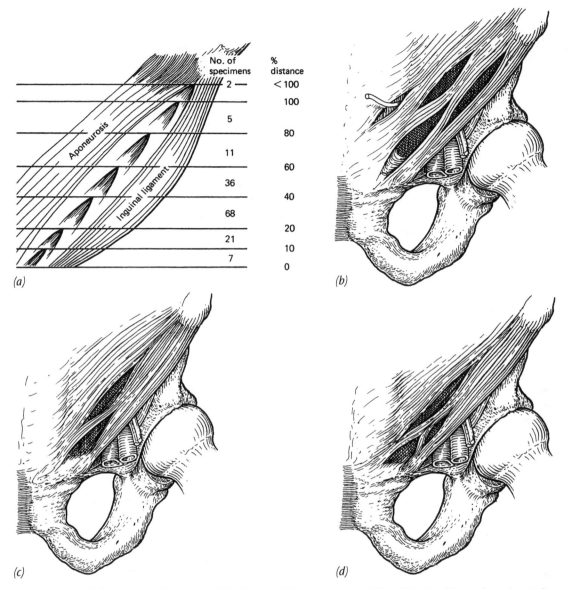

Figure 2.14 *The anatomy and dimensions of the superficial inguinal ring are very variable. The 'ring' is a triangular cleft separating the insertions of the external oblique muscles into the pubic crest and the pubic tubercle. Its base is medial and inferior and its apex superior and lateral. In 80% of subjects the apex lies in the medial half of the lower abdomen, but in the remaining 20% the apex approaches the anterior superior iliac spine (a). In 2% of subjects, there are accessory clefts superior to the main cleft (b,c,d). One of these clefts may transmit the iliohypogastric nerve (b). (From Anson, Morgan and McVay, 1960.)*[39]

There is a defect in the external–oblique aponeurosis just above the pubis. This aperture – the superficial inguinal ring – is triangular in shape and in the male allows passage of the spermatic cord from the abdomen to the scrotum. In the female the round ligament of the uterus passes through this opening. The superficial inguinal ring is not a 'ring'; it is a triangular cleft with its long axis oblique in the same direction but not quite parallel to the inguinal ligament. The base of the triangle is formed by the crest of the pubis and the apex is lateral towards the anterior superior iliac spine. The superficial inguinal ring represents that interval between the aponeurosis of the external oblique which inserts into the pubic bone superiorly and, as the inguinal ligament, inserts into the pubic tubercle inferiorly. The aponeurotic margins of the ring are described as the superior and inferior

crura. The spermatic cord, as it comes through the superficial ring, rests on the inferior crus which is a continuation of the floor of the inguinal canal (the upturned internal margin of the inguinal ligament).

The dimensions of the superficial inguinal ring, or aponeurotic cleft, are of surgical importance. Far from being of standard size and predictable extent it may sometimes be snug around the cord and occasionally extend upward and laterally beyond the anterior superior iliac spine. In 80% of cases the cleft is confined to the lower half of the area between the midline and the anterior superior spine, but in the remaining 20% it extends more laterally. In about 2% of cases there are one or more accessory clefts, usually superolaterally to the main cleft; the accessory cleft may transmit the iliohypogastric nerve[39] (Figure 2.14).

The relationship between the apex of the cleft and the deep epigastric vessels (indicating the lateral margin of Hesselbach's triangle) is of crucial importance in closing the inguinal canal anteriorly and containing a potential direct inguinal hernia. Whereas the canal is usually described as closed anteriorly by the external oblique aponeurosis, in only 11% of cases does the apex of the cleft lie less than halfway along a line from the pubic tubercle to the inferior epigastric artery; in 52% the cleft extends to the level of the epigastric vessels and, most importantly, in 37% the apex of the cleft is lateral to the epigastric vessels[39] (Figure 2.15).

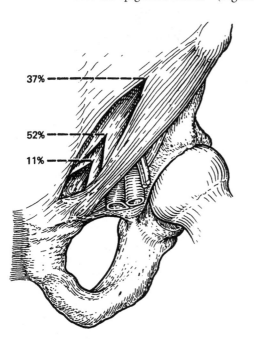

Figure 2.15 *The size of the superficial inguinal ring, the cleft in the external oblique, is crucial in closing the inguinal canal anteriorly. In 11% of subjects the cleft extends less than 50% of the length of the inguinal canal, in 52% it extends as far as the deep epigastric vessels, and in 37% the cleft extends lateral to the deep epigastric vessels. (From Anson, Morgan and McVay, 1960).[39]*

The crura of the superficial ring are joined together by intercrural fibers derived from the outer investing fascia of the external oblique aponeurosis. The size and strength of these intercrural fibers vary. In 27% of specimens these fibers do not cross from crus to crus and, therefore, do not reinforce the margins of the cleft[39] (Figure 2.16).

The external oblique aponeurosis in the region of the groin forms a free border known as Poupart's ligament or the inguinal ligament, which is simply the lower margin of this aponeurosis; it is not a condensed thickened ligamentous structure. The ligament presents a rounded surface towards the thigh where the aponeurosis is rolled inwards back on itself to make a groove on its deep surface. Laterally the ligament is attached to the anterior superior iliac spine and medially to the pubic tubercle and via the lacunar and reflected inguinal ligaments to the iliopectineal line on the superior ramus of the pubis. The inguinal ligament is not straight; it is concave, with the concavity directed medially and upward towards the abdomen (Figure 2.17).

The medial attachment, or continuation, of the inguinal ligament as the lacunar (Gimbernat's) and the pectineal (Cooper's) ligament gives a fan-like expansion of the inguinal ligament at its medial end, which curves posteriorly to the iliopectineal ligament. This expansion has important surgical implications.

The lacunar ligament is a triangular continuation of the medial end of the inguinal ligament. Its apex is at the pubic tubercle, its superior margin continuous with the inguinal ligament, and its medial margin is attached to the iliopectineal line on the superior ramus of the pubis. Its lateral crescentic edge is free and directed laterally, where it is an important rigid structure in the medial margin of the femoral canal. The ligament lies in an oblique plane, with its upper (abdominal) surface facing superomedially and being crossed by the spermatic cord, and its lower (femoral) surface looking anterolaterally. With the external oblique aponeurosis and the inguinal ligament, the superior surface forms a groove for the cord as it emerges from the inguinal canal (Figure 2.18).

The reflected part of the inguinal ligament (Colles') is a broad band of rather thin fibers which arise from the crest of the pubis and the medial end of the iliopectineal line and pass anterosuperiorly behind the superior crus of the subcutaneous inguinal ring to the linea alba. The reflected part of the inguinal ligament is very variable in its extent but it is an important structure closing the potential space in the posterior wall of the inguinal canal between the iliopectineal line and the lateral margin of the rectus muscle (Figure 2.19).

THE INTERNAL OBLIQUE MUSCLE

The internal oblique muscle arises from the lateral half of the abdominal surface of the inguinal ligament, the intermediate line on the anterior two-thirds of the iliac crest and the lumbodorsal fascia. The general direction of the fibers is upward and medial. The posterior fibers are inserted into the inferior borders of the cartilages of the lower four ribs. The intermediate fibers pass upward and medially and end in a strong aponeurosis which extends from the inferior borders of the seventh and eighth ribs and the xiphoid process to the linea alba throughout its length. The lower fibers, from their origin at the inguinal ligament, arch downward and medially: with the lowest fibers of the transversus muscle they pass in front of the rectus muscle, to form the anterior rectus sheath, and insert on the pubic crest and the iliopectineal line behind the lacunar ligament and reflected part of the inguinal ligament (Figure 2.20).

The internal oblique is not invariable in its anatomy in the inguinal region. Its origin may commence at the internal ring or at a variable distance lateral to the ring. The muscle may then insert either into the pubic crest and tubercle or into the lateral margin of the rectus sheath a variable distance above the pubis. There are thus four common combinations of origin and insertion of the internal oblique in the groin. The contribution of the internal oblique to groin anatomy and

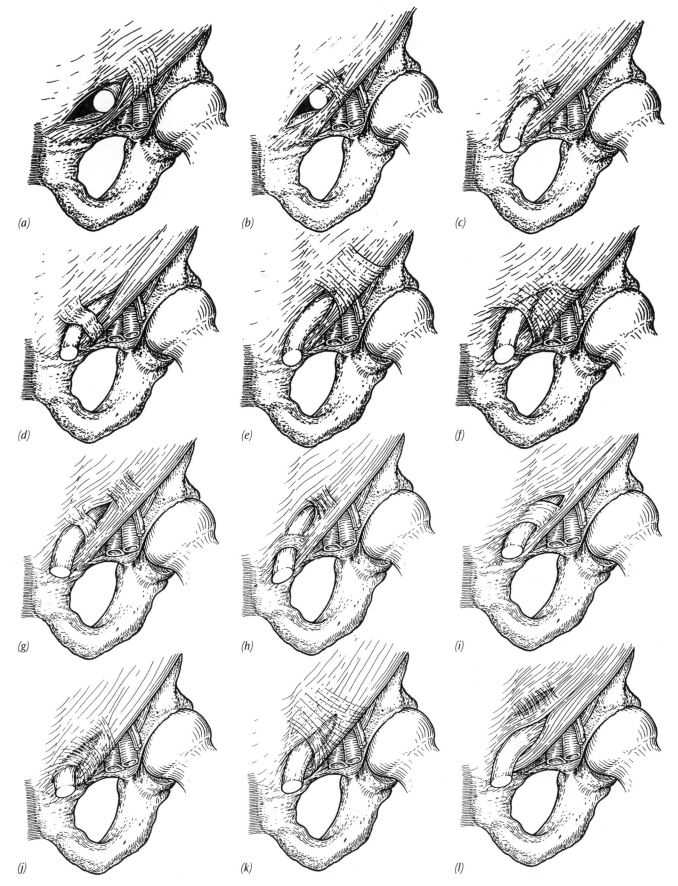

Figure 2.16 (a–l) Variations in the structure of the superficial inguinal ring. The intercrural fibers between the two crura ofige the ring are very variable, in 27% of subjects these intercrural fibers do not cross from one crus to the other. (From Anson, Morgan and McVay, 1960.)[39]

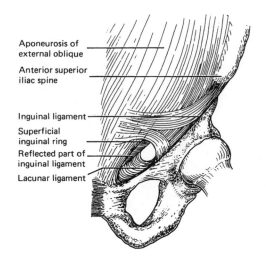

Figure 2.17 *The inguinal ligament is the lower margin of the external oblique muscle. Medially it is attached like a fan to the iliopectineal line (Cooper's ligament) and the tubercle of the pubis.*

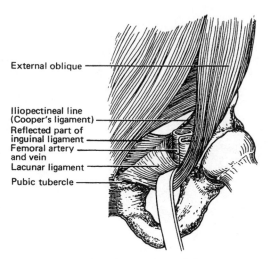

Figure 2.18 *The upper abdominal surface of the attachment of the inguinal ligament to the pubic tubercle is the floor of the inguinal canal which the cord rests on as it emerges from the canal.*

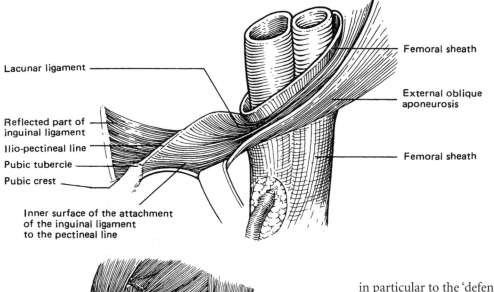

Figure 2.19 *Medially the posterior wall of the inguinal canal is reinforced by the reflected part of the inguinal ligament, a strong triangular fascia arising from the pubic crest anteriorly to the attachments of the internal oblique and transversus muscles and passing medially to the linea alba into which it is inserted.*

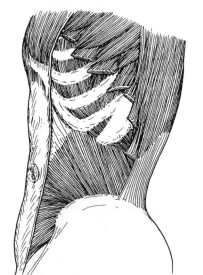

Figure 2.20 *The internal oblique muscle arising from the lateral half of the inguinal ligament and the iliac crest to be inserted into the lower costal cartilage and, via its aponeurosis, continuous with its fellow muscle contralaterally.*

in particular to the 'defences' of the inguinal canal is very variable. There are a number of well-recognized variations in the anatomy of the internal oblique in the groin (see pages 45 and 46) (Figure 2.21).

The detailed anatomy of the semilunar line and rectus sheath, and that of the insertion of the lowermost fibers of the internal oblique into the pubic bone, are of surgical significance and warrant more detailed consideration.

At the lateral margin of the rectus muscle the aponeurosis of the internal oblique splits into two lamellae – the superficial lamella passes anterior to the rectus and the deep lamella goes posterior to the rectus. The anterior lamella fuses with the aponeurosis of the external oblique to form the anterior rectus sheath; likewise the posterior lamella becomes fused with the aponeurosis of the underlying transversus muscle. The detailed anatomy varies but has importance in the causation of umbilical and epigastric hernias (see page 238). In the lower part of the abdomen, in an area inferior to a point about midway between the umbilicus and the pubis, the aponeurosis does not split into lamella but courses entirely in front of the rectus to

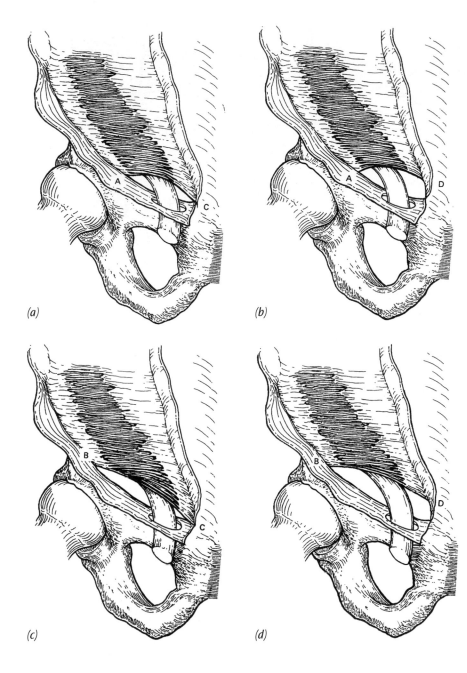

(a)

(b)

(c)

(d)

Figure 2.21 *The origin and insertions of the internal oblique muscle and aponeurosis in the inguinal region are variable. The origin of the red muscle fibers is from the lateral inguinal ligament; this origin may extend as far medially as the deep ring (a), or the muscle may arise more laterally (b). The insertion of the aponeurosis is also variable; it may be inserted into the pubic crest and pubic tubercle (c) or solely into the rectus sheath (d). This gives four variants of the lower margin of the internal oblique in the inguinal canal: A–C, A–D, B–C, B–D.*

fuse with the overlying aponeurosis of the external oblique (Figure 2.22).

The internal oblique muscle in its lateral fleshy part is not uniform in structure; it is segmented or banded. The muscular bands terminate just lateral to the border of the rectus muscle and are most marked in the inguinal and lower abdominal region. The bands are generally arranged like 'the blades of a fan with the interspaces increasing as the medial extremities are reached'.[1074,1238] The bands may easily be separable up to the point where they fuse with the aponeurosis lateral to the rectus muscle. In a fifth of cases there are potential parietal deficits between these bands. Spigelian hernias occur through these defects of the semilunar line, which are more pronounced in the lower abdomen (see page 255).

At the lowermost part of the internal oblique muscle, adjacent to its origin from the inguinal ligament, the spermatic cord passes through or adjacent to the medial margin of the muscle. Laterally the cord lies deep to the fleshy muscular fibers, then as it emerges alongside the muscle it acquires a coat of cremaster muscle from the muscle.

The fascicles of the lower internal oblique muscle follow a transverse or oblique direction. Medial to the cord they convert to an aponeurosis which continues to the insertion of the muscle. There is variation in both the medial and the inferior extent of the muscle fibers of the internal oblique.

The fleshy muscle extends to the inferior margin in only 2% of cases; in 75% the extent is a centimeter or so above the margin, and in 20% there is a broad aponeurotic leaf superior to the spermatic cord. Likewise the fleshy muscle extends as far as the emergent cord in 20%, medial to the cord but not as far medially to the rectus margin in 75%, and medial to the lateral margin of the rectus in 2%.

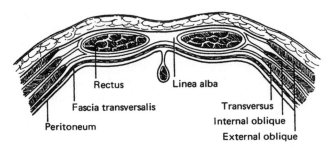

Figure 2.22 *Structure of the posterior rectus sheath in the upper abdomen. The internal oblique divides into two lamellae which enclose the rectus. The line of the fascia transversalis is deliberately emphasized.*

In clinical practice a direct inguinal hernia is never encountered when the lower margin of the internal oblique is fleshy *and* when the fleshy fibers extend medial to the superficial ring. Direct herniation is most frequently found at operation when the internal oblique muscle is replaced with flimsy aponeurosis in the roof of the inguinal canal[39] (Figure 2.23).

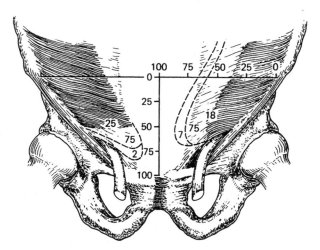

Figure 2.23 *Extent of the muscular fibers of the internal oblique. In only 2% of subjects the muscle extends inferiorly to the inguinal canal (left of diagram). Similarly the medial extent of the fleshy muscle fibers varies (right of diagram). The contribution of the internal oblique to the 'defences' of the inguinal canal is very variable. (From Anson, Morgan and McVay, 1960, by permission of Surgery, Gynecology and Obstetrics.)*

In 52% of cases the lowermost arching fibers of the internal oblique are continuous above with the remainder of the internal oblique muscles but in the remainder a variety of spaces between banding occur. In the medial and lower musculo-aponeurotic plate, defects superior to the spermatic cord may compromise the shutter mechanism of the canal and lead to direct inguinal herniation. Similarly, Spigelian hernia defects can develop between the muscle bands, enter the inguinal canal and present as direct inguinal hernia[1152] (Figure 2.24).

Rarely (0.15% of hernia cases), the spermatic cord comes through the fleshy part of the lower muscle belly so that the

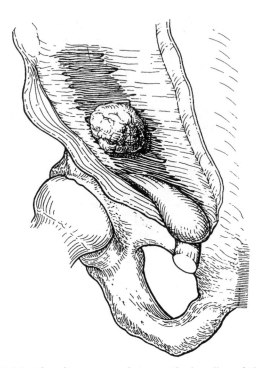

Figure 2.24 *A hernia can occur between the banding of the lower internal oblique muscle. Although this hernia is truly a variant Spigelian hernia, it presents as a direct hernia into the inguinal canal.*

muscle had an origin from the inguinal ligament medial to emergent cord. In these cases there is prominent banding of the muscle in the lower abdomen so that effectively there is a band caudal to the cord (Figure 2.25).

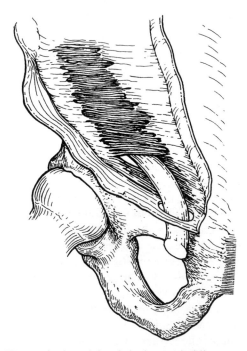

Figure 2.25 *Rarely the origin of the internal oblique extends medially to the deep ring so that the cord passes between bands of the muscle.*

THE TRANSVERSE ABDOMINAL MUSCLE

The transversus abdominis is the third and deepest of the three abdominal muscle layers. The muscle arises from the iliopsoas fascia along the internal lip of the anterior two-thirds of the iliac crest. The iliopsoas fascia is continuous with the thoracolumbar fascia (which is effectively the posterior aponeurosis of the muscle extending its origin to the vertebral column), and the costal cartilages of the lower six ribs interdigitating with the origin of the diaphragm (Figure 2.26).

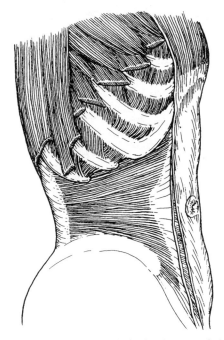

Figure 2.26 *The transversus muscle is the deepest of the parietal muscles; it arises from the iliopsoas fascia and the iliac crest in its anterior two-thirds. The muscle extends to the lowest six costal cartilages and to the linea alba and its contralateral fellow.*

Anteriorly, the muscle fibers end in a strong aponeurosis which is inserted into the linea alba, the pubic crest and the iliopectineal line. For the most part the fibers run transversely, but in the lower abdomen they take on a downward and medial curve so that the lower margin of the muscle forms an arch over the inguinal canal. The lower fibers give way to the aponeurosis which gains insertion into the pubic crest and the iliopectineal line. The insertion of the transverse muscle is broader than that of the internal oblique and consequently its aponeurosis extends further along the iliopectineal line (Figure 2.27).

In the epigastrium and in the lower abdomen, down to a point midway between the umbilicus and the pubis, the transverse aponeurosis fuses with the posterior lamella of the aponeurosis of the internal oblique to form the posterior rectus sheath. In the lowermost abdomen the aponeurosis passes in front of the rectus muscle and fuses with the aponeurosis of the external oblique and internal oblique muscles to form the anterior rectus sheath (Figure 2.28).

The muscle consists of more aponeurosis and much less muscle fibers than either the external or internal oblique muscles.

In 67% of cases fleshy muscle covers only the upper part of the inguinal region. In only 14% of cases are any fleshy fibers found in the lowermost fibers arching over the inguinal canal. Similarly, in 71% of subjects the red fibers do not extend medially to the deep epigastric vessels. The aponeurotic portion of the muscle shows its greatest anatomical variation in the inguinal region, where it is most important in hernia repair.

The lower border of the transversus abdominis aponeurosis is called the 'arch'. Above the arch the transversus aponeurosis forms a continuous strong sheet, with no spaces between its fibers. Below the arch the posterior wall of the inguinal canal is closed by transversalis fascia only. This is a weak area through which direct herniation can occur. The aponeurotic arch is easily identifiable as a 'white line' of aponeurosis at operation (Figures 2.27 and 2.29).

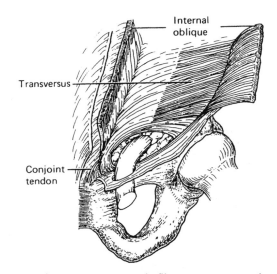

Figure 2.27 *The transversus muscle fibers run transversely, except in the lower abdomen where they form a strong aponeurosis (tendon) which is inserted to the pubic crest and the iliopectineal line. The insertion of the transversus tendon is broader than that of the internal oblique. The extent to which this tendon extends along the iliopectineal line determines its contribution to reinforcing the posterior wall of the inguinal canal. In surgical jargon the lowest fibers of the transversus aponeurosis cross over the cord to form the 'roof' of the canal. These white aponeurotic fibers are referred to as the 'arch' by some surgeons.*

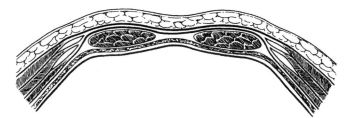

Figure 2.28 *Composition of the posterior rectus sheath in the lower abdomen. In the lower abdomen, inferior to the arcuate line of Douglas, the rectus sheath becomes deficient posteriorly. This is related to the variable anatomy of the internal oblique muscle. The fascia transversalis is stronger in the lower abdomen.*

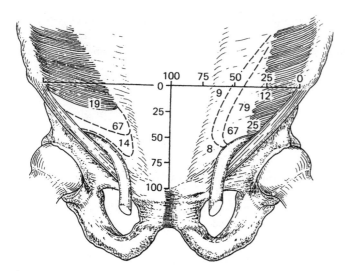

Figure 2.29 *The extent of fleshy red muscle in the transversus muscle is much less than in the internal oblique. Only in 14% of subjects is the lower margin of this muscle in the roof of the inguinal canal composed of red muscle (left of diagram). The medial extent of red fibers is similarly restricted; in 71% of subjects muscle fibers do not extend medially to the inferior epigastric vessels (right of diagram). (From Anson, Morgan and McVay, 1960, by permission of Surgery, Gynecology and Obstetrics.)*

THE CONJOINT TENDON

The transverse fibers of the transversus muscle proceed horizontally to their insertion in the rectus sheath and the linea alba, while the lower fibers course downward, medially and caudally – sometimes to fuse with fibers of the internal oblique as they insert into the anterior pubis and the iliopectineal line.

Only when the aponeuroses of the transversus and the internal oblique are fused some distance lateral to the rectus sheath may the term conjoint tendon be correctly used. Thus the conjoint tendon is the fused aponeuroses of the internal oblique and transversus muscles which is inserted into the anterior 2 cm of the iliopectineal line. The transversus muscle contributes 80% of the conjoint tendon. The conjoint tendon is lateral to the rectus muscle and lies immediately deep to the superficial inguinal ring. It passes down to its insertion deep to the inguinal and lacunar ligaments. The spermatic cord, or round ligament, lies anterior to it as it passes through the superficial inguinal ring.

The conjoint tendon has a very variable structure and in 20% of subjects it does not exist as a discrete anatomic structure. It may be absent or only slightly developed, it may be replaced by a lateral extension of the tendon of origin of the rectus muscle, or it may extend laterally to the deep inguinal ring so that no interval is present between the lower border of the transversus and the inguinal ligament. A shutter mechanism for the conjoint tendon can only be demonstrated when the lateral side of the tendon, that is the transversus and internal oblique muscles, extend onto and are attached to the iliopectineal line.[1237] The

extent of this insertion is very variable. In 8% of cases this attachment does not extend lateral to the rectus muscle, leaving the posterior wall of the inguinal canal (fascia transversalis) unsupported; in 31% the attachment extends to the midpoint of the posterior wall between the pubic spine medially and the deep epigastric vessels laterally; in 40% it extends as far as the deep epigastric vessels. In a minority of cases bands of aponeurosis wind off the main aponeurotic arch and are inserted independently into the iliopectineal line. Sometimes, therefore, the lateral margin of the rectus sheath is formed only from the lowermost fibers of the transversus aponeurosis which curve inferiorly to become attached to the pubis – this is called the falx inguinalis.

A few fibers of the lowermost lateral margin of the rectus tendon may be fused with the fascia transversalis in their attachment to the iliopubic ligament – this has been called Henle's ligament (Figure 2.30).

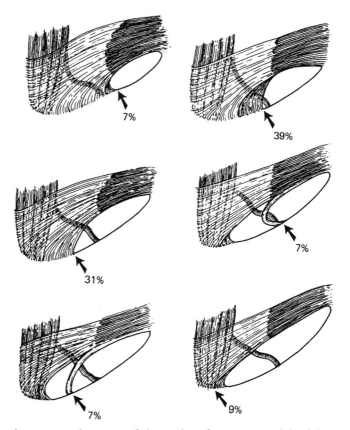

Figure 2.30 *The extent of the tendon of transversus abdominis contributes to the posterior wall of the inguinal canal. The arrows indicate the lateralmost extension in the percentages of subjects. (From Anson, Morgan and McVay, 1960.)[39]*

To understand the importance of the attachment of the internal oblique and transversus aponeuroses to the iliopectineal line, the posterior aspect of the inguinal canal must be visualized from inside the abdomen. If there is full attachment of the conjoint tendon to the iliopectineal line, the posterior wall of the inguinal canal is completely reinforced by aponeurosis. Absence of this attachment removes this reinforcement and there is then the potential to develop a direct or large indirect hernia.

Of all the anatomic layers the external oblique is the least variable; in the inguinal region it is invariably aponeurotic. The internal oblique and transversus layers are very variable; they may be fleshy almost to the midline, aponeurotic or banded fan-like with the space between the musculo-aponeurotic bands occupied only by the flimsiest fascia. If these local weaknesses are superimposed, herniation is facilitated.

Zimmerman and colleagues have drawn attention to the frequency with which defects occur in the internal oblique and transversus muscles in this area. In 45% of their dissections there was a defect in one or other layer and in 6% these defects, of the lower linea semilunaris, were superimposed. These defects predispose to spontaneous ventral hernias either of preperitoneal fat or more extensive hernias with peritoneal sacs.[1237]

THE LINEA ALBA, AND THE RECTUS SHEATH AND ITS CONTENTS

The linea alba is formed in the midline by the decussation of the fibers of the three aponeuroses. The linea alba is a dense fibrous band which extends from the xiphoid process to the pubic symphysis. The linea is broad in the epigastrium, then broadest at the umbilicus, and below the umbilicus it narrows down to become little more than a line between the two rectus muscles at the pubis. The linea alba is pierced by several small blood vessels and by the umbilical vessels in the fetus.

The anterior rectus muscle sheath forms the most important portion of the abdominal wall aponeuroses. When the anterior sheath is gently dissected, during a paramedian incision for example, it is shown to be made of three lamina. The most superficial fibers are directed downward and laterally; these form the external oblique of the opposite side. The next layer, derived from the external oblique of the same side, has fibers at right angles to the first layer, that is they run downwards and medially. Finally, the third component of the anterior rectus sheath is formed from the anterior lamina of the internal oblique muscle of the same side whose fibers generally run in the same direction as, and parallel to, the fibers of the external oblique of the opposite side. This gives the anterior rectus sheath a triple criss-cross pattern similar to plywood.[56] In the lower abdomen the fusion of the external oblique aponeurosis to the internal oblique aponeurosis is very medial, an important anatomical arrangement that allows a tendon slide to be used to release the tension of the internal oblique in direct inguinal hernia repair without compromising the integrity of the anterior rectus sheath.[56] (For further description, see page 22.)

The most important feature from a surgical perspective is that the fibers of the rectus sheath run from side to side. Vertical incisions divide fibers while horizontal incisions down closure with sutures encircling fibers rather than between fibers.

The posterior rectus sheath has a similar trilaminar criss-cross pattern above the umbilicus, where it is composed of the posterior lamina of the internal oblique and the aponeurosis of the transversus abdominis muscle from their sides.

Within the rectus sheath are the rectus muscles, the pyramidalis muscle, the terminal portions of the lower six thoracic nerves and the superior and inferior epigastric vessels (Figure 2.31).

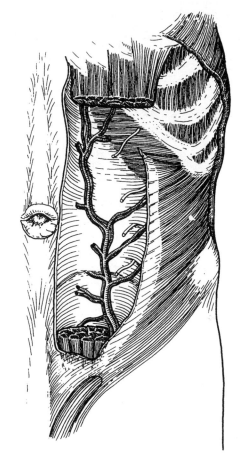

Figure 2.31 *Rectus sheath and linea alba. The contents of the rectus sheath are the rectus and pyramidalis muscles, the superior and inferior epigastric vessels and the terminal branches of the lower six thoracic nerves.*

The rectus muscle is flat and strap-like and extends from the pubis to the thorax. Each muscle is separated from its fellow of the opposite side by the linea alba. The muscle arises by two tendons; the larger and lateral is attached to the crest of the pubis and the smaller and medial mingles with fibers from the opposite side and arises from the ligamentous fibers over the symphysis pubis. The muscle is inserted by broad bundles into the fifth, sixth and seventh costal cartilages and into the xiphoid by a small medial slip. The rectus muscle has three tendinous intersections – one at the xiphoid, one at the umbilicus and one midway between these two. Sometimes a further incomplete intersection is present below the umbilicus. The intersections extend a variable distance across the muscle mass and are intimately adherent to the anterior lamina of the sheath of the muscle, but have no attachment to the posterior sheath.

The pyramidalis muscle is triangular in shape, arising by its base from the ligaments on the anterior surface of the symphysis pubis and being inserted into the lower linea alba. The muscle is absent in 10% of cases (Figure 2.32).

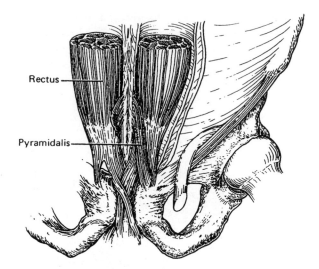

Figure 2.32 *The rectus muscle arises by two tendons – the larger and lateral from the crest of the pubis and the smaller and medial from the pubis of the opposite side and from the ligamentous fibers of the symphysis. The pyramidalis is variable; it arises from the ligamentous fibers of the symphysis and adjacent pubis and is inserted into the linea alba.*

FUNCTION OF THE ANTERIOR ABDOMINAL WALL

Although the anterior abdominal wall is composed of two halves, right and left, it functions in a co-ordinated fashion. The individual muscles cannot work separately. The upper part is the actively mobile respiratory zone, where the rectus sheath – the flank muscles and the rectus muscle through its tendinous attachments to the rectus sheath – functions as an accessory respiratory muscle. The lower part has no tendinous intersections and is a relatively fixed lower belly support zone. This anatomical and physiological configuration has been demonstrated using a transillumination silhouette technique by Askar.[56]

THE FASCIA TRANSVERSALIS – THE SPACE OF BOGROS

The fascia transversalis lies deep to the transverse abdominal muscle plane. It is continuous from side to side and extends from the rib cage above to the pelvis inferiorly.

In the upper abdominal wall the fascia transversalis is thin, but in the lower abdomen and especially in the inguinofemoral region the fascia is thicker and has specialized bands and folds within it. In the groin region, where the fascia transversalis is an important constituent of the posterior wall of the inguinal canal and where it forms the femoral sheath inferiorly to the inguinal ligament, the anatomy and function of the fascia transversalis is of particular importance to the surgeon. As originally described by Sir Astley Cooper in 1807 the fascia transversalis, in the groin, consists of two layers.[238] The anterior strong layer covers

the internal aspect of the transversalis muscle where it is intimately blended with the tendon of the transversus muscle. It then extends across the posterior wall of the inguinal canal medial to the deep ring aperture and is attached to the inner margin of the inguinal ligament. The deeper layer of fascia transversalis, a membranous layer, lies between the anterior substantial layer of fascia transversalis and the peritoneum. The extraperitoneal fat lies behind this layer between it and the peritoneum (Figure 2.33). The deep epigastric vessels run between the two layers of fascia transversalis.

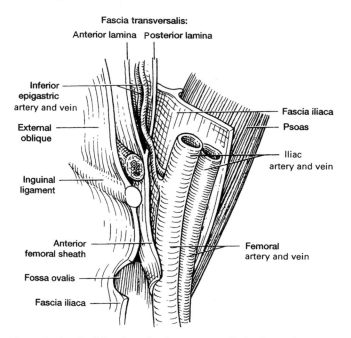

Figure 2.33 *The bilaminar fascia transversalis in the groin. (After Read, 1992; Skandalakis et al., 1996.)[947,1060]*

These two distinct layers of fascia transversalis are readily identified laparoscopically and must be opened separately to allow access to the avascular preperitoneal space (of Bogros) when undertaking an extraperitoneal repair of a groin hernia either laparoscopically or by open surgery. The deeper layer extends down behind the inguinal canal and fuses with the pectineal ligament (of Cooper) before continuing downward into the pelvis. The deeper layer fuses with the spermatic cord at the deep ring and continues into the cord as the internal spermatic fascia.[110,238,947] The existence of the bilaminar structure of the fascia transversalis at the deep ring was confirmed by Lytle[720] and by Cleland,[224] but its nature disputed by the later anatomists Anson and McVay,[39] and its relevance and importance questioned by experienced surgeons.[236]

The dissection of both layers of fascia transversalis from the cord structures at the deep inguinal ring is an important component of hernioplasty; it allows dissection of an indirect peritoneal sac and the divided peritoneal stump to retract at the deep ring in a classic Bassini and Shouldice operation for indirect hernias.

In the lower abdomen it is attached laterally to the internal lip of the iliac crest, along which line it becomes continuous with the fascia over the iliacus and psoas muscles. From these lateral attachments the fascia extends medially as a continuous curtain, which is interrupted only by the transit of the spermatic cord at the deep inguinal ring. The fascia transversalis invests the cord structures as they pass through it with a thin layer of fascia, the deep spermatic fascia. On the medial margin of the deep ring the fascia transversalis is condensed into a U-shaped sling, with the cord supported in the concavity of the ring and the two limbs extending superiorly and laterally to be suspended from the posterior aspect of the transversus muscle. The curve of the 'U' lies at or just above the lower border 'arch' of the aponeurosis of the transverse muscle.

This U-shaped fold, the fascia transversalis sling, is the functional basis of the inguinal 'shutter' mechanism; as the transverse muscle contracts during coughing or straining, the column/pillars of the ring are pulled together and the entire sling drawn upwards and laterally. This motion increases the obliquity of exit of the spermatic cord structures through the ring and provides protection from forces tending to cause an indirect hernia[720] (Figure 2.34). The reconstruction of this sling medially with preservation of the function of the ring laterally is the rationale of anterior inguinal hernioplasty. In front of the ring lies the lower border of the transverse muscle and the internal oblique muscle. Each of these structures supports the internal ring and together they provide a very effective valve when the intra-abdominal pressure rises.

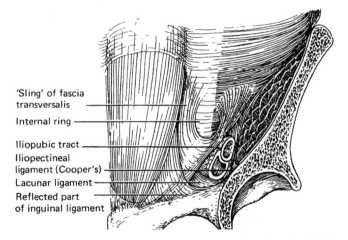

'Sling' of fascia transversalis
Internal ring
Iliopubic tract
Iliopectineal ligament (Cooper's)
Lacunar ligament
Reflected part of inguinal ligament

Figure 2.34 *The fascia transversalis, or endo-abdominal fascia, is continuous with the fascia on the deep surface of the transversus muscle. In the upper abdomen this fascia is thin and featureless; however, in the lower abdomen and pelvis the fascia transversalis has an important role. It is thickened and includes specialized bands and folds. It forms the posterior wall of the inguinal canal, and at the deep ring it has a condensation medial to the cord. This condensation is part of a U-shaped sling through which the cord passes. This sling hitches the cord up laterally when the transversus muscle contracts. Just above the inguinal ligament the fascia transversalis is thickened as the iliopubic tract. (After Lytle, 1945.)*

The 'shutter' action of the internal ring, the fascia transversalis sling, can be demonstrated readily at operation under local anesthetic. If the patient is asked to cough, the ring is suddenly pulled upwards and laterally behind the lower margin of the transverse muscle. In the adult with an obliterated

processus vaginalis, a flat lid of peritoneum covers the ring internally for the spermatic vessels and the vas deferens lie extraperitoneally. The spermatic vessels pass down almost vertically retroperitoneally on the psoas muscle. As they enter the narrow gutter of the groin they are joined by the vas deferens: the spermatic cord thus formed turns obligingly upwards and then hooks around the fascia transversalis sling to enter the deep ring, acquiring an investment of internal spermatic fascia as it traverses the ring (Figure 2.35).

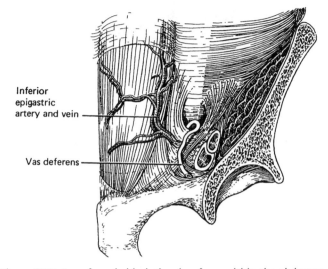

Inferior epigastric artery and vein
Vas deferens

Figure 2.35 *Seen from behind, the view from within the abdomen, the inferior epigastric vessels are deep, on the abdominal side, of this curtain of fascia transversalis. The vas deferens and cord structures ascend to and hook over the sling of fascia transversalis at the deep ring.*

The inferior border of the internal ring abuts on a condensation of the fascia transversalis, the iliopubic tract or bandelette iliopubienne of Thomson. This small fascial band extends from the anterior superior iliac spine laterally to the pubis medially. The band is a condensation of and integral part of the fascia transversalis; it lies on a plane somewhat deeper than the inguinal ligament which can be readily demonstrated as distinct from it at operation. The iliopubic tract bridges the femoral canal medially and then curves inferiorly and posteriorly to spread out fan-wise to its attachment to a broad area of the superior ramus of the pubis along the iliopectineal line (Cooper's) ligament). The iliopubic tract thus forms the inferior margin of the defect in the fascia transversalis in an indirect inguinal hernia and in a direct hernia: it is anterior to the peritoneal sac of a femoral hernia (Figure 2.36).

The fascia transversalis superior to the iliopubic tract extends over the posterior wall of the inguinal canal up to and posterior to the arch of the transverse muscle. Medially the fascia transversalis merges into the rectus sheath and aponeurosis of the transverse muscle or conjoint tendon. The fascia transversalis in the posterior wall of the inguinal canal is supported to a variable extent by the aponeurosis of the transverse muscle as it arches down to its attachment to the pubis and iliopectineal line. Medial to the deep inguinal ring and deep to the fascia transversalis, lying in the extraperitoneal fat between the peritoneum and

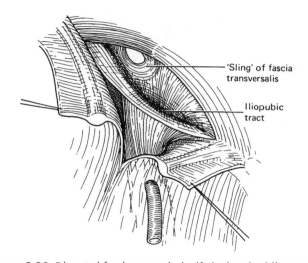

Figure 2.36 *Dissected further anteriorly, if the inguinal ligament is divided, the fascia transversalis can be seen to be continuous with the femoral sheath. The thickening at the junction of fascia transversalis with the femoral sheath is the iliopubic tract. The internal oblique muscle, which arises from the lateral inguinal ligament, acts as a shutter or 'lid' on the deep inguinal ring.*

the fascia, the deep epigastric vessels follow an oblique course upward and medially to the deep aspect of the rectus muscle. This triangular area, bounded by the deep epigastric vessels laterally, the lateral margin of the rectus muscle medially and the inguinal ligament below, is known to surgeons as Hesselbach's triangle; this is the area through which a direct inguinal hernia protrudes.

More exactly, a direct hernia explodes through the fascia transversalis in the area bounded by the iliopubic tract inferiorly, the medial limb of the fascia transversalis sling laterally and the lower margin of the arch of the transversus aponeurosis superiorly.

Condon (1971) has investigated the anatomy of the fascia transversalis using a technique of transillumination of fresh tissue. He clearly shows these anatomic details and defines the margins of the aponeurotic deficiency in the posterior inguinal canal wall through which direct hernia protrudes. This area of fascia transversalis is buttressed anteriorly to a greater or lesser degree by the aponeurosis of the transverse muscle as it inserts to the iliopectineal line. At operation these features – the iliopubic tract, the deep ring and the 'line' of the arch of the transverse aponeurosis – are easily identifiable if the fascia transversalis is adequately dissected. Indeed, the identification of all these features is an essential prerequisite for adequate inguinal hernioplasty[235] (Figure 2.37).

The fascia transversalis in the groin is but a segment of the endo-abdominal fascia. This fascia is distinct in the lower abdomen, but is fused into the fascia on the deep surface of the transverse abdominal muscle superiorly. This composite layer, the transverse muscle and its fascia (the fascia transversalis), is the most important of the abdominal wall strata in solving the problem of inguinofemoral hernia, as the integrity of this layer prevents herniation. Defects in it, congenital or acquired, are the etiology of all groin hernias.

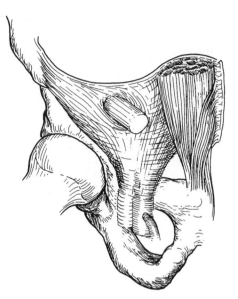

Figure 2.37 *From the front, as the surgeon visualizes the subject, the fascia transversalis in the groin resembles a funnel with a valved side vent. The femoral vessels come out of the funnel below and the cord structures out of the 'side vent' which is 'valved' by the sling of the fascia transversalis at the deep ring.*

The fascia transversalis descends behind the inguinal ligament into the thigh as the sheath of the femoral vessels – this is a funnel-like sheath. Inferior to the inguinal ligament the fascia transversalis attaches to the iliopectineal line medially and posteriorly to the femoral vessels. This funnel of fascia transversalis extends into the thigh as far as the fossa ovalis in the deep fascia. This anatomic arrangement allows for a small 'space' medial to the femoral vein through which some lymphatics pass. When a femoral hernia develops, this 'space' is expanded (Figure 2.38).

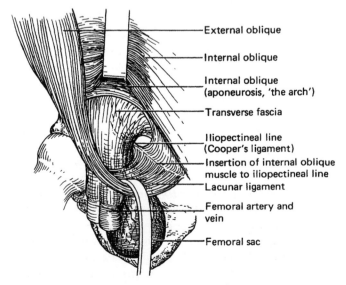

Figure 2.38 *A dissection to demonstrate the anatomy of a femoral hernia. The femoral cone of fascia transversalis is stretched on its medial aspect; the hernial sac extends within this cone of fascia transversalis medial to the femoral vein and lateral to the lacunar ligament.*

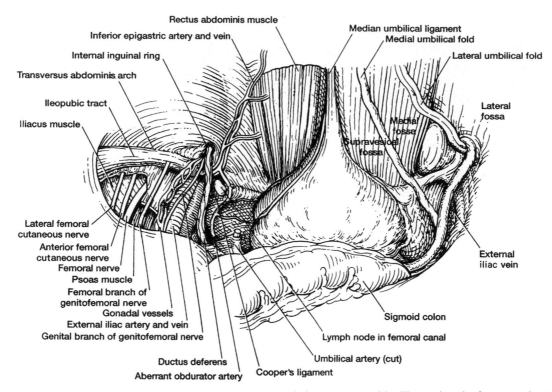

Figure 2.39 *The posterior view of the lower abdomen. The peritoneum is intact on one side, illustrating the fossae projected by the umbilical ligaments. On the contralateral side the peritoneum is reflected to allow visualization of the extraperitoneal structures, the vessels and nerves. (After Van Mameren and Go, 1994.)*[515]

What, then, is the anatomy of the peritoneum relative to the layering of the abdominal wall we have considered previously? In the lower abdomen the peritoneum is thrown up into five folds which converge as they pass upwards to the umbilicus. The median umbilical fold extends from the apex of the bladder to the umbilicus and contains the remnant urachus. To either lateral side the medial umbilical fold contains the obliterated umbilical artery and more laterally the inferior epigastric vessels raise the lateral umbilical fold. These folds create depressions or fossae in the anterior abdominal peritoneum: the supravesical fossae right and left, and the medial and the lateral inguinal fossae right and left. A further depression on either side is below and medial to the lateral inguinal fossa and separated from it by the inguinal ligament. This overlies the femoral ring and is called the femoral fossa.

Hernias egress through these fossae – the femoral through the femoral fossa, the indirect inguinal through the lateral inguinal fossa and the direct through the medial fossa. Internal supravesical hernias can occur in the supravesical fossa (Figure 2.39).

The landmarks are the peritoneal folds, particularly the medial umbilical ligament (containing the obliterated umbilical artery) and the lateral umbilical fold (containing the inferior epigastric vessels). The peritoneum overlying the deep inguinal ring is identified with the testicular vessels and vas deferens clearly visible beneath the peritoneum. The peritoneum is separated from the underlying fascia transversalis by adipose tissue except medial to the deep ring where the peritoneum is more firmly fixed to the subjacent fascia transversalis below

posterior to, the inguinal ligament the genital branch of the genitofemoral nerve is seen joining the cord structures at the deep ring.

The lateral cutaneous nerve of the thigh and the femoral branch of the genitofemoral nerve lie rather deeper in the fatty tissue overlying the iliopsoas muscle. Blood vessels are also found in the adipose tissue beneath the peritoneum, in the extraperitoneal plane branches of the deep circumflex iliac vessels laterally and of the obturator vessels inferiorly and medially. There is an extensive venous circulation (anastomosis) in the extraperitoneal tissues between the inferior epigastric vein and obturator veins. This venous anastomosis lies between the two lamina of the fascia transversalis in the space of Bogros.[110] This space is continuous from side to side and with the pelvic space, the cave of Retzius. The space of Bogros is important for extraperitoneal repair of hernia and is the repository of bleeding in pelvic trauma.

THE PERITONEUM – THE VIEW FROM WITHIN

Hernia sacs are composed of peritoneum and they may contain intra-abdominal viscera. From within they consist of the peritoneum, then a loose layer of extraperitoneal fat, then the deep membranous lamina of fascia transversalis, then the vessels such as the epigastric vessels in the space of Bogros, then the stout anterior lamina of fascia transversalis, then the muscles and aponeuroses of the abdominal wall.[237] The preperitoneal space lies in the abdominal cavity between the peritoneum internally and transversalis fascia externally. Within this space lies a variable quantity of adipose tissue, loose connective tissue and membraneous tissue and other anatomical entities such as arteries, veins, nerves and various organs such as the kidneys and ureters. The clinically significant parts of the preperitoneal space include the space associated with the structural elements related to the myopectineal orifice of Fruchaud, the prevesical space of Retzius, the space of Bogros and retroperitoneal periurinary space.[597] The myopectineal orifice of Fruchaud represents the potentially weak area in the abdominal wall, which permits inguinal and femoral hernias. The preperitoneal space that lies deep to the supra-vesical fossa and the medial inguinal fossa is the prevesical space of Retzius. The space of Retzius contains loose connective tissue and fat but more importantly vascular elements such as an abnormal obturator artery and vein. Bogros' space, which is a triangular area between the abdominal wall and peritoneum, can be entered by means of an incision through the roof and floor of the inguinal canal through which the posterior preperitoneal approach for hernia repair can be achieved. In the groin these muscles and aponeuroses are variously absent over the inguinal and crural canals. The myopectineal orifice of Fruchaud, which is divided into two parts by the inguinal ligament[376,1188] (Figure 2.40). This concept of one groin aperture is relevant for mesh repairs, whether anterior open operation or posterior laparoscopic operation. The boundaries of the myopectineal orifice of Fruchaud are superiorly the 'arch' of the transversus muscle, laterally the

iliopsoas muscle, medially the rectus muscle and inferiorly the pecten of the pubis.[49] The space is utilized in both the trans-abdominal preperitoneal and the totally extraperitoneal laparoscopic approaches to the repair of inguinal and femoral repairs. A thorough understanding of the limits of this myopectineal orifice is necessary to accomplish an effective repair of the inguinal floor with the laparoscopic methodology.

Between the peritoneum and the fascia transversalis there is a loose layer of extraperitoneal fat, used as an important landmark in many surgical operations. Hernial protrusions progress from within outward through deficiencies in the musculo-aponeurotic lamina of the abdominal wall; they carry this extraperitoneal fat with them along the track of the hernia sac. Abundance of this fat at the fundus of an indirect inguinal hernia gives rise to the surgical misnomer a 'lipoma of the cord' – in reality this is no more than extraperitoneal fat around the fundus of a peritoneal hernia sac (Figure 2.41).

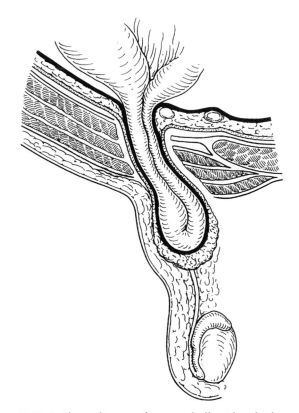

Figure 2.41 *As the peritoneum forms an indirect inguinal hernia it carries with it a covering of extraperitoneal fat. This extraperitoneal fat is given the misnomer 'lipoma of the cord' by many surgeons.*

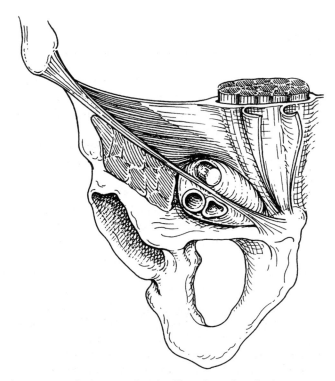

Figure 2.40 *The 'myopectineal orifice of Fruchaud': the area of the groin closed by fascia transversalis with the inguinal canal above and femoral canal below the rigid inguinal ligament. (After Wantz, 1991.)[1188]*

THE UMBILICUS

Between the sixth and tenth week of gestation the abdominal viscera enlarge rapidly so that they cannot be contained within the more slowly enlarging coelom. Viscera are extruded through the broad umbilical deficit into a peritoneal cavity, the exocoelom, which occupies the base of the umbilical cord. At about the tenth week the abdominal cavity has enlarged so much that it can now contain all the extruded viscera, and by the time of birth all the intestines are reduced inside the abdominal cavity proper. At birth the abdominal wall is complete except for the space occupied by the umbilical cord. Running in the cord are the urachus and the umbilical arteries coursing up from the pelvis, and the umbilical vein to the liver. After the cord is ligated the stump sloughs off and the resultant granulating surface cicatrizes and epithelializes from its periphery.

In the normal umbilicus there is a single layer of fused fibrous tissue consisting of the superficial fascia, the rectus sheath and linea alba, and the fascia transversalis. The peritoneum is adherent to the deep aspect of this (Figure 2.42).

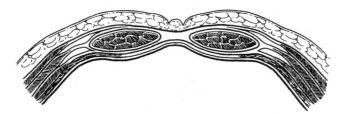

Figure 2.42 *Cross-section through the umbilicus. The aponeuroses of all three laminae are fused in the umbilical cicatrix.*

THE SPERMATIC CORD

The spermatic cord is composed of: (a) the arteries – the testicular artery, the cremaster artery and the artery of the vas deferens; (b) the veins – the testicular veins form the pampiniform plexus of veins within the spermatic cord; (c) the lymphatics; (d) the nerves – the genital branch of the genitofemoral nerve and autonomic nerves; (e) the vas deferens; and (f) the processus vaginalis.

The spermatic cord, as it emerges through the abdominal wall from the deep inguinal ring, receives investments of fascia. The fascia transversalis forms a thin, funicular coat called the internal spermatic fascia: the internal oblique invests it with a tracing of muscle fibers, the cremaster muscle, and most superficially it is coated with external spermatic fascia derived from the external oblique aponeurosis at the subcutaneous inguinal ring. Each of these fascial layers requires opening to identify the processus vaginalis or sac of an indirect hernia. Until birth the processus vaginalis, although minute, remains as an uninterrupted diverticulum from the abdominal peritoneum through the length of the cord to the testis, where it opens out to become the tunica vaginalis of the testis. The processus vaginalis closes in most males soon after birth. More recently the persistence of the processus vaginalis into adult life has been confirmed when hydrocele or hernia has complicated peritoneal dialysis in renal failure patients. The theories and mechanism of testicular descent and the development of the processus vaginalis are described in detail in Chapter 10 (Figure 2.43).

An indirect inguinal hernial sac is a similar peritoneal diverticulum which extends into the spermatic cord and occupies

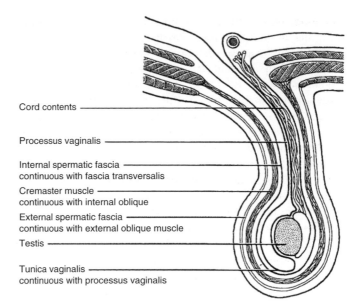

Cord contents

Processus vaginalis

Internal spermatic fascia
continuous with fascia transversalis

Cremaster muscle
continuous with internal oblique

External spermatic fascia
continuous with external oblique muscle

Testis

Tunica vaginalis
continuous with processus vaginalis

Figure 2.43 *Section through the spermatic cord and testis. The importance of the layers is demonstrated. The external spermatic fascia is derived from the fascia over the external oblique muscle at the superficial ring, the cremaster arises from the internal oblique muscle and the internal spermatic fascia is the continuation of the fascia transversalis over the cord structures. Each of these layers needs division in inguinal hernia repair.*

the same position as the primitive processus vaginalis. Often indirect hernias also have extraperitoneal fat at their fundus.

COMPARATIVE ANATOMY

A cool environment for spermatogenesis is a necessity in warm-blooded birds and mammals. Birds, which have high blood temperatures and are invariably cryptorchid, keep their testes cool by an air stream around the abdomen. In some sea-living mammals – whales and sea cows – the testes remain intra-abdominal, but presumably the constant contact with cold water is effective in keeping them cool.

The necessity to have the testes reside in a colder scrotum leads to problems, not only in humans but in domestic and farm animals; the topic of hernia and undescended testicles appears in veterinary textbooks where it has a practical and economic importance of its own. Inguinal hernias are fairly common in pigs and horses, but less common in bovines. The economic consequence of an inguinal hernia in a stallion is considerable; it may incarcerate during mating and forestall full consummation. A similar problem is known in stud bulls. Hernias are relatively common in dogs, but are rather rare in cats. Both male and female dogs are likely to develop inguinal hernias, but the males are more likely to have intestine caught within the hernial sac. When a female dog develops a hernia the usual content is one of the uterine horns and the broad ligament; this can present the danger of strangulation if the bitch becomes pregnant (the content of a congenital hernia in a girl is most likely an ovary and a fallopian tube). In the dog, most veterinary surgeons treat the hernia by orchidectomy (a proposition which is sometimes put forward for the handling of the same situation in the elderly human).

Bats have testicles which are normally intra-abdominal and descend into the scrotum only at the time of mating. In these animals there is a low incidence of hernia and of a patent processus vaginalis. The testicles in bats descend to the scrotum and ascend to the abdomen, although there is no patent processus vaginalis. In small boys with retractile testicles which disappear up to the external inguinal ring, a hernia is rarely present.[803]

RADIOLOGICAL ANATOMY

Precise knowledge of the radiological anatomy is the key to success in the diagnosis and evaluation of groin masses which defy clinical diagnosis. Several diagnostic modalities are available including conventional radiography, ultrasound, CT and MRI scanning.[1160] Herniography can be used in the diagnosis of hernia for patients with equivocal findings or those presenting with groin pain (see Chapter 11). The technique involves intraperitoneal administration of 50 ml of non-ionic contrast medium, a standard series of views of both groins is obtained during straining with the patient prone and in a slightly elevated position, as follows posteroanterior, posteroanterior with caudocranial angulation of the tube (15 degrees), two oblique views and a lateral view. A normal herniogram shows the median medial and lateral umbilical folds and the supravesical, medial inguinal and lateral inguinal fossas (Figure 2.44). A disadvantage of herniorrhaphy is its invasiveness and its inability to depict pathological conditions other than hernias.

or even 3.5 MHz transducers may be used which however result in low resolution images. The entire anterior abdominal wall including the oblique muscles, transversus muscle, rectus abdominus and peritoneum can be appreciated (Figure 2.45). A major advantage is the ability to perform the examination in supine and upright positions as well as at rest and during straining, the so-called dynamic scanning technique. Ultrasound is also non-invasive and allows comparison between the symptomatic and the asymptomatic side. The disadvantage however is its operator dependency and the great variety of imaging quality associated with body habitus.

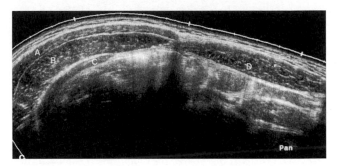

Figure 2.45 *Extended field-of-view ultra-sound image demonstrating the entire anterior abdominal wall. A, external oblique muscle; B, internal oblique muscle; C, transversus muscle; D, rectus abdominis muscle.*

Computed tomography (CT) is usually performed in the inguinal region during breath-hold without straining. The anatomy of the anterior abdominal wall can be delineated clearly (Figure 2.46). Because the inferior epigastric vessels forming the lateral umbilical folds can be clearly identified CT is very reliable at differentiating direct from indirect hernias.

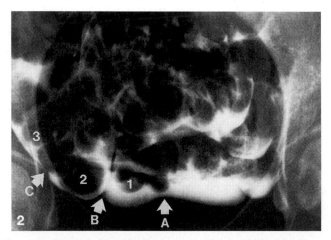

Figure 2.44 *Normal herniography. A, median umbilical fold; B, medial umbilical fold; C, lateral umbilical fold; 1, supravesical fossa; 2, medial inguinal fossa; 3, lateral inguinal fossa.*

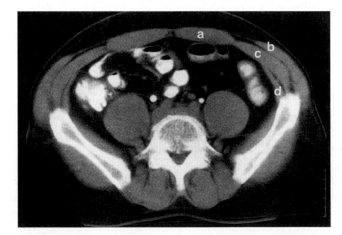

Figure 2.46 *A CT scan demonstrating normal anatomy of the muscles of the abdominal wall. a, rectus abdominis muscle; b, external oblique muscle; c, internal oblique muscle; d, transversus muscle.*

Ultrasonography with a high frequency (7.5–10 MHz), short focused transducer can depict the muscle and fascial layers of the abdominal wall and groin region. In these patients 5 MHz

Magnetic resonance imaging (MRI) has the advantage of being able to obtain images in any plane either by directly

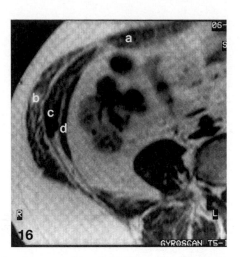

Figure 2.47 *Transverse T2-weighted MR image depicting the muscles of the anterior abdominal wall; a, rectus abdominis muscle; b, external oblique muscle; c, internal oblique muscle; d, transversus muscle; R, right; L, left.*

scanning in different planes or by making multi-planar reconstructions on a work station. MRI can also be performed during straining to gain dynamic images. The layers of the anterior abdominal wall can be delineated and also the transversalis fascia, extraperitoneal fat and peritoneum (Figure 2.47). CT scanning and MRI imaging have approximately the same sensitivity and specificity for correctly diagnosing groin hernias.

3

Epidemiology and etiology of primary groin hernias in adults

The population prevalence (the percentage of a population being studied that is affected with a particular disease at a given time) and the incidence (the rate of occurrence of new cases of a particular disease in a population being studied) of groin hernias has been studied extensively by a variety of authors in the last 100 years.[997] In developed countries the incidence of operations for groin hernia is approximately 2000 operations per million population per year.[96] Nationwide information on the relation between the number of procedures performed per year and the rates of incidence of groin hernia have been more difficult to establish. However, the 1981/82 morbidity statistics from general practice (Third National Study) estimated that approximately the same number of new hernias diagnosed from general practitioners per year as the number of patients consulting their doctors with existing hernias, suggesting that a large number of groin hernias are not being referred to surgeons for definitive treatment and that the prevalence is far higher than the annual incidence of operation. A survey in Somerset and Avon Health Authority in the United Kingdom of a stratified random sample of 28 000 adults age greater than 35 years enquired about lumps in the groin and invited those indicating positive replies to a clinic for interview and examination. The results revealed that of the hernias discovered, one-third of patients had not consulted their primary care physician and of the two-thirds that had seen their primary care physician, less than half had been referred to a surgeon for a decision on definitive management. Interestingly of the third of patients who had not consulted their general practitioner, two-thirds said they would accept an operation if this was advised. Of the patients who eventually reached a surgeon, 20% were advised that operation was not required. This survey indicates that there is an unmet need for groin hernia surgery, many patients were denied access by their general practitioner or primary care physician, surgeons are the gatekeepers and discriminate. Finally, there appears to be a need for patient education in terms of the possible dangers of having a lump in the groin.

Nevertheless it is estimated that the number of groin herniorrhaphies done worldwide every year exceeds 20 million[97] and the lifetime risk of groin hernia is 27% for men and 3% for women.[926]

EPIDEMIOLOGY

Prevalence and incidence data give no indication about the actual or potential demand for hernia surgery. Although incomplete and subject to many pitfalls in interpretation, UK data sources which relate to the need for hernia surgery include: the English Hospital In-Patient Enquiry (HIPE) Data, 1975–1985, the English Hospital Episodes System (HES) Data, 1989/90 and Data on Surgical Activity in Independent Hospitals in the National Health Service (NHS) from local and national surveys.[1211]

There have been no true population or community-based studies of the incidence of groin hernia. The closest estimates for the true incidence of inguinal and femoral hernia can be obtained from the 1981/82 Morbidity Statistics from General Practice (Third National Study).[978] These figures are probably an underestimate because a proportion of patients will fail to seek medical advice. However, based on these figures the annual incidence of inguinal hernia in England will be of the order of 113 000 per year. The 95% confidence intervals are approximately 80 000–160 000.

The published evidence comes from three main sources. Firstly, population prevalence and incidence: there have been few community-based estimates of the prevalence of groin hernias. None have estimated the incidence. Each has been performed in communities where access to surgery was limited, e.g. African populations. Further research defining the population incidence of subjects with groin hernias is required. Prevalence estimates are of local value only; they reflect not only the distribution and morbidity in the community but also the success of past local activity. Secondly, 'demand' incidence rates are based on the number of people who seek medical advice for their problem. However, numerous factors may influence this decision and the data must therefore be treated with caution. Estimates of the incidence of inguinal and femoral hernias (Table 3.1) comes from the 1981/82 Morbidity Statistics from General Practice (Third National Study) based on consultations with 143 volunteer general practice principals caring for 332 000 patients.[978] Figures 3.1 and 3.2 show incidence rates for inguinal and femoral hernia, each of which denotes a consultation where the patient was seeking medical advice concerning a groin hernia

Table 3.1 *Incidence rates (95% confidence limits) of inguinal and femoral hernia per 10 000 persons at risk (1981/82 morbidity statistics from general practice, third national study, Royal College of General Practitioners, 1986)*

Age (years)	Males	Females
Inguinal hernias		
0–4	58 (44.9,74.8)	13 (6.9,22.2)
5–14	7 (2.8,14.4)	3 (0.6,8.8)
15–24	7 (2.8,14.4)	3 (0.6,8.8)
25–44	20 (12.2,30.9)	4 (1.1,10.2)
45–64	70 (55.5,88.2)	6 (2.2,13.1)
65–74	88 (71.5,108.2)	7 (2.8,14.4)
75+	150 (128.2,175.5)	17 (9.9,27.2)
Femoral hernias		
0–4		
5–14		
15–24		
25–44	1 (0.02,5.6)	2 (0.2,7.2)
45–64	1 (0.02,5.6)	2 (0.2,7.2)
65–74	1 (0.02,5.6)	2 (0.2,7.2)
75+	9 (4.1,17.1)	7 (2.8,14.4)

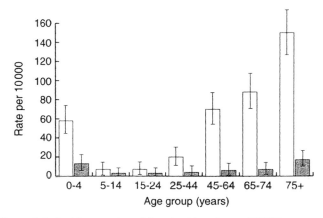

Figure 3.1 *Incidence rates of inguinal hernia per 10 000 persons at risk (1981/82 morbidity statistics from general practice, third national study[978]). □ = Males; ■ = Females.*

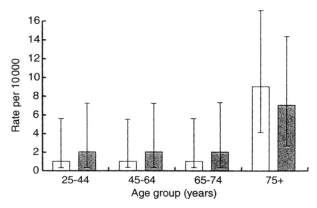

Figure 3.2 *Incidence rates of femoral hernia per 10 000 persons at risk (1981/82 morbidity statistics from general practice, third national study[978]). □ = Males; ■ = Females.*

for the first time during the study year. Again, these data must be interpreted with caution because neither the doctors nor the patients may be representative of the general population, and the diagnoses were not validated. The age-specific incidence rates are given with 95% confidence intervals.

DEMAND FOR GROIN HERNIA SURGERY IN ADULTS

The overall rates for inguinal hernia repair (primary and recurrent) performed in NHS hospitals in England did not change between 1975 and 1990 (Figure 3.3). The total numbers for 1989/90 were 64 998 primary inguinal hernia repairs and 3480 recurrent inguinal hernia repairs (Table 3.2). Age-specific hernia rates have altered considerably since 1975 with a significant increase in the surgical rates for older men. For instance, the age-specific inguinal repair rate for the 65–74-year age group rose from 40 per 10 000 in 1975 to 70 per 100 000 in 1990. This probably reflects improvements in anesthetic delivery and postoperative recovery in high dependency or intensive care units. A more detailed analysis of age-specific inguinal hernia repair rates for males and females is shown in Figure 3.4, which indicates the high rates in infants and men over the age of 55.

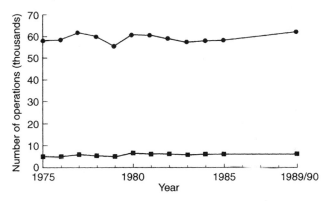

Figure 3.3 *Trends in number of inguinal hernia repairs, NHS hospitals in England, 1975–1989/90.[1002] ● = Males; ■ = Females. (From Williams et al., 1992.)*

Of the approximately 65 000 inguinal and 6000 femoral hernia repairs performed in NHS hospitals in England each year, 10% are emergency operations; these have remained constant for two decades. There has been an expansion in the private sector, which now accounts for 14% of all elective groin operations. Referring to the data in Figures 3.4 and 3.5, it cannot be

Table 3.2 *Number and percentage of single procedure inguinal hernia operations performed in NHS hospitals, England, 1989/90*

Inguinal hernia	Total no. of operations	No. (%) done as single procedure
Primary	64 998	54 090 (83)
Recurrent	3480	2790 (80)

From Williams, 1992, with permission.

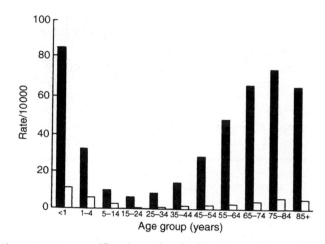

Figure 3.4 *Age-specific primary inguinal hernia repair rates, NHS hospitals, England 1989/90.[1002]* ■ *= Males;* □ *= females. (From Williams et al., 1992.)*

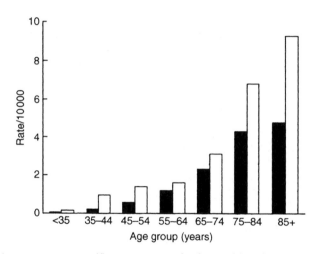

Figure 3.5 *Age-specific surgery rates for femoral hernia per 10 000 for males and females, NHS hospitals, England, 1989/90.* ■ *= Males;* □ *= females. (From Williams et al., 1992.)*

Of more importance is the demographic structure of the population being studied, which may vary widely between regional populations. The demand for emergency treatment of strangulated inguinal hernia is better defined, being estimated at 3.25–7.16 per 100 000 per annum, in Western Europe.[33,248] However, deficiencies of available data arise from three facts: firstly, they are based on Health Service use rather than health-care needs; secondly, patterns of morbidity have an uncertain relationship to indications for treatment; and thirdly patients will seek treatment only if they are aware of the significance of underlying morbidity and the consequences of treatment.

Inguinal hernias are more common than femoral hernias, occurring in ratios of 8:1 or 20:1 depending on the surgical series, and are more common in males, where the inguinal to femoral ratio may be up to 35:1. Seventy percent of inguinal hernias are indirect and 30% direct. Inguinal and femoral hernias may coexist: 2% of males with inguinal hernias also have a femoral hernia and 50% of those with femoral hernias have a coexisting inguinal hernia. This distribution of groin hernias is illustrated graphically in a large series of 4173 hernias operated on in Truro, south-west England by Barwell 1974–1992[1027] (Figure 3.6). Similar figures are reported by Nilsson et al. from Sweden.[850]

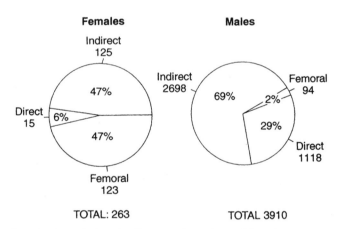

Figure 3.6 *Groin hernia diagnoses in males and females, Truro 1974–1992. (From Williams et al., 1992.)*

assumed that these repair rates approximate to the population incidence of inguinal and femoral hernias, because only 60% of groin hernias are referred to specialists for operation.[978] The implications for the English population will be 112 700 new cases per annum for inguinal hernias, and 6900 for femoral hernias. Because a considerable proportion of patients are not undergoing groin hernia surgery, this may account for the 40 000 trusses sold annually.[208,641]

There is considerable variation in surgical rates for populations of health districts in England, and the weak correlations between these rates and supply factors (e.g. consultants per 1000 population) and demand factors (e.g. waiting lists), suggest that a considerable proportion of the variation is accounted for by differences in medical decision making.[1214]

Demand incidence is based on surgical procedures. In a stable catchment population, the number of people who seek surgery during a defined period can be established.

Age-standardized hernia surgery rates vary considerably worldwide. For instance, the hernia surgery rate per 100 000 population per year in England and Wales is 200, Norway 200, the USA 280 and Australia 180. The actual approximate number of operations performed per year in respective countries is 5500 in Scotland, 100 000 in England, 30 000 in Holland, 25 000 in Belgium, 100 000 in France and 180 000 in Germany.[458,1025,1028] In the USA, where at least 550 000 inguinal hernia operations are carried out per year, the annual costs estimated in 1987 were 2.8 billion dollars, or 3% of the total healthcare budget. These figures are obtained from The National Center For Health Statistics (NCHS) through its National Hospital Discharge Survey, which has compiled data on the number of operations performed annually in the USA, from a 5–8% sample of patient records.[997] In the UK hernia surgery rates peak in the 55–85-year age group, at 600 operations per 100 000 population per year, and the incidence of strangulated hernia is 13 per 100 000 population, with a peak in the 80-year-old age group. A graphical analysis of hospital discharge data and demographic information guided by three hypotheses on urgency of surgery, age and evidence of discordance between population prevalence of disease and rates of surgery has suggested that in the last 10 years in Scotland, the rates of operation have increased in the over 65-year-olds but the rate of elective surgery has decreased in the more socioeconomically deprived areas.[1040] It could be concluded from this data that more hernia surgery is being carried out in an aging population and the need for patient education is particularly required in the lower socioeconomic population group.

In the USA the high rates of hernia surgery may have contributed to the reduction in mortality associated with strangulation. For instance, the mortality for hernia and intestinal obstruction obtained by analysis of statistics data from the NCHS shows a fall in the number of deaths per year per 100 000 population in patients over the age of 15 years, from 5 in 1968 to 3.1 in 1978, and stabilizing at 3.0 in 1988. This was in spite of the fact that hernia patients with intestinal obstruction were on average 15 years older in 1988 than in 1968. In 1971 Medicare discharges for inguinal hernia without intestinal obstruction showed 94% of patients having surgery, with a probability of death at 0.005 (5 per 100 000 population).[790]

INGUINAL HERNIAS IN ADULTS

Inguinal hernias are more common in males than females, in a ratio of 8:1 or 20:1 in different series. However, there is considerable incidence of under-reporting of inguinal hernia, as illustrated by two validity checks in the US National Health Surveys. In both studies half the hernias recorded during the previous year were unreported on interview, and in another study in Baltimore positive reports were received from only 21% of men found to have hernias on clinical examination.

In the literature the incidence varies depending on the source of the count. Approximately 94% of hernias among males are estimated to be in the inguinal region. Ninety-five per cent of inguinal hernia operations are on males. Three times more females undergo femoral hernia operations than males. By the age of 75 years 10–15% of males have already received inguinal hernia surgery. In the period 1975–1990 mortality from inguinal hernia surgery in the UK fell by 22% and for femoral hernia by 55%. In the USA, for inguinal hernia with obstruction, 88% underwent surgery with a mortality rate of 0.05%.[790] Incidence estimates vary widely. A study of World War I British recruits between the ages of 18 and 41 years shows these variations: in Scotland 31 per 1000 were found, whereas in London and south-east England it was 17–56 per 1000; in men aged 16–30 years the rate was 6 per 1000, whereas in men of 40–50 years it was 24 per 1000. In contradistinction, the rate in Stockport and Manchester was 125 per 1000. Sir Arthur Keith, in 1924, estimated the prevalence at 25 per 1000 males.[578]

The figures from recruits in World War II are equally confusing: the prevalence was generally about 26 per 1000, but a range from 6 to 79.6 per 1000 recruits is given – these are in young males so, bearing in mind that most inguinal hernias occur in the later decades, the overall incidence is probably higher.[1238]

Sixty-five percent of inguinal hernias in adult European males are indirect in type. Right-sided inguinal hernias in adult males are slightly more frequent than left-sided; 55% occurring on the right, regardless of whether the hernia is indirect or direct. Bilateral hernias are four times more often direct than indirect. In Western series the peak incidence of groin hernias is in the sixth decade.[530]

A possible genetic link has been postulated in the Inuit living in the Western Arctic of Greenland. Hernia is common in males and thought to be due to a high prevalence of disorders associated with instability of mesenchymal tissues, such as spondylolisthesis, arthritis and heart block. The Inuit have been living in almost complete genetic isolation for 150–200 generations and have a high incidence and frequency of the HLA-B27 allele. Such polymorphism could result in the frequency of hernia in these people.[482]

The difference between the ratio of indirect to direct inguinal hernia in different geographical locations support a polygenic predisposition. In Japan hernias are twice as frequent in twins, in Ghana one in every five live births is a twin, twice the rate found in non-Africans – which may account for the higher incidence recorded.[103]

Comparing the age structure of the patients with inguinal hernia operated in Accra with the age structure found in a field study in Ghana shows that all age groups are equally represented in the Accra hospital population, whereas in rural Ghana the prevalence of groin hernia rises with increasing age.[66,103]

It is impossible to compare these findings. The large-scale surveys of uncomplaining males are drawn from recruits into British and American forces in two world wars and are not, therefore, representative samples of the population. The only field study is from southern Ghana and confirms that inguinal hernias are at least three times more common in Africans than Europeans.

The true prevalence of inguinal hernias can be estimated only by community-based epidemiological studies, the validity of which will depend on the diagnostic criteria used. The presence of a visible, palpable lump may be supplemented by such diagnostic criteria as cough impulse at the internal or external ring and the presence of an incision in the groin. The latter, of course, may represent another form of surgery, such as orchidopexy, rather than hernia. Moreover, recurrent inguinal hernias may not be adequately diagnosed or sub-categorized. These pitfalls are well illustrated by the two studies alluded to above, carried out on British Army recruits in the first and second world wars. The prevalence was 1.6% for groin hernias in recruits aged 30–40 years in World War I and 11% in World War II.[578,1214]

Perhaps the most rigorous epidemiological study carried out was that of Abramson in Western Jerusalem between 1969 and 1971.[2] Males from differing ethnic and social backgrounds were studied, although young males were largely excluded because of national service. The study was performed by interviewing subjects in their homes, where the response rate was

Table 3.3 *Percentage of age group with inguinal hernia (Abramson, 1978)*

	Age (years)						Total
	25–34	35–44	45–54	55–64	65–74	75+	
No. examined	620	438	300	322	156	47	1883
Current prevalence (excluding successful repairs)	11.9	15.1	19.7	26.1	29.5	34.1	18.3
'Obvious' hernias*	1.0	4.8	9.0	14.3	19.2	29.8	7.6
Unoperated swellings	0.7	3.7	5.7	10.9	13.5	23.4	5.5
Recurrences	0.3	1.4	3.7	3.4	5.8	6.4	2.2
Palpable impulse only	11.0	10.3	10.7	11.8	10.3	4.3	10.7
Lifetime prevalence (including successful repairs)	15.2	19.4	28.0	34.5	39.7	46.8	24.3
'Obvious' hernias*	4.7	9.6	18.3	24.2	30.8	44.7	14.5

From Yavetz, 1991, with permission.
*'Obvious' hernias included swellings and repaired hernias and excluded those presenting with a palpable impulse only. The current prevalence of obvious hernias may be less than the combined prevalences of unoperated swellings and recurrences, since a person may have for example an unoperated swelling in one groin and a recurrence in the other.

high (over 86%). Of these, 91% participated in the second stage of physical examination. Interviewers and examiners had been trained in the use of questionnaires and diagnostic criteria. The results are shown in Table 3.3. The prevalence increased with age in all cohorts studied, and the majority were diagnosed on the basis of a visible swelling. An important finding from the Abramson study was the concordance between interview and examination findings: only 50% of men reported a swelling in the groin on interview, which is in close agreement with the 50% under-reporting revealed from validity checks by the US National Health Surveys.[836] It is obvious from these studies that questionnaire-based data must be supplemented by clinical examination if the true prevalence is to be ascertained, although this may be confounded by problems with diagnostic criteria. Suffice to say that all data regarding the incidence statistics of hernia patients are difficult to assure complete accuracy and are probably underestimations.

FEMORAL HERNIAS IN ADULTS

The prevalence and incidence of femoral hernias in the population cannot be determined accurately due to lack of investigation. However, the demand incidence can be estimated as for femoral hernia from the General Practitioner Morbidity Survey of 1981/82, which is summarized in Table 3.1. An incidence figure for England derived from these data is approximately 7000 per year, but the 95% confidence intervals range from approximately 1500 to 24 000.

Femoral hernias are less common than inguinal and account for only 10% of all groin hernias. They are more frequent in females than males in a ratio of 2.5:1 (Table 3.1). There is other data that disputes this statistic, however (see Chapter 16, page 217). Maingot gives femoral hernias in females as eight times more common than in males.[735] Glasgow, from Toronto, reports more males than females in his series, in a ratio of 5:3.[421] Glasgow's series is of patients undergoing

elective operation for inguinal hernia and many of his cases were found as concomitant femoral hernias in men undergoing elective inguinal hernioplasty. Clearly the Toronto series is not representative of wider general surgical practice. In British practice 40% of femoral hernias are admitted as emergency cases with strangulation or incarceration.[930] Females undergo three times as many inguinal hernia as femoral hernia repairs. Femoral hernia is rare in those under 35, is most common in multiparous women and is as common in men as in multiparous women. The ratio of inguinal to femoral hernias is between 10:1 and 8:1. In Accra femoral hernias are rare, accounting for only 1.2%, with an inguinal to femoral ratio of 77:1; in Kampala the ratio is 21.6:1. It is interesting to observe that indirect inguinal hernias outnumber direct inguinal hernias in Accra and in Zaria, Nigeria, whereas in Kampala direct hernias are more frequent. In Kampala there are nine women with femoral hernias to one man, whereas in West African Hausa the male to female ratio of femoral hernias is 1.2:1.[55,67,618,868,1232]

The surgical volume for rates of femoral hernia repair in NHS hospitals in England has remained stable between 1975 and 1990, with 5083 primary femoral hernia repairs and 299 recurrent femoral hernia repairs being performed in 1989/90. The age-specific data indicate an increasing rate of repair through the decades with a peak in those over 85 years (Figure 3.5).

There is considerable variation in surgical rates for both inguinal and femoral hernia for each district in English Regional Health Authorities. The range for primary inguinal hernia repair is 0.57–24 per 10 000 and for primary femoral hernia repair 0.16–2.3 per 10 000. Such wide variations reflect diversity in clinical practice, demand for and supply of treatment.[1214]

ETIOLOGY OF PRIMARY GROIN HERNIA

The pathogenesis of groin hernia is multifactorial. Sir Astley Cooper's 'predispositions' to hernia, in 1827, and the subsequent addition of chronic cough and ascites are now only of historic interest.

Because indirect inguinal hernias are so common in infancy the first surgical speculation was that they were due to a developmental defect. Indirect inguinal hernia arises from incomplete obliteration of the processus vaginalis, the embryological out pocketing of peritoneum that precedes testicular descent into the scrotum. The testes originate along the urogenital line in the retroperitoneum and migrate caudally during the second trimester of pregnancy to arrive at the internal inguinal ring at about 6 months of intrauterine life. During the last trimester they proceed through the abdominal wall via the inguinal canal and descend into the scrotum, the right slightly later than the left. The processus vaginalis then normally obliterates postnatally except for the portion surrounding and serving as a covering for the testes. Failure of this obliterative process results in congenital indirect inguinal hernia. The modern epidemiological support for this hypothesis has already been reviewed, while the differing familial and tribal incidences, and the coincidence of hernias in twins, are supportive.

John Hunter, in the late 18th century, researched the development and descent of the testis in men and domestic animals. He showed that in some inguinal hernias the sac was continuous with the processus vaginalis.[524] Cloquet (1817) observed that the processus vaginalis was frequently not closed at birth.[225] The complete (scrotal) indirect hernia of adult men has the same anatomy as that of the neonate – it is invested by all the layers of the spermatic cord as it transverses the inguinal canal and its sac is continuous with the tunica vaginalis of the testis. Additional support for the congenital theory of indirect inguinal herniation is the finding at autopsy that 15–30% of adult males without clinically apparent inguinal hernias have a patent processus vaginalis at death.[520] A Bedouin mother and her four daughters with indirect inguinal hernia in whom there was no evidence of collagen diseases, normal hormone profile and normal pelvic anatomy suggests that in adult females as well, there is genetic heterogeneity.[445] Such an occurrence in females may be associated with an alteration in the anatomy of the round ligament, which normally terminates in a hernia sac and is attached to the mid portion of the fallopian tube near the ovary.[29]

Review of the contralateral side in infantile inguinal hernias reveals a patent processus vaginalis in 60% of neonates and a contralateral hernia in 10–20%. During 20 years of follow-up after infantile hernia repair, 22% of men will develop a contralateral inguinal hernia, of which 41% occur if the initial hernia was on the left and 14% if the initial hernia was on the right.

The introduction of continuous ambulatory peritoneal dialysis for renal failure has demonstrated that the persistent processus vaginalis, if subjected to intra-abdominal pressure, will dilate to give a hydrocele or hernia.[202,333,1029] This has been reported as late as 2 years in a 61-year-old man recently commenced on continuous ambulatory peritoneal dialysis (CAPD). The development of inguinal hernia in female CAPD patients adds further force to this argument.[241,496,1032]

Russell, an Australian pediatric surgeon, in 1906 advanced the 'saccular theory' of the formation of hernia, a theory that 'rejects the view that any hernia can ever be "acquired" in the

pathological sense and maintains that the presence of a developmental peritoneal diverticulum is a necessary antecedent condition in every case … We may have an open funicular peritoneum and we may have them separately or together in infinitely variable gradations.'[987]

It would be apparent from the above that the problem of indirect inguinal hernia is not simply one of a congenital defect, i.e. a persistent patent processus vaginalis. The high frequency of indirect inguinal hernia in middle-aged and older people suggests a pathological change in connective tissue of the abdominal wall to be a contributory factor. Indeed, simple removal of the sac in adults results in an unacceptably high recurrence rate. Thus the susceptibility to herniation is based on both the presence of a congenital sac and failure of the transversalis fascia. In direct inguinal hernia there is no peritoneal sac and the prevalence parallels ageing and other factors including smoking.[327,943] The absence of an adequate musculo-aponeurotic support for the fascia transversalis and the medial half of the inguinal canal occurs in about a quarter of individuals.[1238] In these men there is deficiency of the lower aponeurotic fibers of the internal oblique muscle, coupled with a narrow insertion of the transversus abdominis onto the superior pubic ramus.[777,778] Because such a congenital anomaly would be symmetric, this explanation is congruent with the clinical finding that direct hernias are frequently bilateral.

The anatomic disposition of the pelvis, and particularly the height of the pubic arch, may be a significant ethnic characteristic predisposing to inguinal hernia. The height of the pubic arch is measured as the distance of the pubic tubercle from the bispinous line between the innermost parts of the two anterior superior iliac spines. African (Negro) people have lower pubic arches than Europeans and a higher incidence of inguinal hernia. In West and East Africa the 'lowness' of the pubic arch is greater than 7.5 cm in 65% of males; in Europeans and in Arabs the arch is less low, 65% of males having a height of between 5 and 7.5 cm (Figure 3.7). In European females 80% have an arch between 5 and 7.5 cm, and they have the lowest incidence of groin hernias.[320,1232,1240]

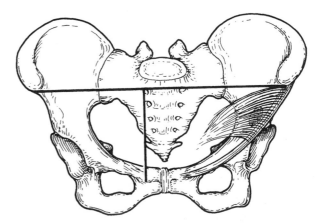

Figure 3.7 *The European pelvis is relatively wide with a less deep arch than the Negro pelvis. This ensures that the internal oblique muscle origin from the lateral inguinal ligament is broad, so that the internal oblique muscle 'protects' the deep ring.*

The low arch is associated with a narrower pelvis and with a narrower origin of the external oblique muscle from the lateral inguinal ligament. With these anatomic variations there is a shorter inguinal canal, the deep inguinal ring may be unclosed by the internal oblique. The canal may then be so short that no muscular 'shutter mechanism' is operative[320] (Figure 3.8).

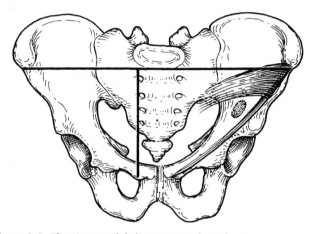

Figure 3.8 *The Negro pelvis is narrower than the European, which means that the lowness of the arch of the pelvis is greater in the Negro and the origin of the internal oblique relatively narrower. Hence the internal oblique will not cover the deep ring during straining and the 'shutter mechanism' of the inguinal canal is deficient. Negroes have a 10 times greater incidence of indirect inguinal hernia than Europeans.*

There is another much rarer form of direct hernia where a narrow peritoneal diverticulum comes directly through the conjoint tendon lateral to the rectus and pyramidal muscles to project at the superficial inguinal ring.

It must be concluded that there are congenital and genetic factors and anatomic variations that render individuals more likely to manifest direct and indirect inguinal hernias.

Sir Arthur Keith (1924)[578] observed: 'There is one other matter, which requires further observation. We are so apt to look on tendons, fascial structures and connective tissues as dead passive structures. They are certainly alive, and the fact that hernias are so often multiple in middle-aged and old people leads one to suspect that a pathological change in the connective tissues of the belly wall may render certain individuals particularly liable to hernia.' He concluded his argument with a statement regarding 'the importance of a right understanding of the etiology of hernia … If they occur only in those who have hernial sacs already formed during fetal life then we must either excise the sacs at birth or stand by and do nothing but trust to luck. But if … the occurrence of hernia is due to circumstances over which we have control then the prevention of hernia is a matter worthy of our serious study.'[578]

Read made the crucial clinical observation which next advanced our understanding of the etiology of inguinal hernia. In 1970 he noted, when using the preperitoneal approach to the inguinal region, that the rectus sheath is thinner and has a 'greasy' feel in those patients who turned out to have direct defects. This observation was confirmed by weighing samples of constant area; specimens from controls weighed significantly more than those from patients with indirect, pantaloon and direct hernias (in that order). Bilateral hernias were associated with more severe atrophy. Adjustment for age and muscle mass confirmed the validity of the primary observation.[943]

Further evidence in support of a collagen derangement in the transversalis fascia has been presented by Peacock and Madden (1974), who observe that satisfactory repair of adult inguinal hernia depends on the local extent of any collagen deficiency. And, if surgical technical failure can be excluded, the logical treatment of recurrent herniation is a fascial graft or prosthetic repair.[892]

This concept was enthusiastically promulgated by Irving Lichtenstein, one of the earliest protagonists of prosthetic repair for primary inguinal hernia.[693] Hydroxyproline, which comprises 80% of the dry weight of collagen, is strikingly decreased in the rectus sheath of hernia patients.[1175] Extraction of the collagen reveals an altered perceptibility and a reduced hydroxyproline: proline ratio. Intermolecular cross-linking is unaffected, but synthesis of hydroxyproline is inhibited and there is variability in the diameter of the collagen fibrils in hernia patients.[1209] Similar electron microscopic findings are present in pericardial and skin biopsies from these patients[1209] and have also been described in connective tissue tumors,[15] pulmonary emphysema[181] and in scurvy.[688] Based upon these observations and the results that have been seen by the passage of time, the prosthetic repair of inguinal hernias has become the standard of care. This has also changed the approach to repair of incisional and ventral hernias such that the majority of these are also repaired with the use of a prosthetic biomaterial.

These observations led Read, in 1978,[950] to the postulate that inguinal herniation is not a localized defect of the groin fascia, but is a manifestation of a generalized connective tissue disorder similar to emphysema, a1-antitrypsin deficiency, osteogenesis imperfecta, scurvy, varicose veins and experimental nicotine deficiency.[181] The actual biomechanical properties of the transversalis fascia and rectus abdominus have been systematically assessed by a computerized suction device to test this hypothesis and measure functional connective tissue abnormalities in the groin.[884] This study, however, was unable to demonstrate any differences in the properties of aponeurosis between hernia patients and controls. There is, however, a difference in collagen ultrastructure when it is examined under an electron microscope and in its physicochemical properties as observed by altered perceptibility and deficiency in hydroxyproline content. It appears that a fundamental problem in the aponeurosis of men with direct inguinal herniation is a failure of hydroxylation of the collagen molecule.

Berliner in 1984 confirmed these findings by studying biopsies from three sites in patients with inguinal hernia.[119] Degenerative changes in the musculo-aponeurotic fibers were found not only in the transversalis fascia/transversus abdominis of patients with direct inguinal hernias, but also in the transversalis fascia at the superior aspect of the internal ring in patients with indirect inguinal hernia and also distant from the hernia site in grossly abnormal transversus abdominis aponeurosis. The main changes observed were reduction in elastic tissue with a paucity and fragmentation of elastic fiber similar to that seen in Marfan and Ehlers–Danlos syndrome. The implication from these findings is that collagen malsynthesis and enzymolysis play a major role in the etiology of both direct and indirect inguinal hernia. Indeed, the in vitro synthesis of type I and III collagens and their procollagen mRNAs was determined in a study of isolated skin fibroblasts from patients with inguinal hernia. Fibroblasts incubated with radiolabelled tritiated proline secreted increased amounts of type III procollagen, which suggested that an altered fibroblast phenotype in patients with inguinal hernia could result in reduced collagen fibril assembly and defective connective tissue formation.[375]

Could an uninhibited elastolytic enzyme system cause groin herniation – a similar mechanism to low serum levels of the protease inhibitor a1–antitrypsin globulin allowing endogenous enzymes to destroy alveoli?[640]

Experimental evidence supports the biochemical hypothesis that the pulmonary connective tissue disorder in emphysema is an imbalance between proteolytic enzyme levels and their inhibitors. Evidence of raised elastolytic enzyme has been found in smokers, and in smokers with inguinal herniation there is a close association between raised elastolytic levels and raised white counts. Leukocytes carry proteolytic and elastolytic enzymes and are actively involved in the lung inflammatory response to cigarette smoke. Could they not also deliver the same proteolytic insult to the transversalis fascia? An association between direct inguinal herniation and aortic aneurysm (as opposed to aortic atherosclerotic occlusive vascular disease) also exists. The prevalence of inguinal hernia (41%) in 119 patients with infrarenal aortic aneurysms was significantly elevated compared with 81 patients with aortic occlusive disease (18.5%) and 293 patients with coronary artery disease (18.1%). Additionally, the number of patients with recent hernia repair (16%) or still awaiting repair (19%) was very high.[679] Also following elective aortic reconstruction for aneurysmal or occlusive aortic disease, at one year follow-up incisional hernias were found in 31% of patients with aneurysm and 12% with occlusive disease and inguinal hernias were found in 19% of patients with aneurysm and 5% with occlusive disease further reinforcing the concept of a biochemical abnormality.[7] Similar findings have been found in patients examined by a magnetic resonance imaging of the abdominal wall following aortic surgery.[829] These findings indicate that up to 66% of patients with non-occlusive infrarenal aortic aneurysm suffer from inguinal hernia. The smoking habits of the three groups were not different, and again the findings support a systemic fiber degeneration.[177] Although the enzymatic elastase content of the wall of abdominal aortic aneurysms is known to be increased, the concept of high levels of circulating elastase has not been confirmed. The term 'metastatic emphysema' has been coined by Cannon and Read (1981) for this generalized connective tissue disorder,[181] which may be due to a leakage of proteases from the lungs of heavy smokers.[948] Read emphasized that the data indicate that more than one factor can cause systemic metabolic disease of collagen leading to abdominal herniation including the genetic expression of collagens type I and III result which has been confirmed in the transversalis fascia of patients with inguinal hernia by measurement of the type I and type III collagens.[603]

We must be cautious in interpreting the experimental data about a proteolytic defect in inguinal hernia patients and then relating it to the proven association with abdominal aortic aneurysm. It is tempting to relate the metastatic emphysema theory of inguinal herniation to Hunt's and Tilson's ideas that aortic aneurysm is a copper transport collagen disorder enhanced by cigarette smoking.[522,1127]

THE GENETICS OF INHERITANCE OF INDIRECT INGUINAL HERNIA

Although there is considerable evidence suggesting the role of genetic factors in the etiology of inguinal hernia, its mode of inheritance remains controversial.[1204] Hypotheses proposed include:

1 Autosomal dominant inheritance with incomplete penetrance.[1068]
2 Autosomal dominant inheritance with sex influence.[813,1198]
3 X-linked dominant inheritance.[800]
4 Polygenic inheritance.[261,1015]

A study of 280 families with congenital indirect inguinal hernia in the Shandong province of China has indicated that the mode of transmission in these families is autosomal dominant with incomplete penetrance and sex influence. There is preferential paternal transmission of the gene, which suggests genomic imprinting in its etiology.[428] In this study the probands had all been operated on by five years of age, the hernia occurring on the right side in 138 probands, and on the left side in 84. This is consistent with the known embryological facts that the right testis descends later than the left, and that the processus vaginalis is therefore obliterated later on the right side than on the left side; hence hernia is more frequent on the right than on the left side. In the study in Budapest,[261] the fathers and mothers of 707 index patients with operated indirect congenital inguinal hernia born during the years 1962–1966 were studied for the frequency of indirect inguinal hernia. There was a 2 and 5.6 times higher incidence respectively in fathers and mothers than in the general population and the rate of affected siblings was higher than that of parents but was generally dependent on the sex of the index patient. In twins the hereditability was 0.77. These data agree with a multi-factorial threshold model involving dominant variance. In a record linkage study of the risk of congenital inguinal hernia in siblings, 1921 male and 347 female cases born during 1970–1986 and who were operated on for inguinal hernia at the ages of 0-15 years, were matched against 12886 male and 2534 female controls.[555] The relative risk for inguinal hernia was found to be 5.8 for brothers of male cases and 4.3 for brothers of female cases, whilst the relative risk was 3.7 for sisters of male cases and 17.8 for sisters of female cases. This pattern of sex dependent risk suggests a multi-factorial threshold modeled for the disease and girls who develop the disease might have a potentially large contribution to susceptibility but genetic or intrauterine risk factors are unrelated to sex.

Indirect inguinal hernia arises from incomplete obliteration of the processus vaginalis, the embryological protrusion of peritoneum that precedes testicular descent into the scrotum. The testes originate along the urogenital line in the retroperitoneum and migrate caudally during the second trimester of pregnancy to arrive at the internal inguinal ring at about 6 months of intrauterine life. During the last trimester they proceed through the abdominal wall via the inguinal canal and descend into the scrotum, the right slightly later than the left. The processus vaginalis then normally obliterates postnatally except for the portion surrounding and serving as a covering for the testes. Failure of this obliterative process results in congenital indirect inguinal hernia.

It is plausible to speculate that morphogenesis may be determined by single genes and complicated by environmental factors. In the case of indirect inguinal hernia, an autosomally dominantly inherited gene with reduced penetrance and sex influence would therefore be susceptible to environmental factors influencing its expression as a clinical inguinal hernia. In most families, however, a monogenic mode of inheritance is not apparent. Therefore the maternal allele may protect against failure of closure of the patent processus vaginalis.

In conclusion, the fact that most affected males have inherited an indirect inguinal hernia gene from their father implicates a role of genomic imprinting in the etiology of the indirect inguinal hernia phenotype.

INTRA-ABDOMINAL DISEASE CAUSING HERNIAS

Ascites due to abdominal carcinomatosis, liver or heart disease can present as recent onset herniation. The mechanism is similar to that already described in CAPD patients, with hydrostatic pressure dilating a pre-existing sac and abdominal contents prolapsing into this enlarged space. The sudden onset of a hernia in middle-aged or elderly patients should arouse diagnostic suspicion. It is a sound policy to subject hernial sacs to histological examination, especially in older patients, where ascites is found or when the sac is thickened. Routine histological examination of 'normal appearance' hernial sacs is not recommended; indeed the chance of an unexpected find of pathology in a 'normal' sac is estimated to be 0.00098%.[569] Histological examination of sacs obtained from children with hernia, hydrocele or undescended testis revealed that in the inguinal hernia patients during childhood smooth muscle was found within the wall of the sac but not in sacs associated with undescended testis. This suggests that this smooth muscle may have played a role in the prevention of obliteration and clinical outcome.[1117] Routine histology is certainly not economically sensible.

Thickening of the sac is not necessarily due to cancer; peritoneum is active tissue and particularly in children and young adults can exhibit over-exuberant tumor-like reaction to mechanical injury to the sac. This mesothelial hyperplasia may follow wearing a truss or occur simply after incarceration.

Microscopically there are atypical mesothelial cells; these may be either free or attached to the wall. Mitoses and multinucleated cells are frequently seen. Mesothelial hyperplasia is reactive and not neoplastic in origin.[968] Abdominal hernias are associated with autosomal dominant polycystic kidney disease.

The development of an abdominal wall hernia may be the initial symptom of decompensated heart or liver disease. Whereas good surgical practice is to repair an uncomplicated hernia, the question of repair in cirrhotics raises other issues. Leonetti *et al.* (1984) report that repair of umbilical hernias in uncontrolled unshunted cirrhotics gave a mortality of 8.3%, a morbidity of 16.6% and a recurrence rate of 16.6%. Umbilical herniorrhaphy in patients with a functioning peritoneovenous shunt was associated with minimal morbidity (7%). These authors suggest that peritoneovenous shunting should be a prerequisite to hernia repair.[683]

Pus can also distend an empty hernial sac, as with any peritoneal recess, during or after general peritonitis. In a review of 32 examples of this phenomenon, 19 were right inguinal, five right femoral, three left inguinal, one epigastric and one umbilical. Acute appendicitis accounted for 16 examples, perforated peptic ulcers for three, one followed pneumococcal peritonitis in a 2-week-old male child, one an acute pyosalpinx and one followed a biliary leak after removal of a common bile duct drain.[254] Every patient with this complication was originally diagnosed as having a strangulated hernia, which is not surprising. If pus is found in a hernial sac, abdominal exploration is mandatory with acute appendicitis being the commonest initial diagnosis, especially in right-sided hernias.[1125]

INGUINAL HERNIA AND APPENDECTOMY

Hoguet, in 1911, first described the development of inguinal hernia in patients who had undergone previous appendicectomy.[509] He found eight right inguinal hernias in a series of 190 patients who had undergone appendectomy; he suggested a causal relationship. Other authors have supported this contention.[47,446]

Right inguinal hernias are more frequent when appendectomy is performed through a lower, 'more cosmetic' incision, which is placed below the anterior superior iliac spine and in which the iliohypogastric nerve is injured. Electromyographic studies have shown conflicting results. While some investigators[46] have shown that denervation of the transversus abdominis muscle in the groin occurs, and could therefore interfere with the shutter mechanism of the deep ring and be a factor in the subsequent development of inguinal hernia, other investigators have failed to detect any abnormality signifying partial or complete denervation of the musculature in and around the right groin.[416]

Using the standard McBurney appendectomy incision (at right angles to a line from the umbilicus to the anterior superior iliac spine, at a point at the junction of its lateral third and medial two-thirds and parallel to the iliohypogastric nerve which is rarely injured if the flank muscles are opened by splitting in their fiber line), there is no evidence that inguinal herniation is a consequence of appendectomy. In a series of 549 patients who had undergone inguinal hernia repair, the percentage incidence of previous appendectomy in right-sided hernias was 8.9% ± 1.7% and in left-sided inguinal hernias 11.2% ± 2.1%.[676]

It is the lower, 'more cosmetic' incisions, which carry a particular hazard to the iliohypogastric nerve and a propensity to subsequent inguinal herniation. The introduction of effective antibiotics, the reduction of wound complications after appendectomy, and the increasing adoption of the laparoscopic appendectomy have also contributed to the lower incidence of inguinal herniation after appendectomy.

HERNIAS RELATED TO TRAUMA AND PELVIC FRACTURE

Abdominal hernias related to trauma and blunt injury are rare and are only reported following lower abdominal and pelvic injuries. To diagnose a traumatic hernia there must be immediate signs of local soft-tissue injury, bruising, hematoma, etc., and then there must be the early presentation of the symptoms of the hernia. The aponeuroses close to their pelvic attachments are most at risk.

Disruption of the inguinal canal and complete ruptures of the conjoint tendon are recorded.[223] Ryan, from the Shouldice clinic, reports five hernias related to pelvic fractures in 8000 hernia repairs.[1005]

Figure 3.9 illustrates an extremely rare case of a patient whose hernia was related to a pelvic fracture: a 40-year-old man developed a 'pantaloon' hernia after fracture of both rami of the pubis in a traffic accident. Hernias related to iatrogenic pelvic fractures, for example osteotomy for congenital dislocation of the hip, are of course well known in the literature. Ryan classifies these fracture-related hernias according to the mechanism of the fracture.[1005]

1 Due to acute anteroposterior forces acting on the pelvis. In these instances there is tearing of the rectus abdominis origin from the pubic crest. The tearing is maximal on the side opposite to that on which maximum bony displacement had occurred. The damage to the muscle is usually more severe medially than laterally, leading to the development of a broad-necked sac just suprapubically from the midline extending laterally across the attachment of the rectus to the pubic crest.
2 Due to lateral or lateral/vertical forces. These fractures involve the superior pubic ramus with consequent tearing of the fascial and aponeurotic attachments of the inguinofemoral region. In these circumstances a direct inguinal hernia develops through the fascia transversalis immediately above the bony fracture line. A repair of the direct hernia corrects the situation.
3 Due to surgical innominate osteotomy. This hernia occurs in children with congenital dislocated hips. The hernia following innominate osteotomy is either a direct inguinal hernia, a prevascular femoral (Narath's) hernia or a combination of the two.[835]

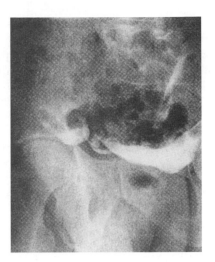

Figure 3.9 *Herniography on a 40-year-old man who had sustained a fracture of both pubic rami. The patient developed a 'pantaloon' inguinal hernia.*

During innominate (Salter's) osteotomy there is a downward lateral and forward displacement of the lower fragment of the pelvis produced by a combination of hinging and rotation at the symphysis pubis.[1010] This procedure leads to an increase in the distance between the edge of the rectus abdominis muscle and the inguinal and pectineal ligaments. There is a consequent weakening in the posterior wall of the inguinal canal. The angle between the midline (and, therefore, the lateral edge of the rectus muscle) and the superior ramus of the pubis is increased by a minimum of 5 degrees when compared to the opposite side, there is also an increase in the distance from the pubic tubercle to the anterior superior iliac spine. These changes alter the anatomy of the inguinofemoral region predisposing to hernia. It must be stressed that a consequent hernia is rare, and undoubtedly compensatory remodeling of the soft tissues occurs as the child develops after the osteotomy operation (Figure 3.10).

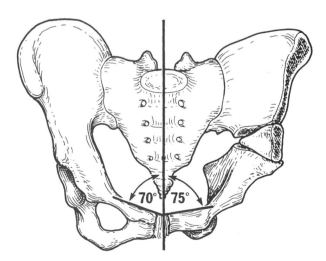

Figure 3.10 *Diagram to show how innominate osteotomy predisposes to inguinal herniation.*

After the removal of autologous bone grafts from the iliac crest, when full thickness grafts are taken from the posterior iliac crest, the inferior lumbar triangle is enlarged predisposing to herniation. These lumbar hernias cause backache and can be complicated by irreducibility and strangulation.[193]

EXERTION AND HERNIATION

There is no evidence that strong muscular or athletic exertion causes inguinal hernia in the absence of a fascial and/or muscular abnormality – either acquired connective tissue disease or congenital anomaly of the abdominal wall. Indeed, inguinal hernia is rare in weightlifters.[271] However, in a study of inguinal hernia and a single strenuous event, in which 129 patients with a total of 145 inguinal hernias were included, in 7% the hernia subjectively was attributable to a single muscular strain.[1066] The authors of this study suggested guidelines to assist in assessing 'cause' in claims for industrial injury in such patients, which involved the following four recommendations:

1 The patient should have made an official report of the incident of muscular strain.
2 Severe groin pain must have been experienced at the time of the strain.
3 The diagnosis of hernia should preferably have been made within 3 days of the incident (or certainly within 30 days).
4 There should be no previous history of inguinal hernia.

At the moment the relative importance of genetic, anatomic and environmental (smoking and heavy manual work) factors cannot be construed in each case. Manual work or strain is never, or very rarely, the sole cause of inguinal hernia.

Recent research suggests that persistent straining and heavy work is relevant to the development of groin hernia. The environment and occupation have an influence on hernia development. Recent European research has stressed these environmental factors rather than congenital defects in hernia development.[186,364] In man and many mammalian quadrupeds there is an absence of posterior rectus sheath below the arcuate line (of Douglas) and an insubstantial transversalis fascia in the groin. Gravitational stress in the erect posture amplifies this hindrance of weakness, which is an involved anatomical defect.[763]

The etiology of groin hernia has an importance in terms of prevention; smoking is a causal agent.

In medico-legal terms, the situation is confused – an accident or heavy strain at work is generally construed as a causal factor in the onset of a hernia and in the English courts damages are usually awarded. Our current understanding of the etiology of inguinal hernias casts doubt on judicial reasoning in many of these instances. The legal foundation for compensating a workman who develops a hernia after an accident at his workplace is the commission of a tort or breach of contract by his employer. The heads of damages awarded are for pain or suffering, loss of amenities (usually sex life), pecuniary loss, medical expenses and loss of earning capacity. The role of a pre-existing disability, patent processus vaginalis or metastatic emphysema, will need offsetting against the damages. This is definitely a task for the judiciary, being largely unrelated to the observations of natural science.[580] This risk of a 'work-related' hernia causes many patients to seek surgical correction of a hernia that is discovered in a pre-employment physical examination (especially in the United States). These hernias must be repaired regardless of the absence of symptomology due to the medico-legal risks to the employer *and* the surgeon.

CONCLUSIONS

- The incidence of primary groin hernia varies in different communities. The exact incidence in adult males is very difficult to estimate, but 16% of adult males will undergo operation for the condition.
- Genetic and acquired factors each interact to allow a hernia to develop; however, we are forced to the conclusion that a failure of the fascia transversalis to withstand the stresses and strains of life is crucial to the development of inguinal hernia.
- A preformed, congenital, peritoneal processus or sac is an important prerequisite of the indirect hernia of childhood or of the indirect sac, which is manifest in CAPD patients or in patients with ascites due to cirrhosis or peritoneal malignancy.
- A tissue defect is demonstrated in adult males with inguinal herniation. This tissue defect is causally related to smoking. Persistent heavy laboring work is associated with hernia development.

4

Logistics of hernia repair

TRENDS IN SURGICAL CARE

Before the Victorian economic miracle in the 1860s allowed extensive hospital construction in the British Isles and simultaneously created the urban deprivation which required hospitals as a haven from a hostile unhygienic environment for the working masses when they were ill, most patients recuperated at home after surgical operations. Only the indigent and members of the armed forces were automatically hospitalized if they required surgery or were wounded. Patients with financial means avoided hospital care. This pattern of surgery was usual in the USA and Europe. The tradition of home surgery lingered on in England where, in the spring of 1951, King George VI had a left pneumonectomy for carcinoma of the lung in a Buckingham Palace room which had been turned into an operating theater.[331]

The regimentation of wartime and the prejudices of officer surgeons on the management of hernias influenced postoperative care in the early days of the National Health Service (NHS). The average time between operation and return to depot in the World War II British Army was 12 weeks: 3 weeks in bed, with exercises commencing on the twelfth day; 3–4 weeks in a convalescent hospital, with exercises conducted under instruction; 4 weeks in a convalescent depot; then a few days' leave. At the end of this time the patient was able to carry out full duties as a 'fighting man'.[327] These orders persisted into peacetime and contributed to conservative surgical practice until Hugh Dudley challenged them in the 1960s.[176]

The British National Health Service (NHS), from its inception in 1948, also encouraged hospitalization for surgery; the 1962 Hospital Plan envisaged all surgery concentrated in one hospital in each district. The 1969 update of that report, like the earlier report, recommended concentrating surgical services but did not recognize the value of day-case or short-stay facilities. Up to the early 1970s the trend to institutional surgery and recuperation as an inpatient continued remorselessly.

Three forces predicated this – the professionalization of the hospital nursing service, the improvements in surgical technology, requiring more and more sophisticated equipment for even the simplest procedure, and the drive by third-party payers (in England the State) to control costs. Costs are most easily controlled in an institution owned by the paymasters, so surgery in hospital becomes normative. Until the 1990s the concept of the NHS contracting out work to an independent day-care facility was unthinkable. By the 1950s it was accepted that for clinical, social and economic reasons surgery and postoperative recovery should take place in hospital, notwithstanding the example of King Emperors and the whimsy of their surgeon knights!

Administrative and governmental influences were not the only conservative forces; the attitudes of the distinguished 'fathers' of modern surgery were conservative too. Billroth believed that rest and protection were essential for the proper repair of coapted tissues.[123] Halsted, writing on the radical cure of hernia in 1889, stated:

'Our patients are kept on their backs for 21 days. Wounds healed thoroughly throughout are not strong in 21 days … are certainly stronger on the fourteenth day than the seventh and certainly stronger on the twenty-first day than on the fourteenth. Just how long wounds of skin and muscle which have healed by first intention … in strength we do not know … I sometimes question the propriety of allowing, as I do, my patients to walk about on the twenty-first day'.[461]

Four years later (1893) Emil Ries, Professor of Gynecology in Chicago, a man who is truly the English-speaking father of early postoperative ambulation, instituted early ambulation and rapid convalescence in his unit. In 1893 Ries had visited Morisani's clinic in Naples and while there he was shown a patient who had risen from her bed and walked across the ward during the evening of the day of symphysiotomy, without detriment to herself or her wound. Not only was early ambulation possible, but Ries soon found that recovery was faster too; these patients commenced on a full diet sooner and they had fewer bowel problems. He concluded that with good asepsis and careful surgery there should be no problems. Ries concluded: 'It means a great deal for the business man or labourer or their wives to be put on their own feet in a short time and to be able to return to their work two or three weeks after an abdominal operation'.[958]

Powers investigated the effect of early ambulation on postoperative complications and return to work following hernioplasty in a New York rural community from 1933 to 1953.

He clearly demonstrated that the duration of hospital stay could be safely lowered from an average of 14 postoperative days to one day, and this allowed a sixfold increase in the number of operations undertaken. Early ambulation was associated with a dramatic lowering of the hernia recurrence rate.[924] This latter improvement in the recurrence rate should not be ascribed to early ambulation alone; the increased experience of the operating surgeon must have improved his technique too.

Surgery, social mores and economics are not static. Advances in anesthesia, newer surgical techniques, lower sepsis rates, a healthier and better nourished population, improved home conditions, co-ordinated home nursing and family doctor services, and inexorable cost containment programs have made us review our indications for inpatient hospital care. High complication rates no longer bedevil anesthesia and surgery. Furthermore, the benefits of self-help and early mobilization are now appreciated.

Today's weltschmerz is cost containment with consumerism, combined with increased longevity, vastly improved medical technology and a quite correct emphasis on efficiency and 'value for money'. Paradoxically, home recuperation after surgery is now the norm often for reasons of patient choice and satisfaction.

Individualizing hernia repair to various clinical, social and economic situations has now become an important concept.[991] In addition to overall rehabilitation (which includes short and long-term postoperative discomfort and return to daily activities and work), four other relevant outcome measures should be incorporated into any evaluation of modern day hernia surgery:

1 technical difficulty
2 complication rates including the overall rate and the seriousness of possible complications
3 recurrence rate and the formidability of repairing it
4 socioeconomic factors, notably cost.

Which of these four outcome measures takes precedence and whether the planners (hospital managers) or the providers (surgeons) decide which is important remains to be resolved. Perhaps with a better health-educated public, patients or their advocates should decide, on the basis of a knowledge of core outcome measures.[163] When studying the logistics and outcomes of hernia surgery, idiosyncratic surgeon-reported data do not often allow meaningful comparison and independent data collection by a nurse research assistant is more reliable. In this respect the short-form (SF) 36 health status questionnaire has been usefully adopted in many clinical trials of hernia surgery technique and allows comparison between clinical trials to become reality. The SF36 questionnaire contains 36 items that measures eight dimensions of health on multi-item scales and a further dimension on a single-item scale that measures change in health over the last year.[643] The eight dimensions of health are physical functioning, social functioning, role limitations caused by physical problems, role limitations caused by emotional problems, mental health, energy/vitality, pain, and general health perception. Raw scores are transformed into a 0 to 100 scale. The SF36 questionnaire has been validated as a useful instrument for the measurement of out come

in inguinal hernia repair.[163,643] More problematic are the conditions-specific questions which relate to a patients expectations and responses to their surgical experience.

VARIATION IN DURATION OF STAY OF ADULT HERNIA PATIENTS

Variations in the length of hospital stay were demonstrated by routine hospital statistics in about 1960. These differences in clinical practice soon began to attract interest. The work of Farquharson and of Stephens and Dudley had alerted managers to the benefits of efficient hospital practice, so it is not surprising that non-clinicians should be attracted to investigate the seemingly inexplicable variations in clinical practice.

Farquharson in Edinburgh (1955) reported 458 outpatient hernioplasties. All his patients were operated under local anesthesia, only 11 developing complications, which required admission. He emphasized the therapeutic advantages of early mobilization and the benefit such rapid turnover brought to others awaiting operation. Farquharson found the system clinically satisfying and continued the practice for the rest of his working life.[344]

Stephens and Dudley (1961) reported a study of outpatient varicose veins and hernia operations, emphasizing that for day-case patients and inpatients the same standards of care must be delivered. They stressed the importance of anesthetic assessment and the organizational rigor that must be instituted.[1087]

Davies and Barr (1965) researched the management of uncomplicated inguinal hernias in adults between 16 and 60 years old by 17 consultant surgical teams in three UK NHS regions – Birmingham, Liverpool and Oxford. Each team provided records of 100 recent patients; in all, 1678 patients were analysed. In the series 80% of the patients were aged between 30 and 59 years of age and 121 (7.2%) were females. One-third were engaged on heavy work, the remainder having light industrial or sedentary occupations. The mean time on the waiting list varied widely; in Birmingham 3.1 months were spent on a waiting list, in Liverpool 3.9 months and in Oxford 6.9 months.[268]

The duration of hospital stay also varied, being shortest in the Oxford region where the waiting list was longest. In Oxford 86% of patients were operated on within a day of admission; in the other two regions there were significantly longer preoperative inpatient stays. In Liverpool, for instance, 27.6% of patients spent 2 days in hospital prior to operation. The greatest degree of correlation was found between the time spent on the waiting list and the duration of inpatient stay: where the waiting list time was short the inpatient duration was long and vice versa. The study also reviewed operative techniques and suture choice and demonstrated that little had changed despite the classic contributions on these topics by Marsden who had reviewed hernia practice in Liverpool in 1958 and 1962.[749]

This three-region study, at a time when earlier studies of ambulant or short-stay inguinal hernia repair had already been published, demonstrates the innately conservative behavior of clinicians. The authors, epidemiologists, concluded that a prospective evaluation of techniques and suture materials was needed and an evaluation of the effect of different lengths of stay was urgently required!

Another study, by epidemiologists, of the duration of stay of men undergoing unilateral inguinal hernioplasty in eight Wessex hospitals from 1970 to 1971, showed that the duration of postoperative hospital stay was related to the hospital, more importantly its size and organization, rather than to other factors. Small hospitals had longer durations of stay. Surgeons operating in two hospitals adopted the normative duration of stay of the hospital rather than vice versa. Pressure of work at larger hospitals may compel shorter stays and modify hospital organization.[438]

These studies do show how helpless the surgeon often is when it comes to implementing good clinical policies, which challenge the accepted practice for the institution. Clinicians, like their patients, can suffer from the institutionalism that stalks hospital corridors!

Clinically oriented studies of short-stay surgery for hernias include those of Morris (1968), Russell et al. (1977), and Ruckley et al. (1978).[809,984,988]

Morris and colleagues randomized patients from the hernia waiting list in Mansfield, Leicestershire, to either inpatient or outpatient surgery. The only problems they reported were postoperative chest infections and some patients' preference for 48 h postoperative inpatient care.[809]

Russell and colleagues in Stockton-on-Tees conducted a prospective randomized controlled study of day-case operation for hernias or hemorrhoids. No surgical adverse effects were seen when day-case hernioplasties were compared with longer stay hernia operations, but in complications with day-case hemorrhoid operations increased twofold. He also found, like Morris and co-workers, that some patients preferred an overnight or 24 h stay.[988]

Ruckley and colleagues reviewed the duration of stay of patients requiring surgery for varicose veins; the patients were preselected for suitability and then randomized to care patterns. A total of 121 were allocated to a 48 h stay in an acute ward, 121 were managed in a convalescent hospital after operation and 117 were discharged directly home to the care of the general practitioner and the community nursing service. Anesthetic and/or surgical problems necessitated keeping five patients (three convalescent and two day-case) in hospital on the day of operation. Two acute ward patients and one convalescent ward patient required readmission for complications; two of these patients had minor pulmonary emboli and one had undiagnosed chest pain. None of the day cases required readmission for any reason.[985]

Day care involved an average of only 8 min more working time, including traveling for general practitioners in the three weeks after operation. Forty percent of patients had no contact whatsoever with their general practitioners during the postoperative period. The average contact times with the community nurse in the three weeks postoperatively were 186 min (for acute ward patients), 204 min (for convalescent ward patients) and 207 min (for day care patients). The saving in day care

compared with 7-day care was a considerable £100 (based on Scottish Hospital Statistics, 1975).[1032]

Customer reaction was tested and day care was the most acceptable of the three options. Women with children at home preferred day care. The average hospital ward compares unfavorably with most home environments in terms of comfort, menu, personal attention, privacy, hygiene and cross-infection risks. It is not surprising that patients undergoing simple surgery, not subject to postoperative risks of a life-threatening nature, should prefer home care.

The development of 'one-day' outpatient surgery for adults with groin hernias has been slow. Enthusiasts in both North America[390] and the UK have published accounts of such surgery, but universal adoption of these policies is perhaps too adventurous for most surgeons. Ambulatory one-day walk-in, walk-out outpatient surgery became a fact of life in the USA when Medicare disallowed reimbursement for hospitalization of those over 65 years undergoing elective inguinal hernioplasty.[1187] Since then in the USA, ambulatory hernia surgery has proved to be safe, convenient, efficient, economical and very popular with patients by softening the emotional impact of the operation and thereby reducing disability by encouraging the patient to get on with their normal life. However the results of ambulatory care are surgeon dependent and what brings success is the enthusiasm for perfection and the painstaking skill with which the hernia care is accomplished.[599] Although Farquharson, in 1955, reported day-case herniorrhaphy in 485 patients treated over a 5-year period in Edinburgh, there can be no doubt that his example did not spread too far afield. In Scotland, in 1967, the median postoperative stay after inguinal herniorrhaphy was 8 days, with a range of 2–12 days.[487,985] In 1974 this remained unchanged at 8 days, with 10% of the patients occupying an inpatient hospital bed for three or more days prior to operation. Indeed, in some hospitals 30% of patients rested in hospital for three or more days before surgery.[1032] In the Northern Region of the NHS in England, in 1981, 18 528 male adults with inguinal hernia underwent operation. The average duration of stay was 6.9 days and 45% were in hospital for longer than 10 days.

Morgan and her colleagues (1987) have analyzed the duration of hospital stay for inguinal hernia repair in adults in the Northern and South East Thames regions of the NHS.[808] In the Northern Region 18% of operations on the under 25-year-old group were performed as day cases; in those 25 years old and over, only 0.6% of inguinal hernia repairs were done as day cases. The mean length of stay for adult inguinal hernia repair in the Northern Region in 1984 was 4.9 days (SD ± 4.5) and in South East Thames Region in 1982 5.4 days (SD ± 4.1). There is a noticeably wide variation. A follow-up study by Morgan in 1992 involved a postal questionnaire completed by 240 staff surgeons (an 85% response rate) in four regional health authorities of the NHS.[807] In this survey only 11% of consultants were regularly undertaking day-case inguinal hernia repair, a further 44% held positive attitudes and 45% were not interested. The major constraints perceived were the lack of hospital facilities and the problems of providing postoperative care in the community due to lack of community services.

Quite clearly durations of stay, particularly preoperative stay, could be reduced without clinical detriment to the patients. There are wide differences between hospitals revealed in these studies. More recently in Plymouth, UK a dedicated Hernia Service was set-up within an NHS public hospital in 1996 that treats over 750 patients with inguinal hernia per year.[595] In the Hernia Service 90.5% of patients receive local anesthesia, 81.4% are treated as day cases, with a saving of 605 inpatient days per annum compared with the pre-Hernia Service performance. Hernia satisfaction questionnaires indicate that patients experience less pain, require less postoperative analgesia and resume normal activity at an earlier stage compared with patients who have been treated on the general surgical service. The economic efficiency of well-organized ambulatory hernia surgery should therefore be obvious, but organizational as well as clinical inertia contributes to its lack of widespread adoption.[808]

Motives other than clinical excellence are likely to encourage short-stay surgery; changing patterns of female behavior and work, with more nursing falling to male nurses and married women, will dictate the requirement for flexible and no-weekend shift systems. The high cost of institutional overheads will optimize single short-stay facilities, which can be closed down completely at weekends. The development of ambulant surgery should reduce the requirement for inpatient facilities. Costs of medical care will continue to remain high and containment of these costs will increasingly become a surgical priority. To date there have been few good prospective studies of short-stay surgery. Such studies need to be adequately controlled to give real comparative data about all the variables, including patient satisfaction. Everyone knows it is possible to remove the appendix on the kitchen table, but is this necessarily a good thing?

To resolve this question a carefully controlled study comparing the social, economic and clinical outcome of the treatment is required. The DHSS commissioned such a study in the early 1970s; however, like so many studies commissioned to bolster administrative policy, it was 'quick and dirty' and did not adequately answer the questions clinicians and their patients find most relevant.[6] The study did not measure the quality of surgical care, although a subsequent report suggests that the 'acid test' of hernia surgery, the recurrence rate of the patients included, was much higher than the best surgery available at the time. Other surgical complications appear to have been above average too. The authors of this study concluded that short-stay hospital care for these conditions saved the hospital and community medical services about £25 per case – this difference is largely accounted for by the difference in the 'hotel costs' of the shorter stay.[6] Herein is the dilemma: any economic or organizational conclusions drawn from a sample in which the clinical and social outcomes are less than optimal are regarded as dubious by both consumers and clinicians.

Day surgery and high quality hernia surgery have been promoted by enthusiasts rather than by administrative decree, day surgery must be of higher-quality and safe. Such attributes evolved at North Tees Hospital in the 1970s. In a prospective series of inguinal hernioplasties in male adults (16 years old and above) from 1970 to 1982, 718 operations were

Table 4.1 *Mean duration of stay for inguinal hernioplasty in England and Wales*

Year	1975	1980	1985	1990	1995
Duration of stay (days)	7.3	5.7	4.9	3.1	2.1

performed, the mean duration of stay was 4.3 days, 28% were day cases (in-hospital stay up to 8 h), 31% overnight stay (<24 h) and 41% greater than 24 h. The recurrence rate, the 'acid test', was under 1%. The problem is how to generalize such results.

In recent years the average duration of stay of inguinal hernia patients has fallen consistently and the proportion of patients being treated on an ambulant day-case basis has increased (Table 4.1).

Overall the development of day-case surgery for adults with groin hernias has been slower in the UK than in the USA, where most inguinal hernioplasties are performed on an ambulant basis. Interestingly, the Shouldice Hospital in Toronto, possibly the owners of the 'gold standard' hernioplasty operation, have not endorsed day surgery for groin hernia. They continue with their 4-day regime for hernioplasty with progressive supervised postoperative ambulation and re-habilitative exercises.[14,1203]

The impact of contemporary socioeconomic pressures on surgical practice in the UK is well demonstrated by inguinal hernioplasty. There are socioeconomic and age-related variations in the uptake of inguinal hernioplasty,[248] and probably related to these there is an increasing uptake of private practice options.[775] Nichol has estimated that repair of hernias in private practice increased by 77% from 1981 to 1986.[845] Private hernia patients in independent hospitals have the longest stay recorded.[1211] This longer stay occurs in all age groups in 1980. A British Private Hospital (The British Hernia Centre) dedicated to hernia surgery has produced some of the best results in terms of complications and recurrence in a series of 1098 cases, 98% of which were repaired on a day-case basis under local anesthesia.[567] In a further effort to keep down costs, the British Hernia Centre advise patients who travel more than 50 miles to stay in a local hotel for their first postoperative night. The relentless drive of cost constraint has clearly not been as potent, except in isolated pockets, in the private sector in the UK as it has in the USA and the NHS.

There is, however, a cost to the community in terms of decreasing lengths of hospital stay.[183] In a prospective study, an evaluation was made of patient satisfaction, time off work and pain scores both before and after re-engineering a surgical service for the treatment of elective inguinal hernia and laparoscopic cholecystectomy. To provide a quality ambulatory hernia service it was necessary to supplement the traditional surgical service with a perioperative unit, a preadmission anesthetic assessment with a self-reported questionnaire, day of surgery admissions, enhanced patient education, clinical pathways and post-acute care. This enhanced set-up did result in shorter length of stay and the supplements to the surgical service resulted in higher patient satisfaction and neither the patients nor the caregivers required more time off work. There was cost saving to the hospital service but increased costs in the community of $200 Australian dollars per patient. This study illustrates clearly that ambulatory surgery is costly both in terms of effort and support systems both in the hospital and the community and does not necessarily save overall costs. Even in the elderly as much as half of the patients can receive their hernia surgery on a day-case basis.[401]

HOSPITAL-BASED OR INDEPENDENT DAY-CARE (AMBULATORY) SURGERY FACILITY?

Early day-case surgery was undertaken from traditional wards, but gradually the concept of a special freestanding unit appeared, the first one in the UK being at the Royal Postgraduate Medical School, Hammersmith, London. Short-stay or ambulatory surgery can be accommodated in three separate settings, each of which has its own advantages and disadvantages. First, patients can be admitted into traditional surgical wards. Secondly, a designated unit can be set up as part of an existing surgical general hospital organization. Lastly, a custom-built, free-standing, independent ambulatory care facility can be built.[287,309,923]

Each of these settings has advantages. Utilization of main inpatient facilities imposes no extra capital cost because facilities are already on site, but the space occupied by short-stay cases will be vacant and wasted at weekends. A designated unit in a general hospital allows for multidisciplinary utilization; it keeps staff on location and also allows weekend closure, thus cutting expensive nursing costs and allowing staffing by married nurses. An additional advantage that has been claimed is that married nurses develop greater empathy and understanding of the special domestic requirements of day-case patients.

Hospital-based dedicated units are the usual model for day-case surgery; they require less capital and they use existing staff, equipment and support services. They allow for flexibility of staffing and can draw on the parent hospital in times of shortage. Furthermore, if complications arise the patients can be handled within the same institution. The disadvantages include surgeons being called away to more pressing emergencies, so that the day-case plan is 'bumped'. Also, patients' morale may be disadvantaged by having to witness other patients receiving critical care or major surgery. As these dedicated units are part of a larger whole their overheads may be unduly high because they have to carry their share of services required in a major hospital but which are not essential to their more restricted role.

It is the problems of capital provision and overhead costs which have led, particularly in the USA, and more recently in Europe, to freestanding Ambulatory Care Centers. American reviews of surgical care provision now seem to give this type of unit, the Surgicenter, more marks than day care located in traditional medical institutions. Separate registration, standardized preoperative and postoperative regimens and an absence of seriously ill incumbents make these units more acceptable to the community. Disadvantages may include the lack of in-house medical staff to deal with the infrequent complication.[369]

Table 4.2 *Preoperative documentation for management of the day-case patient*

Name:	Hospital number:
Date of birth:	Address:
Ward:	
Name of ward sister:	
Ward doctor:	

Date of admission/completion of this form:
Reason for admission:
Occupation of patient:
Past medical history:
Previous operations:
Complications of previous operations:
Current drug therapy:
Is there any history of allergies?
Is the patient taking anticoagulants?
Alcohol intake:
Smoking habits:
Does the patient take any other social drugs?
Female patients:
    Are you pregnant?
    Date of last menstrual period?
    Are you taking oral contraceptives?
    If 'yes', what DVT prophylaxis has been ordered?
Systematic enquiries:
    Cardiovascular system
    Respiratory system
    Other

Active intercurrent illnesses:
Physical examination

Height:	Weight:
Pulse rate:	Blood pressure:
Temperature:	Urinalysis:
Chest examination:	
Cardiovascular examination:	
ASA	grade:

However, in the United States, any complication will be easily managed through the Emergency Department by the emergency physician or, more commonly, by the treating surgeon.

PATIENT MANAGEMENT POLICIES

Day-case and short-stay surgery depend critically on the administrative and nursing, as well as the surgical, protocol. There must be an easy flow from first patient contact through operation to home, convalescence and return to employment. If this flow is to be effortless the entire program must be formalized, repeatable and understood by all concerned – including the patient. It is advisable to have standard printed documentation including details of pre-admission (Table 4.2), operation and postoperative care, nursing and consent all on one form. Details of the organization, management and patient selection are extensively reviewed and protocols set out in the Royal College of Surgeons of England Guidelines for Day Surgery revised edition 1992.[980,981]

Table 4.3 *ASA classification of physical status for surgical patients*[22]

Class 1	The patient has no organic, physiological, biochemical or psychiatric disturbance. The pathological process for which operation is to be performed is localized and does not entail a systemic disturbance. Examples: a fit patient with inguinal hernia; fibroid uterus in an otherwise healthy woman.
Class 2	Mild to moderate systemic disturbance caused either by the condition to be treated surgically or by other pathophysiological processes. Examples: non- or only slightly limiting organic heart disease; mild diabetes; essential hypertension; or anemia. Some might choose to list the extremes of age here, either the neonate or the octogenarian, even though no discernible systemic disease is present. Extreme obesity and chronic bronchitis may be included in this category.
Class 3	Severe systemic disturbance or disease from whatever cause, even though it may not be possible to define the degree of disability with finality. Examples: severely limiting organic heart disease; severe diabetes with vascular complications; moderate to severe degrees of pulmonary insufficiency; angina pectoris or healed myocardial infarction.
Class 4	Severe systemic disorders that are already life-threatening, not always correctable by operation. Examples: patients with organic heart disease showing marked signs of cardiac insufficiency, persistent angina, or active myocarditis; advanced degrees of pulmonary, hepatic, renal or endocrine insufficiency.
Class 5	The moribund patient who has little chance of survival but is submitted to operation in desperation. Examples: the burst abdominal aneurysm with profound shock; major cerebral trauma with rapidly increasing intracranial pressure; massive pulmonary embolus. Most of these patients require operation as a resuscitative measure, with little if any anesthesia.

At the first consultation a diagnosis should be made and a decision to operate (or not) taken. The patient's physical and emotional health and suitability or not for general or local anesthesia are reviewed, as are home and other relevant social conditions and operation day transportation. Important facts to record include age, weight and height for pharmacological reasons, active intercurrent medical conditions, current drug therapy and social drug composition.

In females, day-case surgery could be inadvisable during pregnancy. The use of oral contraceptives and the requirement for deep vein thrombosis (DVT) prophylaxis will need assessing. Preoperative cessation of oral contraceptives may be advised; however, a six-months off dry period is required if the risk of DVT is to be reduced. The frequent use of sequential compression stockings in these patients minimizes this risk. Therefore, this requirement is infrequently enforced. The possibility of pregnancy may be a greater risk to the patient. This will require a decision at the initial consultation.

The American Society of Anesthesiologists' (ASA) grade should be recorded. Only patients of ASA classes 1 and 2 can ordinarily be considered suitable for day-case surgery (Table 4.3).[22]

The date and time of operation, and the date and time of discharge, are set at this initial consultation. All medical and nursing process documentation including the consent form, which can be repetitive, time consuming and wearying for the patient, is rolled up into one document to be filled in at the initial consultation. Completed, this checklist is passport, visa, ticket and boarding pass to surgery. When giving consent the patient must clearly understand that he is to be discharged postoperatively with a newly created surgical wound. Failure to obtain this consent and explain its consequences may lead to difficulties later. Patients need to know what to expect and who to contact if they are concerned when they return home.

A very worthwhile and effective preoperative routine can be a nurse assessment clinic. Such a clinic can undertake much of the routine preoperative check of physical status and additionally verify the social context and suitability of the patient for day surgery.[473]

The patient needs instructions that he can review at home; these may be written or as a tape or video (Table 4.4). 'Going home' is the crucial moment for the patient. The emphasis must be on accurately timed discharge. Planned discharge imposes constraints on all the actors; the commitment to predictable discharge is more demanding than the commitment to admission – hence the term 'planned early discharge'.

In order that arrangements and the patient's status remain unchanged, as short an interval as possible should occur between the various phases. For example, a groin hernia in a child or adult should be processed within a few weeks.

On admission the patient's identity and medical status must be re-checked. It is convenient to use a structured form for this. The site of the operation is checked for cleanliness and freedom from sepsis. It should be indelibly marked, with the patient conscious when this is done.

In the operating room the patient's identity should be checked. Identifying the patient can be most hazardous in children and a fail-safe double-check procedure, with surgeon and anesthetist separately doing the check, is advised.

An excellent booklet containing details for the patient has been published by the British Association for Day Surgery entitled Day Surgery and one on hernia repair Hernia Repair Operation, Questions and Answers published by the Royal College of Surgeons of England. In the USA a similar patient booklet, Hernias of the Groin, by the late Professor George Wantz of New York, can be recommended. It must be stressed again that patient information is vital to successful modern hernia short-stay surgery.[979,981]

A clinical pathway for inguinal hernia repair reduces hospital readmissions for problems such as postoperative pain, wound complications and comorbid conditions such as cardiopulmonary disease.[1216] The reasons for an improvement

Table 4.4 *Instructions to day-case hernia patients*

This letter relates to your admission to hospital for repair of your hernia.

In the morning, before you come into hospital, would you please shave your lower abdomen, groin and pubic/scrotal area completely.

It is expected that you will be discharged about 5 p.m. but would you please advise your family to contact Sister on the ward if you have not arrived home by 7 p.m.

You will be given 20 tablets for pain. You should not have any pain, but if you do one of these tablets should be quite sufficient to relieve it.

You should be fit to get up and about as soon as you get home. We strongly advise you to exercise. If possible, you should go out for a walk each day after your operation. At all costs you must keep fully mobile about the house.

Your hernia has been repaired with modern suture material which is very strong, at least as strong as your tissues; this means you can walk and exercise as much as you want. The only restriction may be imposed by pain in the first few days after surgery.

We do *not* advise heavy lifting for about three weeks after surgery.

You must not drive yourself in a car for 7 days after surgery; your groin will be stiff and this could interfere with your movement of the pedals.

The skin wound has been stitched internally and then the surface closed with spray-on plastic and a dressing. Keep the wound dry during the first four days. On the fifth day have a warm bath or shower, and when the wound is well wetted remove the dressing and discard it. The wound may appear a little red and proud at first, but just keep it clean, washing it each day and drying it carefully. It will heal up to give you a neat red scar in 2 weeks and an almost invisible white scar in 3 months.

You will be fit to resume office work in 3–7 days.

You will be fit to resume heavy work – laboring, gardening, scaffolding, coalmining, etc. – 8 weeks after operation. Swimming can be resumed 4 weeks after operation; violent sports, rugby, soccer or squash, can be resumed gradually after four weeks to full activity at twelve weeks. Sexual activity is best resumed gently from 2–4 weeks after operation. Any activity that does not cause pain is good for you. Early resumption of work enhances wound healing and will reduce the chance of recurrence of your hernia.

If you have any complications you can either contact your own doctor or the ward here.

in outcome by the application of clinical pathways are multifactorial and include improvements in surgeon and staff awareness. The development of care pathways or practice guidelines must therefore be multidisciplinary and based on the results of properly conducted systematic reviews with graded recommendations.[631]

PRE-DISCHARGE CRITERIA

Patients need to be fully conscious prior to discharge. They also must be mobile and able to care for themselves. They must be taking fluids by mouth, not nauseated and 'happy' on oral analgesics and be able to medicate themselves adequately when they arrive home. Voiding urine may be difficult after a hernia repair, especially for the male. Micturition must be accomplished prior to departure from hospital. However, in many centers, even this dictum is less frequently enforced if the patient does not have a predisposing condition that places him or her at risk, such as prostatism or cystocele, respectively. The patients must understand their care plan, the management of the wound and the management of pain and discomfort.

The patient needs to take home with him full details of his operation, whatever medication that he has been advised and what postoperative regimen is planned. These should be given to him so that if something goes awry he can hand all this information to the doctor or nurse who attends the patient in

Simultaneously the patient's family doctor and nursing staff should be advised that the patient has undergone the operation, that he has been discharged, what has been done and what postoperative care is advised. It must again be stressed, however, that postoperative care is properly the responsibility of the operating surgeon.

Cannon and colleagues at the Middlesex Hospital, London, have reviewed the reasons for delayed discharge in a consecutive series of 104 unselected patients undergoing planned repair of an inguinal hernia. It was intended to discharge all of them from hospital within 48 h after operation; however, taking into account social and clinical factors only 54 patients were proposed for 48 h discharge and of these 24 (44%) were discharged on time. Of the 104 patients, 62 (60%) were discharged on the planned day, but only 24 (23%) left hospital 48 h after surgery. The most frequent reason for delaying discharge was persistent postoperative pyrexia, which occurred in 24 patients. In retrospect, Cannon and co-workers report that a raised postoperative temperature did not foreshadow any more important clinical complications and should not therefore be a criterion for delaying discharge from hospital.[102,182] Temperature elevation is such a common postoperative finding that this can usually be ignored if the temperature is less than 101°F and is relieved within 24–48 h. The most common etiology is, of course, atelectasis.

Inner city deprivation is sometimes advanced as an argument against planned early discharge. However, although adverse social circumstances may preclude the inclusion of some patients in such a scheme, the reality is that a well-constructed system can function in most communities.

POSTOPERATIVE CARE

The aim should be minimal care, if possible without professional input. Postoperative pain control should be demand-led and self-prescribed by the patient. Wounds should be doctor and nurse non-dependent. Sutures or clips that need skilled removal should not be used and dressings should easily be removed and, if necessary, replaced by the patient or the caregiver. Techniques used should not impose an additional burden on family doctors. It is possible to construct a surgical system that is free-standing and not transferring its workload onto others that may be caring for the patient.

Postoperative care should not impose costs above expected inpatient costs on the patient or his family. Research has confirmed that the trousseau effect of admission to traditional hospital care, plus the costs of spouses visiting, is at least as expensive as the cost of additional meals, spouse attention and other incidentals of home convalescence.[988]

Day-case surgery is only advantageous if it is well coordinated and free of problems; it is not an excuse to divest oneself of responsibility for postoperative care.[981]

Sleep

Even relatively minor surgical interventions can cause major, though temporary, disruptions of sleep in otherwise healthy individuals. Preoperative sleep is often forgotten; most patients that are admitted to the hospital show evidence of diminished preoperative sleep on the night before surgery. Anxiety, a new environment and clock-fixed nursing routines are important determinants of this. Admitting the patient on the day of operation overcomes many of these difficulties.

For the first two nights postoperatively, sleep is characterized by restlessness, lightness and the almost complete absence of rapid eye movement and delta sleep.[572] The consequences of these postoperative sleep disturbances are uncertain, but there is evidence that sleep deprivation causes psychological instability and may also be a precursor of poor wound healing.

The adverse effect of the hostile ward environment on sleep is again a strong argument for day-care surgery. However, in both day-care and hospital-care surgery the case for adequate analgesics and hypnotics in the perioperative phase must be emphasized.

DAY-CASE SURGERY FOR CHILDREN

As early as 1909 the Royal Glasgow Hospital for Children reported that outpatient surgery was satisfactory for children with inguinal hernias, but 25 years later surgeons were still keeping children in bed for 3 weeks after hernia repairs.[844] This has mostly changed and outpatient herniotomy in pediatric practice is now well-established.[64]

The experience, in Brighton, Sussex, of treating children with hernias, hydroceles and other minor conditions as day cases demonstrates all the advantages of the system. One hundred children were studied; each child was initially diagnosed and recommended for day-case surgery in the surgical clinic. The children were then reviewed in a special anesthetic clinic and finally the parents and the family doctors were asked to complete a questionnaire about the patient care incident.[43]

Of the 100 patients, there were 72 boys and 28 girls, and 64 of them were aged under 5 years old. Four patients were deemed unfit for day-case anesthesia and a further two patients developed respiratory infections just prior to operation, necessitating a rescheduling. One child was detained in hospital with a hematoma, but no child required readmission or intervention by the family doctor for complications.

The family doctors were enthusiastic about the scheme – two even included their own children in the subsequent day-care programme! Ninety-two percent of the parents replying to the questionnaire approved. The low duration of child–parent separation, the involvement of the parents in the day-care admission and the devolution of postoperative nursing to the parents were all considered advantages.

The economic aspects were not quantified, but the programme did relieve the pressure on beds, reduced the night nurse workload and reduced the waiting list. All of these were economic positives. However economically advantageous a day-case programme may be, unless it appeals to patients (and parents) it cannot be regarded as successful. This study illustrates clinical, social and economic success.[814] The organization of day care for children needs to be exact; an outstanding system has been developed in Southampton UK by Atwell.[62] This topic is further explored in Chapter 10. In the United States, the practice of outpatient surgery for the pediatric population is commonplace.

CONVALESCENCE AND RETURN TO WORK

In general, the philosophy of day-case and short-stay surgery should encourage early mobility and a rapid return to work. The rate of healing of fascial wounds dictates how soon the patient can walk and how soon the patient can return to work. Fascial wounds sutured with non-absorbable suture material have 70% of their final strength immediately on completion of the operation (see page 70); in comparison, fascial wounds sutured with catgut lose all the tensile strength imparted by the catgut within one month, at a time when wound healing has only contributed 30% of normal tissue integrity.

These researches provide the experimental basis for permitting early unrestricted physical exertion after surgery. Blodgett and Beattie, in 1947, demonstrated no adverse effects consequent on early mobilization after hernia repair.[130] In a series of over 2000 patients undergoing inguinal hernia repair, Lichtenstein and co-workers demonstrated that the recurrence rate was 0.9%, despite immediate postoperative resumption of normal activity.[691] At the Shouldice clinic the patients get up off the operating table and walk back to their rooms, and their recurrence rate is one of the best in the world.[1203]

Baumber (1971) reviewed the time of return to work in 54 adult males with inguinal hernia: the range of time off was from 3 to 91 days, with a mean of 45 days for indirect and 56 days for direct hernia. He records that occupational physical stress did not influence the recurrence rate.[94]

Glasgow (1976) has pointed out that 12.5% of all surgical admissions to general hospitals in Britain are for hernia repairs. In England and Wales 80 000 hernioplasties are performed each year, nine out of ten of these are for inguinal hernias. Thus if the practice of early return to work at about eight weeks after operation were adopted, 3212 working man-years per year could be gained.[423]

Palumbo has suggested that the loss of defensive reflexes in the immediate postoperative period may predispose to damage if the patient is encouraged to take too much activity before the anesthetic effects have completely worn off. It is general experience in undertaking hernia repairs under general anesthetic that early activity is not contraindicated. All patients can be mobilized as soon as they have regained consciousness and indeed some patients will get up immediately following surgery and go for a walk in the hospital precincts.[880]

Ross reviewed retrospectively 260 adult males who had undergone inguinal hernia repair and found that there was no evidence that a prolonged convalescent period reduces the subsequent hernia recurrence rate. However, he does conclude that many patients restrict their postoperative activities after inguinal hernia repair for much longer than is necessary. He recommends that the patients should be advised to resume their normal activities immediately after discharge and should remain off work for up to four weeks only if they are engaged in occupations which are physically very strenuous. He suggests that this advice should be given to the patient by the surgeon prior to the patient's discharge from hospital.[974]

In a controlled study of the effect of early return to work after elective repair of inguinal hernias, Bourke and co-workers compared early return to work at 48 days after operation with standard return to work 65 days after operation. They note that there is considerable monetary benefit for the workers to return to work at the earlier date. They found no evidence of a higher recurrence rate in patients who resumed even strenuous activities at the earlier date. The self-employed in Bourke's study returned to work 31 days after operation. Their financial incentive to return to work was great. Seventy percent of the self-employed in their study were heavy workers. The most compelling reason to attempt to change attitudes to return to work after hernioplasty is that the workers themselves lose money by prolonged convalescence. This was estimated to be £19.86 per week (at 1978 prices).[137]

Attitudes of management in industry need to alter too: the most depressing fact to emerge from the studies in Nottingham is the negative attitude of a major industry to early re-employment after hernioplasty. The more realistic economic climate prevailing since 1984 may modify this atavism.

In the armed forces the surgeon can control the date of resumption of full duties. An experiment to test the safety of early return to work in the Royal Navy and Royal Marines concluded there was no contraindication or increased recurrence rate to servicemen resuming full physical duty 3 weeks after repair of an uncomplicated unilateral inguinal hernia.[1119]

The Middlesex Hospital, in 1982, published a report of a series of inguinal hernias repaired on a short-stay basis. They advised early return to work after operation and achieved an average time off work of 52 days. In 1985 they published a further series of results, the difference being explicit advice to return to work 28 days after surgery. In this latter series they achieved a mean duration of absence from work of 37 days. An additional one week of work beyond that advised by the surgeon was the norm.[104,182]

Return to work is most often dictated by other factors than the rate of wound healing. Barwell, in a study of 399 hernia repairs using the Shouldice technique, observes that the self-employed returned to work far sooner than those whose employers allowed them generous insurance coverage (this confirms the earlier observation of Bourke and co-workers). He further observes that provided a non-absorbable suture is used for the repair, the likelihood of recurrence is independent of the time off work.[84] Barwell's insight into the economic drive of self-employment and its association with early return to work has, perhaps, more cogency than all the exhortations of doctors![84]

Semmence and Kynch, reviewing the return to work of patients in Oxford, were unable to account for the different durations of time off work. Age, social class, type of operation and amount and duration of sick pay only accounted for part of the variance in time off work. The type of occupation and the amount of duration of sick pay were the only statistically significant contributions. The heavier the job the longer the employee took to return to work. Paradoxically, the more the sick pay and the longer it lasted the less time the men took off work.[1037]

General practitioner attitudes to return to work after hernioplasty have been studied. Questionnaires were sent to 50 family doctors and 38 (76%) were returned. Thirty-one respondents were of the opinion that a period of inactivity after hernia repair helps to reduce the chances of a recurrence of the hernia, five disagreed and one 'did not know'. The mean recommended time off work after operation was 53 days (range 28 days to 26 weeks). All the respondents agreed that a distinction should be made according to the occupation of the patient, a person doing light work and a retired person being advised a shorter convalescence than a heavy worker. The average time off work in the UK after repair of a unilateral inguinal hernia is 70 days.[1037] The observations that general practitioners encourage longer periods off work than the operating surgeons are confirmed by Cannon and colleagues from the Middlesex Hospital, London.[182] Robertson and colleagues sent questionnaires to 100 recently appointed staff surgeons, 400 of their patients and 200 recently established partners in primary care to assess current practices for convalescence after inguinal herniorrhaphy.[962] It was found that surgeons advised a mean of 4.4 weeks off work, general practitioners 6.2 weeks and in both cases the period varied with the nature of the patient's occupation. The patients actually took a mean of 7.0 weeks off work and those in sedentary occupations actually took more time off.

In 1993 the Royal College of Surgeons of England Clinical Guidelines on the Management of Groin Hernias in Adults recommended patients should be fit to return to office work after 2 weeks following an inguinal hernioplasty and back to heavy work after four weeks.[982] These guidelines had a considerable impact on the practice of adult hernia surgery in the UK. A review of such practice several years after publication of the College Guidelines was undertaken by postal survey to all staff surgeons in Wales.[221] The survey received an 85% response rate and indicated that 91% of respondents had read the guidelines and their surgical management of groin hernia had changed in 20%. Meshes (an important recommendation by the Guidelines) had been used by only 20% of surgeons in 1993 and have risen to 79% in 1997. Although there appeared to be a more uniform surgical management of adult inguinal hernia by 1997, only 10% of surgeons had adopted ambulatory surgery, whereas 80% advocated an inpatient stay of 1–2 days. Most surgeons were still advising their patients to return to activity at specific times, commonly light work at 2 weeks and heavy work at 4–6 weeks.

A second questionnaire study sent to patients 6–12 months following their inguinal hernia repair compared the recommendations of the College Guidelines with the actual policies for hernia repair carried out in an English NHS Hospital, including indications, techniques, complications and outcome.[786] This study also indicated lengthy time off work but also found an ambulatory rate of 56% and 72.5% of patients being discharged within 48 h of their surgery. Both these studies indicate that Guidelines need to be updated and reviewed on a regular basis. To illustrate how local practice dictates care pathways in another area of the UK during the same time period, only 22% of groin hernia repairs were carried out on an ambulatory basis in Scotland.[458] In the USA, the majority of inguinal hernia repairs are done on an ambulatory basis.

There are, however, few published randomized studies to support recommendations in the College Guidelines. For instance Shulman has challenged the advice on return to activity, stating that there is no reason for any caution following mesh repair.[1053] Proponents of the mesh repair in the UK have suggested that return to work is quicker after 'their operation'.[567] Rider *et al.* have shown that return to work correlates closely with the patient's preconceived idea.[957] Perhaps the most potent factor preventing return to work is the patients insurance coverage or the ability to receive an income whilst 'convalescing'.[1008] In a matched retrospective case controlled study in a single clinic involving seven surgeons, workers with insurance compensation were more frequently symptomatic postoperatively and had a median duration of postoperative pain of 27 days and 36.5 days off work. Those patients with only commercial insurance had 7.5 days of postoperative pain and took a median of 8.5 days off work. This study shows that pain perceived by the patient is influenced more by socioeconomic factors than by the procedure or the anatomy involved i.e. motivation affects clinical outcome. Education preoperatively by the surgeon would surely be of crucial importance in influencing a patient's decision but this needs to be consistent and evidence-based. Jarrett has undertaken an important study of consultants and general practitioners' attitudes to return to work after surgery. He has demonstrated that the mean time off work recommended by general practitioners is about twice that recommended by surgeons.[547] The most recent surgical literature only adds to confusion about return to work; surgeons continue to advise early return to work while GPs, perhaps for social reasons, delay return to work.[962,982]

The key to early return to work after surgery probably rests with the surgeon: his explanation has more impact than an explanation from the general practitioner. With a carefully controlled care pathway it has been shown that the surgical technique employed does not affect postoperative pain and return to activity.[575] Local anesthesia was the only technical factor which significantly reduced analgesic requirements during the first three postoperative days. An effective care pathway with an enthusiastic surgeon who advises immediate return to unrestricted activity within the limits of the postoperative pain experienced by the patient, is more likely to achieve faster recovery periods.[105] Other more subtle socioeconomic and psychological factors also have a bearing on outcome such as patient educational level, income level, symptoms of depression and disposition.[139,554] The economic advantages of early return to employment clearly have an important role in resuming work after surgery.

Driving should be prohibited for 7 days or so after hernia repair, not for reasons of recurrence but because the foot reaction time does not return to normal before then. The ability to perform an emergency stop in a car simulator before operation and on the 3rd, 7th and 10th postoperative day indicated that on the 3rd and 7th postoperative days patients had significant prolonged foot reaction times that did not return to preoperative levels until the 10th postoperative day.[45] There is, however, no evidence based information on driving after groin hernia surgery and surgeons give a range of advice ranging from no contraindication, to driving the same day of surgery, to waiting for 6–8 weeks, but the most common advice is that the patient should wait 2 weeks.[537] Perhaps the limiting factor is whether the patient is using narcotic analgesics, otherwise they may resume driving once the amount of postoperative discomfort is minimal.[23]

Further research on return to work and social activity is summarized on page 64.

CONCLUSIONS

- Day-case surgery is clinically feasible for most children with hernias and for at least 50% of adults with primary hernias. In most adults without significant co-morbid medical conditions, ambulatory surgery is the chosen course in at least 90% of patients in the USA.
- Day-case surgery requires technical and organizational excellence if the long-term results are going to be worthwhile and if complications are to be avoided.
- After surgery, early return to work should be encouraged. We all need educating in the benefits of modern surgical technology.
- Despite the clear demonstration of the feasibility and clinical excellence of day-case and short-stay surgery for inguinal hernias, it is the behavioral attitudes of the surgeons rather than the social circumstances of the population served that need modification. Clearly, there is a geographic difference in the use of this option.

5

Economics of hernia repair

INTRODUCTION

'It is now recognized that resources will never be adequate to support all that surgery has to offer, and that we must all be conscious of the need to make the most efficient use of what resources there are' (Royal College of Surgeons, 1992).[981]

Economic evaluations of new and existing healthcare interventions are an essential input into decision making. Healthcare systems around the world face steady increases in expenditure resulting from demographic change and improvements in medical technology. Increasingly, payors must choose which interventions will be provided and which will not be reimbursed from limited public or private funds. This creates difficult choices, as systems are no longer limited by what is technically possible to improve the health of patients but by what is practically possible given resource constraints. In a situation where resources are scarce, all choices about who will be treated have an opportunity cost – the value of the benefit foregone. Health economics and the techniques of economic evaluation aim to maximize the amount of health which is produced within the scarce resources available. In the UK the National Institute for Clinical Excellence (NICE) synthesizes evidence and reaches a judgement as to whether on balance the intervention can be recommended as a cost-effective use of NHS resources.[1034] In 2000 NICE published recommendations for the use of laparoscopic hernia surgery and recommended its use, only in centers of expertise for cases of bilateral inguinal hernia or recurrent inguinal hernia. In the UK in 1996 approximately 10% of hernia repairs were carried out laparoscopically[860] and since the publication of the NICE guidelines the figure has decreased dramatically and supports the concept that the application of clinical pathways can reduce costs.[1216] Such measures are important in the UK where the numbers of medical staff and the annual NHS budget is well below that in other countries of Europe, OECD countries and the USA[631] (Tables 5.1 and 5.2).

It is no longer sufficient to consider the clinical or therapeutic effects of healthcare interventions: purchasing choices will be predicated on studies which identify, measure and value what is given up when an intervention is used (the cost) and what is gained (improved patient health outcomes). This requires explicit economic evaluation of healthcare interventions. Purchasers have a fixed budget and are aware of the opportunity costs

Table 5.1 *Cost comparison of out-patient vs. in-patient repair of inguinal hernia (From Devlin, 1985, by courtesy of the Royal College of Surgeons of England)*[293]

Reference	Outpatient costs ($)	Inpatient costs ($)	Savings ($)
Rockwell (1982)	617	1119	502
Coe (1981)	398	1168	770
Flanagan and Bascom (1981)	300	1000	700

Table 5.2 *Theater and ward costs (From Devlin, 1985, by courtesy of the Royal College of Surgeons of England)*[293]

Theater	Open 24 h per day 365 days per year, 168 h per week (£)	Open 8 a.m.–5 p.m. Monday to Friday 45 h per week (£)
Cost per year		
Medical staff	25594	10923
Nursing staff	131367	28860
Total	160961	39783
Cost of 30 min operation	17472 per year[a]	9.21
Cost of 30 min operation (4160 per year[b])	38.69	9.57

[a] The cost of a 30 min operation is similar if the theaters are 100% used for a 'night shift' in addition to 100% occupancy of the daytime. The staffing assumptions of these calculations may be obtained from the author.
[b] Low utilization of fully staffed operating theaters dramatically increases the unit costs of each operation episode.

of interventions. Increasingly they are likely to require evidence of effectiveness and cost effectiveness, and they may develop contracts and enforce protocols to ensure this (Table 5.3).

Economic evaluation values both inputs (costs) and outcomes (consequences) of an intervention, comparing more than one alternative. This builds upon clinical evaluations which assess efficacy (can an intervention work, in experimental circumstances?) and effectiveness (does it work, in normal clinical practice?) to assess efficiency (does it provide the greatest benefit at least cost?). The type of economic evaluation depends upon the outcome measure chosen:

• Cost minimization analysis is appropriate only when the outcomes of two or more interventions have been

Table 5.3 *Health status yield per £ for three selected treatments provided by the NHS, at November 1981 prices (From Hurst, 1984, with permission of the Controller of Her Majesty's Stationery Office)*[526]

Treatment	Health status yield	Cost of treatment (£)	Health status yield per £'000 cost
Home hemodialysis	191.25	160 000	1.2
Successful renal transplant and subsequent maintenance	197.30	35 000	5.6
Uncomplicated hernia repair	5.53	420	13.2

demonstrated to be equivalent, in which case the least costly alternative is the most efficient, and only cost analysis is required.

• Cost effectiveness analysis includes both costs and outcomes using a single outcome measure, usually a natural unit. This allows comparisons between treatments in a particular therapeutic area where effectiveness is unequal, but not between therapeutic areas where natural outcome measures differ.

• Cost utility analysis combines multiple outcomes into a single measure of utility (e.g. a quality adjusted life year, or QALY). This allows comparisons between alternatives in different therapeutic categories with different natural outcomes.

• Cost benefit analysis links costs and outcomes by expressing both in monetary units, forcing an explicit decision about whether an intervention is worth its cost. Various techniques have been used to attach monetary values to health outcomes, but the technique remains rare in health economics.

Considerations in cost-effectiveness are particularly relevant at a time when healthcare costs are disproportionately escalating in relation to gross national product in many westernized countries.[795] The value of any indicated treatment is directly proportional to treatment outcome and inversely proportional to treatment cost. Evaluation of both the numerator (outcome quality) and the denominator (cost) of the equation is subject to many methodologic limitations. The value depends on whether it is viewed from the perspective of the patient, surgeon, hospital, employer, payor or industry. Moreover, cost does not equate with charge. In hernia surgery the total cost includes pretreatment (diagnostics), treatment, post-treatment medical care including complications and recurrence and finally societal and employer costs which include insurance, workers disability compensation, worker replacement costs and loss productivity. Each sector of the treatment process has variable fixed and semi-fixed costs. The trends to eliminate general anesthesia and to perform conventional herniorrhaphy in an ambulatory setting have been cost beneficial. Ideally costs containment could be achieved by performing all elective inguinal hernia repairs at ambulatory surgical centers for a standardized charge (Table 5.1).

Technological innovation in surgery and in other areas (for example diagnostic innovation) is not regulated in the same way as innovative pharmaceutical therapies. A new pharmaceutical product is subjected to rigorous clinical trials to identify evidence of safety and efficacy, before licensing for public use.

Increasingly, new and existing pharmaceutical products are also subjected to well-defined economic evaluation, to show evidence of effectiveness and efficiency. Guidelines issued by the Department of Health state that 'the economic evaluation of pharmaceuticals should become part of taking decisions about treatment', and set out clear guidelines regarding how a high-quality economic evaluation should be carried out.[284]

The careful procedures that control the introduction of innovative pharmaceutical products are essential for innovative surgical and diagnostic therapies. How, then, should technological innovations such as laparoscopic surgery be introduced? All such pioneering innovations should be evaluated in well-designed trials. There are difficulties in implementing randomized controlled trials of surgical techniques due to the difficulties of blinding, but a carefully designed trial can mitigate these problems. Clinical trials protect the safety of patients and ensure that new technologies produce effective healthcare. Economic evaluations ensure that such health gains are purchased at least cost. The guidelines applied to pharmaceutical products, intended to protect society's health and scarce resources, should also be applied to surgical innovations but this is a difficult task to institute.

The principle of evaluating innovative surgical interventions was accepted by the Department of Health in a press release in 1995, which announced that major innovations were to be 'scrutinized, evaluated and then, if approved, fast tracked throughout the health service'.[285] A major advance should, under a new system, be subjected to clinical trials and a central register would give information on approved operations. The register could then be consulted by purchasers as a measure of the effectiveness of various operations and procedures. This register, the Safety and Efficacy Register of New Interventional Procedures (SERNIP), is managed by the Academy of Medical Royal Colleges, and funded by the Department of Health. Doctors are asked to register new techniques which they intend to pilot, and to check the register to discover the current status of new invasive procedures.[138] An advisory committee convened by SERNIP will then assess all known data and assign the procedure to one of four categories:

1 Safety and efficacy unsatisfactory – procedure must not be used.
2 Safety and efficacy established – procedure can be used.
3 The procedure is sufficiently similar to one of established safety and efficacy to raise no reasonable doubts and can be used.
4 Safety and efficacy is not established. Controlled evaluation is needed.

The proposed system is voluntary and clinically controlled and in time economic evaluation of innovative invasive procedures will be required, as is the case for pharmaceutical products. In the majority of other countries, including the United States, such a system does not exist at any level.

ECONOMICS OF HERNIA REPAIR

Hernia repair is an established and effective procedure and its relatively fixed cost and high volume amongst surgical procedures means that economic evaluation of the procedure itself has become a priority. Hernias create pain and discomfort for patients and limit ability to work or carry out other productive activities. While the increased risk of surgical procedures in elderly people means that repair of some small direct hernias may not be mandatory, there would seem to be clear clinical and economic arguments in favor of carrying out hernia repairs amongst the majority of the working population.[982]

Hurst, a health economist, has compared the benefits and costs of hernia repair with the benefits and costs of home dialysis for renal failure, and with the benefits and costs of a successful renal transplant. Drawing on a measure of health status which measures two dimensions of health (disability and distress), and using DHSS cost data, Hurst calculates the health status yield per pound sterling for the three selected treatments. Using this cost–benefit equation, uncomplicated hernia repair comes out better than a successful renal transplant and a renal transplant is better value than continuous home hemodialysis.[526] Memories of Cecil Wakeley's (1940)[1178] aphorism crowd in to confirm that refined clinical judgment may well be as valuable in evaluating the benefits of clinical care as the statistical gymnastics of contemporary health economists!

Innovations in the procedure of hernia repair and the management of patients should, however, be subject to economic evaluation, ideally based upon a randomized controlled trial. The recent development in hernia repair such as the expansion of day-case surgery in Europe require a clinical and economic base. However, the experience from the Shouldice clinic in Canada and the results from the United States support the use of limited hospitalization for the repair of hernias. Laparoscopic inguinal hernia surgery has not been proven to represent an economic benefit for the unilateral primary hernia. There may be some benefit for the patient with bilateral and/or recurrent herniation.

ECONOMICS OF DAY-CASE SURGERY

Reductions in length of stay for many surgical and other inpatient procedures result from improvements in surgical procedures reducing recovery time, changing preferences of patients, and financial and political pressures on hospitals to reduce costs. Day-case surgery is often preferred by patients, and it may encourage early mobilization and reduce the risk of hospital-acquired infection,[984] Day-case treatment for hernia repair

may result in good outcomes for lower costs than other organizational forms of care.[145,985] The Royal College of Surgeons recommends that at least 30% of elective hernioplasties should be performed on a day-case basis.[981] In the United States, on the other hand, all but the most ill or infirm individuals with inguinal hernias are performed as an outpatient operation. Additionally, because of the increasing trend of incisional herniorrhaphy by the laparoscopic method, there are many incisional and ventral hernias that are performed with a length of stay of 23 h or less.[282,665]

Economic appraisal is unlike surgical decision making. Economists analyze the results of their interventions by comparing them within different scenarios: as the scenarios change – employment prospects, labor relations – the economics change too! Surgeons are used to evaluating their outcomes over time with the scenario held constant. For instance, with day-case surgery and a constant surgeon-related scenario, one impact of shortening the patients' stay will be empty beds – which the surgeon will perceive as the currency of an 'efficiency saving'. The economist would not call this a 'saving'; the concept of 'opportunity cost' means that no 'benefit' has accrued until the empty beds (resources) are put to some alternative use. 'Benefit' is thus not necessarily the same to the surgeon as to the economist.

Any economic appraisal of day-case surgery must, therefore, first address the crucial issue of 'benefit'. Are the benefits to be:

- More surgery – using the freed resources to undertake a greater volume of surgery or more complex innovative surgery?
- A redeployment of the freed resources towards a different client group, for example elderly or mentally ill people?
- A reduction in overall health service expenditure by the amount saved?

A day-case surgery policy will need to be appraised in the 'short run' and the 'long run'. Short-run benefits may be very difficult to gain; for instance, a reduction in surgical bed requirements by 15 may confer no benefit since you cannot knock down half a 30-bed ward and reduce staff costs by 50% overnight! While there may be no short-run gains, the long-term gains could be substantial and allow explicit alterations to existing surgical and nursing practice. Consequently new hospital provision could include less traditional inpatient surgical wards and instead have dedicated day-case units.

Stepping through the looking-glass, more day-case surgery will need less capital expenditure on surgical inpatient facilities, and fewer nursing staff will need employing for the same volume of work in the long term.

The quantification of savings accruing from a day-case policy is difficult; four approaches have been advanced:

1 Comparing the bills paid by patients in private practice.[964]
2 The analytical device of holding the level of service constant and estimating the benefits that could be bought with the now unused resources.[988]
3 The technique of comparing average per diem inpatient and outpatient costs.[162] Farquharson (1955) produced

the seminal paper advocating this type of economic evaluation.[344]

4 Comparing and computing the one-year costs of a day-care facility with the one-year costs of a traditional inpatient unit.[980]

Bailey, an economist from the Audit Commission in the UK, has proposed an alternative strategy to determine the resources that might be released as a result of a change from inpatient to day-case while treating an equivalent patient. He states that the costs of day surgery are substantially less than inpatient care but it is misleading to interpret such measures as 'savings'. The resource implications of more day surgery should be estimated directly by looking at precisely what changes are planned to take place.[70]

In conclusion, there is evidence that the unit costs of day-case surgery are much lower than inpatient care of the order of 40–75% per treatment episode, however calculated. These lower unit costs will free resources to do more surgery or for alternative uses. Day-case surgery has been found to be superior to inpatient surgery in terms of wound infection and return to work, although this finding is not statistically significant.[208] Day-case surgery is also becoming increasingly acceptable to patients. A dedicated 5-day care unit allows more resources to be saved compared with day cases in a traditional theater suite and ward where all the resources cannot easily be redeployed, particularly in the short run. This is consistent with the conclusions of a US review of cost-effectiveness of management of hernia by Millikan and Deziel (1996).[795] These authors concluded that the most cost-effective approach to hernia repair would use an ambulatory surgical center with open mesh repair for primary inguinal hernia and failed primary suture repair.[795]

Incentives and day-case hernioplasty

To date, resource savings from day-case surgery in the NHS have largely been used to expand surgical services either quantitatively or qualitatively. Every hospital experienced this phenomenon in the 1970s. It has been quantified and shown that as resources are liberated by day-case work they are used up in other surgical endeavors. This extra work attracts further resources and the overall surgical budget becomes larger.

Increasing the proportion of day cases in the surgical unit mix will lead to a fall in the average cost of each patient treated. This may enable more cases to be operated upon, and even though the marginal costs of doing each extra case within normal working hours are low the aggregated cost to the hospital will be higher, although greater demand will initially be met and the queue reduced. If there is no queue and no excess demand, reducing the costs should allow premises to be closed and staff made redundant, with considerable reduction in fixed and estate costs and in wages. The cost of doing an extra case after-hours in a day-case unit, when staff must be paid overtime, is a very high marginal price – a fact to be remembered when case scheduling is considered.

If day-case surgery is used to cut unit costs and increase the overall volume of surgery, this extra burden of rising productivity

will fall on the surgeons and nurses. There are reports of the proportion of day cases rising to close to 40%, in some units, with consequent increases in surgical throughputs. Ultimately the increased output may demand an alteration on the supply side of the equation, and more doctors and nurses may then need to be employed to cope with increased demand.[293] While the relation between demand and output of a surgical service is elastic in the short term, in the longer term supply inevitably must be increased to allow greater output.

It must be apparent that there is no economic incentive for surgeons and other hospital employees to expand day-case surgery. Substantial savings can only be achieved by maintaining constant the quantity of surgery done, not allowing day cases to increase the output, and by closing premises and dismissing redundant staff. Such a policy is unlikely to make surgeons who take up day-case surgery popular!

RETURN TO NORMAL ACTIVITY AND WORK

There is enormous variation in reported times for return to normal activity and work. For instance, in a socialized system of healthcare where patients' expectations and the insurance system still favor hospitalization, length of hospital stay after hernia surgery may be in excess of 8 days.[443] Even in the USA, where a headlong rush for day-care surgery in ambulatory units has taken place, length of stay may be several days in institutions where reimbursement is not as strictly controlled as the private sector. Customers of the Metropolitan Life Insurance Company surveyed by a nationwide claims questionnaire revealed a length of stay that averaged 2.9 days.[993] In the US Army average hospital stay for hernia surgery is 4.6 days.[485] In reality housing conditions, distance from home to hospital, and availability of home nursing care (spouse, relative or friend) are the major factors affecting early discharge after hernia repair.[791]

The technique adopted has little predictive value for early postoperative pain and analgesic consumption. Kawji and colleagues[575] in a study of 240 patients who had been treated with Lichtenstein GA, Lichtenstein LA, laparoscopic TAPP, Shouldice operation or preperitoneal Wantz procedure, found that the only technical factor significantly reducing analgesic requirement during the first 3 perioperative days was local anesthesia. Lau and colleagues[638] studied postoperative pain by linear analog scores in 239 patients having inguinal herniorrhaphy with a variety of techniques. With multiple regression analysis older age was the only independent factor of pain, a finding in keeping with anecdotal experience of surgeons used to operating on patients under local anesthetic.

The French Association for Surgical Research investigated the feasibility of discharge within 48 h of inguinal hernia repair in 500 consecutive men with unilateral, uncomplicated nonrecurrent inguinal hernias. Of 411 patients suitable for early discharge 107 (26%) eventually stayed longer than 48 h, early discharge was declined by 84 and contraindicated in 42 (these patients had local or general complications), which finally resulted in one-day surgery being performed in only 51 (10%)

of the patients. These results emphasize the need for careful preoperative evaluation, which includes not only the hernia and the patient's general medical condition, but also any social conditions such as isolation, flights of stairs, or lack of a telephone, which may limit the ability to discharge a patient soon after surgery.

Advice concerning return to normal activity has been poorly managed by surgeons.[547] Recent studies indicate that factors limiting a patient's return to activity and work are governed principally by perceived amount of postoperative pain. Socioeconomic factors strongly influence this perception over and above the actual procedure performed or the anatomy involved.[1008] In a case-controlled comparison of patients receiving workers compensation compared with patients having commercial insurance, seven surgeons from a single clinic compared 22 consecutive workers compensation patients with 22 commercial insurance patients. All patients had received open hernioplasty and the duration of postoperative pain and the days off work were compared. The differences between the two groups were striking: the median duration of postoperative pain in the workers compensation group was 27 days, with 36.5 days off work. In the commercial insurance patients the duration of postoperative pain was 7.5 days and they went back to work after only 8.5 days. Personal motivation, therefore, appears to be the most important factor affecting clinical outcome and return to activities. Callesen has demonstrated that well-defined recommendations and improved pain management can shorten convalescence.[171] One hundred patients having elective herniorrhaphy under local anesthetic and managed analgesia were recommended to have one day of convalescence for light/moderate work and 3 weeks for strenuous physical activity. The overall median absence from work was 6 days; the unemployed returning to activities in just one day, those in light/moderate work in 6 days and those in heavy jobs by 25 days. A more detailed prospective study of return to work after inguinal hernia repair has been undertaken by Jones and colleagues.[554] Data were collected by personal interviews, written surveys and medical record reviews in 235 patients, the main outcome measures being actual and expected return to work. Age, educational level, income level, occupation, symptoms of depression, and the expected day of return to work (10 days) accounted for 61% of the variation in actual (12 days) return to work.

Advice given in the UK on driving after groin hernia surgery varies widely because there is no evidence-based information.[537] In a postal questionnaire sent to 200 surgeons the advice ranged from: it was alright to drive the same day (3% of respondents), to patients should wait 6–8 weeks before driving (9%), the most common response being that patients should wait 2 weeks (37% respondents). Amid has stated that the recovery period is solely dependent on the amount of postoperative discomfort, which should be minimal and usually not requiring narcotic analgesia.[23] He recommends that patients can resume driving as early as one week or less after surgery depending on their comfort and whether they are using narcotic analgesics. Those who drive different types of vehicles need different advice.

It must be apparent that there is no economic incentive for surgeons and other hospital employers to expand day-case surgery. Substantial savings can only be achieved by maintaining constant the quantity of surgery done, not allowing day cases to increase the output, and by closing premises and dismissing redundant staff. Such a policy is unlikely to make surgeons, in some areas of the world who take up day-case surgery popular! However, the experience in the USA, where day surgery is quite commonplace, has proven that the patients and their surgeons are quite satisfied with these economics. In fact, many patients are dismayed when they are told that their medical condition dictates a hospital stay of even one night.

ECONOMICS OF LAPAROSCOPIC SURGERY

The introduction and rapid diffusion of laparoscopic surgical techniques since the pioneering laparoscopic removal of a gall bladder by the French surgeon Phillippe Mouret in 1987 was accepted with 'unbridled enthusiasm' and often without question by many surgeons, the media and the general public. The years that have passed have allowed a more rational approach to many of these procedures. The majority of laparoscopic adaptations of the general surgical operations have proven to be cost effective due to the diminution in the length of hospital stay. The great exception is that of the laparoscopic repair of inguinal hernias, which are always more costly.

Some 'economic' arguments have been used to support the rapid diffusion of laparoscopic surgery. Studies often quote reductions in the length of inpatient hospital stay in comparison with standard surgical procedures and imply that this will necessarily save hospitals money. This is, however, not necessarily the case, and hospital managers are increasingly questioning the appropriateness of procedures which involve purchase of sophisticated and expensive capital equipment and considerably increased theater time, resulting in lower patient throughput for surgical procedures. Available time in the operating theater is a scarce resource, and although operating time in laparoscopic surgery declines as experience increases, Cuschieri (1994) estimated that on average it will continue to take about one-third longer than the corresponding conventional operation, with the excess of time over open surgery the higher the more complicated the basic operation.[258] Time, however, has proven that once past the 'learning curve' many of these operations are as long or shorter than that of the open method. Many of these comparisons may be flawed because, as we all know, there are 'slow operators' and 'quick operators.'

The effect of length of inpatient stay on health service resource use is an important issue in many studies. Cuschieri (1994) estimates that discharge may on average be expected to be less than 48 h.[258] This is thought to result in cost savings from earlier discharge and earlier return to normal activities including work; however, economists such as Sculpher (1993) note that this may not always be the case.[1035] Firstly, a reduction in the demand for hospital beds may not result in cash savings, unless it allows ward closures. At one time, this was felt to be unlikely as laparoscopic surgery represented a small proportion of all hospital procedures. Other arguments were that laparoscopy did not release other resources used for surgical procedures, particularly theater time, and that some laparoscopic procedures replaced non-invasive therapies rather than open surgery. It is important to remember that lengths of inpatient stay were falling for many years, and the additional savings from laparoscopic surgery may be lower than anticipated. History, however, has proven that many of these worries have not resulted in a decline in the use of laparoscopic surgery. In most procedures, save inguinal hernia repair, the trend is upward.

Complication rates are an important determinant of the overall costs of any surgical procedure. Complications with laparoscopic surgery procedures, such as bile duct injuries with laparoscopic cholecystectomy, have been well documented – see Table 1 from Soper *et al.* (1994).[1072] Most bile duct injuries have also occurred early in a surgeon's experience, highlighting the need for careful training and accreditation of surgeons, and clinical practice guidelines.[1036] The rate of conversions from laparoscopic operations to open operations ranges from 1.8 to 8.5%, and tends to be highest early in a surgeon's experience.[1072] The cost implications of complication rates include increased operating time, increased length of inpatient stay, increased care burden on families or other carers and increased time for the patient to return to work or normal activities. The current rates of complications, however, have now established the laparoscopic cholecystectomy as the 'standard of care' for gallbladder disease because they are comparable, whether open or laparoscopic.

A recent systematic review of the effectiveness and safety of laparoscopic cholecystectomy showed that effectiveness of this procedure is similar to that of open and mini-cholecystectomy.[316] Complete alleviation of symptoms was achieved in 60–70% of patients. However, safety profiles differ, with more technical support and specialized surgical equipment required for the laparoscopic procedure. Differences in complication rates were difficult to assess because of methodological problems and differences between studies. In particular, studies often do not have sufficient statistical power to identify clinically important differences in outcomes, particularly bile duct injury, because the rate of adverse events is low.

Sculpher (1993)[1035] argues that laparoscopic surgery has a different 'production function' to conventional surgical techniques – i.e. it requires a different mix of inputs to the production process – more inputs of theater and medical staff time, more sophisticated equipment, and less inputs of inpatient bed days (see Figure 5.1). The overall effect on hospital costs and on overall costs to society is unclear, and requires economic evaluation. Evaluation should be long term, in order to include any effects of different readmission rates, and should include not only hospital costs and effects but also the burden on community based services, patients and carers, which may change due to earlier discharge.[1035]

The 'production function' description of surgery is useful in considering other issues. The appropriate level of individual and center specialization should be determined by evidence of economies of scale. If a center specializes in laparoscopic surgery, this may influence costs per patient, as theater time may be reduced as familiarity with the procedure increases. In addition,

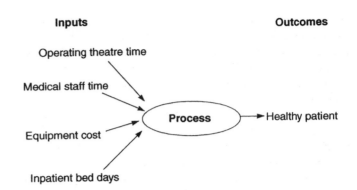

Figure 5.1 *A surgical production function (source: Sculpher, 1993).*[1035]

outcomes may be improved, particularly by reduced complication rates. However, the appropriate level of individual and center specialization requires careful evaluation: could the alleged benefits of centralization be matched by careful training and treatment protocols at local levels? Identification of the conditions necessary for the production of efficient laparoscopic procedures is absent but inhibits neither unsubstantiated assertions by policy makers nor significant investments in new facilities.

The repair of the inguinal hernia with the laparoscopic method continues to raise many questions in terms of economics. Whereas, it is generally accepted that this technique is effective for these hernias, the costs associated with this method cause many surgeons to question the usefulness of this technique. In 1996, the benefits were unclear.[645] In 2002, the clinical efficacy is not generally questioned (see Chapter 15). The cost issues have been resolved for the most part. It is more expensive to perform the minimally invasive method except in a very few areas that have managed to eliminate the use of disposable instruments and tissue expansion balloons.

Evidence-based studies have definitely revealed that the levels of pain and subsequent convalescence are decreased when compared to the open repair.[338] This is particularly true with the comparison of the pure tissue repairs but has also been found with the open prosthetic repairs (see Chapter 7). However, some studies have reported that while these patients experience less pain postoperatively, the return to work interval was not different after TAPP repair. The opinion of these authors was that the increase in costs did not justify the operation unless the operative costs could be reduced.[881] Another study found that laparoscopically repaired patients returned to their usual activities 7 days earlier than those of the open group. The incremental cost for this time frame was £55 548 per quality of life year over the open method. This report showed that there may be specific situations that this laparoscopic repair may be viable alternative particularly when reusable instruments were used rather than disposable because these costs were decreased significantly.[782]

The operative costs that are increased with the laparoscopic approach are the use of disposable instruments, balloon dissection devices, balloon trocars, additional personnel and the length of the operation. One can diminish these to the extent that the operation can approach that of the open procedure. Lorenz has shown that by the deliberate attempt to decrease costs, the laparoscopic approach can be less expensive to the hospital.[709] Beets found the open approach can be more expensive than the laparoscopic approach (open – US$1150 vs. laparoscopic – US$1179).[101] In many centers, however, this has been a stimulus for the surgeon to abandon the procedure altogether (willingly or unwillingly). The insurance industry has refused to reimburse the hospitals and the surgeons for the procedure, leading to its rapid demise. Medicare, in the USA, actually pays the surgeon less to perform the operation laparoscopically than through the open technique.

These realities have resulted in the trend of many centers to utilize this operation only in the bilateral situation and for recurrent hernias. The success for this diagnosis is proven.[1014,1023] The ongoing studies of the MRC Laparoscopic Groin Hernia Trial Group support the move to specialist surgeons to perform this operation.[821] Based upon the experience in the USA, this appears to be the trend.

The data comparing the open versus laparoscopic repair of inguinal hernias are now voluminous. A detailed analysis of all the factors is beyond the scope of this clinical text. Suffice to say that the vast majority of reports have identified the same findings that are commonly known. That is, in general, the operation is more expensive but the postoperative pain is diminished and the return to work notably shorter. The learning curve and the payors of these operations will force this procedure into the hands of a few skilled surgeons with excellent outcomes. Even in this instance, this will be for the bilateral and recurrent hernias. Studies such as that by Lawrence *et al.* (1996) used a UK randomized controlled trial as the basis of an economic evaluation of laparoscopic versus open inguinal hernia repair, on data collected from 104 day-case patients.[645] The mean total health service cost of laparoscopic repair was £1074 vs. £489 for open repair. Linking this additional cost with the additional pain-free days in the laparoscopic group showed an additional cost per pain-free day of £109 (95% CI £41–393). The authors concluded that there were strong arguments against the introduction of laparoscopic hernia repair until evidence on long-term outcomes becomes available. Such studies, though important, are few. Another author, Hekkinnen, conversely proved that the overall societal costs are less with the laparoscopic method.[488] Regardless, the cost–benefit structure of the insurance industry does not appreciate the societal costs as does the individual patient and surgeon. Therefore, this limited use of the laparoscope to repair inguinal hernias will probably be permanent in the USA. In other countries, such as those in Europe, a more critical look at these issues may be possible because of the public nature of the healthcare system. This is needed.

Unlike the data of the laparoscopic inguinal herniorrhaphy, the clinical and economic benefits are rather clearer with the laparoscopic repair of incisional and ventral hernias. There are many papers in the literature that have demonstrated the short period of hospitalization that is seen with this approach to this problem.[247,282,612,665] It is generally believed by those surgeons proficient in this technique that this method does, in fact, lessen the length of hospitalization for the patients. There have been five publications that compared the open and laparoscopic repair of incisional and ventral hernias (Table 5.4). In all of

Table 5.4 *Results of comparative analysis of open and laparoscopic incisional and ventral herniorrhaphy*

	Open repair	Laparoscopic repair
Operative times – range (min)	45–259* (1)	70–211* (1)
	27–148 (2)	45–170 (2)
	60–180 (3)	30–180 (3)
	25–220 (4)	18–225 (4)
	N/A (5)	N/A (5)
Operative time – average (min)	97.6* (1)	128.5* (1)
	78.5 (2)	95.4 (2)
	111.5 (3)	87 (3)
	82 (4)	58 (4)
	N/A (5)	N/A (5)
Range of length of hospital stay (days)	N/A (1)	N/A (1)
	2–26* (2)	1–17* (2)
	3–21* (3)	1–15* (3)
	N/A (4)	N/A (4)
	0.5–14* (5)	0.5–3* (5)
Average length of hospital stay (days)	4.9 (1)	1.6 (1)
	6.5* (2)	3.4* (2)
	9.06* (3)	2.23* (3)
	2.8 (4)	1.7 (4)
	4.4* (5)	0.8* (5)
Complication rate (%)	31 (1)	15 (1)
	36.7* (2)	17.9* (2)
	?? (3)	(3)
	36 (4)	10 (4)
	N/A (5)	N/A (5)
Recurrence rate (%)	12.5 (1)	1 (1)
	34.7 (2)	11 (2)
	2 (3)	0 (3)
	20.7 (4)	2.5 (4)
	0 (5)	4.8 (5)
Range of costs in US dollars	1987–12 611* (1)	3555–5235* (1)
	N/A (2)	N/A (2)
	N/A (3)	N/A (3)
	N/A (4)	N/A (4)
	6574–18 448 (5)	5323–11 223 (5)
Average US dollar cost	7299* (1)	4395* (1)
	N/A (2)	N/A (2)
	N/A (3)	N/A (3)
	N/A (4)	N/A (4)
	12 461 (5)	8273 (5)

*Statistically significant difference.
References – 1: Holzman *et al.*, 1997; 2: Park *et al.*, 1998; 3: Carbajo *et al.*, 1999; 4: Ramshaw *et al.*, 1999; 5: DeMarie *et al.*, 2000.

these series, the laparoscopic repair was associated with fewer complications and fewer days of hospitalization than that of the open method as shown in the table. Only two of these papers evaluated the cost of the repair.[282,511] In both the laparoscopic method was associated with less cost than the open repair. This fact is primarily based upon the decreased length of stay of the laparoscopically repaired patients. This occurred even when the additional costs of any re-admissions were included in the overall determination. Interestingly, the DeMarie paper evaluated the costs based upon an open repair using a polypropylene product versus the laparoscopic repair using an expanded poly-tetrafluoroethylene patch.[282] Therefore, based upon the limited study that has been done on this operation, it appears that the laparoscopic herniorrhaphy for incisional and ventral hernia is the economically preferred choice.

CONCLUSIONS

- It is no longer sufficient to consider only the clinical and therapeutic effects of healthcare: purchasing choices require explicit economic evaluation to identify, measure and value costs and patient health outcomes. Surgical interventions are no exception to this.
- Hernia repair is an established and effective procedure for most patient groups, and its relatively low cost amongst surgical procedures means that economic evaluation of the procedure itself is not a priority. However, innovations in the procedure of hernia repair and the management of patients, such as day-case and laparoscopic hernia repair, should be subject to economic evaluation.
- The unit costs of day-case surgery are lower than those of traditional in-hospital care. Any money saved will enable more operations to be done and more patients to be treated. Alternatively, savings generated could be used to develop other services.
- Laparoscopic surgery has spread rapidly through many surgical specialties but there are still major knowledge gaps about its clinical and economic attributes. The potential clinical and economic benefits of laparoscopic hernia repair are particularly unclear given the need for general anesthesia and the possibility of rare but serious injuries to intra-abdominal organs. This procedure benefited from large-scale clinical trials and economic evaluations for inguinal hernia repair. The use of laparoscopy for incisional and ventral herniorrhaphy seems to have a strong economic benefit, however.

6

Principles in hernia surgery

GENERAL PRINCIPLES

There are three principles which dictate the management of all abdominal wall hernia patients.

1 The patient must be adequately prepared for surgery. The mortality from hernia operations, particularly the mortality and morbidity of strangulated femoral hernias in older women, is almost entirely due to operating when the patient is in a less than optimal physiological condition. Hernias almost never require emergency surgery, although they may require urgent surgery as soon as the patient is rendered fit. To operate before adequate rehydration and renal function is restored, or before the cardiorespiratory status is assessed and stabilized, is to court disaster.[1123] Four or five hours of careful resuscitation may be needed in the most ill patients.[155] Even in the very elderly mortality can be reduced to a minimum; death is usually a result of complications of the strangulated hernia rather than associated diseases which should have been adequately treated before the urgent operation.[386] For elective hernia repair the same golden principle applies – do not operate until the patient has been fully assessed and is in an optimum physiological state. An analysis of 175 patients with ages greater than 66 years, of whom 58% were ASA grade III or higher, revealed that elective or urgent operation can be carried out with zero mortality, provided prompt diagnosis and treatment of primary systemic diseases is performed. Appropriate anesthesia, such as local anesthetic or epidural anesthesia, should be given careful consideration in those not fit for general anesthesia. Thus, severe systemic disease that limits activity but is not incapacitating is not a contraindication for elective groin hernia repair.[404]

2 The contents must be reduced after inspection at open operation and following careful inspection for viability. If strangulation has occurred infarcted contents must be resected. The dangers of forcible reduction of contents into an inadequate cavity when there is 'lack of storage capacity of the abdominal cavity' or when organs have lost the right of domain must be appreciated (see pages 200 and 207).

3 The defect must be repaired. When repairing abdominal wall hernias with the pure tissue repair the principle is to repair each layer of the defect discreetly. One may also reinforce weak layers with mesh to restore the patient's anatomy so that it resembles the normal unoperated condition. The process of repair in aponeurosis is slow. Only tendinous/aponeurotic/fascial structures can be successfully sutured together: suturing red fleshy muscle to tendon or fascia will not contribute to permanent union of these structures. Nor will it reconstruct anything resembling the normal anatomy!

Frequently, particularly with the repair of the larger incisional and ventral hernias, the reconstruction of the patient's anatomy is not feasible. The use of a prosthetic biomaterial is the only option for these individuals. When this is the case, the surgeon must assure that a large overlap of the prosthetic is used so that the resulting repair will be sound and permanent. The use of prosthetic biomaterials in the repair of hernias of all etiologies is now commonplace. In fact, in the USA, its use exceeds 90%.

HEMOSTASIS

Careful hemostasis and tissue handling is most important if hematoma formation and sepsis are to be avoided. Larger vessels, especially the veins in the subcutaneous fat, could be carefully ligated with an absorbable suture, taking care not to leave large stumps of tissue to undergo absorption. Most often the use of effective electrocautery will control these vessels as well. For ligatures, metric 3.5 (3-0) braided polyglycolic acid (Dexon) or metric 3.5 (3-0) braided polyglactin 910 (Vicryl) are used. Chromic catgut is not recommended because of its adverse effect on wound healing (see below). Electrocautery is employed for hemostasis in small vessels.

Hematomas are more likely to occur if local anesthesia with adrenaline is used, and extra care with hemostasis is then advised. Closed suction drains can be used whenever there is extensive dissection, particularly if there is 'dead space' in which hematoma or serum may collect. When large incisional hernias are repaired, suction drains may be necessary, especially in the open repair of these defects. They are no longer considered mandatory in all cases and certainly are rarely used in the laparoscopic repair of these hernias.

SEPSIS

Sepsis is the great hazard to hernioplasty, particularly when non-absorbable suture material is used. With the common use of synthetic prosthetic meshes and devices, the occurrence of an infection can be especially difficult to manage and may require the explant of the prosthesis. The perioperative use of antibiotics has not been conclusively shown to diminish the risk of infection in inguinal hernia repair.[408] Nevertheless, as with all surgical procedures, one must utilize scrupulous surgical technique if infection is to be avoided. The skin may be covered at the site of operation with sterile adherent film, which is not removed until the wound is closed.[323] This is particularly popular during laparoscopic incisional hernia repair.

In the past, it has been recommended that sutures should not be used to close the skin, for by their very nature they have potential for introducing bacteria into the subcutaneous tissue along their tracks.[36] In today's practice, however, there are many methods to close the skin incision(s). These include the use of skin staples, sutures, subcutaneous suturing, skin closure tapes and skin adhesives. None of these options has been shown to be significantly superior to each other such that a definitive recommendation can be made. It should fall upon the individual surgeon to maintain constant vigilance of his or her own patients and base the skin closure choice upon the best results that are obtainable.

It is important that infection rates of laparoscopic hernia repair does not exceed rates reported in the literature for open repair, which is of the order of about 1%.[408] Infection in an inguinal hernia repair increases the incidence of hernia recurrence by a factor of four.[296,418] If an infection develops following the laparoscopic incisional hernia repair that has utilized an ePTFE product, a recurrence is virtually assured because the biomaterial will necessarily require excision to eradicate the infection.

WOUND HEALING

Important variables in hernia repair are the rate at which the aponeurosis regains strength and the stability of the healing process. Many of the factors that regulate wound healing are under the control of the surgeon, and an appreciation of their effects and their clinical significance can aid in the proper care of the patient.

Much of the data on wound healing have been gathered by animal experimentation; there are, however, important species differences in animals and care must be exercised in translating all animal research directly into clinical practice. For example, catgut skin closure in dogs is characterized by a rapid gain in wound strength with little cellular reaction, whereas in rats and rabbits there is a slow gain in strength and a most intense cellular reaction to catgut skin sutures.[1166]

The pioneering work on the maturation and development of tensile strength in wounds was reported by Howes and his group in 1933. They reported the healing of experimental skin, fascial, muscle and gastric wounds in dogs. They observed a lag phase extending from wounding until the 5th or 6th day. During the lag phase the wound appeared quiescent, the wound strength did not increase and wound apposition was maintained by the sutures only (Figure 6.1).[518,519] Next there was a phase of fibroplasia, during which wound strength increased rapidly, reaching a maximum around the 14th to 16th day.

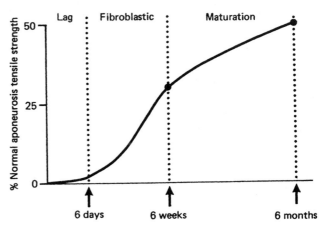

Figure 6.1 *Phases of wound healing. During the initial lag phase the wound is quiescent and during the fibroplastic phase wound strength increases rapidly over a few days; however, it is in the third, maturation, phase that significant and permanent strength gain occurs.*

Howes mentioned a third phase – the maturation phase – which he did not study longitudinally. He attributed much of the restoration of mechanical strength to the fibroblastic phase. In this he was mistaken: had he studied the maturation phase he would have discovered that this late phase, rather than the fibroblastic phase, was critical in the healing of aponeurotic wounds.

Douglas (1952) studied the rate of tensile strength gain of incisions in the lumbodorsal aponeurosis of rabbits. He found that the rate of tensile strength was slow, much slower than earlier reports suggested – about 50% of the original strength was gained at 50 days and only 80% regained at one year postoperatively.[314,315] Mason and Allen (1941) had made similar observations on the healing of tendons. They observed that if the tendon was rested the rate of gain in strength during the maturation phase was slower than if active motion was permitted,[754] this observation providing a sound experimental basis for advocating early ambulation in hernia surgery.

The lag (or latent) phase extends from the time of wounding until the fourth to sixth day in humans. During this phase the inflammatory reaction prepares the wound for subsequent healing by removing debris, necrotic tissue and bacteria. At the same time there is mobilization and migration of fibroblasts and epithelial cells and accumulation of non-collagenous proteins and glycoproteins. During the lag phase only the gluing of the fibrin holds the wound edges together. This point needs stressing. At this stage, wound security is a property of the suture material not the tissue. The initial cellular penetration of any prosthetic biomaterial is also occurring at this time.

At about the 4th to 6th post-wounding day, proliferating fibroblasts begin to synthesize collagen, mucopolysaccharides and glycoproteins. This is the fibroblastic stage of repair. The collagen quickly aggregates into fibers. Once this production of collagen commences there is the most rapid increase in the tensile strength of the wound. Because of this phenomenon, the prosthetics are becoming incorporated into the tissues at this phase. The macroporous meshes will experience a greater degree of collagen deposition during this time interval than the microporous meshes. Recent studies have shown, however, that at the time frame as early as 3 days, the macroporous interstices are filled with fluid rather than cells. The newer microporous meshes are manufactured into such a form that the fibroblasts and macrophages appear earlier in the healing phase, thereby providing greater collagen and tissue attachment.[661]

As the fibroblastic phase runs down, the phase of maturation begins. During this, further wound strength gain is due to intra- and intermolecular collagen remodeling and cross-linking. This remodeling takes 6 months to a year for completion. Probably it is the failure of this remodeling that accounts for the late appearance of incisional hernias in healed laparotomy wounds.[332,468,1167]

To obtain optimal sutured repair in hernia wounds it is necessary to incise the aponeurosis or fascia prior to suturing it. Incised fascial and aponeurotic wounds heal faster and are ultimately considerably stronger than invaginated or infolded aponeurotic or fascial wounds. This is because incision of tissues initiates the normal cascade of healing mechanisms, which ultimately lead to formation of organized collagen and mature strong connective tissue. Invagination with interrupted or running suture causes areas of local ischemia with disorganized healing and defects of collagen formation which can become apparent as areas of weakness with potential for recurrence of hernia. Aponeuroses have weak powers of regeneration and take a long time to repair. The abdominal wall only regains its preoperative resistance and strength at about the 4th postoperative month.[940] Continuous suturing of aponeurosis by spreading tension gives better ultimate healing than interrupted sutures. Aponeurotic wound healing is accelerated if there has been previous recent wounding.

It is often necessary, however, in order to prevent wound failure to close the abdominal wall with prosthetic biomaterial which reinforces the natural tissues.[602] The normal process of wound healing in the presence of a prosthetic biomaterial involves coagulation, inflammation, angiogenesis, and epithelialization. This is then followed by fibroplasias, matrix deposition, and, finally, scar contraction. During this process the cellular components are platelets, monocytes, macrophages, leukocytes, fibroblasts, endothelial cells, and smooth muscle cells. This is accompanied by the activation of a variety of growth factors and cytokines.[523] This prosthetic material, in turn, undergoes maturation with the scar contraction that occurs in all wounds and accounts for the alleged shrinkage of meshes.

The rate of wound healing and the ultimate tensile strength of wounds is adversely affected by severe protein deficiency, vitamin C deficiency, prolonged hypovolemia, increased blood viscosity, intravascular coagulation, cold vasoconstriction and chronic stress. Hypoxia, some drugs, irradiation and other factors can be critical in wound healing. For the surgeon, the most important variables are suture strength to maintain wound apposition until collagen synthesis is well advanced and exercise of the healing tendon or aponeurosis which speeds the entire process.[370,754,1012,1022]

With the use of synthetic meshes and the modern suture materials (in open repairs) or metal fixation devices (in laparoscopic repairs), wound healing has become less of a factor. Many surgeons do not depend as heavily upon these healing processes in the determination of time period to allow patients to resume normal activities. More frequently, this decision is based upon pain tolerance rather than a presupposed number of postoperative days.

SUTURES

'The material used for sutures is probably not very important' observed Aird, in 1957 (Figure 6.2).[11] Nearly 70 years have now passed since Aird summarized in one sentence the choice of a suture for hernia repair.[10] During these years the dynamics of wound healing have been defined and a revolution has overtaken sutures.[52] The modern surgeon should choose a suture according to objective biological data and marry biological science to surgical craft. Naturally occurring sutures – silk, linen and catgut – are obsolete; synthetic fibers are today's choice.[1101]

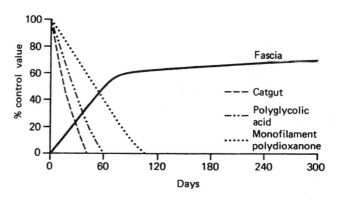

Figure 6.2 *Relationship of wound strength gain to the rate of wound healing in aponeurotic wounds. Absorbable sutures do not survive long enough to ensure wound stability. Polydioxanone occupies an intermediate position between the traditional catgut and the absorbable polymers on the one hand and the non-absorbables on the other.*

In the past the choice of suture material was based on availability and experience. And most importantly the obiter dicta of a former chief decided the acolyte's initial behavior or, as Charles Mayo has stated, experience can consist of doing the same thing wrongly over and over again. Until recently surgeons have concentrated on the mechanical properties of the

Table 6.1 *Sutures (in the sizes available for hernia surgery)*

Suture	Raw material	Type	In vivo tensile strength retention	Trade name
Plain	Sheep submucosa	Absorbable	67% lost in 5–6 days	
Chromic	Sheep submucosa	Absorbable	67% lost in 10–14 days	
Poliglecaprone 25	Copolymer of glycolide and E-caprolactone	Absorbable	70–80% lost in 14 days	Monocryl®
Polyglycolic acid	Polyglycolic acid	Absorbable		Dexon®
Polyglactin 910	Copolymer of lactide and glycolide	Absorbable	60% lost in 21 days	Vicryl®
Polyglactin 910 coated with polyglactin 370	Copolymer of lactide and glycolide coated with same combined with calcium stearate	Absorbable	60% lost in 21 days	Coated Vicryl®
Polydioxanone	Polyester of poly (p-dioxanone)	Absorbable	50% lost in 28 days	PDSII® Panacryl®
Silk	Silkworm larvae	Non-absorbable	Lost in one year	
Nylon	Polyamide polymer	Non-absorbable	15–20% per year is lost	Ethilon®
Stainless Steel	Stainless steel	Non-absorbable	Fatigue fractures at one year	
Braided Nylon	Polyamide polymer	Non-absorbable	15–20% per year is lost	Nurolon®
Polypropylene	Polymer of propylene	Non-absorbable	Two years or longer	Prolene®
Polyester	Polyethylene terephthalate	Non-absorbable	Lasts indefinitely	Mersilene®
Coated Polyester	Polyethylene terephthalate coated with polybutilate	Non-absorbable	Lasts indefinitely	Ethibond® Extra
Expanded polytetra-fluoroethylene	Polytetrafluoroethylene	Non-absorbable	Lasts indefinitely	Gore-tex®

suture and often paid scant attention to the interaction of the host tissue and the suture. Three postulates summarize the mechanical and biological relations of suture and tissue.[1166]

1 Sutures should at least be as strong as the normal tissue through which they are placed.
2 If the tissue reduces suture strength with time, the relative rates at which the suture loses strength and the wound gains strength are important.
3 If the suture alters the biology of wound healing, the impact of this alteration is important.

If these postulates are accepted, and then applied to the healing wound, the surgeon requires information about the normal strength of the tissue, the rate of gain of strength in the wounded tissue, the strength of the suture, the rate at which the suture loses strength when embedded in tissue, and about the interaction of suture and tissue. Only after considering these factors can the surgeon proceed to account for the handling and knotting properties, the 'memory', ease of sterilization and shelf life of the suture.

Sir Berkeley Moynihan, at the inaugural meeting of the Association of Surgeons in 1920, set out the essential conditions for sutures and ligatures which must remain within the wound.[819] Such material should ideally: (a) achieve its purpose – be sufficient to hold parts together, close a vessel, etc.; (b) disappear as soon as its work is accomplished; (c) be free from infection; (d) be non-irritant. These principles are still important today.

Sutures are either absorbable or non-absorbable and made from natural or synthetic products, distinctions that are increasingly blurred by modern polymer chemistry.

Tissues that are mainly formed of collagen/fascia/aponeurosis tend to heal slowly, so that only about 50% of their original tensile strength has been recovered at 3 months; thus most older absorbable sutures, whether natural or synthetic, do not generally persist long enough for adequate structural integrity to be restored. However, the healing curve of these tissues, a curve that reflects the laying down of collagen, is initially steep, so that fascia aponeurotic wounds of the abdominal wall closed with absorbable sutures or, more particularly, the modern synthetics, may just have enough strength to withstand disruption unless there are major forces, such as coughing, applied to them. In contrast, tissues which do not contain much structural collagen heal and gain their initial tensile strength much more rapidly, the gut being a particular example of this.[1164]

The suture material must retain its strength for long enough to maintain tissue apposition and allow sound union of tissues to occur. In aponeurotic wounds a non-absorbable or very slowly absorbable suture material must therefore be employed. The inherent disadvantageous properties of non-absorbable suture materials – proneness to sepsis, adverse tissue reaction and sinus formation – have led surgeons to seek compromises for hernia repair.

Table 6.1 lists the properties of natural and synthetic suture material.

Synthetic absorbable sutures

The first polymer possessing reasonable physical and biological properties was synthesized in the 1960s by Du Pont Research Laboratories. It was a braided polyester suture made of poly-L-lactide. The first commercially available absorbable synthetic suture was also a braided polyester, polyglycolic acid (PGA, Dexon), introduced in 1971. In 1974 another braided polyester suture, polyglactin 910 (Vicryl), a copolymer of lactide and glycolide, was introduced.[1113]

The basic ingredients of these polymers and their eventual breakdown products are lactic acid, glycolic acid or a combination of the two. Compared with catgut and collagen these biodegradable polymer sutures have some interesting properties. Catgut and collagen are digested by cellular enzymes and, therefore, excite an intense cellular reaction, which prolongs the lag phase in wound healing. The new polyester sutures degrade by hydrolysis and do not excite cellular activity; indeed they will hydrolyze similarly in vitro if placed in buffer solution at body temperature. Consequently they do not delay wound healing. Because they are synthetic materials produced under tight manufacturing controls they are also much more uniform and predictable in their dimensions and tensile strength than the biologically made natural fibers formerly used.

There are disadvantages. The polymer sutures, while they possess greater and more predictable strength than catgut or collagen, are also much harsher and stiffer fibers. These sutures have to be braided to provide good handling characteristics and carefully tied to avoid slippage on the first throw when tied. Because of their stiffness only extremely fine monofilaments can be used in surgery, their usefulness being confined to microsurgery and ophthalmology.

In order to overcome the abrasive quality of these fibers and to improve tying, coated polymer sutures have been introduced. The coating decreases the 'drag' through tissues and allows sliding of knots for better control.

Polydioxanone (PDS) is a newer more flexible polyester suture, introduced in 1981. Its greater flexibility, compared with PGA and polyglactin 910, allows it to be used as a monofilament. Like all the polyesters it degrades by hydrolysis and excites little tissue reaction; however, its rate of degradation is much slower than that of PGA or polyglactin 910. Polydioxanone suture was completely absorbed from rat muscle by 180 days versus 60–90 days for polyglactin 910 and 120 days for PGA suture. In vivo polydioxanone retains its strength for longer than other synthetic absorbable sutures: 58% versus 1–5% at 4 weeks and 14% versus 0% at 8 weeks.[684,942]

The place of synthetic absorbable sutures in hernioplasty is unclear. There were early favorable reports of the use of PGA sutures (Dexon) for laparotomy closure. Irvin et al. (1976)[536] compared PGA, polyglactin and polypropylene in a randomized clinical trial. They reached the conclusion that there was little to choose between these sutures. The trial was small: 161 cases randomized equally to each suture, a layered closure was used – the wound failure rate was 5.8% for polyglactin, 9.6% for PGA and 8.8% for polypropylene. Wound failure was closely related to wound infection.[536] When PGA was compared with nylon mass closure the rate of wound failure was 12.5% in the PGA group, compared with 4.7% in the nylon group. It was concluded that closure of abdominal wounds with absorbable sutures does not appear to be justified.[157] Polyglactin and polydioxanone sutures have prolonged tissue integrity compared with PGA's and may therefore be more

satisfactory for laparotomy. Polydioxanone is as good as a non-absorbable.[651] It does need stressing that it takes years to assess the final outcome of a wound closure technique and until this assessment is made by enthusiastic clinical researchers, ordinary regular surgeons should continue to use tested and proven suture techniques.[650,651] In many parts of the world, at this time, the laparotomy wound is commonly closed with either polyglactin or polydioxanone (where these are available). In the majority of cases, the fixation of the prosthetic biomaterial in open inguinal hernia repair is done with a longer lasting absorbable suture, particularly polyglactin.

Non-absorbable sutures

For closure of aponeurosis a non-absorbable monofilament flexible material with good knotting properties has been considered the ideal in the past. Of the suture materials available, stainless steel wire provides the greatest strength and knot security by a wide margin. However, the poor handling characteristics of wire limits its usefulness, despite its additional advantage of minimal tissue reaction. Silk has long been considered the standard non-absorbable suture material and has enjoyed widest use. Silk was recommended by Halsted and by Whipple.[461,1208] In terms of strength and knot security silk is distinctly inferior to many other materials, and the tissue reaction to silk correlates with the incidence of granuloma and sinuses in clinical use. Cotton was introduced in 1940 during World War II when silk was relatively unobtainable. Its strength is similar to silk, but its handling characteristics are inferior – again it has a high incidence of granuloma and sinus formation. Cotton is similar to linen in many properties.

Nylon was developed by the Du Pont Company and introduced as an alternative to silk in 1943. Compared with silk, nylon has distinct advantages: it can be used as a monofilament, it loses less strength when wet (15% versus 25%), it is stronger, and it causes much less tissue reaction. However, it is not as flexible, it is difficult to handle and to knot, and the knots have a tendency to slip. Monofilament nylon undergoes both plastic (irreversible) and elastic (reversible) elongation when subjected to tension. When nylon is stretched using a force of 5 kg, the total elongation produced is 22.5%, of which 6.9% is irreversible. When aponeurotic wounds are closed with nylon and then the sutures are tightened to 5 kg to produce 'compression' of the wound, the suture stretches by 27.7%.[760] This plastic irreversible elongation has an importance in closing fascial wounds: unless the nylon is tightened adequately, its elongation when the patient breathes and moves will lead to loss of apposition of the wound edges and ultimately to wound failure.

Monofilament polypropylene is an alternative to nylon. The advantages of polypropylene are greater flexibility and easier handling characteristics. It knots better than nylon.[497,499] The 'memory' characteristic of this suture does make this material difficult to use in certain circumstances, however.

Braided non-absorbable sutures have distinctly better handling and knotting characteristics than monofilaments, but they give the least good results for suturing aponeurosis and repairing hernias. The particular problems are infection and the persistent sinuses and so braids should be abandoned. If infection occurs in a wound repaired with a non-absorbable braid, there is no alternative to removing the suture. With monofilaments, infection can be controlled and suture removal is not needed. Others have confirmed the unsuitability of braided non-absorbable sutures in hernia repair.[553]

MECHANICAL FACTORS IN ABDOMINAL WOUND CLOSURE

Wounds are not set in their dimensions, but undergo change as they heal. Not only do the wounds themselves change, but the cavities or tissues they contain alter, and these alterations critically vary the dimensions of the wound.

The events of wound healing lead to edema of the wound and then to the development of a healing ridge and fibroblast proliferation as collagen placement gets under way. Edema of the wound by increasing wound bulk increases the tension in each suture bite. If suture bites are initially tight this increase in tension may lead to (a) suture breakage, (b) knot failure or (c) cutting out. These same three consequences develop from changes in body compartments beneath suture lines. In the abdomen, extreme examples of this phenomenon occur. In voluntary inspiration, pregnancy and abdominal distension, mean alterations of girth of 6%, 18% and 27% have been measured, while simultaneously the mean xiphoid to pubis distance increases by 12%, 15% and 37%, respectively (Table 6.2). In these circumstances an abdominal wound will increase in length by an estimated 30% overall.

The alterations in wound length that occur during healing have a critical impact on the technique of suturing an abdominal wound. Jenkins has analyzed this geometrically[549] and concluded that the ratio of suture length (SL) to wound length (WL) is critical to aponeurosis repair.

An SL:WL ratio of 4:1 or more is optimum; if the SL:WL ratio decreases below 2.5:1 the risk of wound disruption increases geometrically. Wound disruption is inevitable as the SL:WL ratio approaches 1:1. This mathematical analysis (Jenkins' rule) is confirmed when tested in clinical practice. These findings have been corroborated by Israelsson 30 years later.[539,540] In two studies examining cohorts of over a 1000 patients from 1989–1991 and 1991–1993 respectively, Israelsson showed that a suture length to wound length of less than 4 was the greatest risk factor for wound failure and predictor of later incisional hernia with lesser risks associated with age, obesity and wound infection. The surgeon was also an important risk factor in that incisional hernia rates varied from 5–26% between individuals. Interestingly in overweight patients (BMI > 25) there was no increase in wound infection rate if the suture length to wound length was between 4.0 and 4.9 although incisional hernias developed in these patients in 15% of cases after 12 months.

Surgical practice, however, continues to rely largely on tradition rather than high-quality level 1 evidence when choosing the ideal method of abdominal fascial closure.[506] Hodgson and colleagues carried out a systematic review and meta-analysis to determine which suture material and which technique reduces the odds of incisional hernia. They studied only randomized controlled trials with a Jadad quality score of >3. (Jadad Quality Scale is the only validated instrument available to assess the quality of randomized controlled trials.) There were two independent reviewers masked to the study site, authors, journal and date. The results showed the following:

1 There was a low occurrence of incisional hernia with non-absorbable sutures.
2 Suture technique favored non-absorbable, continuous suturing.
3 Sinus tract formation and wound pain were lower with absorbable sutures.
4 There was no difference in dehiscence rates or wound infection rates with respect to method of closure or material used.

Abdominal fascial closure with a continuous non-absorbable suture had a significantly lower rate of incisional hernia. The ideal suturing technique is therefore non-absorbable and the ideal technique is continuous. The data for this study drew information from 13 randomized trials including a total of 5145

Table 6.2 *Increases in girth and xiphoid–pubis distance caused by abdominal distension (From Jenkins 1976, with permission)*

Abdominal distension associated with:	Type of measurement	Percentage increase in distension	
		Mean value	Extreme value
Voluntary inspiration (*n* = 18)	Girth	6	11
	Xiphoid–pubis	12	18
Cesarean section (*n* = 27)	Girth	18	94
	Xiphoid–pubis	15	36
Gut obstruction or paralytic ileus (*n* = 5)	Girth	27	53
	Xiphoid–pubis	37	67

patients and utilizing nine different suture materials with a continuous or an interrupted technique, mostly in vertical midline incisions. This meta-analysis provides the most powerful evidence yet for informing surgeons on the optimal technique for abdominal fascial closure.

In the pure tissue hernia repair it is important to take deep bites of aponeurosis, to place the sutures close together, observing Jenkins' rule, to make the suture bites irregular to avoid splitting between the strands of aponeurosis and to tighten the sutures to allow for plastic elongation of the suture polymer in the postoperative period. A relatively simple abdominoplasty method to avoid the use of prosthetic mesh is the component 'separation' technique in which the external oblique is separated from the internal oblique in an avascular plane 1 cm lateral to the Spigelian line which allows the formation of a medial advancement flap consisting of the rectus muscle, the anterior rectus sheath and the internal oblique-transversus.[938] An advancement of 10 cm can be achieved at the umbilicus.

Certain principles should be adhered to when implanting any prosthetic biomaterial. It is important to provide secure fixation of the prosthesis so that it does not move and to ensure that there will be no or minimal deformation of the biomaterial during the healing process. The laparoscopic repair of inguinal hernias frequently can be performed without the use of any fixation of the prosthesis at all. This cannot be said for the laparoscopic incisional herniorrhaphy which mandates secure transfascial fixation with non-absorbable sutures.[492,657]

Knots

The knot is the weakest part of a suture and knot efficiency is a crucial component of the suture technique. Conventional knots cause a 40% decrease in the strength of most suture materials except for nylon (and probably polypropylene). Self-locking knots permit the end of a continuous suture to slide inside the knot, thus absorbing some of the energy which would otherwise be transmitted to the knot and cause it to break.[889] Additionally, self-locking knots are less bulky than more conventional knots, thus diminishing the risk of infection and sinus formation.[899,1141]

Suture manipulation

Generally, little thought is given to the handling of the suture material during its use and implantation into the tissues. Most of the modern synthetics can tolerate considerable manipulation as they are placed. One should be cognizant of the fact that some of these materials can be frayed and weakened when they are secured in the jaws of a needle holder, forceps or hemostats, etc. Sometimes the surgeon does not recognize this newly created weakness. This can result in an early fracture of the suture material, which, in effect, results in a cut suture that no longer is intact. This can result in failure of healing of the tissues that are held with that suture. Similarly, this can result in a hernia recurrence if that suture is the method of fixation of a prosthetic biomaterial. Therefore it is incumbent upon the surgeon to be careful in handling any portion of a suture that will remain within the tissues so that this will not become a problem that is manifest by a new or recurrent hernia.

SKIN CLOSURE

Sutures, penetrating the skin and then tied on the surface, are the traditional closure method for wounds. Alternatives include subcuticular sutures, skin clips, which do not penetrate the full skin thickness and plastic tape adherent to the skin. Recently a new product, Dermabond® tissue adhesive, has become available that can be used without the need for sutures. This acts like glue that maintains good approximation of the skin edges.

The requirements for adequate skin closure are that the skin edges should be held together in apposition for sufficient time to allow the skin to grow together. To promote rapid healing, the edges should not move in relation to each other and tension should be minimal to prevent necrosis. Careful suturing should prevent the introduction of sepsis. Lastly, but perhaps of overriding importance to the patient, a good cosmetic result is needed.

Clean or contaminated surgery demands different regimens for wound management. One of the oldest surgical principles is that a frankly contaminated wound should be left open. The wound which is expected to be compromised by early (reactionary) hemorrhage is managed by delayed primary suture. If localized infection is anticipated, interrupted sutures may allow early drainage. These are the traditions of wound care. Hernia operations nowadays are clean operations – we are searching for quick uncomplicated healing with the best functional and cosmetic results. Hence we should review our methods of skin closure and optimize skin healing as far as possible.

Conventional (traditional) skin suturing techniques do have certain disadvantages – the needle passing through the skin on either side carries fragments of both epidermis and skin organisms down its track and into the depths of the subcutaneous tissue. This causes an increased wound infection rate than when skin closure by a sutureless technique is used. The complications of suture track infection are greater when a multi-strand suture is used and when the tension upon the wound edges is too great. Poor technique in inserting the sutures and subsequent edema after suturing lead to localized ischemia and a poor cosmetic result.

Clips avoid the problem of introducing deep infection into the wound. Michel-type clips may produce localized tension and cause local pressure necrosis. Unless they are removed within 24–48 h, this local ischemia can cause tissue necrosis and a permanently poor cosmetic result. Consequently, these are seldom used in modern surgical theaters. Currently available disposable applicators for the introduction of wire skin clips with a rectangular configuration of the closed clip give excellent results. Closure with adherent tape gives excellent healing.[323,896,1118]

A randomized controlled clinical trial comparing skin closure using vertical mattress sutures of monofilament nylon and steel clips in laparotomy incisions has confirmed the significant advantage of avoiding skin sutures. In a consecutive series of 341 wounds (182 skin sutured and 159 closed with clips), the infection rate in the sutured wounds was 17.0% versus 6.3% in those closed with clips ($\chi^2 = 9.26$; $P < 0.01$).[911] Subcutaneous absorbable sutures may be the favorite method with surgeons, nurses and patients. In a randomized trial four different methods of thigh wound closure after removal of the saphenous vein for coronary artery bypass grafting were used.[36] Continuous nylon vertical mattress sutures, continuous subcuticular absorbable PGA sutures, metal skin clips and adhesive sutureless closure (Opsite) were compared. Assessment of the healing showed subcuticular PGA to be more effective than skin clips or vertical mattress nylon sutures. The final cosmetic result showed subcuticular PGA to be superior to sutures or skin clips and as effective as sutureless adherent closure. Subcuticular absorbable sutures do not require removal; this is an economic saving.[936] Subcuticular skin closure for open inguinal hernia repair using polydioxanone or polyglactin 910 is recommended. The results of these sutures have been excellent. The suture does not require removal. Wound healing is quick and neat and, most importantly, the lack of through-skin sutures has removed much of the postoperative pain. Closure of laparoscopic trocar skin incisions is performed with interrupted polyglactin 910 and/or skin tapes.

TECHNIQUES OF PLACEMENT OF PROSTHETIC BIOMATERIALS

The open prosthetic mesh repair of abdominal wall defects can be accomplished by the following techniques[635,636,1157,1158] (a) extra-aponeurotic–subcutaneous; (b) subaponeurotic and extraperitoneal or preperitoneal; (c) subaponeurotic and intraperitoneal (Figure 6.3). Additionally, intraperitoneal placement of the mesh can be supported by an extra-aponeurotic stent (Figure 6.4).

The laparoscopic method of prosthetic mesh placement will always place the prosthetic material in the subaponeurotic plane. In the inguinal hernia repair this will be placed in the preperitoneal space using the transabdominal or the totally extraperitoneal approaches. There are only a few centers that

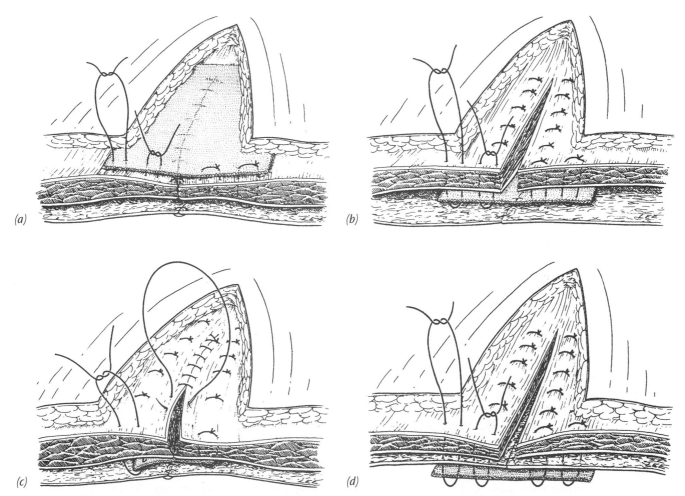

(a)   (b)   (c)   (d)

Figure 6.3 *Prosthetic repairs of abdominal wall defects. The prosthesis can be placed extraparietally or subcutaneously (a), subaponeurotically, extraperitoneally, or preperitoneally leaving any aponeurotic defect open superficial to the prosthesis (b), subaponeurotically with closure of the defect (c), or intraperitoneally (d).*

have chosen to place the prosthesis in the intraperitoneal position with this method of inguinal hernia repair. The laparoscopic repair of the incisional and ventral hernias, on the other hand, will generally always put the prosthesis in the intraperitoneal position. Conversely, there are a few centers that utilize either an extraperitoneal or transabdominal preperitoneal approach to this procedure. This, however, is considerably more difficult to perform.

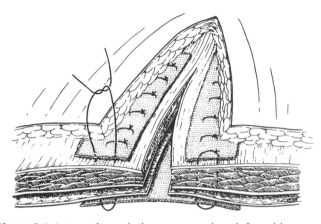

Figure 6.4 *Intraperitoneal placement can be reinforced by an extra-aponeurotic stent.*

There are now numerous varieties of prosthetic pre-shaped or preformed devices that have been designed for the repair of inguinal hernias. In some cases, these have been used for the repair of incisional or primary ventral hernias as well. These are too numerous and their methodologies so variant that these are discussed in detail in Chapter 7. One point that must be emphasized continuously, however, is that all of these products are inserted with an individual technique specific for that prosthetic device. Deviation from this methodology may subject the patient to an increased incidence of complications or recurrence.

SUMMARY – RECOMMENDATIONS

- The patient must be fully resuscitated, when necessary, before any operation is undertaken.
- The aponeurosis must be closed by a method which maintains tissue strength in excess of 3 months – a method that causes little tissue reaction and does not cause persistent sinuses, if infected. A monofilament non-absorbable synthetic suture may be preferred. If this is selected, a large size monofilament polypropylene is recommended. The technique of deep irregular close bites (to avoid splitting the aponeurosis) is employed. It is important to knot the suture carefully. A double throw double tie square knot is the minimal requirement if knot failure is to be avoided. Careful use of instrumentation on the portion of the suture that remains in the patient is necessary to avoid early suture failure.
- If the subcutaneous fatty layer is closed the suture material employed must cause little, if any reaction, and be absorbed fairly rapidly. Polyglactin or PGA sutures are suitable for this layer.
- Closed suction drains may be used if there is any possibility of hematoma formation. Only in the largest of hernias is this necessary, however.
- In the skin, desirable features of the skin closure technique include a neat scar with no skin markings from sutures on it, a minimal reaction to material used in suturing and, above all, a low instance of infection and subsequent sinus formation. If the material does not require removal it has advantages. Subcuticular clear PDS or polyglactin 910 suture is recommended.

The synthetic prosthetic biomaterials can be divided into the absorbable and non-absorbable products. The absorbable biomaterials (polyglycolic or polyglactic acid) have been used to cover polypropylene prosthetics used to repair a fascial defect in an effort to protect the viscera from that product or as a temporary closure of the abdominal wall for intra-abdominal sepsis. While these materials may appear to have a role in the prevention of adhesions, they may, in fact, enhance their development because of the inflammatory response that develops as a natural consequence of the use of these materials. There is no clinical data to support this type of usage of the absorbable biomaterials. Recent laboratory studies have shown that this technique does not achieve its intended result.[1173]

There has been a recent introduction of non-synthetic biomaterials that are designed to be used for the repair of hernias. Three are based upon the use of porcine tissues to produce a collagen matrix while another is based upon cadaveric skin. All of these products are not truly absorbable as they are intended to provide a scaffold for the native fibroblasts to incorporate natural collagen to repair a fascial defect.

The synthetic non-absorbable biomaterials are of many types, sizes and shapes. The use of these products is commonplace in the repair of inguinal hernias. The current use of the prosthesis in the tension free concept of a repair of the incisional hernias has gained widespread acceptance within the last several years. More than 90% of incisional and ventral hernias in the USA are repaired with the use of some type of prosthetic biomaterial. Outside the USA, however, the repair of these hernias is frequently performed without their use, cost being a prime hindrance to this adoption. With the exception of the very smallest of hernias, every laparoscopic approach employs a prosthesis.

The materials that are presented are given in an arbitrary format. We have attempted to identify all of the currently available products that are used in most parts of the world at the time of publication. Additionally, some of these materials have either no clinical data or very scanty information as to the performance characteristics. Therefore, it is certain, however, that some products and/or details have been overlooked despite our efforts to present all that we can identify.

ABSORBABLE PROSTHETIC BIOMATERIALS

There are only a few of the prosthetic materials that are not permanent (Table 7.6). The general purpose of these is the temporary replacement of absent tissue. The strength of these materials and the lack of permanency make most of them unsuitable for the permanent repair of any hernia. They are particularly helpful in the smaller infected wounds that develop after abdominal surgery.

Table 7.6 *Absorbable biomaterials and their manufacturer*

Knitted Vicryl® mesh, Ethicon, Inc., Somerville, NJ, USA
Woven Vicryl® mesh, Ethicon, Inc., Somerville, NJ, USA
Dexon®, US Surgical Corp./Davis and Geck, Norwalk, CT, USA

The Vicryl® and Dexon® meshes are primarily polydioxone (Figure 7.1). They can be affixed onto the fascia directly with sutures but are generally not of sufficient strength to formally repair a defect. Most frequently these are used to provide a buttress of support for the temporary closure of an infected incisional wound of the abdomen or in the patient with intra-abdominal sepsis or abdominal compartment syndrome. There have been a few reports of the use of such materials used to cover a polypropylene prosthesis in the laparoscopic repair of incisional hernias.[77] There is experimental evidence that this does not achieve the desired result.[1173]

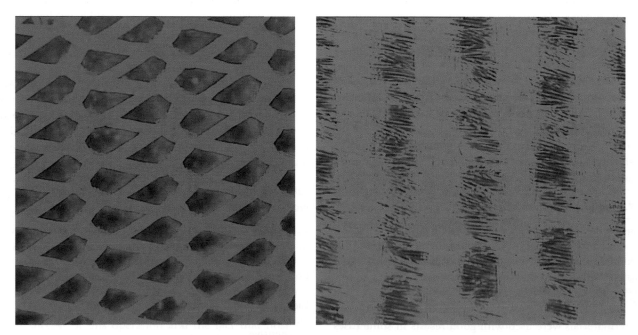

Figure 7.1 *Knitted Vicryl absorbable mesh and woven Vicryl absorbable mesh. (Ethicon, Inc., Somerville, NJ, USA.)*

COLLAGEN-BASED PRODUCTS (Table 7.7)

These products represent a new concept in hernia repair. They are based upon a collagen matrix that is manufactured into sheets of tissue-engineered materials that can be used to repair defects in the abdominal wall. The concept of these materials is that the bioengineered patches will allow the migration of the patient's own fibroblasts onto them so that collagen will be deposited to form a 'neo-fascia'. This is not true technically as some of these biomaterials act as their own tissue replacement in the same manner as the synthetic products. Studies have shown that the extracellular matrix scaffolds from these materials show rapid degradation that is associated with remodeling to a tissue with strength that exceeds that of the native tissues.[69]

Table 7.7 *Collagen matrix materials*

Surgisis ES® and Surgisis Gold®, Cook Surgical, Inc., Bloomington, IN
FortaPerm™, Organogenesis Inc., Canton MA
FortaGen™, Organogenesis Inc., Canton MA
Permacol™, Tissue Science Laboratories plc, Covington, GA, USA
Alloderm®, Lifecell, Inc., Branchburg, NJ

Surgisis® is a different concept of a synthetic biomaterial as it is not truly absorbed (Figures 7.2 and 7.3). This product is available in one, four (Surgisis ES®) or eight layers (Surgisis Gold®) of porcine small intestinal submucosa. The 4- and 8-ply

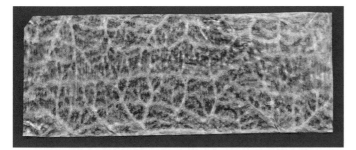

Figure 7.2 *Surgisis ES. (Cook Surgical, Bloomington, IN.)*

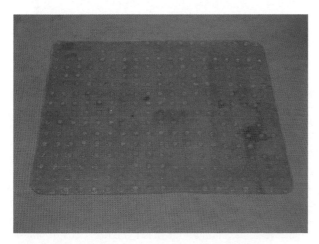

Figure 7.3 *Surgisis Gold. (Cook Surgical, Bloomington, IN.)*

products are designed for the repair of inguinal, incisional, and hiatal hernias. The 1-ply material is too thin to be used in the repair of hernias but the 4-ply has been used successfully for the open repair of inguinal and diaphragmatic hernias. The thicker product is recommended for the larger abdominal wall defects such as an incisional hernia. This product represents a collagen matrix (Figure 7.4). This is stated to allow this surface to act as a scaffold for the encroachment of fibroblasts onto the product. In this manner, the prosthesis will be replaced with a 'neo-fascia' thereby replacing the fascial defect. It may be particularly helpful in infected fascial defects from any etiology that does not involve a fistula of the intestine. The contents of the fistulous drainage will denature the collagen of the biomaterial and result in the digestion of the protein.

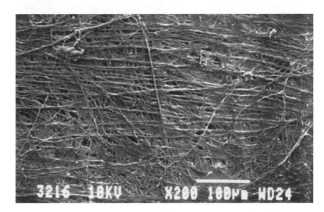

Figure 7.4 *Scanning electron microscopic (SEM) view of the collagen matrix of Surgisis.*

FortaPerm™ and FortaGen™ are based upon FortaFlex™ technology from porcine small intestinal submucosa as is the Surgisis above. These products are collagen that is engineered into laminated sheets that are cross-linked to increase strength and control the persistence of these biomaterials in the body. The FortaGen material (Figure 7.5) is a five-layer construct

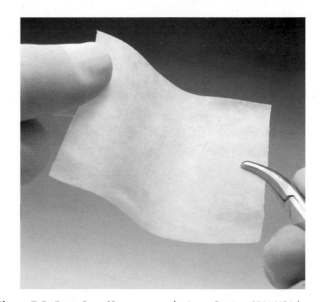

Figure 7.5 *FortaGen. (Organogenesis, Inc., Canton MA, USA.)*

with a low level of cross-linking that allows cellular infiltration and remodeling, as does Surgisis. This will be replaced by the native tissue and is recommended for hernia repair. The FortaPerm product resists cellular infiltration and is therefore more suitable to applications other than hernia repair such as mastopexy (Figure 7.6). Permacol is another porcine-based product but it is produced from porcine dermal collagen (Figure 7.7).

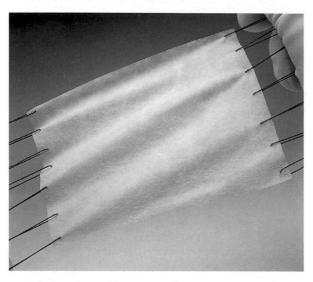

Figure 7.6 *FortaPerm. (Organogenesis, Canton MA, USA.)*

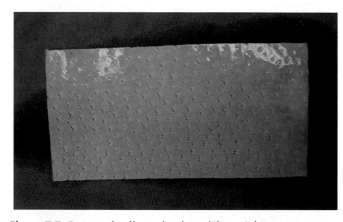

Figure 7.7 *Permacol collagen implant. (Tissue Science Laboratories, Covington, GA, USA.) This is also a collagen implant but it is based upon porcine skin.*

Alloderm® is not like the above materials in that it is based upon human cadaveric tissue (Figure 7.8). As the other two products listed immediately above, it must be hydrated prior to use. While it is available in several sizes, the larger 4 × 12 cm product is produced in a thickness that is for use in the repair of hernias (≥0.78 mm thickness). There are few studies on the use of this biomaterial in hernia repair.[1054]

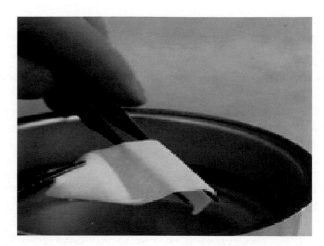

Figure 7.8 *Alloderm. (Lifecell, Branchburg, NJ, USA.)*

FLAT PROSTHETIC BIOMATERIALS

The currently available products in use today are polypropylene (PPM), polyester, expanded polytetrafluoroethylene or a composite material of these materials. All are available in a variety of sizes and can be cut to conform to the dimensions that are necessary. There are currently so many products on the market today that it is quite difficult to become well versed in all of these materials. In fact, the similarities of these biomaterials may result in many of them to be considered a 'commodity' type of a product, whereupon only the pricing of the material will influence the use of it. The most prominent and commonly used PPM biomaterials that are available for the surgical repair of hernias are listed in Table 7.8.

Table 7.8 *Polypropylene biomaterials and manufacturer*

Angimesh, Angiologica, S. Martino Sicc., Italy
Atrium (Prolite), Atrium Medical Corporation, Hudson, NH, USA
Biomesh P1, Cousin Biotech, Wervicq-Sud, France
Biomesh P3, Cousin Biotech, Wervicq-Sud, France
Biomesh 3D, Cousin Biotech, Wervicq-Sud, France
Hertra 1, 2, HerniaMesh, S.R.L., Torino, Italy
Hermesh 3,4,5, HerniaMesh, S.R.L., Torino, Italy
Intramesh NK1, NK2, NK8, Cousin Biotech, Wervicq-Sud, France
Marlex, C.R.Bard, Inc., Cranston NJ, USA
Parietene, Sofradim International, Villfranche-sur-Saône, France
Prolene, Ethicon, Somerville, NJ, USA
Prolene Soft Mesh, Ethicon, Somerville, NJ, USA
Prolite Ultra, Atrium Medical Corporation, Hudson, NH, USA
Surgipro (Monofilament), United States Surgical Corp./Tyco, Norwalk, CT, USA
Surgipro (Multifilament), United States Surgical Corp./Tyco, Norwalk, CT, USA
Trelex, Meadox Medical Corporation, Oakland, NJ, USA

Angimesh is available in three different products. These are also differentiated by the thickness and the weave of the meshes (Figure 7.9). Atrium (now called Prolite) mesh has been used for many years as a single flat mesh (Figure 7.10). *Biomesh P1* and *P3* products are also differentiated from each other on the

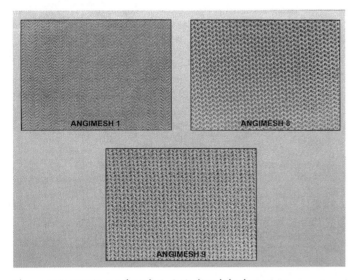

Figure 7.9 *REPOL Angimesh 1, 8, 9. (Angiologica, S. Martino Sicc., Italy.)*

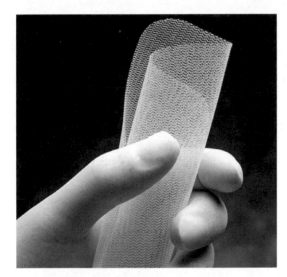

Figure 7.10 *Prolite. (Atrium Medical Corporation, Hudson NH, USA.)*

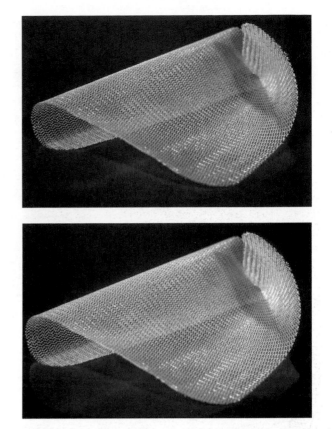

Figure 7.11 *Biomesh P1, P3. (Cousin Biotech, Wervicq-Sud, France.)*

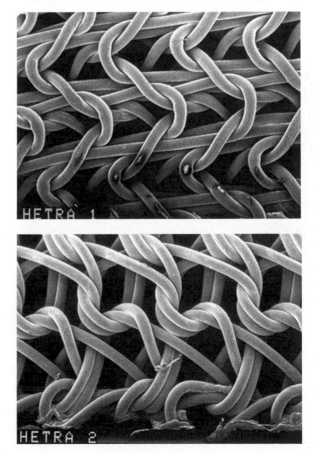

Figure 7.12 *Hetra 1 and 2. (HerniaMesh, S.R.L., Torino, Italy.)*

basis of the weight of the material (Figure 7.11). All of the products from HerniaMesh differ in weight, porosity and thickness. *Hetra 1* and *2* are both a two course knit that are 0.68 mm and 0.53 mm thick respectively (Figure 7.12). *Hermesh 3*, *4*, and *5* are 0.48 mm, 0.45 mm, and 0.42 mm respectively (Figure 7.13). The *Marlex* and *Trelex* are similar meshes and are only produced in a single individual product (Figures 7.14 and 7.15). The former, of course, is considered the original product of all of these hernioplasty products. The current *Prolene* is the second generation of material and is slightly softer than the original (Figure 7.16). The *Parietene* and *Biomesh 3D* are products that have a three-dimensional weave of PPM and represents a new concept in mesh design (Figures 7.17 and 7.18).

Surgipro was originally introduced as a multifilamented mesh. Because of the demand for a monofilamented product,

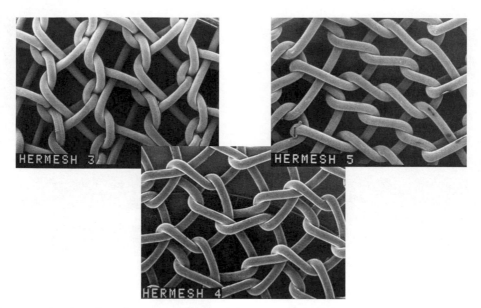

Figure 7.13 *Hermesh 3, 4, and 5. (HerniaMesh, S.R.L., Torino, Italy.)*

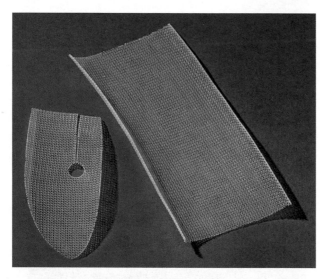

Figure 7.14 *Marlex. (C.R.Bard, Inc., Cranston NJ, USA.) This product is currently marketed as Bard mesh.*

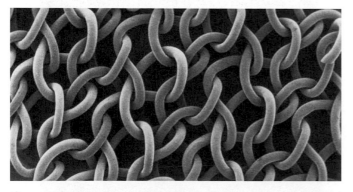

Figure 7.15 *Trelex. (Meadox Medical Corporation, Oakland, NJ, USA.)*

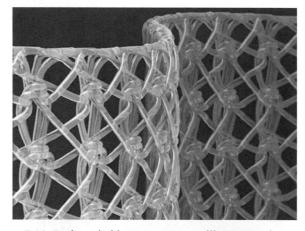

Figure 7.16 *Prolene. (Ethicon, Inc., Somerville, NJ, USA.)*

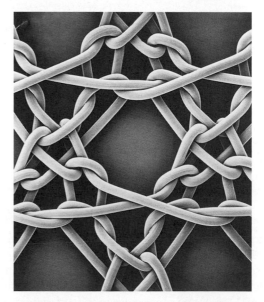

Figure 7.17 *Parietene. (Sofradim International, Villfranche-sur-Saône, France.)*

the second-generation product was released (Figure 7.19). The multifilament material is noticeably softer than the monofilamented one and may have less predisposition to the formation of intra-abdominal adhesions.[653,654]

Newer products have begun to decrease the amount of synthetic biomaterial in the construction of the meshes. One such

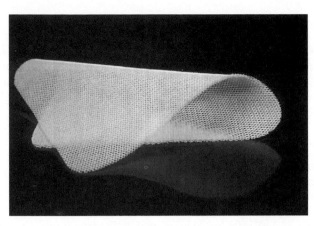

Figure 7.18 *Biomesh 3D. (Cousin Biotech, Wervicq-Sud, France.)*

product is the *Prolite Ultra*™ that is manufactured by Atrium Medical Corporation (Figure 7.20). It is a low profile mesh that is quite thin and malleable. Similarly, the *Prolene Soft Mesh* has thinner biomaterial with larger interstices (Figure 7.21). Additionally, this latter product has blue lines that cross the mesh so that the alignment during laparoscopic inguinal hernia repair is facilitated.

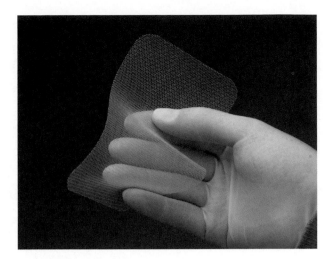

Figure 7.20 *Prolite Ultra. (Atrium Medical Corporation, Hudson, NH, USA.)*

Biomesh NK1, *NK2* and *NK8* are distinctly different from the other PPM products that are described above. These are a polypropylene mesh that is non-woven and non-knitted (Figure 7.22). They are quite soft and are suitable for both open and laparoscopic hernioplasties.[365] They are distinguished from each other by their different thicknesses. Interestingly, NK2 is the thinnest (0.25 mm) and NK8 is the thickest (0.36 mm). NK1 is 0.3 mm.

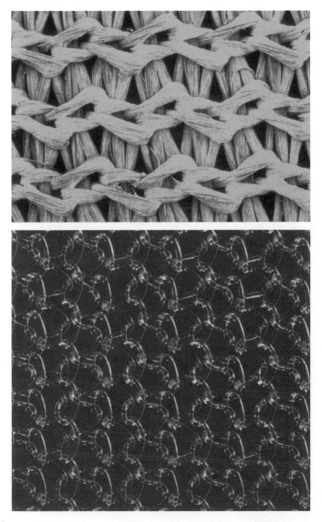

Figure 7.19 *Surgipro multifilament (top) and monofilament (bottom) meshes. (United States Surgical Corp/Tyco, Norwalk CT, USA.)*

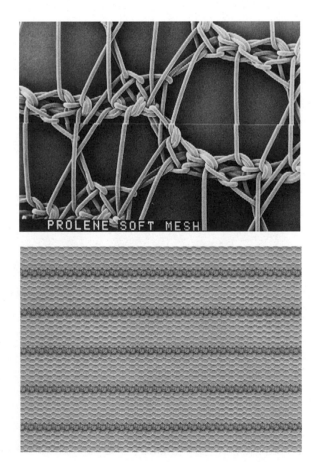

Figure 7.21 *Prolene Soft Mesh. (Ethicon, Inc., Somerville, NJ, USA.)*

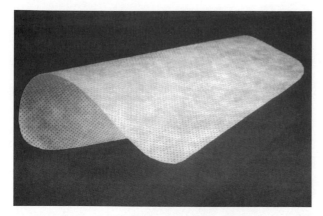

Figure 7.22 *Biomesh NK1, NK2, NK8. (Cousin Biotech, Wervicq-Sud, France.)*

The scanning electron microscopic views of some of these products are shown in Figure 7.23. The differences in the appearance of the prosthetics are easily seen in these photos. The size of the pores of these materials as well as the thickness of the product will have a significant impact on the stiffness. These factors affect the degree of scarring within the tissues. Additionally, the pore sizes vary greatly from each of these products. This will also have a significant impact in the amount of scarring and adhesion formation that is seen following implantation. Generally, the monofilament weaves with larger interstices will result in more adhesions that are more tenacious than the multifilamented weaves with smaller pore sizes.[653,654,666]

Polyester biomaterials have had relatively limited usage in the United States as opposed to the extent of the implantation in Europe, particularly France. Like the PPM biomaterials there has been an increase in the number of products that are available today. Also, like the PPM, these products can be associated with fistula formation. Some of the currently available products are listed in Table 7.9.

Table 7.9 *Polyester prostheses and manufacturer*

Biomesh A1, Cousin Biotech, Wervicq-Sud, France
Biomesh A3, Cousin Biotech, Wervicq-Sud, France
Biomesh 3D, Cousin Biotech, Wervicq-Sud, France
Mersilene, Ethicon, Inc., Somerville, NJ, USA
Parietex® TEC, Sofradim International, Villfranche-sur-Saône, France
Parietex® TECR, Sofradim International, Villfranche-sur-Saône, France
Parietex® TET, Sofradim International, Villfranche-sur-Saône, France

Biomesh A1 and *A3* are multifilamented biomaterials that are of different knits (Figure 7.24). The tensile strength of the former is much greater than that of the latter. Therefore the A1 can also be used for rectal and genitourinary prolapse. For many years the only material that was commercially available was *Mersilene* (Figure 7.25). Consequently, the largest experience with the polyester biomaterials is that of this product. *Parietex®* TEC is similar to these products because all of these three

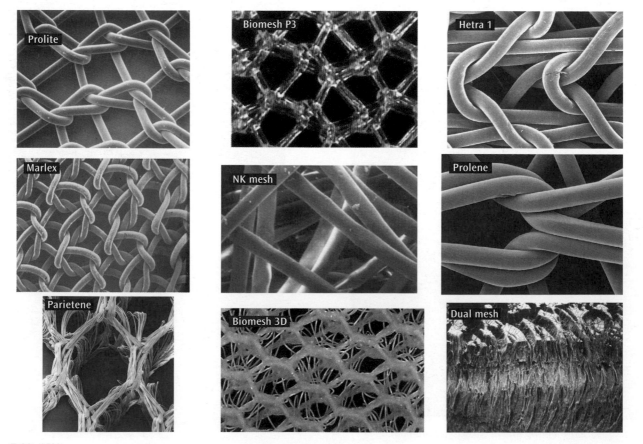

Figure 7.23 *SEMs.*

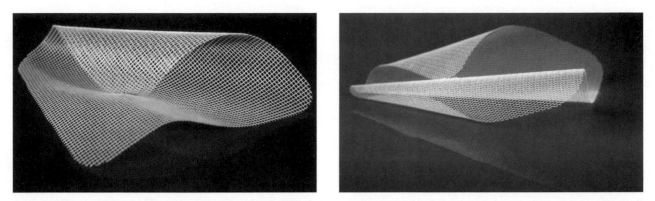

Figure 7.24 *Biomesh A1 (left) and A3 (right). (Cousin Biotech, Wervicq-Sud, France.)*

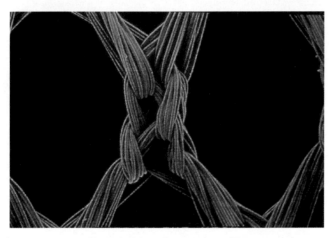

Figure 7.25 *Mersilene. (Ethicon, Inc., Somerville, NJ, USA.)*

meshes are bi-dimensional (Figure 7.26). *Parietex® TECR* is also a bi-dimensional flat polyester mesh that is similar to the TEC but is more rigid than the TEC biomaterial (Figure 7.26).

Parietex® TET and *Biomesh 3D*, in contrast, are a newer three-dimensional form of polyester (Figures 7.27 and 7.28). It

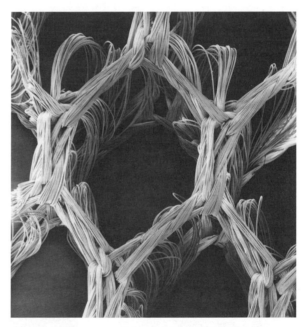

Figure 7.27 *Parietex TET and pre-shaped TET. (Sofradim International, Villfranche-sur-Saône, France.)*

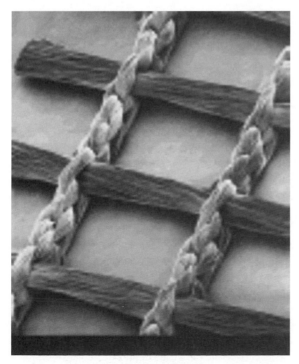

Figure 7.26 *Parietex TEC and TECR. (Sofradim International, Villfranche-sur-Saône, France.)*

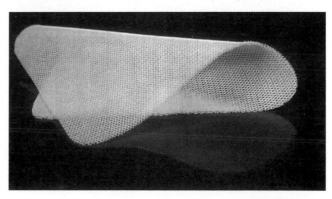

Figure 7.28 *Biomesh 3D. (Cousin Biotech, Wervicq-Sud, France.)*

is stated that this newer knit allows good flexibility with high suture and staple retention. The Parietex® TET is available as a pre-shaped product for the repair of inguinal hernias as TET (Figure 7.27).

Expanded polytetrafluoroethylene (ePTFE) prostheses are listed in Table 7.10. The earliest of these was the *Soft Tissue Patch* (Figure 7.29). Its use has waned because of the development of the other products that are listed in Table 7.10. The *Reconix* patch

is visually indistinguishable from that of the Soft Tissue Patch (Figure 7.30). It is slightly stiffer in handling. There are very distinguishable differences in these two products when viewed in the scanning electron microscope. There is a shorter distance in the nodes of the PTFE in the Reconix when compared with the other product (Figure 7.31). Additionally, this material is laminated rather than the structure of the Soft Tissue Patch (Figure 7.32).

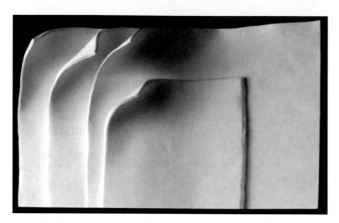

Figure 7.29 *Soft Tissue Patch. (W.L. Gore and Associates, Flagstaff, AZ, USA.)*

Table 7.10 *ePTFE Biomaterials and manufacturer*

DualMesh, W.L. Gore and Associates, Flagstaff, AZ, USA
DualMesh Plus, W.L. Gore and Associates, Flagstaff, AZ, USA
DualMesh with Holes, W.L. Gore and Associates, Flagstaff, AZ, USA
DualMesh Plus with Holes, W.L. Gore and Associates, Flagstaff, AZ, USA
Dulex, C.R. Bard, Inc., Cranston NJ, USA
Mycromesh, W.L. Gore and Associates, Flagstaff, AZ, USA
Mycromesh Plus, W.L. Gore and Associates, Flagstaff, AZ, USA
Reconix, C.R. Bard, Inc., Cranston NJ, USA
Soft Tissue Patch, W.L. Gore and Associates, Flagstaff, AZ, USA

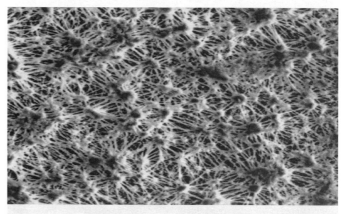
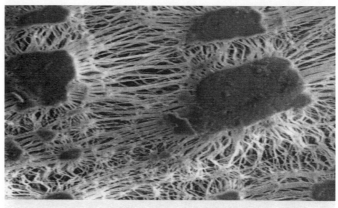

GORE-TEX® Soft Tissue Patch

Bard® Reconix™ Patch

Figure 7.31 *Scanning electron microscopic views of the surfaces of Soft Tissue Patch and Reconix.*

The current *DualMesh* products are very similar in construction. These represent the second generation of this biomaterial. These all have two distinctly different surfaces. One side is very smooth and has interstices of three microns (Figure 7.33), while the other has the appearance of corduroy with an approximate 'ridge to ridge' distance of 1500 microns (Figure 7.34). This prosthesis is designed for use in the intraperitoneal space. The smooth side must therefore be placed facing the viscera as this inhibits the potential for adhesion formation. The rough surface is applied to the abdominal wall so that maximum tissue penetration will occur. In the studies of the author (KAL) it has been shown that the penetration of fibroblasts and subsequent collagen deposition occurs throughout the entire biomaterial with the exception of the smooth surface (Figure 7.35). Further studies have shown that the level of tissue penetration and difficulty of extraction of the biomaterial from the tissues exceeds that of Marlex at 3 days.[661] Follow-up operations in patients that have undergone

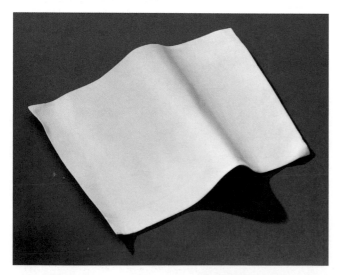

Figure 7.30 *Reconix. (C.R. Bard, Inc., Cranston NJ, USA.)*

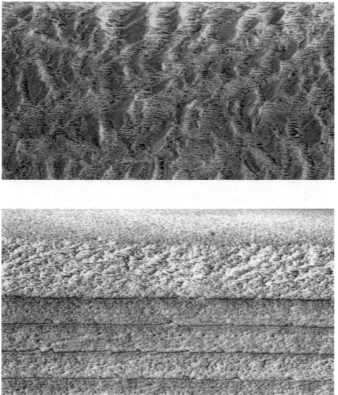

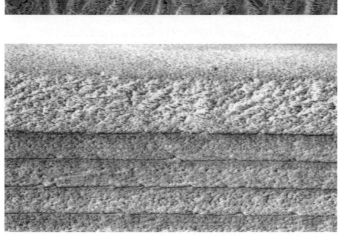

Figure 7.32 *Scanning electron microscopic views of the cross-sectional appearances of the Soft Tissue Patch (top) and the Reconix (bottom).*

laparoscopic repair of incisional hernias have confirmed that there is very little incidence of adhesions to the product.[611]

DualMesh is available in one and two millimeter thicknesses. It is also available with or without the impregnation of silver and chlorhexidine as *DualMesh Plus* (Figure 7.36). These two chemicals are antimicrobial agents that are added to decrease the risk of infection. One study evaluated the possible side effects of these products to the patients but there were no adverse events noted.[273] *DualMesh with holes* is of the same construction as that of the DualMesh (Figure 7.37). The penetration of the holes requires that this product is 1.5 mm in thickness. The concept of the addition of these perforations is

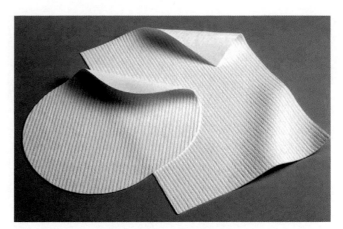

Figure 7.34 *Surface view of the 'corduroy' surface of DualMesh. (W.L. Gore and Associates, Flagstaff, AZ, USA.)*

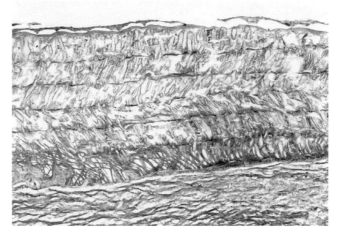

Figure 7.35 *Histologic view with trichrome stain of the collagen deposition (blue) throughout the entire biomaterial of DualMesh. (W.L. Gore and Associates, Flagstaff, AZ, USA.)*

that there may be greater penetration of the fibroblasts and other cells across the material. This has not been shown to be of any clinically significant benefit, however. DualMesh with holes is also available with and without the silver and chlorhexidine as *DualMesh Plus with holes* (Figure 7.37).

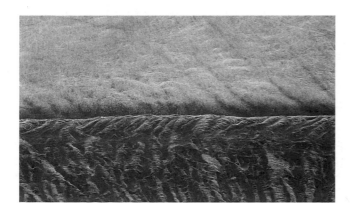

Figure 7.33 *Surface view of the smooth side of DualMesh. (W.L. Gore and Associates, Flagstaff, AZ, USA.)*

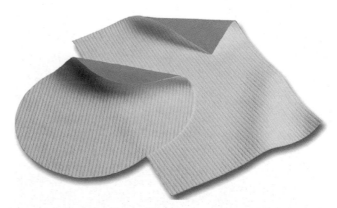

Figure 7.36 *DualMesh Plus. (W.L. Gore and Associates, Flagstaff, AZ, USA.)*

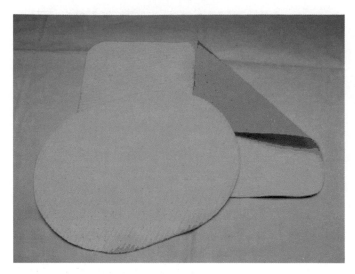

Figure 7.37 *DualMesh Plus with holes. (W.L. Gore and Associates, Flagstaff, AZ, USA.)*

Dulex is a newer product that has only been available for about 2 years (Figure 7.38). Its construction is similar to that of Reconix in that the ePTFE is laminated (Figure 7.39). One surface of the material, however, is studded with numerous outcroppings as seen on the scanning electron microscopic view that are approximate 400 microns apart (Figure 7.39).

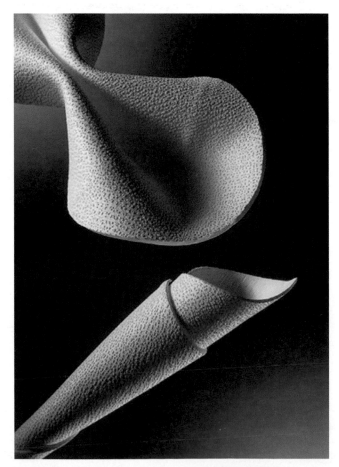

Figure 7.38 *Dulex. (C.R. Bard, Inc., Cranston NJ, USA.)*

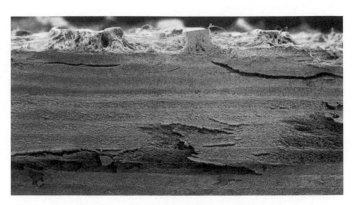

Figure 7.39 *Dulex cross-sectional view. (C.R. Bard, Inc., Cranston NJ, USA.)*

This gives the product the appearance of sandpaper (Figure 7.40). The intent of this surface is to provide for greater fibroblastic attachment and subsequent greater collagen deposition. Further studies are needed to evaluate its effectiveness.

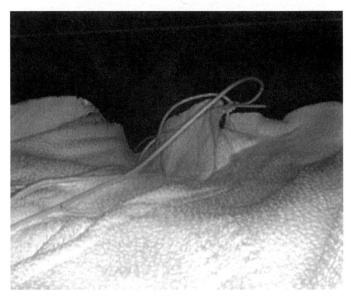

Figure 7.40 *Dulex laparoscopic view. (C.R. Bard, Inc., Cranston NJ, USA.)*

Mycromesh. This is available with (as *Mycromesh Plus*) and without silver and chlorhexidine. This is also a dual-sided prosthetic with one surface of three microns and the other of 17–22 microns. The latter surface is textured. This material is perforated for reasons that are similar to that of the DualMesh Plus with holes. It is only available as a one millimeter thick, however (Figure 7.41).

FLAT MESH DEVICES FOR INGUINAL HERNIOPLASTY

There are a few 'new' concepts in the use of the flat mesh to repair the inguinal floor. While each of these products differ slightly in their intended purpose, all use two separate flat

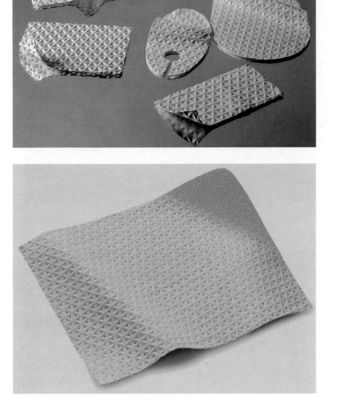

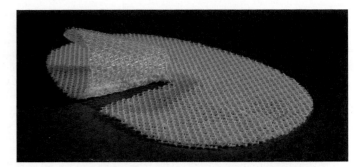

Figure 7.42 *EaseGrip. (Sofradim International, Villfranche-sur-Saône, France.)*

Figure 7.41 *Mycromesh and Mycromesh Plus. (W.L. Gore and Associates, Flagstaff, AZ, USA.)*

Table 7.11 *Flat mesh devices and manufacturer*

EaseGrip®, Sofradim International, Villfranche-sur-Saône, France
LHI mesh, C.R. Bard, Inc., Cranston NJ, USA
Protesi Autoregolantesi Dinamica®, Ethicon S.P.A., Pomezia, Italy
Sperma-Tex, C.R. Bard, Inc., Cranston NJ, USA
T4 Pre-shaped Mesh with Hertra onlay mesh, HerniaMesh, S.R.L., Torino, Italy
T5 Pre-shaped Mesh with Hertra onlay mesh, HerniaMesh, S.R.L., Torino, Italy
Wings®, Angiologica, S. Martino Sicc., Italy

meshes (except for the LHI mesh). These products are listed in Table 7.11.

EaseGrip®. This product is composed of the three-dimensional polyester of Parietex (see above) and is manufactured with a left and a right mesh (Figure 7.42). It is elliptical in shape with a colored marker on the median edge of the prosthesis to indicate the location of the suture that is placed at the pubic tubercle for fixation. There is a self-gripping flap that is designed to overlap the slit that is precut into the biomaterial, which allows for the exit of the cord structures through the mesh. This flap is placed in the inferior position of the inguinal floor. The manufacturer recommends that the external oblique

fascia be closed below the cord structures so that there is no direct contact with the polyester fabric.

The concepts of the *T4* and *T5* meshes are similar (Figure 7.43). As can be seen in the figures, both of these products have a 'pre-shape' shape that includes a circular defect. Both of these meshes are designed to be inserted in the preperitoneal space with the spermatic cord placed within the defect. The larger T5 mesh is meant to be used when there is a significant loss of tissue strength of the transversalis fascia, as in a large Gilbert type III inguinal hernia. The T4 would be used in the small indirect inguinal hernia. Both repairs require the additional Herta onlay mesh (see above) to be placed over the transversalis fascia to complete the repair of the hernia.[1138]

LHI mesh. This is a flat mesh that is preconfigured into the shape of the inguinal area based upon the concepts of the Lichtenstein repair. This was developed according to the requirements of the Lichtenstein Hernia Institute (LHI). This device has a dome that is to be placed adjacent to the pubic tubercle to allow for the increase of the size of this area with normal abdominal wall movements (Figure 7.44). The concept of the dome, however, is actually to allow more prosthetic coverage in that area. This is placed so that the contraction of the tissues during the healing process will not result in a repair that becomes less tension-free because of the expected 'shrinkage' of the mesh. Because of the positioning of the dome, there is a left and a right mesh.

Protesi Autoregolantesi Dinamica (PAD). The English translation is the dynamic self-regulating prosthesis and is an interesting hypothesis. This prosthesis is designed to reduce tension, torsion, wrinkling or dislocation of the prosthesis that is used in the repair of inguinal hernias.[1159] The smaller prosthesis is placed at the point that the internal oblique fuses with the rectus sheath. The larger pre-shaped flat mesh is placed above the initial prosthetic (Figure 7.45). Only the superior and inferior of the respective meshes are affixed with sutures. In this manner, it is said to allow the meshes to assume the correct orientation and thus be self-regulating (see Figure 13.53).

Sperma-Tex. This product is designed specifically for the repair of inguinal hernias. There is a preformed PPM that has an additional piece of ePTFE that is attached on the surface that will contact the cord structures (Figure 7.46). This is placed in that position to prevent adherence of the contents of the inguinal cord to the PPM. Little is known of the effects of this device.

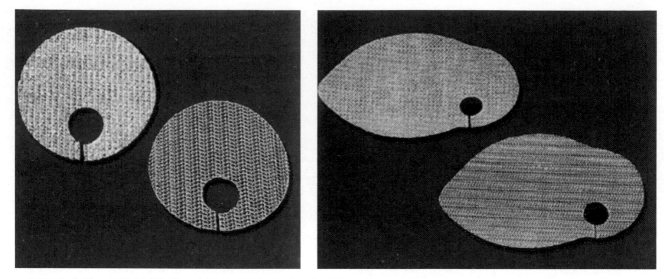

Figure 7.43 *T4 (left) and T5 (right). (HerniaMesh, S.R.L., Torino, Italy.)*

Wings®. This is a similar concept to that of the EaseGrip that uses a single dimension of polypropylene mesh in which there is a precut portion (Figure 7.47). There is a circular defect in a portion of the device to allow for egress of the cord. This two-layer product then has an oblique slit in each of the meshes in opposition to each other. This allows the surgeon the ability to place the mesh around the cord structures allowing the 'wings' to hold the mesh in place around the cord. It is stated that this allows the prosthetic placement to be sutureless.

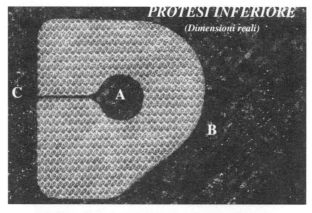

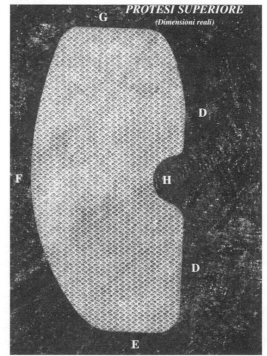

Figure 7.45 *Protesi Autoregolantesi Dinamica (PAD). (Ethicon S.P.A., Pomezia, Italy.)*

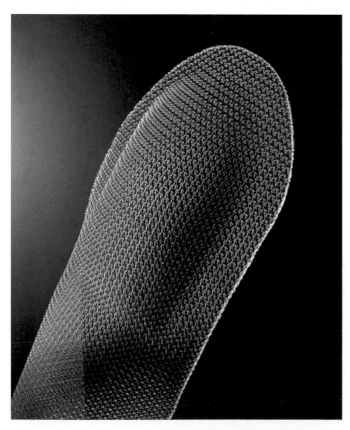

Figure 7.44 *LHI mesh. (C.R. Bard, Inc., Cranston NJ, USA.)*

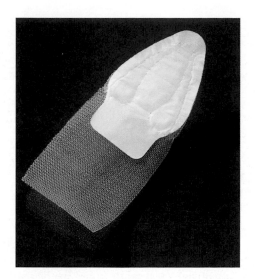

Figure 7.46 *Sperma-Tex. (C.R. Bard, Inc., Cranston NJ, USA.)*

COMBINATION PROSTHETIC BIOMATERIALS FOR HERNIOPLASTY

There are relatively few such materials available for the surgeon to use in the repair of hernias. This material has been available

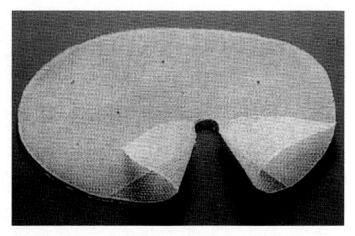

Figure 7.47 *Wings. (Angiologica, S. Martino Sicc., Italy.)*

in Europe for the most part. This concept has been promulgated because of the diminution in the 'weight' of the synthetic mesh that remains following the implantation of this product and once the absorbable product has been resorbed.[1204]

These biomaterials, *Vypro* and *Vypro II* are actually a combination of PPM and the absorbable polymer polydioxone (Vicryl®, Ethicon, Somerville, NJ). As is readily evident in Figure 7.48, these materials are distinctively different than all

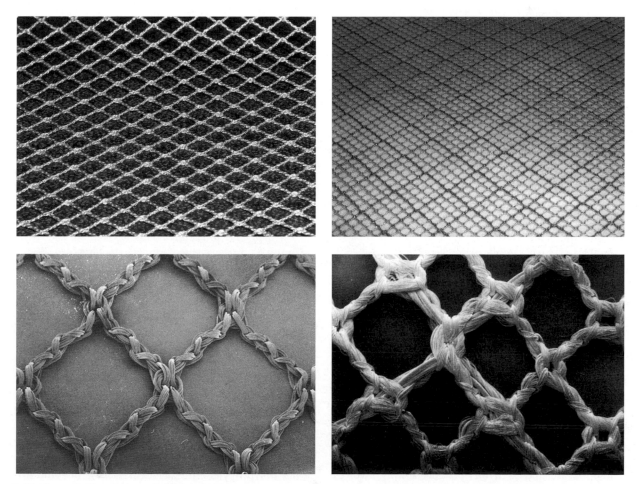

Figure 7.48 *Vypro (left) and Vypro II (right). (Ethicon.)*

of the other synthetic biomaterials that are currently available. The combination of these materials results in a very pliable and malleable material. Once the polydioxione has been absorbed, the PPM that remains has very large interstices into which the fibroblasts and collagen are deposited (Figure 7.49). This results in an abdominal wall compliance that is more normal in function than that of the polypropylene materials that has been available in the past.[560,1204]

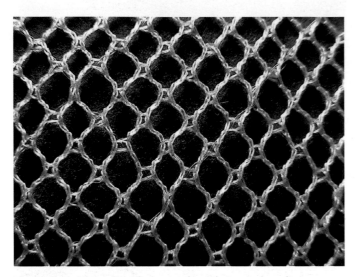

Figure 7.49 *View of the polypropylene that remains after absorption of the polydioxanone.*

PREFORMED PROSTHETIC DEVICES FOR OPEN HERNIOPLASTY

There has been a significant amount of interest in the repair of inguinal and femoral hernias utilizing one of the many preformed prosthetic devices in the last several years. The manufacturers of these prostheses have developed several ingenious products for this use. All are of a polypropylene biomaterial. There is currently an increasing interest by a few surgeons in the application of some of these for the repair of other hernias of the abdominal wall such as umbilical and ventral hernias.[827]

The first such devices were plugs. Lichtenstein first reported the use of cylindrically coiled mesh plug to repair recurrent femoral and inguinal hernias in 1974.[692] Bendavid described the use of a mesh umbrella to repair primary femoral hernia in 1987.[107] This was followed by the report of Gilbert in 1992 on the use of a polypropylene plug that was configured into the shape of an umbrella to treat indirect hernias.[407] They all abandoned the use of these 'home-made' devices because of shrinkage of the inserts, which lead to recurrences of the hernias. A similar device that was called a 'dart' was also used with this concept. It, too, was abandoned. The first commercially successful device was that of the Perfix plug and patch. The devices that are currently available are shown in Table 7.12. The repair of inguinal hernias with this product simply involves the insertion of the plug into the fascial defect, which is then

Table 7.12 *Plug type prosthetic devices and manufacturer*

Atrium® Self-Forming Plug, Atrium Medical Corporation, Hudson, NH, USA

Atrium® Pro-loop Plug, Atrium Medical Corporation, Hudson, NH, USA

Biomesh Plug and Patch, Cousin Biotech, Wervicq-Sud, France

HerniaMate®, US Surgical Corporation/Tyco, Inc., Norwalk, CN, USA

Obtura Mesh®, Cousin Biotech, Wervicq-Sud, France

Perfix® Plug and Patch, C.R. Bard, Inc., Cranston NJ, USA

REPOL Plug Flower, Angiologica, S. Martino Sicc., Italy

REPOL Plug Cap, Angiologica, S. Martino Sicc., Italy

T2 and T3 Plugs, HerniaMesh, S.R.L., Torino, Italy

secured to the edges of the fascia. Additionally, they also employ the use of an overlay of an additional piece of mesh to complete the repair. There are structural differences with these products that alter the concept of each one.

Atrium Self-Forming Plug. While representing a plug-like product, this device is not quite the same as most of the other devices. The concept with this product is that it will conform to the hernia defect upon insertion. Rather than a stiff fluted cone the Atrium plug is made of three circular flat meshes constructed of Atrium mesh (Figure 7.50). These are bonded together with a tab on one surface to allow for the grasping of the product by forceps during insertion. This is soft and pliable so that it assumes the shape of the defect rather than forcing itself into the defect. It, too, is available in different sizes. Additionally, this plug is available in the Prolite Ultra™ mesh construction which makes this very soft and pliable. Due to this softness, it may be associated with the least amount of postoperative pain that has been seen in other plug devices.[427]

Atrium Pro-loop Plug. This is an extension of the other type of plugs but this product has a very unique appearance (Figure 7.51). As shown in the photo, this product is quite different in appearance from the other plug devices. Although preformed into a cylindrical shape, it is very supple and conforms to the defect into which it is inserted. This is a new product and there is little clinical information at this time.

Biomesh Plug and Patch. This device, like the Atrium self-forming plug attempts to configure the plug into the size that is appropriate to the hernia defect. This product differs in that there is a purse-string suture that is pre-placed (Figure 7.52). The surgeon tightens the suture to the size deemed necessary and inserts the plug (this can be done without the use of the suture, however). The suture can then be tied or removed once the plug has been inserted.

HerniaMate®. This product is very similar to the Perfix® device but it is structurally based on the monofilament of Surgipro® rather than that of Marlex® in the Perfix®. It also contains internal petals that can be removed to modify the plug to fit the fascial defect (Figure 7.53).

Obtura Mesh®. This device also attempts to plug the hernia defect but is a hollow configuration or cone fabricated from a flat polypropylene mesh (Figure 7.54). The 'mouth' of the product has a flat piece of mesh to seal the upper portion so

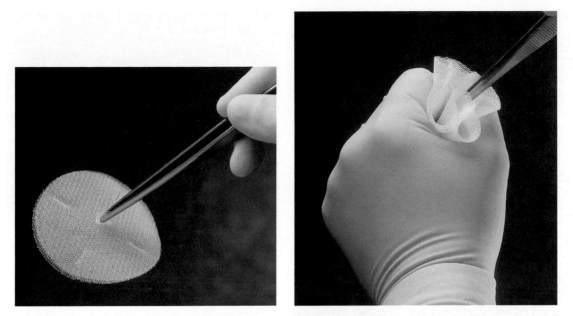

Figure 7.50 *Atrium Self-Forming Plug. (Atrium Medical Corporation, Hudson, NH, USA.)*

that this repair is similar to the plug and patch within one product device. Obtura is a relatively new device at the time of this printing and little is known of the long-term results of this newer concept in the plug-type devices.[304]

Perfix® Plug and Patch. This product is available in three different sizes (Figure 7.55). This is the most mature of the commercial products. This has become a very popular method for repair of inguinal hernias that has been easy and rapid to

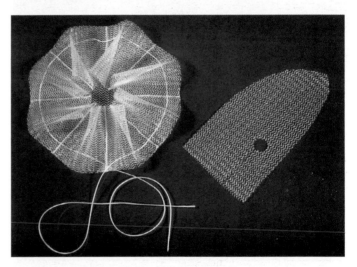

Figure 7.52 *Biomesh Plug and Patch. (Cousin Biotech, Wervicq-Sud, France.)*

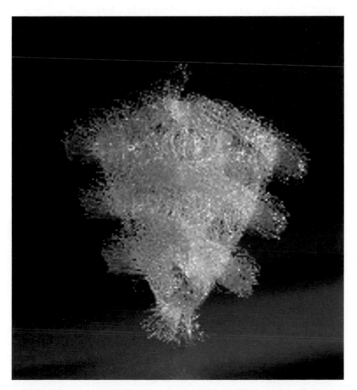

Figure 7.51 *Pro-loop Plug. (Atrium Medical Corporation, Hudson, NH, USA.)*

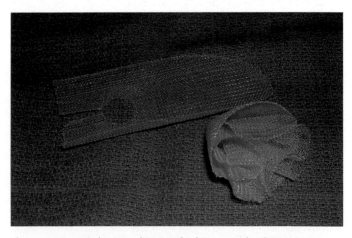

Figure 7.53 *HerniaMate. (US Surgical Corporation/Tyco, Inc., Norwalk, CN, USA.)*

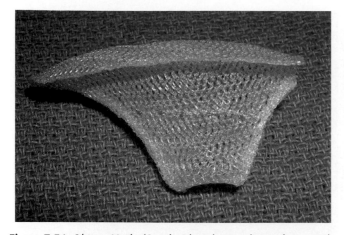

Figure 7.54 *Obtura Mesh. (Cousin Biotech, Wervicq-Sud, France.)*

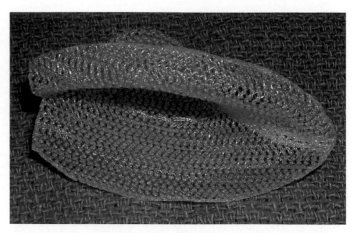

REPOL Plug Flower. This product closely resembles the Perfix® plug (Figure 7.57). It has six 'petals' that are to be inserted into the hernia defect as do the other plugs.

REPOL Plug Cap. This product closely resembles the T2 plugs of HerniaMesh S.R.L. It has a three 'pedalled' plug device with a circular piece of polypropylene mesh attached to the top of the product (Figure 7.58).

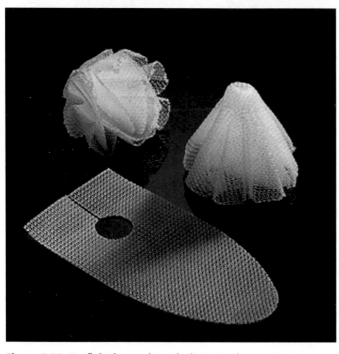

Figure 7.55 *Perfix® Plug and Patch. (C.R. Bard, Inc., Cranston NJ, USA.)*

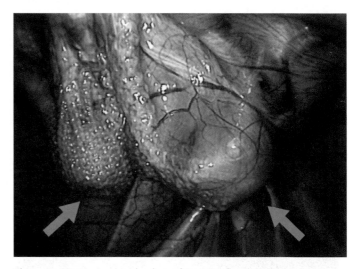

Figure 7.56 *Laparoscopic view of two Perfix plug at the internal ring.*

perform. The published reports of the use of this device have shown acceptable results.[828,996,997] One report details success with a modification of the configuration of the plug.[794] There are a few recognized outcomes with these plugs, the most frequent of these is persistent chronic pain in about 6–10% of the patients.[878] In many individuals, this has necessitated another operation for the removal of the device in as many as 7% of the patients.[594] Other complications have included migration, small bowel fistulization and deep venous thrombosis.[656] This may be related to improper surgical technique, 'shrinkage' or the fact that this device is quite stiff and has a significant protrusion into the abdominal cavity. Figure 7.56 shows the laparoscopic appearance of such a device. Complications have not been reported with the use of the other 'plug' type devices but this may be related to the fact that there is a paucity of literature detailing the use of them.

T2 and T3 Plugs. These devices are also significantly different from all of the other plugs. The T2 plugs have a circular piece of flat mesh that has a rounded plug portion affixed to it whereas the T3 plugs have a rectangular piece of mesh affixed to it (Figure 7.59). There are differing sizes that are chosen based upon the size of the defect. The concept is still that of the plug and patch but the rounded plug may be associated with fewer complications than the cone-shaped ones. There are no clinical data to support this idea, however.

The commonality of all of these devices is the use of an onlay of a flat mesh onto the transversalis fascia. There are differences in the size of the patch as well as the type of

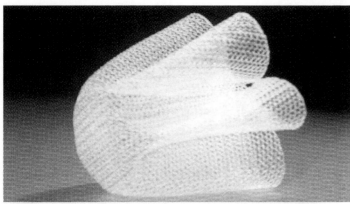

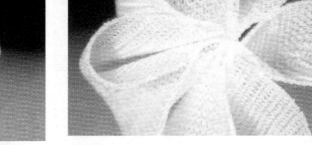

Figure 7.57 *REPOL Plug Flower. (Angiologica, S. Martino Sicc., Italy.)*

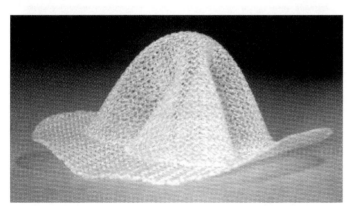

Figure 7.58 *REPOL Plug Cap. (Angiologica, S. Martino Sicc., Italy.)*

polypropylene weave and thickness of the mesh. The popularity of this type of repair is based upon the ease of use and the rapidity of the operation itself. While the majority of use of these devices has been in the repair of inguinal hernias, there are scattered reports of the use of some of them in the repair of umbilical and ventral hernias.

EXTRAPERITONEAL PROSTHETIC DEVICES FOR OPEN INGUINAL HERNIORRHAPHY

The posterior repair of inguinal hernias is based upon the approach in the preperitoneal space. The use of a preformed prosthetic device in this space represents an emulation of the Stoppa repair and the giant prosthetic repair of the visceral sac of Wantz. The products that have been manufactured for this concept are not 'giant' prostheses, however. There currently are three such products (Table 7.13).

Table 7.13 *Flat devices and their manufacturer*

Kugel Patch, C.R. Bard, Inc., Cranston NJ, USA
Prolene Hernia System, Ethicon Inc., Somerville, NJ, USA
Prolene 3D Patch, Ethicon Inc., Somerville, NJ, USA

Kugel Patch. This product consists of two oblong circular flat meshes of Marlex® mesh. Near the edge of the device is a polyester ring that maintains the shape of the device after insertion into the preperitoneal space (Figure 7.60). There are

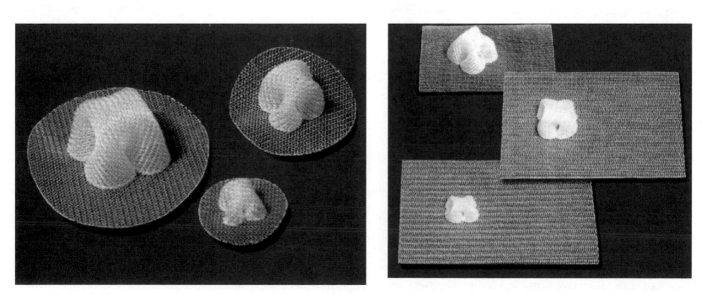

Figure 7.59 *T2 (left) and T3 (right) Plugs. (HerniaMesh, S.R.L., Torino, Italy.)*

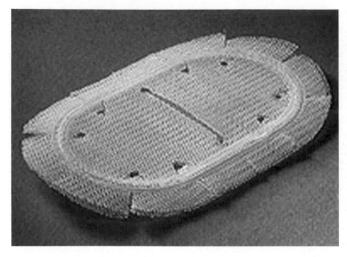

Figure 7.60 *Kugel Patch. (C.R. Bard, Inc., Cranston NJ, USA.)*

several sizes of this product as well as those that are in the circular configuration.[622] The latter materials have seen increasing usage in the repair of ventral hernias.

Because of the increasing use of this product in the preperitoneal or extraperitoneal position, a layer of ePTFE has been placed on one surface of the device (Figure 7.61). This has been added in an effort to shield the bowel from the PPM surface. This product has also had a few anecdotal reports of its use for ventral and incisional hernias.[626]

Prolene Hernia System. This product also represents a departure from the traditional concepts in the use of prosthetic biomaterials in the repair of hernias. It is based upon the best

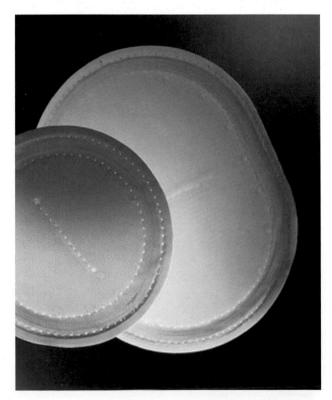

Figure 7.61 *Composix Kugel Patch. (C.R. Bard, Inc., Cranston NJ, USA.)*

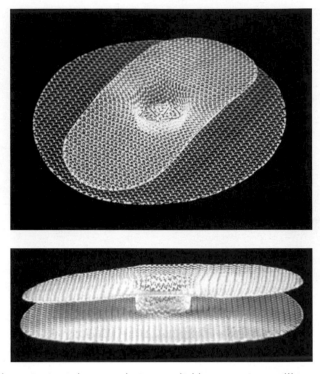

Figure 7.62 *Prolene Hernia System. (Ethicon Inc., Somerville, NJ, USA.)*

aspects of the 'tension-free' repairs, which include the placement of the onlay prosthetic patch, the placement of prosthesis in the preperitoneal position, and the use of a device to fill the fascial defect. In that regard, the PHS product consists of a rounded underlay mesh that is connected to an oblong overlay mesh by a cylindrical portion of mesh. The entire product is constructed of Prolene® mesh.

This product is available in three sizes: medium, large, and extended (Figure 7.62). As shown the differences in these are the size of the underlay and/or the size of the overlay portions of the device. The use of this product has been associated with few complications[594] and an exceedingly low rate of recurrence seen in only two of 3000 patients.[410,411] There are anecdotal reports of the use of this product in the repair of umbilical and smaller incisional hernias.

Prolene 3D Patch. This is a new three-dimensional device for the repair of inguinal hernias. As seen in Figure 7.63, there are two portions to this product. The diamond shaped portion is inserted into the preperitoneal space. A single pull of the suture causes the diamond to flatten out underneath the tranversalis fascia (Figure 7.63). The overlay portion is then secured as in the tension-free repairs. It is available in two sizes of the diamond portion and with or without a pre-shaped overlay.

PRE-SHAPED PRODUCTS FOR LAPAROSCOPIC INGUINAL HERNIORRHAPHY

The history of laparoscopic repair of inguinal hernias involved flat meshes of one type or another. This continues to be the

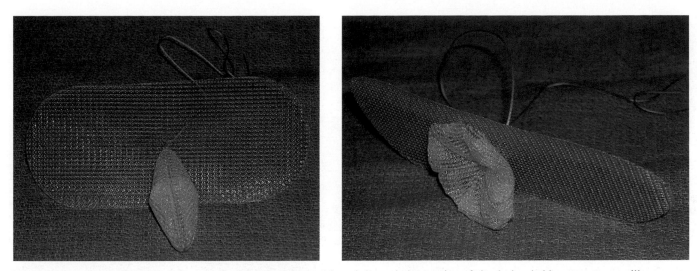

Figure 7.63 *Prolene 3D Patch before and after fixation of the position of the underlay portion of the device. (Ethicon Inc., Somerville, NJ, USA.)*

most frequently used prosthetic product for this operation. There are, however, a number of devices that have been constructed for this procedure (Table 7.14). These all attempt to ease the placement of the prosthetic over the myopectineal orifice or serve to conform to the anatomic surfaces at that site of the repair.

Table 7.14 *Pre-shaped products and manufacturer*

3D Max, C.R. Bard, Inc., Cranston NJ, USA
Anatomical Mesh (TECT), Sofradim International,
   Villfranche-sur-Saône, France
Folding Mesh, Sofradim International, Villfranche-sur-Saône,
   France
Folding Rigid Mesh, Sofradim International,
   Villfranche-sur-Saône, France
Visilex, C.R. Bard, Inc., Cranston NJ, USA

3D Max. This product represents a rather unique concept for the laparoscopic inguinal hernia repair in that the prosthesis is in two preformed sizes but with a similar configuration (Figure 7.64). Upon insertion into the patient, the device opens to conform to the convexity of the myopectineal orifice. Because of this shape there is a left and a right product for the appropriate placement. It is made of PPM and, as such, exhibits the typical 'stickiness' of such a material. Because of this fact, it is felt by many surgeons who use this device that there is no need for the use of any fixation of the product. The reports thus far have shown favorable results with this prosthesis.[876] There can be some difficulty with the deployment of the device in the thinner or smaller patient due to the shape of the product and the lack of an identifiable landmark on the prosthesis itself to assist in orientation. This typically can be overcome with experience or the use of the smaller product (which requires fixation).

Anatomical Mesh (TECT). This represents another attempt to conform to the configuration of the myopectineal orifice.

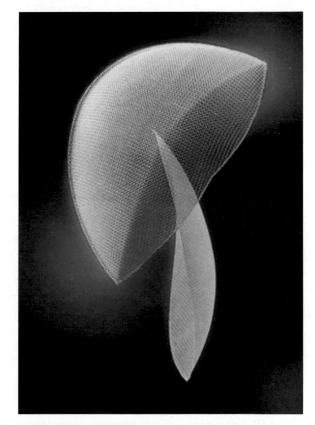

Figure 7.64 *3D Max. (C.R. Bard, Inc., Cranston NJ, USA.)*

There is a large flat piece of Parietene® (PPM) that is to lie on the undersurface of the inguinal floor. This has an attached piece of Parietex® polyester that is designed to lie over the iliac vessels. This latter material is pre-shaped to conform to that anatomy (Figure 7.65). There is limited use for this device that has been reported thus far.

Folding Mesh (TEC). The Parietex® TEC mesh is shaped as a flat mesh with rounded edges that is 10×14 cm in size. To aid in the insertion and deployment of this mesh in the preperitoneal

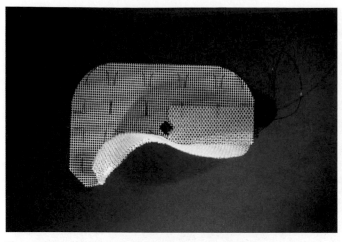

Figure 7.65 *Anatomical Mesh (TECT). (Sofradim International, Villfranche-sur-Saône, France.)*

space during the laparoscopic repair there is a suture that is woven through the material (Figure 7.66). This suture is placed such that when it is pulled tight the mesh will be drawn into a small somewhat cylindrical shape (Figure 7.66). It is then placed into the preperitoneal space whereupon the suture is cut, allowing the mesh to resume its original shape. It can then be positioned appropriately. This device is also available with a slit if one desires to place the cord structures within it.

Folding Rigid Mesh (TECR). This product is identical to the one above except that it is made of the TECR polyester mesh and is, therefore, more rigid.

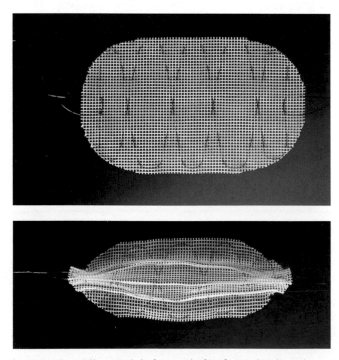

Figure 7.66 *Folding Mesh before and after formation into the cylindrical shape. (Sofradim International, Villfranche-sur-Saône, France.)*

Visilex. There is a rigid edge of the PPM, which is meant to ease the manipulation of the mesh in the preperitoneal space during laparoscopic inguinal hernia repair (Figure 7.67). It is estimated that it is used in approximately 4% of these operations.

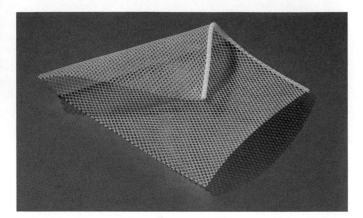

Figure 7.67 *Visilex. (C.R. Bard, Inc., Cranston NJ, USA.)*

BIOMATERIALS FOR INCISIONAL AND VENTRAL HERNIORRHAPHY WITH AN ABSORBABLE COMPONENT

Somewhat surprisingly, most of the currently available products for this operation are modifications of older materials or a composite type material of the older synthetic biomaterials. However, recently newer composite materials have been introduced. While the driving force behind the development of these products has been the upsurge in popularity of the laparoscopic methodology, in general, all of these prosthetic devices can or have been used in both open and laparoscopic incisional herniorrhaphies. All of these have the common purpose to repair the hernia and eliminate or prevent the development of adhesions with the attendant complications associated with this result of the healing processes. Only a few of these products have long-term follow-up data to support the idea that there is a lack of problems related to adhesion formation.

These products incorporate an absorbable layer or an integral portion into a non-absorbable product (Table 7.15). The resorption of that substance leaves a permanent layer of mesh that will incorporate into the tissues of the patient. The intent of the product combination is the diminution of the development of intestinal adhesions that will predispose the patient to the risk of obstruction or fistulization. The confusing part of this idea is the fact that the problems that are related to the development of adhesions following the implantation of a synthetic biomaterial do not become manifest for many years post-implantation. Therefore, the late effects of these products will necessitate many years of follow-up to validate these claims.

Parietex® Composite. This is the same polyester biomaterial (Parietex®) that is described earlier in this chapter. It has an

Table 7.15 *Composite biomaterials with an absorbable component and manufacturer*

Parietex® Composite, Sofradim International, Villfranche-sur-Saône, France
Parietene® Composite, Sofradim International, Villfranche-sur-Saône, France
Sepramesh®, Genzyme Corporation, Cambridge, Massachusetts, USA
Glucamesh, Brennen Medical, Inc., St. Paul, MN
Glucatex 3D, Brennen Medical, Inc., St. Paul, MN

incorporated hydrophilic layer of a mixture of oxidized Type I atelocollagen, polyethylene glycol and glycerol, which is absorbable (Figure 7.68).

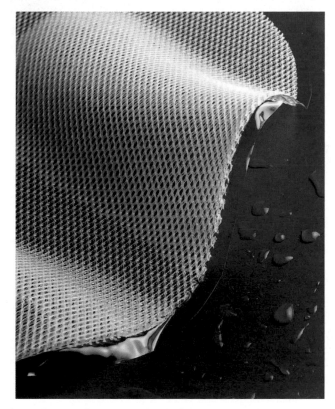

Figure 7.68 *Paritex Composite. (Sofradim International, Villfranche-sur-Saône, France.)*

Parietene® Composite. This likewise is the same as the polypropylene Parietene® biomaterial noted above but which also has the absorbable film incorporated within it. These materials will experience resorption of the collagen within a few weeks. There are a few reports that have had a favorable experience in limited numbers of patients.[74,106,806]

Sepramesh®. A single layer of polypropylene is covered by the previously released Seprafilm® which is marketed as an anti-adhesive biomaterial (Figure 7.69). The 'barrier' is a combination of carboxymethylcellulose and hyaluronic acid. This portion of the product is stated to last approximately 7 days, at which point, it has been resorbed by the inflammatory cells that are present in reaction to the product. One

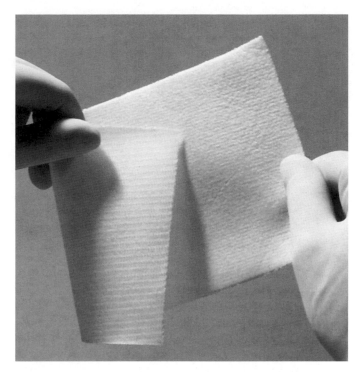

Figure 7.69 *Sepramesh. (Genzyme Corporation, Cambridge, Massachusetts, USA.)*

must be careful in the use of this product so that the foam is not dislodged during implantation. Additionally, the manufacturer recommends that the omentum should be placed under the material to protect the bowel. There are only reports regarding the Sepramesh® product in the use in the experimental animal.[435] Clinical trials and long-term studies are in process.

Glucamesh. This is a non-woven mesh that is composed of polypropylene thermally bonded together and impregnated with oat beta glucan (Figure 7.70). Oat beta glucan is a purified complex carbohydrate that is isolated from the cell wall of oats. This product has been studied as a potential biological response modifier.[337] It has an interesting microscopic picture (Figure 7.71). It was available in France at the beginning of 2001 and was released for use in the USA at the end of 2002. It is also available in a pre-shaped mesh that has a slit to be used around the spermatic cord in the repair of inguinal hernias. Clinical studies are ongoing.

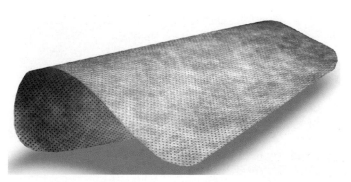

Figure 7.70 *Glucamesh. (Brennen Medical, Inc., St Paul, MN.)*

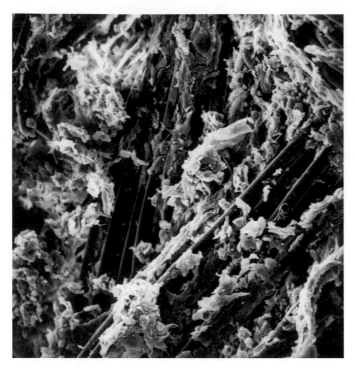

Figure 7.71 *Microscopic view of Glucamesh. (Brennen Medical, Inc., St Paul, MN.)*

Glucatex 3D. This product also contains the oat beta glucan as an absorbable component that has been bonded to a three dimensional polyester biomaterial. It, too, is designed to be used in either open or laparoscopic hernia repair. It has not been released for use at the mid-year of 2002 but should be available in the future.

PERMANENT BIOMATERIALS FOR INCISIONAL AND VENTRAL HERNIORRHAPHY (Table 7.16)

These products can be used in either the open or the laparoscopic repair of these hernias with the exception of the Parietex® TEL prosthesis. The choice of methodology will be dictated by the location and size of the hernia as well as the surgeon's preference. The DualMesh and Dulex prostheses were described earlier in this chapter (pages 89 and 90)

Table 7.16 *Permanent prostheses for LIVH and manufacturer*

Composix, C.R. Bard, Inc., Cranston NJ, USA
Composix EX, C.R. Bard, Inc., Cranston NJ, USA
Composix Kugel Patch, C.R. Bard, Inc., Cranston NJ, USA
DualMesh, W.L. Gore and Associates, Flagstaff, AZ, USA
DualMesh Plus, W.L. Gore and Associates, Flagstaff, AZ, USA
DualMesh with holes, W.L. Gore and Associates, Flagstaff, AZ, USA
DualMesh Plus with holes, W.L. Gore and Associates, Flagstaff, AZ, USA
Dulex, C.R. Bard, Inc., Cranston NJ, USA
Intramesh W3, Cousin Biotech, Wevicq-Sud, France
Parietex TEL, Sofradim International, Villfranche-sur-Saône, France

(Figures 7.33–7.40). These products are more easily deformable than those below. In fact, because the structure of the Dual-Mesh is not laminated (as is the Dulex) and it is 50% air by volume, even the largest of the sizes can be inserted into the abdomen via a five-millimeter port site. These products and those described below are available in a variety of sizes.

Two composite materials incorporate polypropylene with an anti-adhesive material. The first of these to be introduced was *Composix*® mesh (Figure 7.72). This material uses the PPM Marlex® with a very thin layer of ePTFE that is heat sealed onto the PPM. This biomaterial is stiff as it is two layers of Marlex® rather than one flat mesh. The ePTFE layer is easily perforated and can separate from the PPM in the surgical manipulation that is necessary for its implantation. Care must be exercised in its use. Additionally, it is impossible to roll this product into a sufficiently small roll so as to permit its introduction into the abdominal cavity via a 5 mm trocar site. It is, in fact, difficult to place it through 10 mm ports as well. There are, however, several centres that have used this product for laparoscopic repair. There are currently no clinical data that has been reported regarding the long-term use and benefits of this biomaterial. However, one experimental study found that 70% of the animals had adhesions to this material.[435]

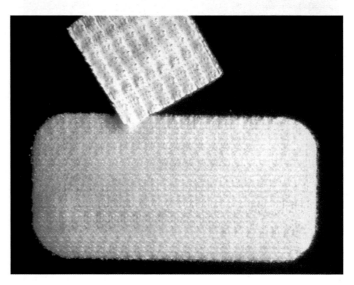

Figure 7.72 *Composix. (C.R. Bard, Inc., Cranston NJ, USA.)*

Many of the difficulties in the use of the original Composix mesh have been improved with the introduction of the *Composix EX* (Figure 7.73). This is a single layer of Marlex® that has ePTFE on one surface that is sewn to the PPM portion. As such this product is more pliable but must still be introduced with the larger port sizes. The ePTFE layer is more stable as it is sewn rather than heated onto the PPM. It also overlaps the PPM layer to prevent the contact of the edge of the mesh to the intestine. Some surgeons do not use any transfascial sutures with this product in the laparoscopic repair of incisional hernias but there are no short- or long-term studies that validate this method of fixation.

Composix Kugel Patch. The Kugel patch that is described on page 98 above has been adapted for use in the repair of

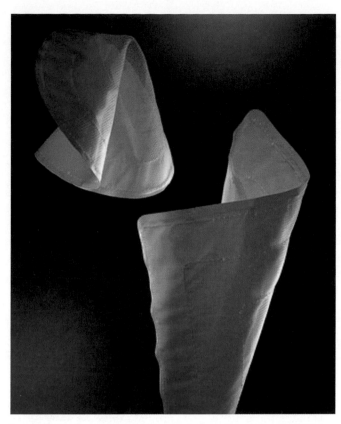

Figure 7.73 *Composix EX. (C.R. Bard, Inc., Cranston NJ, USA.)*

incisional, ventral and umbilical hernias. The smaller hernias can be repaired with the standard Kugel patch but if the peritoneum has been violated there is a need to protect the bowel from the polypropylene component. This product is a hybrid of the standard Kugel patch with a layer of ePTFE similar to that of the Composix EX (Figure 7.61).

Intramesh® W3. A polyester material that is neither woven nor knitted is combined with a silicone surface to lessen adhesions. This is also perforated with 0.8 mm micro-perforations that are placed to allow for fluid exchange (Figure 7.74). Little is known about the use of this prosthesis in the repair of hernias.

TEL. This is another adaptation of the Parietex® TEC mesh. This product has an 'X' shape. It is designed so that the

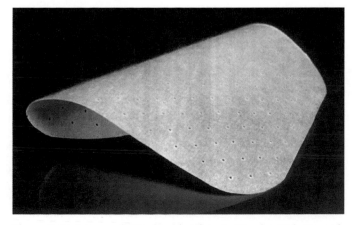

Figure 7.74 *Intramesh W3. (Cousin Biotech, Wervicq-Sud, France.)*

prosthesis is placed in the fascial defect with the wings of the device to be placed anterior and posterior to the anterior wall musculature. The stated preferred use of this biomaterial is in the open repair of larger incisional hernias.

COMMENT ON ADHESIONS AND BIOMATERIALS

It is common knowledge that there are risks of adhesions with the use of any prosthetic biomaterial within the abdominal cavity in contact with the intestines. In fact, adhesions can be commonly seen in the inguinal area resulting from an anterior inguinal hernia repair despite the fact that the peritoneum was never violated. These result from the intense inflammatory response that some of these meshes generate. Therefore, not all adhesions can be prevented. The newer products that are available, and undoubtedly those that will become available in the future, are trying to address this difficult and undesirable phenomenon. While there are many anecdotal experiences in re-operation of patients that have had implantation of all of these meshes, laboratory data is also available to assist the surgeon in the decision of the choice of a prosthetic biomaterial for the repair of hernias. There is one article that showed favorable outcomes at unrelated re-operation following prior laparoscopic implantation of DualMesh® in the repair of incisional hernias.[611]

The findings that are noted in the laboratory are that the larger the pores and the thicker the biomaterial the greater the increase in the amount of adhesions as well as an increase in the tenacity of these adhesions. Laboratory studies involving both rabbit and porcine models have demonstrated the differences in the adhesive potential in these different products.[653,654,666] In these experiments the amount of adhesions and the difficulty that was encountered in the dissection of them off the biomaterial at 30 and 90 days after implantation were evaluated. These explants were scored as an 'adhesion score'. The extent of the prosthesis covered by adhesions was given a number from 1–4 based upon 25% points of coverage. A score of one indicated that 25% or less of the biomaterial was covered by adhesions, two indicated 50% or less, etc. The tenacity was graded from 1–3 based upon adhesions that were easily pulled off, bluntly dissected off or excised with scissor dissection. A score of three reflected the need for scissor dissection to release the adhesions. These values were added together so that the combined scores ranged from 1–7 (seven being the worst possible score). The percentage of the prosthetic that was covered by adhesions was noted and is shown in Figure 7.75. The score from 1–7 divided by the number of animals provides the adhesion scores shown in Figure 7.76. It was apparent that stiffer biomaterials with larger pore sizes produced a corresponding increase in the amount of adhesions seen as well as increasing the difficulty in the removal of them from the prosthesis (i.e. a higher adhesion score). The greatest extremes are noted between Marlex® and first-generation DualMesh® as used in these studies.

The results of these studies are borne out in the clinical situation. The adhesions that are encountered with reoperation of

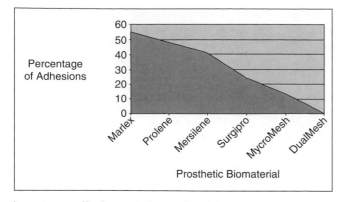

Figure 7.75 *Adhesions noted to various biomaterials.*

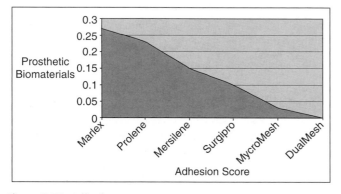

Figure 7.76 *Adhesion scores.*

the patients that have had a PPM implant are quite tenacious and frequently difficult to remove. This results in significant risk of adhesions and potential fistulization and has been seen in polyester products as well.[374,652] The Koehler study noted above found little adhesions with ePTFE. To overcome the problems with adhesions to the omentum and bowel as well as the risk of fistulization, manufacturers have responded with new materials. The need for this type of material is particularly acute with the laparoscopic repair of incisional hernias.

COMMENT REGARDING SHRINKAGE OF MESHES

There has been and there continues to be a significant amount of discussion regarding the 'shrinkage' of the prostheses that are use in the repair of hernias. One of the concerns about shrinkage is that the implanted product will not continually cover the areas necessary to prevent a recurrence of the hernia defect. The data that has been advanced now identify this 'shrinkage' as scar maturation. As such, this represents a normal event in the healing phase of a wound. Therefore, a change in the size of all of the prosthetic biomaterials following implantation should be expected. This phenomenon has been one of the reasons that have resulted in the recommendation that a minimum of 3 cm of overlap of the prosthetic biomaterial is necessary to repair incisional hernias laparoscopically.

One of the findings that was noted in the animal studies above was that if the mesh were not flat on the abdominal cavity at the edges of the mesh, there were a higher proportion of adhesions in those animals. This finding should encourage the surgeon to place the prosthetic material as flat as feasible during the repair so that the potential for adhesions will be lessened. This will be influenced by the method of fixation that is utilized.

CONCLUSIONS

- The use of a prosthetic biomaterial for all hernia repairs is the norm rather than an isolated event. In fact, because of the common use of these products there are some individuals that now question if there is too much use of synthetic products to repair some hernias.[853] The purpose of this chapter is to identify and differentiate the products that can be used in hernioplasties. It is as complete as we could make it at this time. Undoubtedly by the time of the printing of this textbook others will have become available. The surgeon should choose carefully.

- We believe that the ideal material has not yet been developed. There are, however, many that have been described above that do function quite well for the surgeon and the patient. Perhaps in the future, the use of genetic engineering will produce a product that is based on human protein from the patient and will allow the patient to incorporate a 'natural' and 'native' product into the tissues without fear of infection or adhesions. A permanent solution to the quest of the perfect biomaterial may be the result.

8

Anesthesia

CHOICE OF ANESTHESIA: GENERAL, REGIONAL OR LOCAL ANESTHETIC

Even though local anesthesia with sedation (so-called monitored anesthesia care) is a more cost-effective anesthetic technique for inguinal hernia repair,[1071] general and regional anesthesia remain the most popular techniques in most district general hospitals. Interestingly, specialized hernia centers use local infiltration anesthesia in more than 90% of these cases.[26,169,423,595,961] The few audit data that exist indicate that on a national and regional scale, general anesthesia is used in 60–70% of cases, regional anesthesia in 10–20% and local infiltration anesthesia in only 5–10% of cases.[97,459,849,860]

General, regional, or local anesthesia is suitable for the repair of most hernias and the type of anesthesia employed may depend on the preferences and skills of the surgical team rather than the wishes of the patient. In socialized systems of healthcare there are no effective incentives for the widespread adoption of cost-effective techniques and for this reason in Europe general anesthesia and regional anesthesia predominate. In contrast in the USA where market forces prevail and the payor can demand that the less expensive local anesthesia is utilized for herniorrhaphy, local anesthesia is employed on a much larger scale.

Only rarely nowadays is the patient totally unfit to undergo a suitably judged general anesthetic. Local anesthesia for hernia repair does have particular advantages – organizational and economic as well as clinical. Local anesthesia can be administered by the operator, thus no medical anesthetist is required; the patient does require shared care during an operation performed under local anesthetic and local practice and clinical governance guidelines will dictate whether the monitoring of the local anesthetic with sedation is undertaken by a medical anesthetist, a nurse anesthetist, an operating department assistant or even in some healthcare environments no specialist monitor.[169] Except in a few areas of the USA, when local anesthesia is used for hernia repair, the use of an anesthesiologist is the norm. This is reflective of the medicolegal climate rather than clinical necessity.

Where a nurse is dedicated to the patient throughout a local anesthesia operation, a qualified medical anesthetist should be available to give assistance at short notice. In the setting of a dedicated ambulatory care unit this will mean that the medical anesthetist is not required to be dedicated to one operating room, but is required to be present in the building of the ambulatory unit or if this ambulatory unit is in continuity with the main hospital building, then a medical anesthetist or the 24-h on-call anesthetist can provide anesthetic cover from the main hospital building. As stated above, the standard practice will include the active presence of the anesthesia personnel at the operating table. Peripheral oxygen saturation must be monitored with a pulse oximeter, especially if intravenous sedation is being used. In addition intravenous access should be established in order that the complications of inadvertent intravascular injection of local anesthetic agents, which may result in cerebral and cardiovascular side effects, can be counteracted. Blood pressure should be recorded on arrival in the operating theater and after the injection of local anesthetic, and preferably monitored throughout the procedure. This may be done by connecting the patient to a cardiac monitor supervised by the anesthetic nurse throughout the operation and regularly recording pulse, blood pressure, and respiratory rate. Emergency resuscitation equipment, including the requirements for endotracheal intubation, must be available in the event of severe respiratory depression needing intubation. The side effects of inadvertent intravenous injection of local anesthesia include systemic excitation of the central nervous system with excessive anxiety, convulsions, hypotension or severe dysrhythmias.

The clinical advantages of local anesthetic include the decreased blood ooze when local anesthetic solution with adrenaline is employed, the prolonged analgesia provided (without any central effects), enhanced definition of tissue planes afforded by the hydrodynamic dissection by the local anesthetic distending the tissues, and lastly the patient co-operation possible in testing and identifying anatomic defects, particularly in inguinal hernioplasty. The patient is saved the anxiety of general anesthesia and the hangover effect of recovery.

Surgery under local anesthesia is more demanding for the operator: he or she must be more precise and less traumatic to tissue than in the unconscious patient. Hemostasis must be more secure and the surgeon must not be overheard demanding too many swabs to wipe away uncontrolled bleeding. Above all, when surgery is completed the subject may be asked to cough or strain so that any deficiencies in technique are immediately observed.

Local anesthesia is not a cheap option for the careless surgeon to administer. Good local anesthesia requires knowledge and skill; it demands careful preoperative assessment, intraoperative monitoring and adequate facilities for recovery from its effects. The complications of the local anesthetic drugs – convulsions, dysrhythmias, hypotension and respiratory failure – are as life-threatening as those of general anesthesia. These complications are invariably caused by intravascular injection, which is the most important technical error the operator must avoid. The management of these complications is as demanding as the conduct of a general anesthetic. Unless the surgeon understands these complications and unless the facilities are on hand to manage them, the single-handed surgeon–local anesthetist is putting the patient to hazard. Prudence dictates that surgeons should not uncritically indulge in major local anesthetic administration.

A Systematic Review examined 11 prospective studies including eight randomized controlled trials and three prospective cohort studies that have compared the use of general, local and regional anesthesia in the treatment of inguinal hernias.[208] Eight compared local (LA) and general anesthesia (GA) and three compared GA with regional anesthesia (RA). Summarizing the results of this systematic review, there was evidence that local anesthesia has less adverse effects on respiratory function than both GA and RA. Contrary to popular belief, operations under LA are shorter than those conducted under GA. Wound complications are less common in patients undergoing repair under LA. Studies looking at postoperative pain have yielded differing results: of the four studies that looked at analgesic consumption, one found significantly more analgesia was used by patients who had surgery under LA, two found they used significantly less, and one found no difference. There was evidence that these results may have been influenced by the length of activity of the local anesthetic agent used. Three studies have looked at return to work and found no significant difference between patients treated under LA or GA.

Hernia surgery requiring extensive dissection, major intra-abdominal manipulation, fluid shifts or blood transfusion is rarely advisable under local anesthetic. When the diagnosis is in doubt, or subject to revision during surgery, it is best to avoid local anesthesia. It follows that incarcerated or strangulated hernias should rarely be operated under local anesthesia. The 'poor risk patient' requires that the risk of operation be shared by the surgeon with a skilled anesthetist; for instance, local anesthesia is not automatically safer than general anesthesia after a myocardial infarct. All local anesthetics have cardiovascular effects. Similarly, the patient with liver failure or hepatitis is not immune from the toxic effects of those local anesthetic agents, which are degraded in the liver. The use of local anesthesia is rarely appropriate during laparoscopic repair of inguinal hernias.[324] Even in this series, the bupivacaine was supplemented with the use of a laryngeal mask anesthesia.

Patient preference in the choice of anesthetic cannot be discounted; the Canadian and American literature suggests that patients prefer local anesthesia, or are at least indifferent in the choice, when they undergo surgery for a simple uncomplicated hernia.[203,390,423] This preference is not universally expressed by British patients nor in certain geographic regions of the USA. Whereas there are enthusiasts for local anesthesia in the UK, experience and research suggests that if patients are given an entirely free choice the majority prefer to sleep throughout the procedure. A surgeon should not be carried away by his enthusiasm for local anesthesia; in a dedicated ambulatory unit undertaking inguinal hernia repair under unmonitored local anesthesia, 1000 patients were sent a questionnaire after the surgical intervention.[169] The questionnaire was returned by 940 patients of whom 124 expressed dissatisfaction with the local anesthesia, the day-case set-up or both. The primary reason for complaint by the patients was because of intraoperative pain (7.8%). This is a relatively high rate of dissatisfaction and suggests that the local anesthetic care pathway still has room for improvement in the intraoperative phase.

Modern general anesthesia makes it possible for safe operations to be performed on patients who are to go home 2 h or so later. The need for tracheal intubation is no longer a contraindication to day surgery. The speed of recovery from general anesthesia is paramount to facilitate full and rapid recovery to consciousness and a degree of physical performance commensurate with returning home by private car or taxi. The introduction of new anesthetic agents that are either exhaled without degradation or excreted or metabolized rapidly has extended to selection of patients for general anesthesia at both ends of the age range. General anesthesia may be provided by inhalational or intravenous drugs, or a suitable combination. Propofol is accepted by most anesthetists as the intravenous agent of choice for use in outpatient surgery: it provides the swiftest recovery (compared with barbiturates such as methohexatone), less excitatory phenomena, and smoother induction.[486] There is little to choose between the inhalational agents (halothane, enflurane and isoflurane), particularly in terms of safety. In most patients optimal general anesthesia for day-case inguinal hernia surgery will comprise propofol infusion supplemented with isoflurane and nitrous oxide inhalation for maintenance. Such a regimen provides a stable technique and rapid recovery and return to 'street fitness'.[279]

The time taken to infiltrate the local anesthesia sufficiently to gain satisfactory analgesia has been thought to add significantly to the length of the operative procedure, but this is not so. Two randomized studies have investigated this.[19,605] In one study, a small study with 45 patients in each arm of the randomization, the operating time was significantly lower in the local anesthetic group. In the other (earlier) study it was claimed that local anesthesia needed 3 min more operative time. Certainly, enthusiasts for local anesthesia have never claimed that it takes significantly less time than general anesthesia.

There are disadvantages in introducing opioids such as fentanyl or alfentanyl into the anesthetic sequence because of the incidence of nausea and vomiting, apnea, occasional awareness, and muscle rigidity. Benzodiazepines have proved useful for sedation; however, recovery from intravenous midazolam is not as rapid as recovery from intravenous propafol, which may be used during general anesthesia.

Finally, the administration of a general anesthetic should not be underestimated, irrespective of technique there is a high incidence of side effects that may persist for up to 24 h, such as drowsiness, headache, cognitive effects, muscle pain, nausea and vomiting. Whatever the type of anesthesia, the recurrence rate is low and the long-term outcome is uninfluenced by whether local or general anesthesia is used. The advantages of early ambulation to prevent thromboembolism are negated by the speed of recovery, and hence early ambulation, that can be achieved with modern general anesthesia.

Patients for both general and local anesthesia are transported to and from the operating room on trolleys. The walk to the operating table and the walk away after local anesthesia is dramatic, but does not necessarily confer any benefit on the patient.

Thus, while the advantages and disadvantages of local or general anesthesia must be considered for each and every patient, for open operations the patient's views should not be overruled by the surgeon's personal preference.

LOCAL ANESTHESIA

History

The use of local anesthesia for the repair of groin hernia has a rather exciting history. Cocaine was isolated as a pure alkaloid from the leaves of the coca plant, *Erythroxylum coca*, by Niemann in 1860. It was then exploited by the Austrian Karl Koller in 1884 when he installed it into the eye of a rabbit. This latter discovery is attributed by some to Sigmund Freud, who had been experimenting with cocaine but who deserted his experiments, and the reporting of them, for his fiancée.[745] Freud later wrote:

'In the Autumn of 1886 I began to practise medicine in Vienna and married a girl who had waited more than four years for me in a distant town. Now I realize it was my fiancee's fault I did not become famous at that time. In 1884 I was profoundly interested in the little known alkaloid of coca, which Merck obtained for me to study its physiological properties. During this work, the occasion presented itself of going to see my fiancée, whom I had not seen for two years. I hurriedly finished my work with cocaine, confining myself in my report to remarking it would soon be put to new use. At the same time I suggested to my friend Konigstein, the ophthalmologist, that he should experiment with cocaine in some eye cases. When I came back from holiday, I found it was not to him but to another friend, Karl Koller, that I had spoken about cocaine. Koller had completed the research on the eyes of animals and demonstrated the results to the ophthalmological congress in Heidelberg. Quite rightly the discovery of local

anesthesia by cocaine, of such importance in minor surgery, was thereafter attributed to Koller. But I bear my wife no grudge for what I lost!'

William Stuart Halsted, in 1885, demonstrated that cocaine could block impulses through nerves and in the process became a lifelong cocaine addict himself. He underwent sanatorium treatment for his addiction before his translation to the chair of surgery at Johns Hopkins. He apparently was never truly cured of this addiction, for he continued to require daily cocaine until his death in 1922. Halsted's resident, Harvey Cushing,[259] pursued the development of local anesthesia for groin hernia repair and in 1900 published the original authoritative paper on the nervous anatomy of the inguinal region and his experiences of local anesthesia in the repair of these hernias. Local anesthesia is mentioned in many treatises on hernia, but it has never become as popular in the UK as elsewhere. It is difficult to discover why this is so. Ogilvie's influential book *Hernia*, published in 1959, devotes only two sparse pages to the topic and describes a technique, which would have given the patient little comfort throughout some of the extensive surgical repairs. Ogilvie goes on to elaborate. Perhaps the brevity of Ogilvie's description of local anesthesia can be forgiven in the light of his qualifying sentence: 'Operations for inguinal hernia must often be undertaken urgently in patients whose age or general condition would prohibit such a step were it not for the greater danger of some threatened complication. The risks are largely eliminated by the use of local anesthetics'.[864]

More recently, Glassow has recorded the experience of local anesthesia from the Shouldice clinic in Toronto, an experience beginning in 1954 and including over 25 000 patients.[425] Barwell and Kingsnorth have described similar results using local anesthesia in the UK.[86,595] The use of local anesthesia in the fit patient for hernia repair is associated with few complications, and if the anesthetic is carefully administered no complications attributable to it should occur.

Less experienced hernia surgeons should be introduced to the technique of local anesthesia with caution. Unless the novice is well supervised and fully conversant with the subtle refinements in technique required to operate under local anesthesia, recurrence rates may escalate.[592,810] In a retrospective review Kingsnorth and colleagues demonstrated that the factor most strongly influencing recurrence was the experience of a particular surgeon with local anesthetic technique.[592] A trainee surgeon should master the dissection and reconstruction of the posterior inguinal wall required for inguinal herniorrplasty before adding to this the skills of local anesthesia. Britton and Morris have reviewed the international data and conclude that inguinal hernia repair under local anesthesia should enable any careful surgeon to achieve low recurrence rates at low cost.[148]

Local anesthesia is becoming more popular for two reasons. First, the prolonged analgesia which persists if bupivacaine is employed has enabled patients to walk sooner and go home sooner than after a general anesthetic. Secondly, convalescence for patients with severe cardiorespiratory decompensation, or patients with liver disease for whom an inhalational anesthetic would be inadvisable, is easy. A qualitative Systematic Review of incisional local anesthesia for postoperative pain relief after abdominal operations has been undertaken.[799] Using the Cochrane library issue 4 and Medline, five randomized controlled trials were evaluated comparing local anesthesia versus placebo after open inguinal hernia repair. Outcomes included pain score, analgesic consumption and time of first analgesic. All the five studies showed a 2–7 h duration of clinically relevant improved pain relief with the use of incisional local anesthetic. A study that compared wound infiltration with 0.5% bupivacaine or saline in the first 24 h after hernia repair showed less analgesic consumption and a longer time to first analgesic.[477]

The concept of pre-emptive analgesia has long been debated. This concept envisages that effective postoperative pain relief benefits the patient by providing comfort in the period after surgery as well as modifying the autonomic and somatic reflexes to pain which delay recovery.[1206] The theory is therefore, that effective treatment of acute pain facilitates early rehabilitation and recovery and that pre-emptive analgesic nerve blocks may prevent central sensitization and secondary hyperanalgesia after tissue damage. In a double-blind randomized trial however, utilizing a field block with bupivacaine as preemptive analgesia for inguinal herniorrhaphy, there were no differences in pain scores or analgesics consumptions up to 7 days after surgery when comparing patients who receive the block either at induction but before surgery, or after surgery but before the end of anesthesia.[413]

A further concept in optimal management of postoperative pain relief is that of balanced analgesia.[576] This concept takes the advantage of multimodal additive and synergistic effects of a combination of analgesic drugs including non-steroidal anti-inflammatory agents given preoperatively, incisional local anesthesia and postoperative oral analgesics. Acting at different points on pain pathways, this approach allows low doses of individual drugs to be used thus decreasing the risk of side effects and maximizing the analgesic effect.[170]

Local anesthetic agents

Two local anesthetic agents are widely used. In the 1970s lignocaine (lidocaine) was the drug of choice but since 1980 lignocaine (lidocaine) has been superseded by bupivacaine. However, some surgeons use a combination of both agents in order to achieve the advantages of rapid onset of action and longer duration of anesthesia. Adrenaline is used with both drugs to protract their duration of activity. Bupivacaine is available in concentrations of 0.25%, 0.50%, and 0.75%. Its onset of action is approximately 20 min. The half-life is 2–3 h therefore providing a length of action of about 3–6 h.

The maximum safe dose of lignocaine is 3 mg/kg body weight and with adrenaline 7 mg/kg. For bupivacaine the maximum dose is 2 mg/kg body weight and 4 mg/kg with adrenaline. Bupivacaine is more potent and longer acting than lignocaine and maintains the analgesic block for 8–10 h, which is a major advantage in day-case surgery.[44] The safety margin in

the recommended maximum safe dose is wide, as illustrated by serial postoperative plasma concentrations following doses approaching the maximum recommended for lignocaine or bupivacaine. For instance, administering lignocaine with adrenaline to the maximum dose of 7 mg/kg, peak lignocaine concentration ranged from 0.23 to 0.9 mg/l, the toxicity threshold being 5 mg/l.[566] The administration of 20 ml of 0.5% plain bupivacaine resulted in peak venous plasma concentrations of 0.07–1.14 m/l, the cardiovascular toxicity occurring at plasma concentrations greater than 4 mg/l.[570]

Prolongation of the duration of local anesthesia by the addition of agents designed to prolong absorption from the local tissues has been explored by several investigators. Loder recommends 1% lignocaine in 10% dextran 150 with 1:250 000 adrenaline added to the solution.[704] He reports that the large numbers of big molecules (10% dextran of average molecular weight 150 000) retards the absorption of the local anesthetic. Others have evaluated 0.25% bupivacaine with dextran 40 without adrenaline and have reported no enhancement or prolongation of the local anesthetic effect.[704] Simpson and colleagues in a small study comparing initial general anesthesia with field infiltration to control postoperative pain, suggest that the addition of heavy dextran to bupivacaine and adrenaline solution prolongs its effect.[1056] This confirms the earlier work of Loder. However, their conclusion, 'It would seem prudent, therefore, in clinical work to combine bupivacaine with high molecular weight dextran and adrenaline', is perhaps a little too enthusiastic on the basis of their small experience. In their series of 40 patients this mixture was only administered to five subjects, casting doubt on the clinical validity of the study. Kingsnorth and colleagues in a similar study could not confirm this recommendation and conclude that the addition of heavy dextran to bupivacaine confers no benefit. More recently, in a study of 30 men undergoing inguinal hernia repair under general anesthesia, postoperative pain, patient rating score or morphine consumption did not differ between patients who had preoperative inguinal nerve block with bupivacaine 0.5% plain and those who received a similar block with bupivacaine 0.5% plain supplemented with 40 mg triamcinolone acetanide. For the present, therefore, it is recommended that local anesthetic agents are used plain or with adrenaline, and not supplemented with additional agents which are of no proven advantage in prolonging their duration of action.[598] Newer local anesthetics with improved safety and anesthetic equivalence have been tested in inguinal hernia surgery. In a study testing the efficacy of ropivacaine, 32 patients operated under general anesthesia were randomized to receive subcutaneous infiltration with 40 ml of ropivacaine or bupivacaine.[334] There was no difference in pain or analgesic requirements after surgery as assessed by visual analog score and pressure algometry (which tested pain–pressure threshold using a handheld electronic algometer and recording the minimal pressure which induced pain). Pain assessments were recorded at 2, 4, 6, 8, 10 and 24 h after the skin incision. In a double-blind study comparing the efficacy of levobupivacaine with bupivacaine in elective inguinal herniorrhaphy in 66 patients, Kingsnorth and colleagues concluded that levobupivacaine exerted similar analgesic effects in the early postoperative period compared with bupivacaine, the theoretical advantage of levobupivacaine being its increased safety margin regarding cardiotoxicity and neurotoxicity.[596]

Barwell, who has the largest UK series of repairs of inguinal hernias under local anesthetic, uses 0.5% lignocaine without adrenaline. He reports 2066 patients operated on under this local anesthetic, two of whom had to be converted to general anesthetic in the early days of his program. He has had no cases of anesthetic toxicity and perhaps the worst complication is 'the occasional hematoma at the site of injection for the field block'.[84] Glassow, reporting the experience of the Shouldice clinic in Toronto, recommends 150 ml of 2% procaine without adrenaline,[423] whereas Ravitch from Pittsburgh recommends 0.5% lignocaine[941] and Wantz a mixture of lignocaine and bupivacaine with adrenaline.[425] Wantz also claims that the burning pain caused by the administration of local anesthesia can be eliminated by neutralizing the agent.[1188] The addition of 1 ml of 8.4% sodium bicarbonate solution to 9 ml of plain local anesthesia brings the pH to a comfortable 7.5, which also enhances the anesthesia and reduces the quantity required. The pH of local anesthetic with adrenaline is 4, and therefore 2.5 ml of the sodium bicarbonate solution is required for neutralization. Ponka and Sapala[917] conclude that bupivacaine is superior to chloroprocaine. They report that 0.25% bupivacaine provides anesthesia consistently lasting longer than 6 h, and as a result of this sustained release the requirement for postoperative analgesia is reduced. Chloroprocaine with 1:200 000 adrenaline was a safe agent, but its action lasted only up to 2 h.

Flanagan and Bascom, initially using 0.25% lignocaine with 1:400 000 adrenaline and currently using bupivacaine 0.125% with 1:400 000 adrenaline, have reported detailed results from Eugene, Oregon. In a prospective study 170 patients, adults with an age range of 12–82 years, with groin hernia, were given local anesthesia as outpatients and 163 were given general anesthesia. They found good patient satisfaction with local anesthesia, few complications and enormous economic and social benefits.[362] Baskerville and Jarrett reported a study of local anesthesia for day-case inguinal hernia repair undertaken in Kingston, UK in 1980.[88] One hundred and thirty-five patients were operated on using 40–60 ml 0.25% bupivacaine

with 1:200 000 adrenaline. There were no complications of the local anesthesia. Patient acceptance of the regimen was high, with 96% of patients stating that they would have another hernia repair performed in the same way. Acceptance of this regimen by the family doctors was also tested and 100% of the family doctors expressed satisfaction with this management of their patients.

Nicholls (1977),[846] reporting his experience from the Seychelles Isles, which are geographically isolated, has commented on the economics of ambulatory surgery under local anesthesia for groin hernia. He reports 136 adult male and female patients treated using 80 ml of 0.5% lignocaine in saline solution as a field block. He administers 70–100 mg of pethidine 1 h before surgery and 5–10 mg of diazepam intravenously at commencement of the operation. His results are impressive and confirm the acceptability and adequacy of local anesthesia. The complications attributable in part to the local anesthesia include a thrombosis of the dorsal vein of the penis during infiltration of the local anesthetic. There are savings in anesthetic gases and the salaries of anesthetists. These, together with the high costs and difficulties of transportation to the Seychelles, are seen as distinct benefits. Patient acceptability was also recorded and found to be high.

Third World experiences are reported by Wijesinha and Agbakwuru. In Wijesinha's study 100 patients in a military hospital were operated on over a 3-year period under local anesthesia.[1210] The stated advantages are less work for nursing staff, less morbidity for patients and less strain on scarce health resources. Patients included soldiers, sailors, airmen, and persons from such diverse trades as cooks, clerks, nurses, drivers, bandsmen, and even the army barber! Agbakwuru had less success in Nigeria. Of 130 patients in whom local anesthesia was attempted for inguinal herniorrhaphy, 32 did not tolerate the field block; 20 of these patients were women. Tolerance of local anesthesia was lower in the younger age group, which is a universal finding in other studies.[8]

Ponka lists the advantages and disadvantages of local and general anesthesia[913] (Table 8.1). Local anesthesia is specific in his experience for some patients with poor cardiorespiratory function, and hepatic or renal disease. General anesthesia is equally specific for the young, the psychotic, the neurotic and

Table 8.1 *Advantages and disadvantages of local anesthesia after Ponka, 1980*[913]

Advantages	Disadvantages
1 Safer for poor risk patient, especially those with severe active cardiac and pulmonary disease	1 Some patients dislike being conscious during surgery; neurotic and psychotic patients, and children, may be unsuitable for local anesthesia
2 Postoperative respiratory disorder and coughing are rare	2 Surgery under local anesthesia takes longer and demands more patient and gentle surgical technique
3 Patient is conscious and can co-operate in testing the repair during surgery	3 Wound complications, hematoma and skin necrosis may occur if care is not taken
4 Urinary retention is rare because voiding reflexes are undisturbed by anesthesia	4 Drug toxicity and sensitivity may occur. All patients should be screened for these risks and monitored throughout the procedure
5 Earlier mobilization decreases the risk of deep vein thrombosis and pulmonary embolization	5 If a complicated surgical problem is found, it is more difficult to deal with under local anesthesia

the nervous. Lastly, some surgeons prefer one or other anesthetic technique. Local anesthesia is only successful if the surgeon is gentle and patient and has confidence in his ability to maintain the patient's morale throughout this procedure. Don't ask, for example, 'Is that hurting?' or mention 'pain'; instead, ask the patient 'Are you quite comfortable?'

Although complication rates are low and hernia recurrence rates lower in many reported series using local anesthesia, it is difficult to suggest that the anesthetic has a direct effect on the recurrence rate, which is governed so much by surgical and technical factors.

There is no consensus on the optimal local anesthetic agent – procaine, lignocaine and bupivacaine each have their devotees. The addition of adrenaline is practised by the majority of operators. With bupivacaine, the anesthesia lasts some 8–10 h; the inadvertent infiltration of the femoral nerve with prolonged paralysis delaying discharge has been reported.[1111] If lignocaine is employed, it is wise to administer atropine preoperatively to reduce the chance of bradycardia.

Local anesthesia for inguinal hernia repair is well recorded in the literature. It has been shown to be satisfactory for the patients and their carers in the community.[26,27]

TECHNIQUE

The recommended local anesthetic agent is a mixture of bupivacaine and lignocaine with the addition of adrenaline 1:200 000. The benefits of this mixture are the rapid onset of action of the lignocaine solution, the prolonged action of the bupivacaine and the possibility of reduced local hemorrhage with the addition of adrenaline. In practice 3×10 ml ampoules of bupivacaine 0.25% solution with adrenaline 1:200 000 are admixed with 3×10 ml ampoules of 1% lignocaine to produce 3×20 ml anesthetic solutions. This 60 ml volume of local anesthetic is suitable for most patients except the excessively lean or excessively obese patient where the volume may be reduced or increased by up to 10 ml. The technique of application of the inguinal block can be achieved by a variety of techniques including the one described in the foregoing section of this chapter. If a preoperative inguinal block is applied, the surgeon should have handy on the scrub nurses trolley a 5 ml supplement of 1% lignocaine which can be used intraoperatively should the need arise. Many experienced operators will use this supplementary local anesthetic around the pubic tubercle before attempting dissection of the spermatic cord in this area. Amid has given an account of the step-by-step, infiltrate-as-you-go procedure of local anesthesia for inguinal hernia repair, which will not be described here.[26] Care must be taken to avoid direct intravascular injection during the infiltration, which is a very rare event since the only major vein in the region is the femoral vein, which should be far from the wandering tip of the infiltrator's needle.

Although pre-anesthetic drugs are unnecessary, patient morale is improved by giving midazolam intravenously just before the start of the procedure. In most patients the dose should be no more than 2 mg midazolam, except for young anxious patients where the dose required may be up to 4 mg, and in elderly patients with comorbid cardiorespiratory disease when sedation is contraindicated or unnecessary. It is essential to monitor the patient carefully throughout injection of the local anesthetic; reading the blood pressure before and after injection of bupivacaine is mandatory, and a pulse oximeter and an electrocardiograph monitor should be used throughout. The importance of monitoring the patient's oxygen saturation, blood pressure, and ECG, particularly as the bupivacaine is injected, must be stressed. An experienced anesthetic nurse (or anesthesiologist, depending upon local custom) should supervise the patient throughout the surgery. The surgeon should not do this and operate. Equipment for tracheal intubation should be available and skilled anesthetic support must be on hand should the patient require it.

Monitoring

Because oxygen desaturation is common in procedures carried out under sedation[204] oxygen supplementation and measurement of arterial oxygen saturation by a pulse oximeter is mandatory. Oxygen saturation and clinical monitoring should be supplemented by devices that continuously display the heart rate, pulse volume or arterial pressure and electrocardiogram.[59] The patient must be able to respond to commands throughout the procedure: if they are unable to do so the sedationist has become an anesthetist. The same standards should be applied to sedative techniques (and regional anesthesia), when there is depression of consciousness or cardiovascular or respiratory complications. Pulse oximetry monitoring should continue until the patient meets the criteria for discharge from the recovery area. Oxygen saturation should not be permitted to fall below 90% (arterial oxygen tension of 7.9 kPa) as below this value a minor fall in oxygen tension results in a rapid fall in oxygen content.

APPLIED ANATOMY

Free nerve endings are distributed throughout the skin; stretch and pain receptors occur in each of the aponeurotic layers and in the parietal peritoneum. The skin and subcutaneous tissue are sensitive to all noxious stimuli. Pin-prick, pressure and chemical stimuli (e.g. hypertonic solutions) cause pain in these tissues. The parietal peritoneum is sensitive to pin-prick, stretching and chemical stimuli. In contrast, the visceral peritoneum and hollow organs are insensitive to touch, to clamp, to knife and to cautery, but the visceral arteries to these organs are sensitive. There is no pain when viscera are handled under local anesthesia, until a clamp is placed on the vascular pedicle.

Abdominal wall

Knowledge of the fundamental physiology and neuroanatomy of pain in the abdomen is essential if adequate local analgesia is to be obtained. Local anesthesia should achieve the following:

1 Ensure skin anesthesia in the line of incision. Remembering the overlap and connections between the rich plexus of epidermal nerve endings, this is best accomplished by a skin weal.
2 Block the nerve supply to the aponeurotic layers, which must be dissected and manipulated.
3 Ensure anesthesia of the parietal peritoneum of the hernia and especially of the neck of the sac, which is very sensitive.

The distribution of the cutaneous nerves to the abdomen, groin and thigh is familiar to all surgeons. The anterior portions of the six lower intercostal nerves are continued forward from their respective spaces onto the anterior abdominal wall, and are accompanied by the last thoracic (subcostal) nerve. Additionally the iliohypogastric and ilio-inguinal nerve (T1 and L1) supply the lower abdomen. The genitofemoral nerve (L1 and L2) via its genital branch supplies the cord structures and anterior scrotum and via its femoral branch the skin and subcutaneous tissue in the femoral triangle. All the nerves of the anterior abdominal wall communicate with each other and thus their cutaneous distribution overlaps (Figure 8.1).

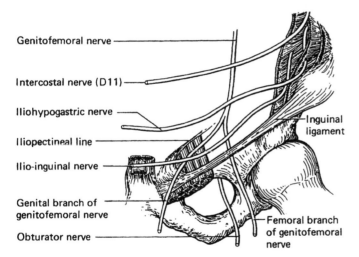

Figure 8.1 *Sensory nerve supply of the inguinal, femoral and obturator regions.*

The intercostal nerves run from their intercostal space forwards between the internal oblique and transversus muscles to the lateral margin of the rectus sheath. They enter the sheath on its posterior aspect, supply the rectus muscle, pierce the anterior sheath and then ramify in the subcutaneous tissue and supply the adjacent skin. Each of these nerves gives a lateral cutaneous branch, which pierces the flat muscles and becomes subcutaneous in the midaxillary line. Once subcutaneous, this lateral cutaneous branch gives anterior and posterior branches to supply the skin and subcutaneous tissue.

For local anesthesia nerve block to be successful, the intercostal nerve must be blocked before the lateral cutaneous branch is given off. The site of election for the local anesthetic

injection is in the posterior axillary line. If the intercostal nerve is blocked too far anteriorly, the anterior division of the lateral cutaneous branch will remain sensitive (Figure 8.2).

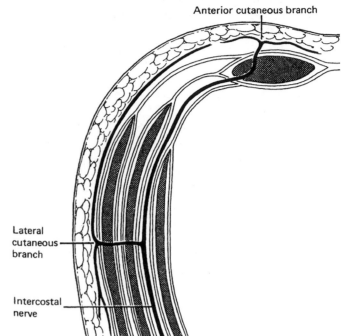

Figure 8.2 *Transverse section through the abdominal wall. The lateral cutaneous branch of an intercostal nerve gives an anterior and posterior division; the anterior division must be blocked for effective abdominal wall anesthesia.*

It should be remembered that the intercostal nerve is tucked under the lower border of the rib in its posterior third and in the center of the intercostal space more anteriorly (Figure 8.3).

When the hernia is exposed, it is important to infiltrate the neck of the hernial sac (parietal peritoneum) to ensure adequate anesthesia while the sac is dissected, incised, emptied and closed (if this is the done rather than mere reduction into the preperitoneal space).

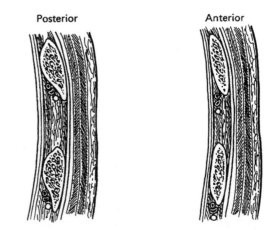

Figure 8.3 *The relative positions of the ribs and the intercostal nerves vary. Posterior to the midaxillary line the intercostal nerves and vessels are tucked under the rib next above, anteriorly they lie midway between the ribs in the mid-intercostal space.*

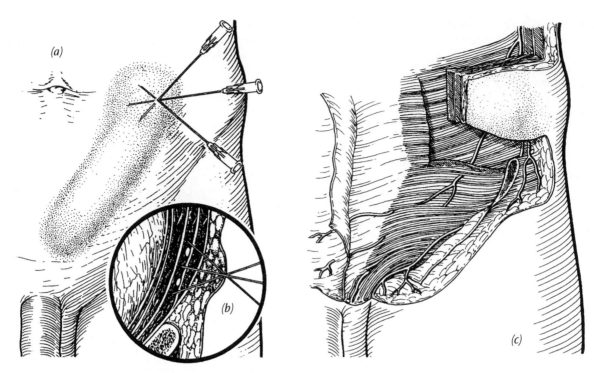

Figure 8.4 *(a,b) At the upper end of the previous weal, at a point approximately 1 cm above and medial to the anterior superior iliac spine, some 3 ml of the anesthetic solution is injected deep to the aponeurosis of the external oblique. The needle is pushed in until the external oblique aponeurosis is felt as a firm resistant structure. (c) The needle is pushed through the aponeurosis and the anesthetic solution distributed to block the ilio-inguinal and iliohypogastric nerves which run between the external and internal oblique muscles at this point.*

The groin

Inguinal and femoral hernias lie in the borderland between the regular anatomy of the abdominal wall and the complex anatomy of the lower limb. However, the same technical sequence ensures adequate regional anesthesia:

1 An injection is made between the internal oblique and transversus muscles about 1 cm superior to the anterior superior spine in an endeavor to block the ilio-inguinal and iliohypogastric nerves. To do this the needle is pushed in vertically; the 'give' as the needle penetrates the aponeurosis of the external oblique allows easy estimate of the depth of the injection. Twenty milliliters of local anesthetic are injected at this site (Figure 8.4).
2 A local weal is raised in the line of the incision. This weal starts 2 cm above and medial to the anterior superior iliac spine. Long spinal needles may be used to deliver this 20 ml infiltration (Figure 8.5).
3 The medial end of the oblique subcutaneous weal is now 'topped up' with 2 ml of local solution, taking care to carry the injection down to the pubic tubercle and the origin of the rectus muscle from the pubis.
4 The final 20 ml syringe of local anesthetic mixture is infiltrated along the direction of the spermatic cord and adjacent peritoneal sac, beginning at the deep ring. To achieve this the tip of the infiltration needle is inserted into the skin at the surface marking of the deep ring, traversed

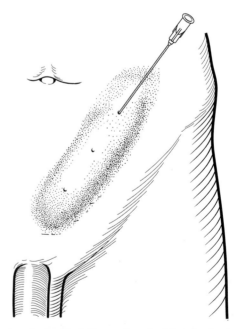

Figure 8.5 *Local anesthesia for an inguinal hernioplasty: using a long spinal needle a weal of local anesthetic solution is made in the line of the groin incision.*

through the skin, subcutaneous fat and external oblique aponeurosis (the 'give' is felt as the needle penetrates the aponeurosis), the syringe aspirated to ensure that the pampiniform plexus has not been penetrated and the content of the syringe is then gently injected obliquely along the direction of the spermatic cord towards and including the pubic tubercle. This solution will anesthetize the deeper structures including the sac and the genital branch of the genitofemoral nerve (Figure 8.6).

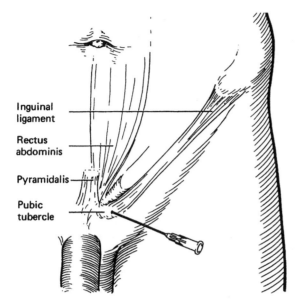

Figure 8.6 *The medial end of the oblique groin (incision) weal is topped up down to the pubic tubercle and origin of the rectus.*

5 This anesthetic block can conveniently be applied by the surgeon or anesthetist under strict aseptic conditions but before scrubbing up and gowning. In the 5 or 10 min between application of the block, scrubbing, gowning and preparing the skin and draping the patient, the infiltration will have become completely effective.
6 Patients should be informed that the slightest discomfort will be supplemented with additional local anesthetic solution. This event is the patient's greatest anxiety and the nature of previous anesthetic experience is the prime determinant of any anxiety preoperatively.[727]

The preoperative inguinal block and the infiltrate-as-you-go technique essentially achieve the same results in experienced hands. Postoperative pain and analgesic requirements are similar in groups of patients given preoperative or intraoperative nerve blocks for groin surgery.[1142]

COMPLICATIONS OF LOCAL ANESTHETICS

Complications of local anesthetics are systemic and local:

1 Systemic: (a) excitation of the nervous system, nervousness, nausea and convulsions – these are very rare; (b) depression of the cardiovascular system with hypotension and arrhythmias; (c) hypersensitivity reactions are very rare with lignocaine and bupivacaine.

2 Local: (a) ecchymoses and bruising; (b) local ischemia and tissue necrosis if too much adrenaline is injected at one site; (c) these local complications can compromise wound healing.

The systemic side effects are life-threatening, hence patients undergoing local anesthesia should be questioned about previous side effects from local anesthetics. Most importantly, they should have their CNS and CVS state monitored throughout the procedure and for up to 30 min after surgery. Increased patient excitability and garrulousness, a rising pulse rate and an increasing blood pressure are the early signs of CNS intoxication. If these signs are observed, an anesthetist, if not present, should be summoned without delay.

SEDATION

A small dose of intravenous midazolam (2–4 mg) reduces anxiety and makes the patient more relaxed and co-operative. In addition the useful side effect of retrograde amnesia will reduce the impact of the unfamiliar surroundings of the operating theater following the procedure. Although recovery from intravenous midazolam is not as rapid as recovery from intravenous propofol, surgeons should not dabble with unfamiliar intravenous agents. Anecdotal evidence suggests that administration of propofol reduces local anesthetic requirements.[204] Nevertheless, the benzodiazepine antagonist flumazenil (Anexate) should be available and used to improve recovery or combat unexpected narcosis caused by benzodiazepines. Recovery should be advanced before reversal to eliminate the likelihood of sleep reoccurring as the antagonist action wears off.

Some surgeons will ask the anesthesia personnel to supplement the above with an intravenous injection of a narcotic. This is particularly useful if the patient continues to experience pain despite what is felt to be an adequate blockade or if the maximum or near maximum dose of the local anesthetic has been administered. In many centers, this is done in nearly every case to assist in the analgesia.

Postoperative analgesia

Effective postoperative pain relief benefits the patient by providing comfort in the period after surgery as well as modifying the autonomic and somatic reflexes to pain which delay recovery. Treatment of pain facilitates early rehabilitation and recovery.[1206] Patients given general anesthesia do not differ in pain scores or analgesic consumption whether given inguinal field block before the surgical incision or after wound closure.[303] Spittal and colleagues have demonstrated that local anesthetic procedures can be simplified still further in that instillation of bupivacaine into the wound provided the same degree of postoperative analgesic effect as a formal inguinal field block in patients undergoing inguinal hernia repair under general anesthesia.[1082] The benefits of supplementary bupivacaine local anesthesia are so well documented that omission of this step should be considered suboptimal care.

Further improvements in postoperative pain relief can be achieved by the use of balanced analgesia or managed anesthetic care (MAC). The combination of non-steroidal anti-inflammatory drugs, opioids and local anesthesia acting at different points on pain pathways can maximize analgesic effects and minimize side effects. The non-steroidal anti-inflammatory drug diclofenac sodium (Voltarol) can reduce postoperative opioid requirements by 15–60% and reduce nausea. A suppository of 100 mg diclofenac sodium administered 1 h before surgery has now become an established part of balanced analgesia regimens. However, this drug should be used with caution in patients with previous gastrointestinal ulceration, asthma, renal failure, heart failure or bleeding diatheses. Another such drug is ketolorac (Toradol).

Previously, dextropropoxyphene 32.5 mg and paracetamol 325 mg (Distalgesic) was recommended as a self-administered analgesic after day-case hernia repair. This policy has been reviewed and abandoned on account of the toxicity of this drug combination. However, perhaps the most important reason for no longer prescribing Distalgesic or its equivalent is that powerful postoperative analgesia is never required after routine repair of an inguinal hernia using current modern techniques. Regular oral paracetamol for up to one week should be recommended to supplement local anesthetic wound blockade, intravenous midazolam and preoperative diclofenac. Narcotics are frequently necessary and used routinely in some areas of the world.

There has been a recent introduction of infusion pumps that perfuse the wound with local anesthetic, usually bupivaine. At the completion of the hernia repair a small catheter is introduced via a separate needle puncture beneath the external aponeurosis and situated in the superior aspect of the wound. This is connected by tubing to one of at least seven types of infusion pumps. The duration of this infusion is 2–3 days. There are ongoing studies of this technique but one has shown that the use of such a portable infusion pump does reduce postoperative pain following a tension-free inguinal hernia repair.[861]

In the early 1970s the use of skin clips, with the attendant removal of them, caused troublesome wound pain. Subcuticular sutures of fine absorbable suture material have eliminated this problem and most patients require minimal postoperative analgesics.

Kehlet and the Hvidovre hospital hernia group have shown that 98% of patients with a reducible hernia referred to a large university hospital for elective repair can safely be operated upon as an ambulatory procedure under local anesthetic with a median postoperative hospital stay of 85 minutes.[168] Gianetta and colleagues have shown that similar results can be achieved in elderly patients with 45% being discharged on the day of surgery and 25% the day after, with a mean hospital stay after surgery of 1.8 days.[401] There is a high rate of co-morbid disease in these elderly patients and it has been demonstrated that 5% of these patients suffer long-term clinically significant decreases in cognitive function when operation is performed under general anesthesia.[1215]

LOCAL ANESTHESIA – INCISIONAL, SPIGELIAN AND OTHER ABDOMINAL WALL HERNIAS

The same concept of local anesthesia – a combination of regional block and field infiltration – can be employed for incisional, Spigelian and epigastric hernias. Important points are to adequately infiltrate the subcutaneous layer, especially cranial to the proposed incision, and then to adequately anesthetize the intercostal nerves, which run deep to the internal, oblique/rectus sheath aponeurosis to within 2 cm of the midline. If a regional block is required, to repair a large incisional hernia, the intercostal nerves must be infiltrated in the posterior axillary line before they give their lateral cutaneous branch. The incidence of urinary retention following inguinal herniorrhaphy, which is the single most common cause of unplanned hospital admission, is significantly reduced by carrying out the operation under local anesthesia.[357,905]

CONCLUSIONS

- Either general, regional or local anesthesia is suitable for hernia repair. Patient and surgeon preference are indications for one or the other.
- Balanced analgesia should be employed.
- Preoperative diclofenac sodium is recommended in selected patients.
- A local anesthetic field block (described here) or infiltrate-as-you-go are the recommended local anesthetic techniques.
- A mixture of 0.25% bupivacaine with adrenaline 1:200 000 and 1% lignocaine is the recommended anesthetic agent.
- Careful intraoperative supervision and monitoring of the patient is essential for safety.
- Local anesthetic wound blockade should be performed in patients receiving general or regional anesthesia.
- The use of postoperative portable infusion pumps may further reduce the amounts of postoperative pain in these patients. Further results of on-going studies are needed.

9

Complications of hernia in general

The complications of hernia include:

- Rupture of the hernia – spontaneous or traumatic.
- Involvement of the hernial sac in the disease process: (a) mesothelial hyperplasia; (b) carcinoma; (c) endometriosis and leiomyomatosis; (d) inflammation – peritonitis, acute appendicitis.
- Incarceration, obstruction and strangulation. Reductio-en-masse.
- Maydl's hernia and afferent loop strangulation. Strangulation of the appendix in a hernial sac. Richter's hernia. Littré's hernia.
- Herniation of female genitalia. Pregnancy in a hernial sac.
- Urinary tract complications, hernia of the bladder, the ureter and of a urinary ileal conduit.
- Sliding hernia.
- Testicular strangulation in: (a) infants; (b) adults with large giant inguinoscrotal hernias; (c) Africans.

SPONTANEOUS AND TRAUMATIC RUPTURE

Spontaneous rupture (dehiscence) of hernia is a well-recognized though rare complication. Helwig (1958), in a comprehensive article, reported 47 cases of spontaneous exteriorization of hernial contents; of these 17 were through incisional hernia, while the remainder were through inguinal, femoral, umbilical or epigastric hernia or through recurrences of these.[491] Spontaneous rupture of an umbilical hernia with evisceration is a very rare event. The complication is so rare that it should not influence the accepted surgical practice of initial conservative management of infantile umbilical hernia.[739]

Four such cases are described in the British literature and one in India. In two cases there was no precipitating cause,[774,1102] in one a bout of severe coughing precipitated rupture and evisceration,[72] in another damage to the overlying skin and trauma,[481] and in the remaining case umbilical sepsis may have been to blame.[205] All of the children were under 4 months at the time of rupture. Damage to the bowel did not occur in any of the four British cases and complete recovery followed reduction of the bowel and standard umbilical hernioplasty.

Further cases of spontaneous rupture of hernia have been described but such ruptures all follow previous surgery; they are all failures of incisional hernia scars. Such cases are described by O'Donoghue (1955) (a 56-year-old woman 13 years after a gynecological operation);[859] Hartley (1962) (two cases – a 74-year-old man 12 years after a suprapubic prostatectomy and an 84-year-old woman 13 years after an appendicectomy through a right lower paramedian scar);[481] Hamilton (1966) (a 76-year-old woman presenting 6 years after a bilateral salpingo-oophorectomy);[467] and Senapati (1982) (a 45-year-old woman who had undergone two cesarean operations 12 and 15 years previously).[1038]

The majority of spontaneous hernia ruptures are in lower abdominal, inguinal and incisional hernias. Many develop insidiously and present in emergency departments some time after an apparently painless disruption. Others are associated with episodes of straining or coughing. The dehiscence would appear to be a degenerative process, with the relatively avascular and thin hernial sac undergoing progressive stretching, becoming increasingly ischemic and finally giving way. This process is accelerated in some cases by skin ulceration due to tight corsets, or to intertrigo and skin infection in pendulous sacs.

Surprisingly, the mortality is low and is only potentially fatal in remote areas where medical assistance is far distant.[865] The main peritoneal cavity is uncontaminated, the tight neck usually preventing reduction of the contents and contamination of the main peritoneal cavity.

Spontaneous rupture leading to fistula and then 'cure' was of course described by Cheselden (1784) (Figure 1.2).[211] A more remarkable example of a spontaneous cure of an incarcerated right inguinal hernia in a 7-week-old Chinese male child whose hernia remained irreducible for 10 days and who then developed a cecal fistula is reported by Stock (1951).[1093]

Rupture of the intestine in an unreduced hernia in a male subjected to trauma is not excessively rare; deaths from this cause appear in nineteenth-century literature.[10] Except in one case in which the colon was damaged in a sliding hernia, the perforated loop of small intestine is invariably found in the general peritoneal cavity. There is an association between small bowel rupture due to blunt trauma and inguinal hernia. Small bowel perforation is more likely to have occurred if the trauma was sustained when a hernia is 'down', or in the presence of a voluminous incarcerated inguino-scrotal hernia.[755]

Where the violence is applied directly to the hernia the explanation is simple – the intestine is damaged locally where it lies unprotected in the hernial sac. Alternatively the force of the blow first opposes the walls of the incoming and outgoing bowel, sealing the loop. Then additional pressure that is applied will raise the loop's intraluminal pressure to the point that traumatic perforation occurs.[955] When blunt trauma is applied to the abdomen, loops of mobile gut slide around to absorb the violence. Fixed gut is most at risk; hence the duodenum and terminal ileum are most frequently damaged. A hernia which is 'down' is another fixed point contributing to gut immobility and predisposing to serious injury.

A number of cases have been reported of sudden rupture of an indirect inguinal hernial sac with extravasation, in patients on continuous ambulatory peritoneal dialysis (CAPD).[935] It is recommended that when patients with inguinal hernias require long-term peritoneal dialysis, even when the inguinal hernia is asymptomatic, repair should be carried before CAPD is commenced.

INVOLVEMENT OF HERNIAL SAC IN DISEASE PROCESS

Nodular mesothelial hyperplasia and mesothelioma

The peritoneum has a great capacity to undergo metaplasia, to form papillary projections, pseudo-acini, squamous nests and even cartilaginous nodules in response to repeated mechanical trauma.[3] Cirrhotic ascites and collagen vascular disease are associated with marked mesothelial hyperplasia. Nodular mesothelial hyperplasia can develop in hernial sacs, particularly those subject to trauma. A truss can be an initiating factor. Nodular mesothelial hyperplasia has been described in hernial sacs in infants and children and in these cases is associated with repeated episodic incarceration or strangulation. A total of 1494 inguinal hernia sacs were pathologically evaluated from 1077 pediatric patients by Partrick and colleagues.[888] Nodular mesothelial hyperplasia was a rare and incidental finding, not affecting clinical management.

The pathological features are the presence in the sac of cellular nodules up to 1.0 cm in diameter. These nodules are composed of cells with a pale acidophilic cytoplasm derived from the peritoneum. The cells show a moderate to severe pleomorphism; most are round cells when lying free in the intercellular fluid, but they are polygonal when compressed together by neighboring cells to form the characteristic nodules.[969] The nodules may coalesce to form cystic spaces grossly resembling a pseudomyxoma.[969]

If injury to the hernial sac is sustained and of sufficient intensity, the mesothelial proliferation can exceed the simple needs of regeneration and acquire pseudomalignant cytologic features. The consummate ability of mesothelial cells to simulate carcinoma should be remembered and pathologists need to be cautious in interpreting the microscopic features of hernial sacs.[969]

Nodular mesothelial hyperplasia is more common in infants and children and in them it exhibits its most exuberant characteristics. The condition is entirely benign – no radical surgery is required and follow-up data confirms the harmless nature of the lesion. It is important to make the correct diagnosis to avoid pointless and potentially dangerous therapy. Ordonez and colleagues (1998)[869] have suggested that the term nodular mesothelial hyperplasia should be replaced by the term nodular histiocytic hyperplasia because the lesions are primarily reactive histiocytic proliferations and occur in other locations aside from the serosal membrane. If any doubt exists in the diagnosis of these histiocytic proliferations because of mitotic activity or cellular atypia, then staining for keratin or the histiocytic marker CD68 may be appropriate. By this means lesions, which present high mitotic activity, can be differentiated from malignancy.

On the other hand, genuine peritoneal mesothelioma has been encountered within a hernial sac.[141] The mesothelioma may be found by chance or alternatively the patient can present with a mass in the hernial sac wall. Rarely, the diagnosis of peritoneal mesothelioma has been made during transabdominal preperitoneal laparoscopic inguinal hernia repair.[662] While mesothelioma generally arises in the main peritoneal cavity, it can arise from the hernial sac itself or from the cord or the tunica vaginalis. If the mesothelioma arises from the cord structures or from mesothelial remnants in them, in addition to the mass the patients usually also feature a hydrocele.

Malignant mesothelioma has been encountered in hernial sacs in patients with no history of exposure to asbestos, further evidence for a relationship with local trauma and the occurrence of mesothelial hyperplasia. Grove and colleagues describe three histologically and immunohistochemically well documented cases of mesothelioma of the tunica vaginalis testis and hernia sac.[444] Analysis and follow-up of these three patients and a review of 30 previously reported cases revealed a varied and often unpredictable clinical course. A classification into high and low-grade malignant tumors was suggested based on clinical and pathological findings. In the high-grade variety intraperitoneal deposits appear and intestinal obstruction and other complications then ensue.[141]

Solitary fibrous tumor (SFT) is a further tumor of mesenchymal origin, which is classified as a variant of fibroma and has been found arising in abdominal wall hernia sacs.[674] SFT of the peritoneum has also been called fibrous mesothelioma and the site of origin is felt to be a submesothelial mesenchymal cell. Two primary tumors arising in hernia sacs were reported by Lee and colleagues associated with copious myxoid material mimicking pseudomyxoma peritonei. Wide local surgical excision is the treatment of choice with the degree of resectability being a powerful predictor of outcome.

Carcinoma as a complication of hernial sacs

Malignancy involving inguinal hernial sacs is uncommon but not rare. Suspicion should always haunt the surgeon's mind, particularly when he is confronted with an elderly patient with the recent onset of a groin hernia.[354,973] If the sac is thickened or ascitic fluid is present in it at operation, it should be subjected to histological evaluation and the ascitic fluid to full cytology. The hernial sac offers a unique opportunity for peritoneal biopsy, which should not be missed. If a suspicious sac is found at hernioplasty, immediate frozen section may elucidate the pathology, while digital palpation through the hernial orifice may give more information. The index of suspicion should be particularly high for male patients of advanced age and especially those who have previously undergone surgery for colorectal carcinoma.[757] Immediate laparotomy is not advised: repair the hernia and subject the patient to early elective operation after bowel preparation and antibiotic prophylaxis.

Lejars (1889)[681] classified malignant involvement of inguinal hernial sacs into three varieties: extrasaccular, saccular and intrasaccular. While this classification has merit it does not easily fit contemporary concepts of pathology and surgery. A better classification is:

- Primary carcinoma: (a) extrasaccular; (b) intrasaccular.
- Secondary carcinoma – predominantly intrasaccular: derived, by metastatic spread from lung, breast, stomach, colon, ovary or any other intraperitoneal viscus.

Extrasaccular carcinoma can arise from the bladder or from a diverticulum of the bladder that is sliding into the medial side of a direct hernia. Similarly, a carcinoma may occur in the colon, which is a component of the wall of a sliding hernia. Such a carcinoma may obstruct, and a mistaken diagnosis of a strangulated hernia be made. Careful history taking can avoid this error. In the six examples recorded in the literature, all the hernias were large and scrotal and all had been present and irreducible for some considerable time before they presented with intestinal obstruction.[677] The carcinoma is usually bulky, locally advanced and may be palpated in the sac, which is not so discreetly tender as the sac containing strangulated small bowel.[437] A liposarcoma of the cord, which invaded the adjacent hernial sac, is reported reminding surgeons that not all malignancy in groin hernias is derived from the peritoneal cavity.[973]

Intrasaccular carcinoma is a primary carcinoma arising from an organ which is a permanent denizen of a hernial sac. The most frequent examples are colon or cecal cancers. Malignant tumors arising from an appendix in a hernial sac also occur.[841]

Carcinomas in hernial sacs are often locally fixed and advanced when the diagnosis is made. This should not prevent wide local excision being successfully undertaken.

Intrasaccular carcinoma can also occur in Spigelian, umbilical and incisional hernias.

Routine histological examination of hernial sacs is not recommended. Kassan and colleagues routinely examined 1020 hernial sacs after surgery; the incidence of unexpected findings, the discovery of an occult tumor, in those specimens, which appeared normal to the surgeon at operation, was 1 in 1020 (0.098%). The incremental cost per unexpected finding was $49 041 and the only unexpected and abnormal finding in the series was one atypical lipoma.[569] If at operation the hernial sac is seen to be abnormal or if it is thickened, then histology should always be performed. However, there is no positive benefit to be gained by the patient from routine histological examination of an apparently normal sac. However, in some areas of the world (notably the USA), the hernia sac, if it is removed, is sent for pathologic examination for documentation of its removal as a medico-legal issue.

Gynecological tumors – endometriosis and leiomyomas

Endometriomas are not infrequently encountered in incisional hernias related to cesarean section. These can also be seen in inguinal or femoral hernia sacs. The characteristic cyclical pain should enable a preoperative diagnosis. Endometriosis in the hernia sac may be the only evidence of the disease and may mimic incarceration.[929,1234] Leiomyomas arising from uterine fibroids are also encountered in inguinal, femoral, obturator[716] and umbilical hernial[228] sacs in women.

Acute inflammation – peritonitis and appendicitis as complications of a hernial sac

Intraperitoneal sepsis producing pus and presenting as a painful distended hernial sac is an important differential diagnosis of strangulated hernia; in these circumstances the hernia is behaving as a peritoneal recess in which pus can loculate. Zuckerkandl first described this phenomenon in 1891. His patient was a 55-year-old male with a 6-day history of a painful irreducible right inguinal hernia. At operation the hernial sac contained pus only and the perforated appendix lay in the peritoneal cavity just above the sac. The appendix was not removed and the patient recovered.[1242] Cronin and Ellis reported five patients from Oxford in which a pus-filled hernia misled surgeons into a preoperative diagnosis of strangulated hernia.[254] This complication of pus in a hernial sac most frequently occurs in right inguinal,[114] then right femoral,[389] then left inguinal and, least often, in left femoral hernias.[1192] The syndrome has been encountered in epigastric and umbilical hernias. Underlying pathologies include acute appendicitis (the most common), perforated peptic ulcer, pneumococcal peritonitis, acute pyosalpinx, acute pancreatitis and biliary peritonitis.[254,329] At least one instance of pus in a left inguinal hernia sac secondary to a periurethral abscess has been found. This patient has had a prior penectomy for ischemic necrosis secondary to diabetic vasculopathy.[671]

In acute appendicitis the appendix may itself be contained in an external hernial sac. Ryan, in 1937, collected 537 cases. An overall incidence of 0.3% of cases of acute appendicitis was found to occur in a hernial sac.[1006] Although the appendix is frequently encountered within an inguinal or femoral hernial sac, it is rarely inflamed. The first reported case of appendicitis in a femoral hernial sac is that of De Garengeot in 1731.[276] Doolin (1919) described a case in which a tender femoral hernial sac was found to contain pus and the gangrenous tip of the appendix. In this patient there were no abnormal findings in the abdomen above the inguinal ligament.[311] Hernial appendicitis usually occurs in a right inguinal or right femoral hernia[686] and in cases of perforated appendix is often misdiagnosed as a strangulated groin hernia.[706,517] Claudius Amyand performed the first successful appendectomy in 1736, which was contained in a right inguinal hernia.[870] Amyand, a Huguenot, was a pioneer of smallpox vaccination and surgeon to King George II at St George's Hospital, London – the appendix had given rise to a fistula in the right groin where it had been perforated by a pin and was discharging through an inguinal hernia. The patient was an 11-year-old boy and the operation was done without anesthesia: it is not surprising that the hernia recurred. However, Amyand deserves the title of pioneer of surgery of the vermiform appendix, having carried out the operation of appendectomy successfully 144 years before Lawson Tate removed an inflamed appendix through the abdomen in 1880.[1048] Most reported cases of appendicitis are in femoral hernias of postmenopausal women or in inguinal hernias in males of all ages from 6 weeks to 88 years. Appendicitis has been reported in a left inguinal hernia,[187] in an umbilical hernia,[310] in an obturator hernia and in incisional hernias.[187,1125]

The diagnosis of acute hernial appendicitis has been reported preoperatively only once, by Gray in 1910. Before the advent of modern radiology, the preoperative diagnosis of acute hernial appendicitis was rarely made.[431] Luchs and colleagues reported two cases of Amyand's hernia which were clinically thought to be incarcerated inguinal hernias but were correctly prospectively diagnosed as having Amyand's hernia on the basis of preoperative computed tomography (CT) examinations. These cases show the utility of CT of the acute abdomen and pelvis in revealing a previously unsuspected diagnosis and rapidly triaging patients to the appropriate management. Laparoscopy is an alternative diagnostic modality, which can be turned to therapeutic advantage to perform the appendicectomy and repair the hernia.[76] The history usually suggests a strangulated hernia with local peritonitis. The differential diagnosis is a Richter's hernia or strangulated omentum. The pain in both these conditions is classically continuous and penetrating, whereas in early appendicitis periumbilical colic is a typical feature.[242]

Treatment is operation, if possible appendectomy via the hernial sac, with repair of the hernia. In a series of seven cases, four femoral and three inguinal, from Bristol and Exeter (England), the preoperative diagnosis was a strangulated hernia in each instance; appendicitis was not suspected. Appendectomy via the sac and hernioplasty was performed in each. All the patients recovered, although wound infection created postoperative problems in three patients. Preoperatively only three patients had right iliac fossa pain, but all had histories lasting longer than 24 h before the diagnosis was reached.[1125] Acute appendicitis in a hernial sac must be distinguished from acute strangulation of the appendix in a hernia (see below).

Where there is sepsis due to inflammation or strangulation of the appendix, the hernia repair should be undertaken without the use of synthetic mesh either laparoscopically or through a preperitoneal open incision that gives access to the peritoneal cavity and the inguinal region.[706]

INCARCERATION, OBSTRUCTION AND STRANGULATION

Incarceration is the state of an external hernia, which cannot be reduced into the abdomen. Incarceration is important because it implies an increased risk of obstruction and strangulation. Incarceration is caused by (a) a tight hernial sac neck; (b) adhesions between the hernial contents and the sac lining – these adhesions are sometimes a manifestation of previous ischemia and inflammation; (c) development of pathology in the incarcerated viscus, e.g. a carcinoma or diverticulitis in incarcerated colon; (d) impaction of feces in an incarcerated colon.

Incarceration is an important finding. It should urge the surgeon to undertake operation sooner rather than later. If reduction of a hernia is performed it should be gentle; forcible reduction of an incarcerated hernia may precipitate reductio-en-masse (see below). If bowel with a compromised blood supply is reduced, stricturing and adhesions between gut loops will follow. This will lead to intestinal obstruction some weeks or months later.[732,802] The best policy is to operate on incarcerated hernias and check the viability of the gut at operation.

Incarceration in an inguinal hernia is the commonest cause of acute intestinal obstruction in infants and children in the UK. In adults, postoperative adhesions account for 40% of cases of obstruction, external hernias for 30% and malignancy for 25% of cases. In tropical Africa, strangulated external hernia is the commonest cause of intestinal obstruction in all age groups.[266] In West Africa, strangulated inguinal hernia is the commonest cause of obstruction, with indirect inguinal hernia accounting for 85% and direct hernias 15% of these cases. In the African experience, Richter's hernias are more common with direct than with indirect sacs.[66] Incarceration of the distal stomach and pylorus in an inguinal hernia can give symptoms of gastric outflow obstruction.[266]

All patients presenting with symptoms of intestinal obstruction should have all the potential hernial sites very carefully examined. The sites of obstruction are inguinal, femoral, umbilical, incisional, Spigelian, and obturator and perineal hernial orifices in that order.

A partial enterocele (Richter's hernia) is a particularly treacherous variety of hernia, especially in infancy (see below). Partial enterocele is a potentially lethal and easily overlooked complication of 'port site' hernia following laparoscopy.[620]

Strangulation is the major life-threatening complication of abdominal hernias. In strangulation the blood supply to the hernial contents is compromised. At first there is angulation and distortion of the neck of the sac; this leads to lymphatic and venous engorgement. The herniated contents become edematous. Capillary vascular permeability develops. The arterial supply is occluded by the developing edema and now the scene is set for ischemic changes in the bowel wall.

The gut mucosal defenses are breached and intestinal bacteria multiply and penetrate through to infect the hernial sac contents. Necrobiosis and gangrene complete a sad and lethal cycle unless surgery or preternatural fistula formation save the patient. Hypovolemia and septic shock predicate vigorous resuscitation if surgery is to be successful.[1172]

Strangulated external hernia

The incidence of strangulated hernia has not altered significantly in the UK over the past 15 years. The average annual incidence of strangulated external hernia is 13 per 100 000 population.[930]

There are significant seasonal variations in the incidence of strangulation, the condition being most prevalent in the winter months (October to March). In the summer 6 months (April to September) the incidence (5 per 100 000 population) is less than half the rate for the winter.[33] Perhaps this is associated with coughing related to respiratory tract infections which are more prevalent in winter.

During the period 1991–1992, 210 deaths occurring following inguinal hernia repair and 120 deaths following femoral hernia repair, were investigated by the UK National Confidential Enquiry Into Perioperative Deaths.[177] This enquiry is concerned with the quality of delivery of surgery, anesthesia and perioperative care. Expert advisers compare the records of patients who have died with index cases. In this group of 330 patients many were elderly (45 were aged 80–89 years) and significantly infirm unfit; 24 were ASA grade III and 21 ASA grade IV. Postoperative mortality was attributed to pre-existing cardiorespiratory problems in the majority of cases. Clearly this group of patients requires high-quality care by an experienced surgeon and anesthetist with skills equivalent to that of the ASA grade of the patient. Postoperative care should necessarily take place in a high dependency unit or intensive therapy unit; this may necessitate transfer of selected patients to appropriate hospitals and facilities. In these patients, the surgery should be performed in the hospital setting initially, rather than subjecting the patient to transfer from one facility to another. Sensible decisions must be made in consultation with relatives of extremely elderly, frail or moribund patients to adopt a humane approach, which may rule out interventional surgery.

The age incidence shows a peak in the very young (see Chapter 10), then a low incidence rising to a peak in the eighth decade. Males predominate until the 75th year, after which females present more frequently. Right-sided hernias strangulate more frequently than left-sided hernias; this is possibly related to mesenteric anatomy (Table 9.1). Therefore, age is the main risk factor and determinant for strangulation.

Table 9.1 *Strangulated hernias: effect of hernia type on rate of bowel resection and morality in adults. (From Andrews 1981, with permission)[33]*

Hernia type	Resection (%)	Mortality (%)
Primary inguinal	9.5	13.6
Femoral	18.0	15.0
Umbilical	25.0	4.0
Incisional	22.0	0.0
Recurrent	40.0	18.0

Neuhauser, who studied a population in Columbia where elective herniorrhaphy was virtually unobtainable, found an annual rate of strangulation of 0.29% for inguinal hernias.[842] There is no previous history of hernia in 10% of cases of strangulation.[373] Strangulation in adults is more likely in femoral, incisional and recurrent inguinal hernias rather than primary inguinal hernias and is associated with a high morbidity and mortality. Therefore, however reluctant surgeons may be to tackle femoral, incisional and recurrent inguinal hernias electively,

the greater risk of strangulation and the high complication rate when these hernias strangulate necessitate elective repair whenever this is possible[33] (Figure 9.1).

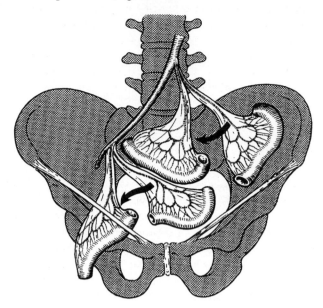

Figure 9.1 *The mesenteric anatomy determines that right-sided inguinal, femoral and obturator hernias strangulate more frequently than left-sided ones.*

A report from the Korle Bu teaching hospital in Ghana reviewed data on intestinal obstruction over a 50-year period. External hernias as a cause of intestinal obstruction decreased from 78% to 60% and the overall caseload of hospital admissions with intestinal obstruction reduced by 50%.[42] The change paralleled a rise in elective hernia day-case surgery for inguinal hernia, which the authors credited for this changing pattern of intestinal obstruction.

Forty percent of patients with femoral hernia are admitted as emergency cases with strangulation or incarceration, whereas only 3% of patients with direct inguinal hernias present with strangulation. This clearly has implications for the prioritization on waiting lists when these types of hernia present electively to outpatient clinics. A groin hernia is at its greatest risk of strangulation within 3 months of its onset.[380,803] For inguinal hernia at 3 months after presentation the cumulative probability of strangulation is 2.8%, rising to 4.5% after 2 years (Figure 9.2). For femoral hernia the risk is much higher, with a 22% probability of strangulation at 3 months after presentation rising to 45% at 21 months (Figure 9.3). McEntee *et al.* in Limerick, Ireland, questioned patients presenting to hospital with strangulated hernias about their previous history.[803] Fifty-eight percent had noted the hernia for one month, 23% of these had not reported the hernia to their family doctor, 24% were known by their family practitioner to have the hernia and a non-surgical approach advised, and 11% had been assessed in secondary care with a view to elective herniorrhaphy (of these half were considered fit for operation and the others were on a waiting list). A further survey indicates lack of uniformity in the approach to elective surgery in patients at high risk of strangulation.[16] A questionnaire sent to 406 senior physicians, geriatricians, surgeons and

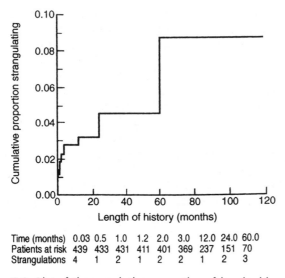

Time (months)	0.03	0.5	1.0	1.2	2.0	3.0	12.0	24.0	60.0
Patients at risk	439	433	431	411	401	369	237	151	70
Strangulations	4	1	2	1	2	2	1	2	3

Figure 9.2 *Plot of the cumulative proportion of inguinal hernias strangulating versus length of history. (Redrawn with permission from Gallegos et al., 1991.)*

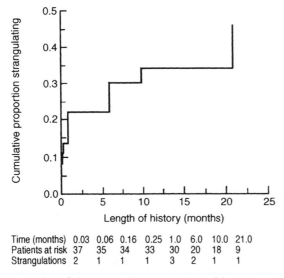

Time (months)	0.03	0.06	0.16	0.25	1.0	6.0	10.0	21.0
Patients at risk	37	35	34	33	30	20	18	9
Strangulations	2	1	1	1	3	2	1	1

Figure 9.3 *Plot of the cumulative proportion of femoral hernias strangulating versus length of history. (Redrawn with permission from Gallegos et al., 1991.)*

general practitioners asked if they would advocate elective surgery for a small, painless, reducible inguinal hernia in a 79-year-old man or an asymptomatic femoral hernia in a frail 80-year-old woman. The percentage of positive answers for elective surgery in the elderly man ranged from 10% (physicians) to 29% (surgeons) and for the elderly female from 38% (general practitioners) to 78% (surgeons). These figures indicate that general practitioners, and to a lesser extent hospital specialists, are wrongly exercising a selective policy at the expense of the elderly. In a patient over the age of 60 years a strangulated hernia has a 20-fold increased risk of death compared with elective repair. The American College of Surgeons in the USA is currently conducting a prospective study in non-operative treatment of selected hernias. This multicenter trial should provide us with a better understanding of the outcomes of such therapy.

In both the UK and the USA the annual death rate due to inguinal and femoral hernia has decreased in the last two to three decades.[790,1214] In the UK deaths for inguinal and femoral hernia declined from 22% and 55% respectively from 1975 to 1990. The annual deaths in the USA per 100 000 population for patients with hernia and intestinal obstruction decreased from 5.1 in 1968 to 3.0 in 1988. For inguinal hernia with obstruction 88% of patients underwent surgery with a mortality rate of 0.05%. These figures could be interpreted as showing that elective groin hernia surgery has reduced overall mortality rates. In support of this contention is the fact that strangulation rates are lower in the USA than in the UK, which could be a consequence of the three times higher rate of elective hernia surgery in the USA. Even so, the available statistics show that rates of elective hernia surgery in the USA per 100 000 population fell from 358 to 220 between 1975 and 1990,[790] although this may be an artefact of the data collection systems rather than a real decline.[993]

The conclusion from these studies is that the general public, especially the elderly, should be aware of the potential dangers of a lump in the groin. The most easily missed of these lumps in the groin is a femoral hernia in an obese patient in whom the consequences of a missed diagnosis carry a high morbidity and mortality.[839] Hospital physicians and general practitioners should be encouraged to refer patients with groin hernias promptly to *surgeons*, particularly those patients with a lump that has been present for 3 months or less. Indeed, patients referred with an inguinal lump or hernia (as opposed to a femoral hernia) should receive an early outpatient appointment with a surgeon because of the doubt in diagnosis.[199]

Obturator hernias are very prone to strangulation; however, their elective repair is rarely feasible and a high index of suspicion particularly in elderly, emaciated female patients with symptoms of intestinal obstruction is required. Clinical suspicion combined with preoperative ultrasonography or CT scan can correctly diagnose obturator hernia preoperatively and result in successful surgery.[414,433,1230] Recently, the magnetic resonance imaging of these patients has identified these hernias readily.[1130] To avoid confusion, primary inguinal hernias in adult males, particularly the direct spontaneously reducible 'dome' hernias, are not at significant risk of strangulation and may not always warrant an elective operation (this is discussed further in Chapter 12).

Management of strangulation

Diagnosis is based on symptoms and signs supplemented by abdominal radiographs when indicated. Pain over the hernia site is invariable and obstruction with strangulation of intestine will cause colicky abdominal pain, distension, vomiting and constipation. Physical examination may reveal degrees of dehydration with or without CNS depression, especially in the elderly if uremia is present, together with abdominal signs of intestinal obstruction. Femoral hernias can be easily missed, especially in the obese female, and a thorough examination should be performed in order to make the correct diagnosis. Frequently, however, physical examination alone is insufficiently accurate to confirm the presence of a strangulating femoral hernia versus lymphadenopathy versus a lymph node abscess. In these instances, one may elect to perform radiographic studies such as an ultrasound or a CT scan on an urgent or emergent basis.

Preoperative laboratory investigations should include full blood count, to assess leukocytosis as an indicator of intestinal infarction and hematocrit to assess hydration. Blood biochemistry may reveal features suggestive of dehydration, such as electrolyte imbalance or raised creatinine and urea. A period of resuscitation is essential to bring these laboratory parameters in line for safe anesthesia. In the elderly a chest radiograph and electrocardiograph will complete the preoperative workup and may indicate the need for additional peroperative monitoring, such as venous pressure monitoring or atrial wedge pressure. Treatment begins with nasogastric suction, bladder catheterization and intravenous fluid replacement. Broad spectrum antibiotics to cover both Gram-negative and Gram-positive organisms should be instituted. The period of resuscitation must be finely judged: the merits of optimizing the patient's state of hydration, electrolyte balance and cardiopulmonary status, must be balanced against the systemic toxic complications of unresected, infarcted bowel.

The choice of anesthetic is dependent upon the general fitness of the patient, patient preference, and the skills of the surgeon or anesthetist. Nevertheless, a bowel resection and anastomosis is always more safely performed through a peritoneal route; this operation should be carried out under general anesthesia. Alternatives include regional anesthesia (epidural or spinal) and, rarely, local anesthetic. Inflamed skin and tissues overlying strangulated hernial sacs have a low pH and local anesthetic solutions may be ineffective. This should be borne in mind when selecting local anesthesia.

The choice of incision will depend on the type of groin hernia if the diagnosis is confident. When the diagnosis is in doubt a half-Pfannenstiel incision 2 cm above the pubic ramus, extending laterally, will give an adequate approach to all types of femoral or inguinal hernia. The fundus of the hernia sac can then be approached and exposed and an incision made to expose the contents of the sac. This will allow determination of the viability of its contents. Non-viability will necessitate conversion of the transverse incision into a laparotomy incision followed by release of the constricting hernia ring, reduction of the contents of the sac, resection and re-anastomosis. Precautions should be taken to avoid contamination of the general peritoneal cavity by gangrenous bowel or intestinal contents. In the majority of cases, once the constriction of the hernia ring has been released, circulation to the intestine is re-established and viability returns. Intestine that is initially dusky, aperistaltic or dull in hue may pink up with a short period of warming with damp packs once the constriction band is released. If viability is doubtful resection should be performed. A small Richter's hernia resulting in ischemia of a limited area of the intestinal circumference may be adequately treated by over-sewing with a serosal suture, taking care not to reduce the bowel lumen circumference.

A viable alternative to this approach for the laparoscopic surgeon is the use of a diagnostic laparoscopic examination. The patient could be given a general anesthetic and the laparoscope can be used to inspect the inguinofemoral quite easily. If a Richter's hernia, as noted above, is found, then this too can be over-sewn with the laparoscopic techniques. Conversion to either an open inguinal approach or a laparotomy could still be performed if there is a need to do this maneuver.

Intestinal resection in children with strangulated hernias is rarely required. Resection rates are highest for femoral or recurrent inguinal hernias and lowest for inguinal hernias. Other organs, such as bladder or omentum, should be resected as the need requires. After peritoneal lavage and formal closure of the laparotomy incision, specific repair of the groin hernia defect should be performed. In this situation prosthetic mesh should not be used in an operative field that has been contaminated and in which there is a relatively high risk of wound infection. The hernia repair should follow the general principles for elective hernia repair. For recurrent groin hernias and femoral hernias, the preperitoneal approach is the preferred method.

Reductio-en-masse

Mass reduction of a hernia is nowadays a great rarity in Western nations, where elective operation is the treatment of choice and where incarcerated or strangulated hernias are subjected to early open operation. Mass reduction is, therefore, not a complication with which surgeons are well acquainted and for this reason the diagnosis may be overlooked. Pearse, in 1931, calculated that it occurred in 0.3% of strangulated hernias treated by taxis (gentle external reduction of the hernial contents).[895]

Reductio-en-masse (mass reduction) refers to reduction of the external herniation with continued incarceration or strangulation of the internally prolapsed hernial contents. The most commonly reported instances followed reduction of inguinal, more frequently indirect than direct, and femoral hernias. However, examples of reductio-en-masse of obturator and other rare hernias have been reported.[687]

The condition was first described by Saviard, in 1702, who reported a post-mortem examination of a patient who had died following successful taxis for a femoral hernia. Barker and Smiddy reviewed the topic in 1970 and added considerably to our understanding of the condition. More importantly, they were able to describe additional clinical signs to enable more accurate diagnosis.[79]

Reductio-en-masse is not a single anatomical entity. There are at least three varieties encountered:[895]

1 The sac still containing its strangulated contents can be forced away from the parietal muscles and come to lie in the abdominal cavity – 'arrachement de collet'.[895] For this to occur, the neck of the sac must be small, fibrosed and unyielding, and once irreducibility has occurred, must grip the contents preventing their reduction. The neck of the sac must also be surrounded by a weak internal ring to which it is not adherent (Figure 9.4). Enthusiastic manipulation by the patient or his attendants can then force the sac and its contents from their moorings and reduce them intact inside the abdominal wall. Reduction of the hernia in these circumstances causes traction on

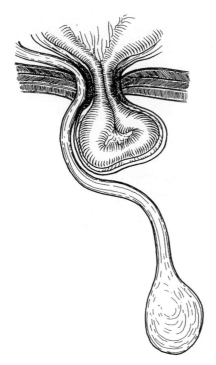

Figure 9.4 *Reductio-en-masse. An incarcerated inguinal hernia with a tight unyielding neck which is not attached securely to the parieties at the deep ring can be forcefully reduced into the abdomen.*

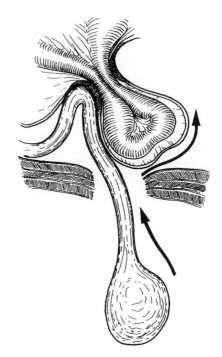

Figure 9.5 *The bowel remains incarcerated; the sac and its contents are 'reduced' into the abdomen where they remain as a tender mass in the inguinal region. The spermatic cord is dragged in by its attachment to the neck of the sac at the deep ring and consequently the testicle is retracted. Attempts to reposition the testicle (traction on the cord) will elicit pain (Smiddy's sign).*

the spermatic cord with retraction of the testis. In these circumstances the reduced mass may still be palpable in the iliac fossa, the testis will be retracted on the same side and gentle traction on the testis and spermatic cord will elicit pain – 'Smiddy's sign'[79] (Figure 9.5).

2 The sac may separate but the constriction ring at the neck remains intact, so that although the external hernia reduces into the extraperitoneal plane, the obstruction/strangulation remains. This is the most commonly reported type, accounting for 92.8% of recorded cases[895] (Figure 9.6).

3 The contents could be reduced from an external sac into a preperitoneal communicating sac if one were present. Moynihan described apparent mass reduction of an incarcerated inguinal hernia into an associated preperitoneal sac, the obstruction at the neck of the sac where it joined the main peritoneal cavity remaining unaltered. This complication can only occur in bilocular sacs. Bilocular sacs are rare, except in patients who have worn a truss for many years and developed adhesions of the superficial inguinal ring. Hence, Moynihan's type of reductio-en-masse is also very rare nowadays[819] (Figure 9.7).

In all cases of reductio-en-masse, although the external hernial mass has gone, palpation of its egress site will demonstrate the empty ring. Usually there is adjacent tenderness around the egress ring and careful gentle palpation of the nearby abdomen will reveal the globular obstructed viscera in it. More importantly, the symptoms of obstruction will persist. Central colicky abdominal pain, increasing distension, vomiting, constipation

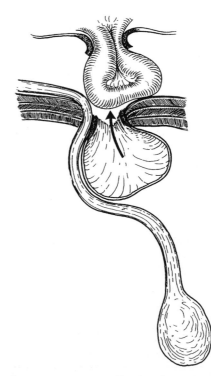

Figure 9.6 *The sac may rupture allowing the contents, still strangulated by the constriction of the neck, to be reduced into the abdominal cavity. The obstruction remains, and additionally there will be extensive local bruising and tenderness.*

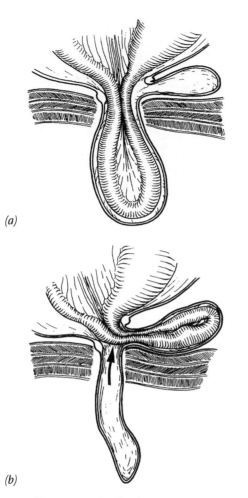

(a)

(b)

Figure 9.7 *Moynihan reported reductio-en-masse as a phenomenon associated with a bilocular inguinal hernial sac. The strangulated bowel was moved from the external component of the sac to another preperitoneal component, the common neck remaining as the site of the constriction. Review of the literature suggests this is the least common form of reductio-en-masse.*

and hypovolemia should alert the clinician. Abdominal radiographs will point up the stigmata of intestinal obstruction, dilated loops and fluid levels.

Operation through an extraperitoneal approach to the groin will allow simultaneous hernia repair if the hernia is inguinal, femoral or obturator in type. The use of preoperative CT scanning may obviate the need for the extraperitoneal approach in this manner. Certainly the use of diagnostic laparoscopy may provide excellent visualization of the reduced bowel. Additionally, the surgeon could then proceed with a laparoscopic hernia repair of his or her choosing.

MAYDL'S HERNIA AND AFFERENT LOOP STRANGULATION

In 1895, Maydl[759] described the hernie-en-W or double loop hernia, in which segments of bowel proximal and distal to an infolded loop become incarcerated within a hernial sac but

without loss of viability. However, the infolded or intra-abdominal loop may become infarcted by strangulation even in the presence of viable loops incarcerated in the hernial sac. When more than one loop is gangrenous it is always the intra-abdominal loops rather than the intrahernial loops that are involved. Isolated gangrene of an intrahernial loop without gangrene of the intra-abdominal loop has not been reported (Figure 9.8).

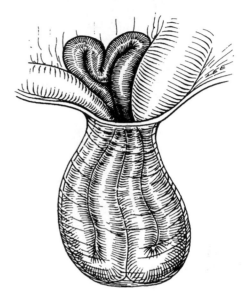

Figure 9.8 *Maydl's hernia or W or 'double-loop' hernia. The infolded, intra-abdominal, loop is strangulated. It is important when operating on a strangulated hernia to inspect in continuity all the loops of gut in the sac so that an infolded loop is not overlooked.*

Maydl's hernia is commonest in men and commonest on the right side. Both small bowel and large bowel are found in these hernias of course; Maydl originally described the strangulated appendix vermiformis in a hernial sac (see below). On the left side the sigmoid colon and transverse colon have been described in the hernia.[383] One patient in whom all the loops were large bowel has been reported. This patient needed a right hemicolectomy because the loops of cecum, ascending colon and hepatic flexure were all gangrenous.[817]

Maydl's hernia is rare in Western series of strangulated hernias. Frankau (1931)[373] reviewed 1487 strangulated hernia from centers in the British Isles; there were 654 strangulated inguinal hernias and in four of these a Maydl's hernia was found (0.6%).[373] In West Africa, where strangulated inguinal hernia is the commonest cause of intestinal obstruction, Maydl's hernia accounts for 2% of all cases.[66,95]

In Korle Bu Teaching Hospital, Accra, Ghana, Maydl's hernia has been reported as frequently as five times in a consecutive series of 26 strangulated inguinal hernias. In this series, four sacs contained a double loop of intestine and the fifth contained three loops. All five patients were male adult Ghanaians. In three of these patients the cecum and part of the ascending colon were lying free in the hernial sac, not sliding intraperitoneally in the lateral posterior wall as is so frequent in European patients. This arrangement allows loops of small intestine to prolapse into the sac behind and lateral to the cecum as well as anterior and medial to it[95] (Figure 9.9).

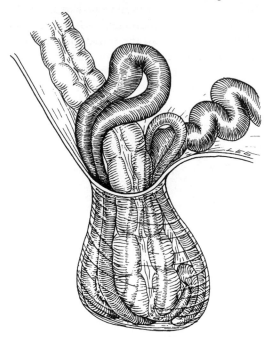

Figure 9.9 *Double Maydl's hernia; described in ethnic West Africans. The cecum, appendix and terminal ileum and two loops of ileum are incarcerated in a giant inguinoscrotal sac. The two intervening loops of small intestine lying within the abdominal cavity are strangulated. Laparoscopy or a laparotomy is essential to assess the extent of bowel viability in a case of double W hernia.*

Afferent loop strangulation is a complication in which intra-abdominal strangulation of small intestine occurs proximal to an obstructed inguinal hernia. It is a common complication of right inguinal hernia obstruction in East Africa. The afferent loop is imprisoned behind the cecum, which is obstructed in the inguinal hernial sac. The internal herniation of the loop of ileum passes from medial to lateral, behind the pendulous cecum, which is fixed in the hernial sac. The cecum retains its circulation from the iliocecal vessels, which form the anterior component of the constriction, imprisoning the loop of ileum and infringing its mesenteric marginal blood vessels. At operation for strangulation, if the cecum when released is pendulous and free, not sliding, the ileum for at least 1 meter proximal should be checked to ensure it has not suffered entrapment and infarction. This advice is most relevant in ethnic East African patients[907] (Figure 9.10).

Davey draws attention to these variations of strangulated hernia when the sac contains the cecum in Africans. As a precaution the surgeon should always count the loops in the sac and inspect the gut for 1 meter proximal and distal. The use of the laparoscope in this type of patient would relieve any doubt about the viability of the bowel if this exists. A diagnosis of strangulated middle or afferent loop Maydl's hernia should be suspected in any patient who presents with a painful but not tender inguinoscrotal swelling, a tender mass in the lower abdomen and a scaphoid empty upper abdomen.[265] Here

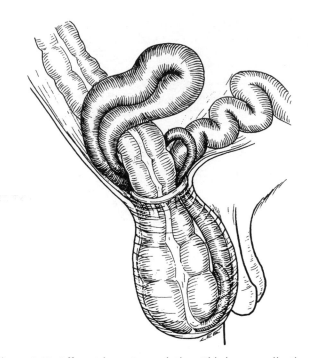

Figure 9.10 *Afferent loop strangulation. This is a complication of large inguinoscrotal hernias in Africans who have a long pendulous scrotum. The cecum is incarcerated in the hernial sac; a loop of small bowel passes behind the ascending colon and is strangulated to the right of the colon. Formal laparotomy is required.*

again, the diagnostic laparoscopy will assist in the determination of the intestinal strangulation.

In small tight-necked indirect inguinal hernia in infants, a Maydl's hernia of the appendix can occur. Appendectomy at herniotomy is appropriate surgery[1194] (Figure 9.11).

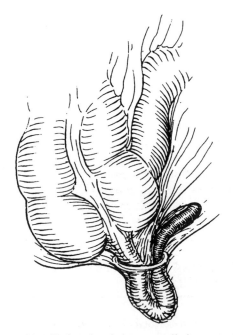

Figure 9.11 *A Maydl's hernia of the appendix is a complication of an incarcerated inguinal hernia in an infant.*

Maydl's hernia can also occur after laparoscopic operations by herniation of small bowel through a trocar site.[112]

STRANGULATION OF THE APPENDIX IN A HERNIAL SAC

The appendix is seen frequently, in an inguinal or femoral hernial sac. Strangulation (as opposed to appendicitis) is rare. On clinical and histological grounds separation of the two diseases should not present difficulties. In strangulation, inflammation is accompanied by venous infarction; it involves all coats of the appendix and is clearly delimited proximally where the constriction is applied.[759] In acute appendicitis, suppuration begins in the mucosa and spreads outwards. It is associated with intracavity purulent distension. A strangulated appendix behaves clinically like a Richter's partial enterocele.[254]

RICHTER'S HERNIA

Partial enterocele, the eponymous Richter's hernia, was not first described by Richter! And the condition has a variety of other names in the English and American literature: nipped hernia, pinched hernia, Lavator's hernia, etc.

Partial enterocele was first observed by Fabricius Hildanus in 1598 and clearly described by Lavator in 1672.[1194] Littré reported cases in 1700 and 1714, Morgagni in 1723, De Garengeot in 1743 and Ruysch in 1744. The most important paper was by Richter in 1785, but it was Sir Frederick Treves who gave an excellent overview on the topic and proposed the title Richter's hernia;[1086] hence the hernia is named after him. Richter's hernia has recently again come into prominence, this time as a complication of CAPD, used in the treatment of renal failure,[333] and as a complication of 'port site' hernias following laparoscopy.[484] There is a significantly greater risk of the development of such a hernia when 10 mm (or larger) trocars are used. The cutting type of trocar can predispose the patient to this possibility, however this is an infrequent occurrence. This risk can be greatly reduced if the surgeon sutures the fascia closed after the completion of the laparoscopic procedure. This risk can also be decreased if the surgeon uses a non-cutting trocar or a dilating type of trocar.

In the partial enterocele the antimesenteric circumference of the intestine becomes constricted in the neck of a hernial sac without causing complete intestinal luminal occlusion (Figure 9.12).

Richter's hernia is most frequently found in femoral or obturator hernias, although the condition has been described at other sites[840] and there is an increasing incidence at laparoscope insertion sites, therefore awareness of this special type of hernia with its misleading clinical appearance is important.

According to localization and the mode of herniation and entrapment, the clinical picture and course can vary considerably. Steinke and Zellweger (2000)[1086] have described four main groups: (i) The obstructive group, in which early diagnosis and therapy leads to an excellent prognosis. (ii) The danger group, in which symptomatology is vague and subsequent delay in surgery is responsible for a high death rate. (iii) The postnecrotic group in which local strangulation and perforation leads to formation of an enterocutaneous fistula (similar to the noblewoman described by Fabricius in 1606); the fistula may close spontaneously ('the miracle cure') or remain chronic. (iv) The 'unlucky' perforation group, in which the postnecrotic abscess, as a result of unlucky anatomical constellations, accidentally finds its way into another compartment, resulting either in a large abscess with severe septic/ toxic load or in peritonitis; both of these would lead to a high death rate.

Richter's hernias occur in infantile indirect inguinal hernias. Colic and distension occur, but absolute constipation for feces and gas is a late phenomenon. Vomiting is also often absent. On physical examination there is tenderness but no palpable lump at the hernial site. Strangulation and gangrene of the bowel wall nipped in the hernial sac sets in rapidly and perforation of the gut into the sac may occur without immediate catastrophic

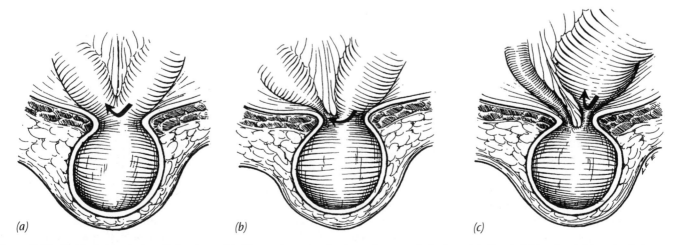

(a)   *(b)*   *(c)*

Figure 9.12 *Richter's hernia (partial enterocele). The antimesenteric circumference of the bowel is first held by the rigid neck of the hernial sac, usually a femoral or obturator hernia. The situation is progressive: from (a) partial involvement of the bowel circumference without obstruction, to (b) subacute obstruction; to (c) complete obstruction and strangulation of the incarcerated bowel.*

peritonitis. It is important to recognize the condition at operation – to return the non-viable bowel to the peritoneal cavity is to precipitate disaster.

LITTRÉ'S HERNIA – HERNIA OF MECKEL'S DIVERTICULUM

Alexis Littré, in 1700, reported three cases of an incarcerated femoral hernia containing an ileal diverticulum. Littré interpreted the ileal diverticulum as a secondary phenomenon related to the hernial ring and arising from the intestine opposite it. Johann Meckel, in 1809, identified the embryological origin of the distal small intestinal diverticulum, which was henceforward to bear his name. Meckel recognized that his diverticulum was a partial persistence of the omphalomesenteric duct communicating between the fetal midgut and the yolk sac.[781] It was only after Meckel's paper that it was realized that the diverticulum in the hernia described by Littré was the diverticulum described by Meckel. The clear elucidation of these facts we again owe to Sir Frederick Treves.[1140]

Meckel's diverticulum is the most common congenital anomaly of the gastrointestinal tract arising as a result of incomplete dissolution of the vitello-intestinal duct. Approximately 4% of patients with Meckel's diverticulum develop complications, Littré's hernia being one of the least common.[31] A Meckel's diverticulum may be a chance finding in an inguinal hernia. It has been described in incarcerated inguinal hernia in infants: in infants the diverticulum frequently becomes adherent to the sac and as a consequence the hernia becomes irreducible. This can be diagnosed when after taxis of a right inguinal hernia in an infant, part of the hernia remains unreduced.[71]

Meckel's diverticulum has also been described in an umbilical hernia. This is not unsurprising when it is recalled that the omphalomesenteric duct is a component of the normal fetal umbilicus.[194] Meckel's diverticulum in femoral hernia is also described; a most unusual variant is the presentation of the diverticulum as a small bowel fistula resulting from strangulation of the diverticulum progressing to a groin abscess which discharged externally with a persistent small bowel fistula[685] (Figure 9.13).

HERNIA OF OVARY, FALLOPIAN TUBE AND UTERUS

The first case of hernia of the ovary was reported by the Greek physician Soranus of Ephesus about AD 97. Hernia of the pregnant uterus (hysterocele gravidarum) was reported by Pol (1531) and another case by Semmentus (1610). Watson (1938) reports two cases and comments that the uterus may become impregnated while in the hernial sac or the pregnant uterus may enter the sac and become irreducible as the pregnancy proceeds.[1194]

The tube and ovary may also enter the hernial sac. Ectopic pregnancy in a hernial sac is reported in these circumstances.[1194]

In contemporary practice, internal genitalia are frequently found in inguinal hernia in baby girls. The frequency with

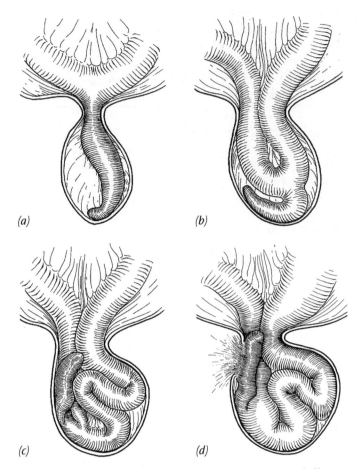

Figure 9.13 *Meckel's diverticulum in a hernial sac. A Meckel's diverticulum may be the only occupant of the sac (a); alternatively, adjacent loop ileum may be in the sac too (b). A Meckel's diverticulum may become adherent to the sac (c) or form a fistula (d).*

which they occur warrants caution to open and inspect each hernial sac to exclude their presence.

In older females the tube and ovary are sometimes the contents of inguinal, femoral or obturator hernias, usually as components of sliding sacs. Pathology may complicate these hernial contents, hydrosalpinx being common in irreducible inguinal hernia.[1164]

A uterus has been described in a male intersex with inguinal hernias. Routine examination of the scrotum for normal testicles should be the drill in all boys with inguinal hernias. If developmental anomalies are then found in the wall of a hernial sac, they can be excised.[124]

URINARY TRACT COMPLICATIONS

The bladder is a very frequent component of the medial wall of direct inguinal and of femoral hernias (Figure 9.14). Herniation of the bladder proper is a rare phenomenon; the involvement of a small part of the organ, often a diverticulum, is more frequent and usually associated with hypertrophy of the prostate.[189] This

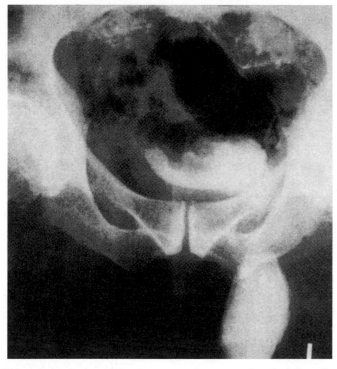

Figure 9.14 *An intravenous urogram demonstrating the left wall of the bladder in a femoral hernia sac in a man with bladder neck obstruction.*

partial bladder herniation is rarely diagnosed preoperatively but in cases where there is a strong suspicion, preoperative cystography is indicated.[385] Usually the bladder is easily identified during dissection, but when difficulty is encountered the obliterated umbilical artery is a useful landmark. If the bladder is near the protrusion of the hernia or part of the hernia, the risk of injury is particularly high during a laparoscopic repair. This situation is even more problematic in the recurrent hernia repair. The inexperienced laparoscopist should not attempt these difficult repairs and should either refer the patient or perform a careful open hernioplasty. The bladder is a very common finding in the medial wall of indirect inguinal hernias in boys (see pages 136, 141 and 142).

Care will protect the bladder from trauma during surgery. If the bladder is injured, closure with two layers of absorbable polymer suture is required and then catheter drainage should be employed for several days.

Herniation of the ureter is a rare and often misdiagnosed event and serious surgical complications are possible. Two types of the uretero-inguinal hernia can be identified: paraperitoneal (more frequent, acquired, always presenting a peritoneal hernia sac, frequently associated with other herniated abdominal structures) and extraperitoneal (very uncommon, congenital, never associated with a true peritoneal sac, always composed only of ureter).[403] The paraperitoneal type usually presents in the lateral wall of giant sliding inguinal hernias. Knowledge, suspicion and care are all that are needed to avoid damaging the ureter. The ureter should be identified, dissected away preserving its blood supply and returned to the abdomen. If the ureter is injured or its vasculature. In doubt, a pliable ureteric catheter

for several days is best advised.[901] Preoperative intravenous urogram and micturating cystogram are advisable before operation on giant inguinoscrotal hernias, to exclude ureteric complications or bladder diverticula in the hernial sac.[912]

Prolapse of an ileal conduit into an indirect inguinal hernia is described.[937] The patient presented with an ischemic blue stoma and anuria. The ileal loop was twisted around its distal fixed point (the stoma) and prolapsed into the hernial sac.

SLIDING HERNIA

Sliding hernia, hernie-en-glissade, 'landslip hernia' or 'landslide of the large intestine' are the various names for this hernia. With hindsight we can discover cases of sliding hernia in much ancient and Renaissance medical literature; however, it was Scarpa in 1819 that published the classic description of these conditions.[1017] Carnett, in 1909, classified sliding hernias,[188] while Watson (1938) reviewed the literature comprehensively and included outstanding diagrams of the anatomic types of sliding hernias of the large intestine.[1194] The most frequent sliding hernias are the cecum and appendix in indirect right inguinal hernias[970] (Figure 9.15) and the sigmoid colon in indirect left inguinal hernias[1005] (Figure 9.16).

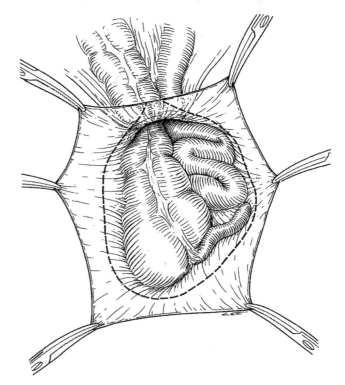

Figure 9.15 *Sliding hernia. The cecum and appendix forming part of the wall of a right inguinal hernia.*

Although Cloquet in 1817[225] and Lockwood in 1893[702] had described the bladder in the medial wall of hernial sacs, it is surprising that not until 1942 did this common problem of the sliding hernia of the bladder receive detailed attention by Zimmerman and Laufman.[1239] Sliding bladder hernias in infants, so-called 'bladder ears', were described by Allen and

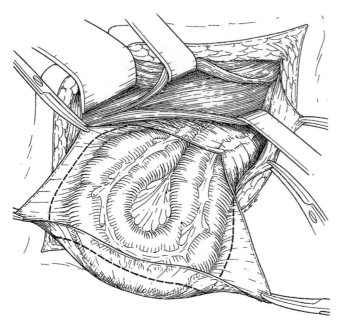

Figure 9.16 *Sliding hernia. The sigmoid loop of colon in a left inguinal hernia. These hernias are sometimes very difficult to reduce and close. A muscle-splitting incision 5 cm or so above and parallel to the inguinal ligament can facilitate mobilization. The hernia is delivered through the higher incision, excess sac is trimmed away and the sac closed. Care with the colon and its blood supply is needed. The repair of the defect is described elsewhere.*

Condon in 1961.[17] The problem of congenital sliding genital hernias in females was highlighted by Gans in 1959.[384] This, despite the fact that sliding hernias were mentioned by Sir Percival Pott, who also described a woman with bilateral sliding ovarian hernias in his treatise of 1757.[922] The woman ceased menstruating when Pott moved both hernial sacs including the ovarian tissues in their walls.

Moschowitz described the two most common intraoperative mistakes that bedevilled surgical intervention for sliding hernias;[816] Ponka described the third.[914] These are:

1 Designating a hernia to be sliding when it is merely a simple hernia in which a loop of intestine is adherent to the sac.
2 Hemorrhage caused by attempting to dissect the viscus (colon or bladder) from its blood supply. This occurs during attempts to 'create' a sac on the extraperitoneal aspect of the viscus.
3 Accidental entry into the bladder or the viscus, particularly during mobilization of the sac wall.

The solution to the management of sliding hernias owes much to the experience of the Shouldice clinic in Toronto and to the sound principles derived from this experience. Earle Shouldice, Ernest Ryan, Donald Welsh and Frank Glassow are the contributors to our knowledge. Until the Toronto group started analyzing their results the series of sliding hernias published had all been small, reflecting the rarity of the problem.

Nearly all the recurrence rates were high and reports had concentrated on technical innovation, usually without adequate follow-up data.

Zimmerman and Laufman described their technique in 1942, with no recurrences in a series of 24 cases.[1239] In 1956, Ryan reported the results of 313 cases repaired at the Shouldice clinic prior to 1952, with one indirect recurrence.[1004] In 1961, Maingot reported his experience in 64 cases with no recurrences.[736] Welsh reported 2300 sliding hernias repaired at the Shouldice clinic with only 11 recurrences.[1202]

All these authors report the same principles. The hypertrophied cremaster is removed from the sac, the cord structures are carefully dissected away from the sac up to and into the peritoneal cavity, and excess peritoneal sac is excised and closed. The hernia and its contents are then returned to the abdominal cavity. The transversalis fascia is carefully reconstructed to contain the hernia and refashion the deep ring around the cord. It is not necessary to 're-peritonealize' the viscera before they are returned to the abdominal cavity. The critical maneuvers are to return the viscera to the abdomen and to contain them within the confines of the abdomen/fascia transversalis.

Once again, the use of the laparoscope should be considered in this situation. It is relatively easy for the laparoscopist to make the diagnosis of a sliding hernia. The TAPP method of repair is sometimes preferred to the TEP method because of the occasional difficulty in reducing a particularly large sliding inguinal hernia with the latter approach. In either case, the hernia is returned to the abdominal cavity and a standard laparoscopic extraperitoneal placement of a prosthetic biomaterial will effectively repair the hernial defect. Typically, these defects are quite large and one may consider the use of a slightly larger prosthetic than would usually be used for the routine hernia repair.

TESTICULAR STRANGULATION

The testicular blood supply is compromised when a tight strangulation compresses it in its passage from the abdomen to scrotum. This may occur in three circumstances:

1 In male infants with incarcerated inguinal hernias, the venous drainage becomes obstructed at the rigid external ring. This is a not infrequent complication of infantile incarceration; it is discussed in detail on page 132.
2 In giant inguinoscrotal hernia, spontaneous infarction of the testicle has been described.[722]
3 In Africans with strangulated indirect inguinal hernia, testicular infarction due to vascular obstruction at the deep ring is reported. At operation the gangrenous testicle should be excised.[722]

The site of the vascular damage in these instances, the superficial ring in infancy and the deep ring in adulthood, emphasizes the different anatomy and structure of the inguinal canal in the pre- and post-pubertal male. It is important to differentiate the diagnosis from that of testicular torsion. In either event, however, surgery is required.

10

Groin hernias in babies and children

Inguinal herniotomy is the operation most frequently performed in pediatric practice.[439] There is an increased incidence of inguinal hernias in premature babies and in boys with cryptorchid testicles.[897,1218] Other predisposing factors are other abdominal wall defects, cystic fibrosis, increased peritoneal fluid volume, connective tissue disorders, and intersex conditions.

Although inguinal herniotomy appears to be a simple operation, it is technically demanding and great harm may be done if it is incorrectly performed. It is not an operation for the occasional pediatric surgeon; there should be no occasional pediatric surgeons. Inguinal herniotomy will probably be the child's and the child's parents (as parents) first encounter with surgery; consequently the experience may color their attitudes to surgeons for many years. Therefore, it behooves us not only to provide expert surgical and anesthetic care, but also to make the entire experience as pleasant as possible.

All elective inguinal herniotomies in children can be undertaken as day cases (i.e. outpatient).[64,226] However, because of the risk of post-anesthetic apnea in premature infants, overnight observation may be preferred in these patients.[1090] Parents should accompany their child to hospital, nurse him or her themselves and thus eliminate any psychological trauma to the family unit. Inguinal hernias in children should be operated on as soon as possible after first diagnosis to avoid the hazard of incarceration.

Preterm and low birthweight babies present special risks of postoperative apnea and bradycardia. Inguinal hernias are among the most commonly encountered surgical problems in infants with very low birth weight (less than 1500 g) with a reported incidence of 16%. A trend towards earlier operation has emerged in recent years with most now being repaired before discharge from the neonatal intensive care unit. The risk of incarceration, anesthetic management, frequency of bilaterality, the higher incidence of undescended testis and technical problems presents special concerns in these patients.[275,797] For these reasons they need appropriate specialist operative and perioperative monitoring;[784] emergency herniotomy for incarcerated inguinal hernia in infants is one of the most difficult operations and should not be undertaken lightly; it is an operation for an experienced surgeon only. Sedation and taxis will

reduce most incarcerated inguinal hernias.

Strangulation, or strangulation of a partial enterocele (Richter's hernia), sometimes complicates incarceration.

ETIOLOGY AND ANATOMY

The testicle appears at the end of the first month of intrauterine life as a ventromedial swelling at the caudal end of the genital ridge. It enlarges rapidly and by the end of the sixth week has a mesentery and bulges into the peritoneum, which invests it anteriorly. The trunk of the embryo is elongating rapidly at this time, resulting in an apparent caudal shift of the gonad, so that at about 10 weeks it is found just above the groin. This is the 'internal phase' of gonad descent. The testicular blood supply directly from the aorta is stretched out by the rapid elongation of the aorta and spine which 'carries' the kidneys cephalad. From the lower pole of the testicle a finger-like column of condensed mesenchymal cells, the gubernaculum, extends behind the peritoneum down through the layers of the body wall to the scrotum.[1218]

At about 8 weeks a pouch of peritoneum begins to bulge down in front of and alongside the gubernaculum, pushing the surrounding muscle layers ahead of itself and stretching them all the way down into the scrotum. The stretched out layers in turn each become the 'coverings' of the cord (the internal spermatic fascia, cremasteric fascia and external spermatic fascia from the fascia transversalis, the internal oblique and the external oblique muscles serially). It is suggested that at this phase of development, when gut is forced out of the abdomen into the embryological umbilical hernia, there is raised intra-abdominal pressure due to the rapid growth of intra-abdominal organs. This raised intra-abdominal pressure forces the processus vaginalis through the abdominal wall into the scrotum, which enlarges to accommodate it.

There are two theories to explain the extra-abdominal descent of the testis. Either the gubernaculum pulls the testis down or the gubernaculum remains always the same size and the testis is pulled down by elongation of the baby. Both these theories are difficult to substantiate. The first because muscle tissue has never been demonstrated in the gubernaculum and the second because rather than a short unchanging stocky fibrous cord the gubernaculum is quite long and rambles through the inguinal canal from the testis to the base of the scrotum. Furthermore, even in normal children who have scrotal testicles at birth, they are retractile and will disappear up into the inguinal canal if appropriate stimulation is applied.

At the end of the seventh intrauterine month the gubernaculum swells markedly, owing to increase in the intracellular matrix probably brought about by hormonal influence. This enlargement dilates the internal ring and the canal then the intra-abdominal pressure probably propels the testicle along the track previously formed by the processus vaginalis through the muscle tunnel and into the peritoneal sac preformed in the scrotum.[1030,1218] Boys with the 'prune belly syndrome' have undescended testicles which are not only high but look grossly abnormal, suggesting that intra-abdominal pressure (muscle tone) is needed to push the testis through the canal and into the scrotal space.[1212] A further characteristic of cryptorchism is a small processus vaginalis or sometimes its complete absence; a further manifestation of intraperitoneal pressure failing to 'push out' the testis into the scrotum.[1048]

The stimuli to the process of normal descent of the testicle and the causes of its failure or erring in its target are ill understood. It is a fault of this process that leaves the processus vaginalis, which is finely patent in 60% of normal infants at birth, as a preformed congenital hernial sac. Few, if any, of the children who present with inguinal hernia have any fascial defect. The patent processus vaginalis is a potential hernial sac but it must not be confused with a clinically evident inguinal hernia.

Normal testicular descent depends upon several factors which include: (a) a normal hypothalamic–pituitary–testicular hormone axis; (b) normal testicular production of androgen; (c) normal end organ response to androgen; (d) a normal gubernaculum; (e) a normal intra-abdominal pressure; (f) spermatic vessels of adequate length; (g) an adequate vas deferens; (h) a normal inguinal canal.[1030,1048,1218]

Primary anatomic abnormalities are probably less common causes of cryptorchism than is dysfunction of the hypothalamic–pituitary–testicular hormone axis.[589,1048] Maternal estrogen levels in early pregnancy may be a factor in determining the function of the embryonic hypothalamic–pituitary–testicular hormone axis.[216] Anecdotal clinical evidence associates vomiting in early pregnancy with cryptorchism and inguinal hernia formation.

CLASSIFICATION

Inguinal hernia in childhood can be divided into two types:[501]

1 Complete scrotal – total funicular hernia of Herzfeld (1938).
2 Incomplete bubonocele – partial funicular hernia of Herzfeld.

Complete hernias are present at birth, but are much rarer than incomplete hernias. About 5% of all inguinal hernias in male infants are of the complete variety.

So far we have only considered the occurrence of a hernia; remnants of the processus vaginalis, however, can remain in the inguinal canal, giving rise to an encysted hydrocele of the cord in the male or a hydrocele of the canal of Nuck in the female.

Figure 10.1 shows the following variants of the processus vaginalis: normal, hydrocele, encysted hydrocele, partial funicular hernia (bubonocele), and complete funicular hernia (scrotal hernia).[501]

INCIDENCE – PATHOLOGY

Some 3% to 5% of full-term babies are born with clinically apparent inguinal hernias, in preterm babies this incidence is substantially increased up to 30%.[73,476,897] Inguinal hernia is the commonest indication for surgery in early life.

The processus vaginalis was found to be open at birth in 94% of infants examined at autopsy by Camper in the 1750s. However, 94% of newborn infants do not have demonstrable inguinal hernias.[976] Robin (1995)[963] studied the natural history of the patent processus vaginalis, reviewing 2764 patients operated on for inguinal hernia at the Children's Hospital, Columbus, Ohio: 280 (10%) had clinically apparent bilateral hernias, 83 (3%) had had a contralateral hernia repaired and 2401 (87%) had a single unilateral hernia. Of the patients with unilateral hernias, 1965 had the contralateral explored in search of a patent processus; positive explorations occurred in 946 (48%) of these patients. This number is lower than reported in most series. The usual figure of children with inguinal hernia having a patent processus on the opposite side is about 60%, but in the Ohio series some patients already had had a bilateral exploration.[590] The highest incidence of patency of the contralateral processus vaginalis occurred in the first 2 months of life (63%); after this there was a steady fall in incidence, until 2 years when the incidence was 41%, at which a levelling off developed to 16 years when a 35% incidence is recorded. Between 15% and 30% of adults without clinical evidence of an inguinal hernia have a patent processus at post-mortem.[1069] Inguinal hernia presenting as a complication of CAPD confirms the incidence of persistent processus vaginalis in adulthood. Females with unilateral inguinal hernias more commonly have a contralateral patent processus vaginalis than males (57% vs. 42%); the incidence of clinical bilateral hernias is the same in both sexes (about 15%), suggesting that the presence of a patent processus is not the sole determinant of development of an inguinal hernia (Figure 10.2). Bilateral inguinal hernia is significantly more common in premature infants (about 30%) and young children. Metachronous bilateral hernia develops in approximately 10% of normal births at a median interval of 1 year, although the incidence is higher in premature infants and up to 30% in children with an incarcerated hernia.[1112] Male infants have a higher incidence of hernias (3:1) compared with female infants (10:1).[1005]

The incidence of inguinal hernia in children in England has fallen in this century. Sir Arthur Keith, in 1924, reported the incidence of inguinal hernia in the first year of life to be 44 per

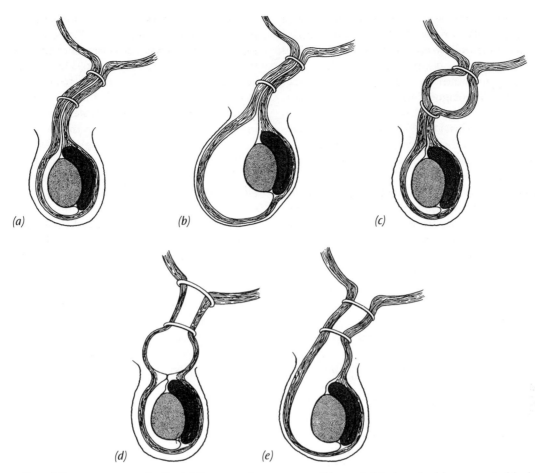

Figure 10.1 *Anomalies of the processus vaginalis: (a) the normal appearance, (b) a scrotal hydrocele, (c) an encysted hydrocele of the cord, (d) an incomplete inguinal hernia, bubonocele The sac extends part of the way along the cord. (e) A complete, funicular or scrotal hernia. The sac includes the tunica vaginalis covering of the testicle in the scrotum. (After Hertzfeld, 1938.)*

1000 live births, from the second to fifth year 9 per 1000, from 6–10 years 6 per 1000, and from 11–15 years 9 per 1000, giving an overall incidence of approximately 60 per 1000 children up to the age of 12 years.[578] Among children of Newcastle upon

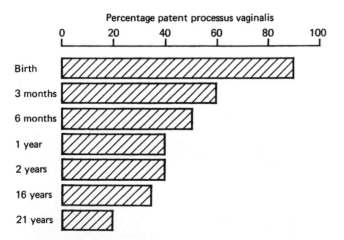

Figure 10.2 *The incidence of a patent processus vaginalis falls during the first year of life; nevertheless 15–30% of adults have evidence of a patent processus vaginalis which can dilate if these persons go on to CAPD.*

Tyne, Knox found that operation for primary inguinal hernia was performed on 10.2 per 1000 children surviving at the age of 12 years. The ratio of boys to girls was 12:1, so that the incidence of inguinal hernia in boys in this community was 1.9%.[606]

Approximately 20–25 live births per 1000 require operation for inguinal hernia of which some 10% require emergency admission for incarceration and strangulation. The ratio of boys to girls is 9:1, which yields an incidence in male children of 4.2%. Similar statistics are recorded by Thorndike and Ferguson (1938),[1126] by Lynn and Johnson (1961),[717] by Daum and Meinel (1972)[264] and by Harvey, Johnstone and Fossard (1985).[483]

The incidence of inguinal hernia is increased in preterm infants.[476,897] Hernias occur with increased frequency in infants under 32 weeks' gestational age or below 1250 g birth weight. Among infants below 32 weeks' gestational age, intrauterine growth retardation significantly increases the risk for development of inguinal hernias, especially in male infants. Thirty per cent of surviving premature infants weighing less than 1000 g develop inguinal hernias. There is an association between neonatal inguinal hernia and intrauterine growth retardation. A small prospective study of eight clinically apparent inguinal hernias in preterm infant girls has suggested that hernias containing intestinal loops regress spontaneously after the girls reach the ages of 2–6 months post-partum. This was confirmed by ultrasonography and at follow-up 2–6 years later there had been no recurrence.[872]

The incidence of inguinal hernias is higher in twins, especially in early infancy.[73] This higher incidence in twins persists throughout the childhood years and is higher in males than females: dizygotic female twins do not have the same high incidence. Inguinal hernias have a higher incidence in children with other birth defects. Inguinal hernias show a familial incidence, suggesting a polygenic defect.

A case–control study carried out by Jones and colleagues estimated the sex specific risks of inguinal hernia in siblings of children with this condition. There were 1921 male and 347 female cases born during 1970–1986 operated on for inguinal hernias at ages 0–5 years during 1970–1987, compared with 12 886 male and 2534 female control subjects. The relative risk of inguinal hernia was 5.8 for brothers of male cases and 4.3 for brothers of female cases. The relative risk was 3.7 for sisters of male cases and 17.8 for sisters of female cases.[553]

The incidence of inguinal hernia in African children is higher than in European children but there is no significant association of the incidence of inguinal hernias with race in a sample of American premature babies studied.[897] Scorer and Farrington,[1030] in common with most other authors,[439] report that there is a marked preponderance of right-sided hernia in boys – 70% right-sided, 26% left-sided and 4% bilateral – whereas in girls the incidence of right-sided hernia is 50%. Of the children who develop a right-sided hernia before reaching one year, 50% will develop a contralateral hernia; in contrast when the hernia develops after one year of age only 10% will develop a contralateral hernia.

Left inguinal hernias are associated with contralateral hernia twice as often as right-sided ones. Atwell, reviewing 3107 cases from Oxford and from Great Ormond Street Hospital, London, reports that the male to female ratio is 10.3:1. Of his personal series of 262 patients, 31% presented a groin lump in the first year of life, 60.6% were right-sided and 15% bilateral. After simple herniotomy, no cases of recurrence were found at follow-up.[63]

INCARCERATION AND STRANGULATION

Ten percent of children with inguinal hernias present as emergencies with incarceration or strangulation. Incarceration or strangulation has its highest frequency in the first three months of life; thereafter the incidence falls off so that incarceration is very rare after the sixth birthday. The incidence of incarceration is higher in premature and low birthweight children. Incarceration or strangulation is 10 times more frequent in male than in female children. Seventy-five percent of the incarcerated hernias in the first 3 months of life present in children in whom no hernia had previously been noted.[39,269,379,442,877,930,1079] Hernias which appear after birth are more likely to strangulate than those present at birth, the presumption being that hernias present at

birth have wider necks than those that develop later by opening of the processus vaginalis.

Incarcerated and strangulated hernias are five times more frequent on the right than the left side.[35,269,877,930] In boys, small gut is the most frequent viscus to be incarcerated. In girls the frequency of incarceration is the same for right and left-side hernias and the ovary and fallopian tube are most likely to be incarcerated. Adhesions between the sac and its contained viscus are very rare, except in Littré's hernia.

While incarceration is not infrequent, strangulation (an irreducible hernia containing viscera with a critically compromised blood supply) is very rare. All series report very low resection rates: Nussbaum (1913)[852] reported two cases of strangulation in 54 000 children cared for, Maclennan (1921–1922) four in 1038.[728] Thorndike and Ferguson (1938) reported five in 1740 (106 of which were incarcerated),[1126] Smith (1954) two in 50 872[1067] and Harvey, Johnstone and Fossard (1985) none in 71 emergency presentations.[483]

Cases of strangulated hernia requiring resection of small bowel have been recorded at 12 days[501] and at 25 days.[1067] Spontaneous cure by cecal fistula after 10 days' strangulation in a 7-week-old Chinese infant is reported.[1093]

Strangulation, or strangulation of a partial enterocele (Richter's hernia), can complicate incarceration. Infants with incarceration require hospital observation for at least 24 h after reduction of the hernia, in case strangulation has occurred and complications of intestinal gangrene become apparent later.

Treatment by sedation and gallows traction (Solomon position) is recommended initially. Eighty percent of incarcerated hernias reduce spontaneously if the child is adequately sedated.[826] The incidence of testicular infarction and atrophy (see below) is less with this form of treatment than with emergency surgery on the day of operation. However, if the incarceration does not reduce spontaneously, after 4 h of gallows traction with good sedation, or if the testicle is persistently tender (ischemic orchitis) and the scrotum edematous, surgery should be undertaken (Figure 10.3).

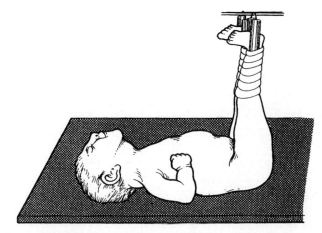

Figure 10.3 *Gallows traction in the 'Solomon position' allows most incarcerated inguinal hernias in children to reduce spontaneously.*

It is unlikely that strangulated, as opposed to incarcerated, bowel will reduce on non-operative suspension treatment. At the induction of anesthetic, incarcerated bowel will reduce spontaneously. If taxis under anesthetic is needed, the operation should proceed and the bowel be inspected for viability. The extraperitoneal approach allows scrutiny of the intestine without the necessity of a second laparotomy/incision and is, therefore, strongly recommended for all irreducible hernias.[556,1148]

Prompt elective operation for inguinal hernia in infants is recommended, the probability of incarceration being 1:4 for hernias in male children diagnosed under 12 months of age. There is some confusion and overlap in the literature between the terms 'irreducible', 'incarceration', 'strangulation', 'infarction' and 'gangrene'. An irreducible or incarcerated hernia in a child is one whose contents cannot be replaced back into the abdomen even with sedation ... these are common in practice. Strangulation and infarction are terms that imply interruption of the blood supply to the organs in the irreducible or incarcerated hernial sac. This is rare in children (except to the testicle – see below). Gangrene is tissue death; tissue death of viscera contained in an irreducible or incarcerated hernial sac is very rare in children. Gross records 63 incarcerated hernias in 3874 treated in one decade, with a single mortality from strangulation.[442]

The vascular compromised gonad

The blood supply to the testicle can be compromised in the male child with an incarcerated or strangulated inguinal hernia.[785,927] Similarly, in female children the ovary and tube may prolapse into the hernia or be a sliding component of it and undergo a similar hazardous sequence. In males, the risk of strangulation of the testicle is due to pressure on its vessels at the superficial ring and in the canal when the testicle is incompletely descended. The duration and completeness of the strangulation influence the viability of the testicle. If incarceration is known to have been present for a long time, greater than 12 h, emergency operation is probably indicated. Interestingly the incarcerated hernia in a female carries greater risk to the gonad, the ovary, than a similar situation in the male.

Infarction of the testicle in a 6-week-old child with an incarcerated inguinal hernia was reported by Sturdy (1960)[1105] and in a 3-month-old male child with incarcerated hernia by Deshpande (1964).[286] Murdoch (1979) reported 120 boys with incarcerated inguinal hernia treated in a 3-year period.[826] In his series, there were six instances of testicular strangulation related to the hernia; strangulation of the testis occurs almost exclusively in infants aged less than 3 months. The strangulation is due to hernia pressure on the cord vessels as they pass through the rigid boundaries of the superficial inguinal ring.[781] When a strangulated testis is discovered at operation, it should be left undisturbed. Full recovery of most strangulated testes can usually be anticipated, although up to 5% of strangulated testicles may ultimately atrophy.

Although the outlook for both incarcerated gut and the ischemic testicle in an irreducible inguinal hernia is good, strangulation and gangrene of the gut and testicle is recorded.[121]

Operation is mandatory for the persisting irreducible hernia. If vomiting and obstruction are present, extra careful resuscitation is needed prior to operation.

CLINICAL DIAGNOSIS OF INGUINAL HERNIA IN A CHILD

A lump in the groin of a child is a common condition that presents to surgeons. In making a diagnosis, the sex and age of the patient and the history of the onset of the lump are critical determinants. Physical diagnosis usually only confirms what can be discovered by careful history-taking.

Sixty percent of inguinal hernias are apparent within the first 3 months of life; the remainder are discovered in well baby clinics or at school medical examinations. Few inguinal hernias are first noticed after 5 years of age.

Inguinal hernias may present at birth or at any date after that, and they are more frequent on the right side than the left side. Their early history often distinguishes them from other lumps. In the infant or child the lump is most often noticed by the mother. The lump is more prominent when the child screams or moves about vigorously, whereas it often disappears in the relaxed child; indeed when the child is brought to be examined in the clinic it may not be apparent. The mother's word alone is enough to make a diagnosis. The lump appears initially as a 'bulge' at the medial end of the groin. It increases in size and may progress down into the scrotum. Episodes of irreducibility are frequent.

The lump disappears in the sleeping child. Persistence of the lump, associated with screaming and local pain, should raise the specter of incarceration.

The inguinal hernia in the male child should be distinguished from the hydrocele. The symptoms are similar, except that with hydrocele the mother will have noticed the swelling in the scrotum before there was a swelling in the groin. She may notice that the swelling is only in the scrotum.

On clinical examination the hernia extends from the superficial ring to the scrotum. The hydrocele extends from the scrotum towards the superficial ring; it may not extend as far as the groin crease and external ring. The hernia is reducible and if it contains gut it will reduce with a gurgle. In older children the cord will be thickened after the hernia is reduced – the 'rolled silk sign'.[149] The hydrocele is readily transilluminable. Some hernias in the newborn are said to be transilluminable (Figure 10.4).

Male and female children both present diagnostic pitfalls. In either sex the lump may come and go, it may be unilateral or unilateral on the right at one time and on the left at another time, or it may be synchronously bilateral. It may appear at any moment after birth, and there may or may not be associated pain. If there is pain the child usually has screaming fits, during which the lump becomes more prominent and tender. The lump we are describing is a congenital indirect inguinal hernia. Early operation should be recommended for all cases that are clinically apparent. If the hernia is discovered in the premature infant, operation should be performed as soon as the patient is

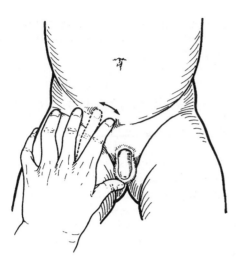

Figure 10.4 *The 'rolled silk' sign. The hernia is reduced; the examining index finger rolls the cord over the pubic bone. If a hernial sac is present, its thickened walls can be felt rubbing against each other like silk in a fine garment.*

medically stable. This is best performed immediately prior to discharge.[934,798]

The problem of the inguinal 'bulge', usually associated with screaming which causes great alarm to the parents, must be mentioned. Sometimes it is impossible to demonstrate a hernia in the clinic, but in many of these cases if a hernia is present careful palpation will demonstrate a thickened cord. The index finger is placed over the cord as it emerges over the pubic bone; the cord is rolled and the thickened sac is felt rubbing against itself with a sensation like two layers of silk rubbing together. This is the 'rolled silk' sign. It is suggestive, rather than pathoneumonic, of an inguinal hernia and its reliability as the sole indication for groin exploration for hernia is questionable.[440] If there are no clinical findings, but the mother's description of the hernia is convincing and accurate, the groin is best explored.

It is important to examine both sides of the scrotum in male children to ensure that concomitant undescended testicles are not overlooked. An overlooked undescended testicle has bleak prospects because the scarring of the herniotomy will compromise subsequent operation.

DIFFERENTIAL DIAGNOSIS

Always examine both groins and both sides of the scrotum with the child relaxed and supine, and then with the child upright (standing or held by the mother). An inguinal hernia in a child must be distinguished from:

- Inguinal lymphadenitis. The irregular 'matted' nature of enlarged inguinal nodes should give the true diagnosis. Examination of the watershed area may reveal the cause, especially in acute lymphadenitis.
- Femoral hernia. Careful delineation of the anatomy – an inguinal hernia is cephalad and a femoral hernia caudal to the inguinal ligament.

- Undescended testicle (in the male).
- A hydrocele of the cord (in the male).
- Hydrocele of the canal of Nuck (in the female). A 'communicating' hydrocele that comes and goes can be confused with a hernia. Many communicating hydroceles communicate with a hernial sac. In both male and female cord hydroceles the swelling has a definite upper limit and is translucent. Hydroceles vary in size.
- Lipoma.
- Psoas abscess. This generally appears lateral to the femoral artery.
- Cystic hygroma.
- Varicocele. The 'bag-of-worms' is the classic finding that should differentiate this entity.

Additionally, if the swelling is tender and the child complains of pain:

- Torsion of an undescended testicle can closely resemble a strangulated hernia. This condition usually appears very suddenly with no previous history of a lump. Usually the absent testicle has been noticed previously. Torsion of an undescended testicle can complicate birth in low birthweight and preterm boys. Local examination reveals a tender lump with edema adjacent to it, and there is no testicle in the ipsilateral scrotum. The gastrointestinal symptoms of strangulation, persistent vomiting and constipation are absent. The acuteness and severity of symptoms in a case of torsion tend to decrease with time, in contrast to the progression of symptoms from incarceration to strangulation.
- Torsion of an appendix of the epididymis can give a swollen inguinoscrotal area, which can be mistaken for a strangulated hernia. The onset is sudden. However, the acuteness of the symptoms settles fairly rapidly. No swelling is palpable in the cord above the scrotum.
- Appendicitis can occur in an inguinal hernial sac in a child.

THE BILATERALITY QUESTION

Because inguinal hernias in children are not uncommonly bilateral, should both groins be routinely explored? In newborn children with unilateral inguinal hernia, a patent processus vaginalis is found on the contralateral side in 60%. The processus vaginalis undergoes a progressive obliteration from birth to 2 years, so that after 2 years only 40% of children with demonstrable unilateral inguinal hernias have a contralateral patent processus vaginalis.[132,544,1056] Whether contralateral exploration should be routinely undertaken when a left hernia is found is a moot point, remembering that a contralateral hernia is twice as likely to be found with a left hernia as with a right-sided one. It must be clearly understood that there is a hazard to the vas and vessels whenever an inguinal hernia is explored. Steigman and colleagues performed histopathological examinations of 7314 hernia sacs at a tertiary care children's hospital.[1085] Seventeen cases contained vas deferens

(0.23%), 22 had epididymis (0.3%) and 30 had embryonal rests (0.41%). Either vas deferens or epididymis was present in 0.53% of patients. Of the 65% of boys who had bilateral hernia repair, there were no cases containing bilateral vas deferens, bilateral epididymis or vas deferens in one side with epididymis in the contralateral side. This study provides useful information for surgeons for preoperative counseling regarding potential injury to the vas deferens or epididymis. Other researchers have demonstrated that the incidence of atrophy or testicular trauma can be as high as 2 or 3% respectively in uncomplicated hernia repair.[546,772,1108]

The actual risk of a metachronous contralateral hernia development has been shown to range from 1–13%.[796,934,1108,1121] Do the risks outweigh the advantages of exploration? In children over 2 years old the case against routine contralateral exploration has been powerfully made.[144,589] On the other hand, the opposite argument has been advanced powerfully, too. Ballantyne and colleagues undertook a retrospective study of 165 boys under 1 year of age undergoing unilateral herniotomy, which was right sided in 83%.[75] Follow-up ranged from 5–10 years and a contralateral hernia or hydrocele developed in only 14 infants (7.7%) none of which were incarcerated. The median time from operation till closure of the contralateral hernia was 18 months.

In infants less than 6 months old, and especially in girls, who have a left inguinal hernia when the right side is explored a sac is almost always found, and because so many infants present with complications of the sac some surgeons routinely explore the right side. In boys who are older, over two years old, the risks of damage to the vas and spermatic vessels probably outweigh the advantages of the inexperienced operator performing a prophylactic dissection.[412] A survey of pediatric surgeons found that 35% of the surgeons routinely explored the groin in boys under two years of age regardless of the side of presentation or age or prematurity. In female patients, however, 84% of surgeons explored the opposite side up to the age of 4 years.[1198]

Burd and colleagues have suggested a strategy for the optimal management of metachronous hernias in children.[159] A decision analysis tree was constructed with three approaches:

1 Observation and repair of a contralateral hernia only if it later becomes apparent
2 Routine contralateral groin exploration
3 Laparoscopy to evaluate the contralateral groin for a potential hernia.

The results indicated that observation was favored over laparoscopy, and laparoscopy over routine exploration, with respect to preventing spermatic cord injury and preserving future fertility. Although observation was the favored approach with respect to cost, laparoscopy was less expensive when the expected incidence of metachronous hernias was high. It was concluded that observation is the preferred approach to metachronous hernia repair because it results in the lowest incidence of injury and costs, and in most patients and is associated with a minimal increase in anesthesia related morbidity and mortality. Laparoscopy may be advantageous for patients of high risk for development of a contralateral hernia.

ULTRASONOGRAPHY AND HERNIOGRAPHY

The use of intraperitoneal herniography is advocated to decide on contralateral exploration. The radiological diagnosis of inguinal hernias using intraperitoneal contrast media was first described in Canada in 1967.[317] Using a midline infra-umbilical injection with an 18-gauge Surgicath under local anesthesia, water-soluble contrast is instilled.[412,451] Sodium diatrizoate (Hypaque M60) is an appropriate contrast medium.

The contrast is injected, the child 'shaken gently' and then prone radiographs taken. In a series of 562 inguinal hernias in children, 335 were clinically unilateral, 210 on the right and 125 on the left; with herniography, 77 (22.9%) of the patients were found to have significant contralateral hernias.[454] Kiesewetter and Oh (1980)[589] compared transperitoneal exploration of the contralateral side by a bent Bakes' choledochal dilator with herniography. They found the technique using the Bakes' dilator unreliable and difficult to use, whereas they found herniography accurate and easy to use. They recommend routine herniography.[590] Clinical complications, including abdominal wall cellulitis, septicemia, hematoma and intestinal obstruction, are reported. Routine use of herniography is not necessary and not recommended.

Ultrasonography is now the preferred radiological investigation and can correctly diagnose up to 95% of sacs based on criteria of a greater than 4 mm internal ring in conjunction with fluid or an intestinal organ in the inguinal canal at rest or on straining.[218] Ultrasonography can also diagnose over 90% of hernia sacs on the asymptomatic side and determine the advisability of exploration.[210] In girls the risk of contralateral hernia is similar to the risk in boys: in a study by Ulman 19% of girls developed a contralateral hernia within 1 year when the original operation was left sided compared with 6% who developed a contralateral hernia when the original operation was right sided.[1153]

LAPAROSCOPY FOR THE DIAGNOSIS OF BILATERAL HERNIAS

The use of laparoscopy in this diagnosis represents an extension of the Goldstein test. In this test, the abdomen is insufflated intraoperatively to identify an undiagnosed contralateral hernia. In practice this technique has been found to be fraught with too many false positives. The ability to laparoscopically view the contralateral side of the patient allows an accurate assessment of the possibility of bilaterality of the hernias. It is very slightly more accurate than preoperative ultrasound (96% vs. 95%).[218] The appeal of this technique is that it does not subject the patient to an unnecessary negative groin exploration. This avoids the risk of injury to the testicular vasculature or the vas deferens. It does not appear to add any additional time to the operation to identify the absence of a hernia than the negative exploration of the groin.[966] The accuracy of this technique is verified by the lack of the development of a subsequent hernia in these patients in up to 57 months of follow-up.[873]

The reluctance in the use of the methodology is the concept of additional trocar incision sites or risk of injury to intra-abdominal organs, especially if the umbilical port is utilized. Today, however, the most common method in which to view the contralateral side is through the open hernia sac of the original hernia through which the abdomen is insufflated from 5–10 mm Hg. This is usually done by placing a small trocar or sheath into the sac and closing the sac around the trocar with a suture. This study will be hampered if there is a tear in the hernia sac or if there is a distended urinary bladder. The typical laparoscope varies from a 2–5 mm diameter with either a 30° or 70° viewing angle. One center places a 1.2 mm laparoscope (0°) through a 14-gauge above the asymptomatic side so that the view is 'in-line' to inspect the inguinal floor.[873]

The findings in these methods have been positive for a contralateral hernia in 12.8%, 32%, 33%, 39% of patients.[217,218,966,1224] This is in marked contrast to the expected rate of approximately 15% reported in the 'open' technique of contralateral exploration. This raises the question of the intra-operative interpretation of the anatomy (see below). However, the series reported by Rogers that compared traditional versus laparoscopic inspection, found that 77% of the 'explored' patients had a contralateral hernia.[966] There have been no reported intraoperative complications with this technique.

There is some difficulty, however, in the interpretation of the findings at laparoscopy because there is variation in the definition of a hernia as reported in the literature. Some of the reports describe the hernia as 'appearing to be a hole', 'a visibly patent processus vaginalis', 'bubbles in the processus', 'the same size as the original hernia', or 'if one cm of depth'.[218,873,1020,1224] Consequently, there does not appear to be a standardized terminology for the diagnosis of a hernia when viewed laparoscopically. Despite this difficulty, many authors, in addition to those above, acknowledge the accuracy of this technique. It is relatively easy to distinguish between the presence (Figure 10.5) or absence (Figure 10.6) of a hernia versus a patent processus vaginalis (Figure 10.7). In some centers, this method is offered to all pediatric hernia patients for both diagnosis and

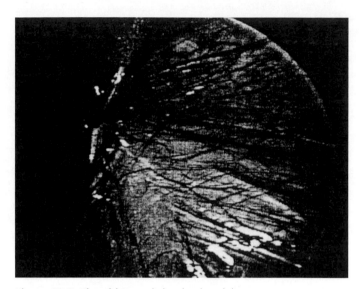

Figure 10.6 *Closed internal ring (no hernia).*

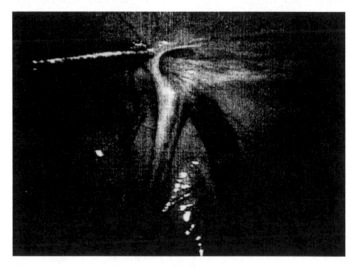

Figure 10.7 *Open processus vaginalis.*

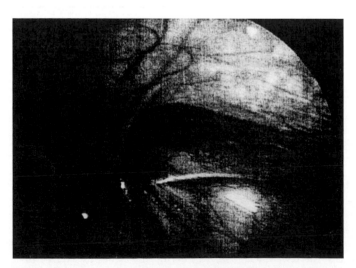

Figure 10.5 *Open internal ring (indirect 'hernia').*

treatment.[1020] The laparoscope may be particularly suited for suspected recurrent pediatric hernias. It can accurately identify indirect or direct recurrent inguinal hernias as well as missed femoral hernias.[903]

INGUINAL HERNIA IN GIRLS

Inguinal hernia in girls should raise the surgeon's suspicions about the child's nuclear sex, particularly if the condition is bilateral. Approximately 1.6% of these children, presenting with inguinal hernia and having apparent female genitalia, prove to be of male nuclear sex, with intra-abdominal testes but female external genital appearance and endocrine function – the 'testicular feminization syndrome'.[62,563,811,848] All female children with inguinal hernia should have their nuclear sex ascertained, and skilled pediatric and genetic counseling advice should be sought where anomalies are found. Testicular feminization is a misnomer because the testes do not feminize the child. The reality is that the affected male has a metabolic disorder – complete androgen insensitivity syndrome (CAIS) – making him resistant to the action of testosterone and dihydrotestosterone. Binding of androgen to receptors is deficient at the cellular level so that a phenotypically female with breasts, external genitalia and clitoris develops.

The chromosome karyotype is 46 XY. Hyperactivity of the testes with high estrogen and testosterone levels, and raised plasma gonadotrophins, lead to female sex characteristics and orientation at puberty.

Most cases of testicular feminization are sporadic mutations. The incidence is 1:62 400 live births, the probable method of inheritance being a sex-linked recessive gene transmitted through the female. Because affected persons are sterile, the syndrome is partially self-limiting. The real surgical problem is what to do with the gonad? Orchidectomy is not indicated in infancy or childhood because removal of gonad function will compromise development of secondary sexual characteristics. The gonads may be intra-abdominal and the condition will go unnoticed. If a unilateral hernia is present, laparotomy with biopsy of the contralateral gonad should be performed to examine the internal genitalia and exclude other varieties of intersex.[902]

With bilateral hernia, the gonads should be saved and placed subcutaneously in the suprapubic fat. Orchidectomy should then be performed after development of the secondary sexual characteristics. After maturity the incidence of malignant change in the abnormally placed gonad, whether intra or extra-abdominal, outweighs the advantages of its endocrine function. An incidence of 8% malignant change has been recorded in one series.[811] Maintenance of secondary sexual appearances can be achieved with hormone therapy.

SLIDING HERNIAS IN CHILDHOOD

In both sexes transitory lateral extraperitoneal protrusions of the bladder occur as a sliding component of the medial wall of indirect hernias. These protrusions ('bladder ears') have been demonstrated on excretion urography in 9% of infants under one year old who have hernias.[17,1041] It is important to recognize the bladder in the medial wall, or the colon in the lateral wall, and to modify the operation technique to avoid damage to these structures. In girls, many indirect congenital sacs are sliding hernias containing genital structures, ovaries, fallopian tubes or even the uterus in the walls. In a series of 262 inguinal hernias in female children, an ovary and/or fallopian tube was found in 41% of those undergoing operation under 2 years old.[63] A primitive uterus has been described in a male child with intersex.

LITTRÉ'S HERNIA IN INFANCY

Littré's hernia, the hernial sac containing a Meckel's diverticulum, has been described in neonates. This condition can be diagnosed

preoperatively; the hernia can be reduced by taxis but after reduction 'a smaller firmer mass remains below the external ring'. This residual mass resists all attempts at taxis and is sometimes tender. There are often adhesions between the Meckel's diverticulum and the sac. These prevent reduction and suggest that closed-loop obstruction may complicate this type of hernia.[71]

RELATION BETWEEN TESTICULAR TUMORS, UNDESCENDED TESTICLES AND INGUINAL HERNIA

There is no doubt that testicular tumors occur more frequently in maldescended testicles, but the quantification of this increased risk is difficult. Campbell (1959) came to the conclusion that the undescended testicle is 48 times more likely to undergo malignant change than the normal testis,[175] whereas Wobbes *et al.* (1980), reviewing experience in Groningen, North Netherlands, estimated the risk to be increased about 17 times.[1219] Are inguinal hernias in infancy similarly associated with an increased testicular cancer risk? Previous inguinal herniotomy was found in 3.4% of the patients with testicular tumor reported from Groningen: this figure is in accord with the usual incidence of infantile inguinal hernia. Consequently there seems to be no increased risk of testicular tumor in patients who have had an operation for inguinal hernia, although Morrison (1976) estimated that infantile inguinal hernia was associated with 2.9 times as high risk of subsequent malignant testicular tumor.[812] Another controversy!

If a testicular tumor develops after inguinal herniotomy, will inguinal node metastases occur? Inguinal node metastases develop in patients who develop testicular tumors after childhood orchidopexy, so that it seems unlikely that childhood herniotomy will influence or limit the spread of a testicular tumor.

Inguinal hernias are frequently associated with other anomalies of the testicle in male children. Chilvers *et al.* (1984) have reported an apparent increase in undescended testicle diagnoses by a factor of 2.3 for the period 1962–1981, the diagnosis of undescended testicle to the age of 15 years rising from 1.4% for the 1952 birth cohort to 2.9% for the 1977 birth cohort.[216] The significance of this change is unclear. Whether there is a similar increase in the incidence of inguinal hernias is also unknown. However, the higher incidence of inguinal hernia in male infants in Stockton-on-Tees from 1970–1979, when compared with the earlier findings of Knox (1959),[606] may reflect a change in the epidemiology of the condition.

INCREASED INTRAPERITONEAL FLUID AND INGUINAL HERNIA IN CHILDREN

With chylous ascites or ascites due to liver disease, or following the insertion of a ventriculoperitoneal shunt for hydrocephalus, or in peritoneal dialysis for renal failure, there is an increased incidence of indirect hernias and hydrocele.[333,441,447] If an inguinal hernia develops in these circumstances in a child, early rather than delayed surgery is indicated.

RECURRENCE

Almost all recurrences of childhood inguinal hernias are due to technical failure at operation. The majority of recurrences are apparent within 12 months of operation. The most likely technical mistakes are a failure to isolate the sac completely at the neck or failure to ligate it high enough flush with the parietal peritoneum. Ligation of the sac with absorbable material, such as catgut, leads to recurrence. The sac should be sutured/closed off with one of the newer, slowly absorbable polymers. Other causes of recurrences are an unrecognized tear in the posterior aspect of the hernia sac, damage to the floor of the inguinal canal causing a direct recurrence, infection, or increased intra-abdominal pressure. Reported recurrence rates vary from 0.1% for elective operation to 5.6% for emergency surgery. Recurrence rates are very closely related to the skill of the operator, being lowest in series operated by skilled pediatric surgeons and highest when junior general surgeons operate.[483] In a series of 118 operations for childhood hernias performed by non-pediatric surgeons in a Swedish community hospital over a 10-year period, the recurrence rate in boys was 3.8% and testicular atrophy complicated 7.5% of the operations in males.[534] Many hernias in neonates nowadays are in premature babies and skilled experienced surgeons are needed to manage them. Inexperience in dealing with diminutive structures, unfamiliarity with the anatomy, sliding hernias in girls and the bladder close by the internal ring in both sexes can cause difficulties. Connective tissue disorders and raised intraperitoneal pressure also predispose to recurrence.[441] As in most areas of surgery, the best results are obtained by surgeons who address the problem regularly. Some studies, however, have found that the incidence of recurrence can be as disappointingly high as 20% in preterm infants.[906]

Laparoscopy is a particularly useful technique to accurately identify the nature of the defect in children with recurrent groin hernias. The defect may be an inguinal recurrence, a femoral hernia or no recurrence is found.[903] In this latter series, positive findings were noted in 44% of the patients that underwent laparoscopy. In many cases, a femoral may actually be misdiagnosed as an inguinal recurrence.[675] One series of 225 patients found recurrence of an inguinal hernia in 10 patients (4.4%) following standard open herniotomy. All of these were successfully repaired laparoscopically.[335]

ARRANGEMENTS FOR SURGERY AND ANESTHESIA

Most children with inguinal hernias can be treated on an outpatient basis. Only for compelling medical or social reasons does the child need to be admitted to hospital. In any case,

the mother should be encouraged to accompany the child to hospital and to nurse him or her after recovery from the operation.

To operate on children with inguinal hernia effectively as day cases requires good hospital organization and excellent hospital-to-community communications. It is essential to have printed advice and instructions for the parents and a 'safety net' system, which can cope with unpredictable situations.

The following American quotation encapsulates all the benefits of day surgery for children: 'It is relatively simple for the parents to drive to the Surgicenter … and park … and enjoy the highly personalized services'.[226]

The operation should be performed as soon as possible after the diagnosis has been established. Young, even newborn and preterm, children tolerate this surgery well, and the parental anxiety and risk of incarceration of the hernia are minimized by early operation.

Day-case surgery in young children is best performed between 10.00 a.m. and 3.00 p.m. Before 10.00 a.m. there may not be time for travel, unhurried preparation and sedation. A screaming child and an anxious mother are not the ideal prelude to elective surgery!

Hypoglycemia and dehydration are of rapid onset when small children are starved unnecessarily. These physiological 'complications' should be prevented by giving the child a normal morning feed and then a preoperative drink of maltose and metoclopramide, and by operating as early after the morning feed as is safe.[64,378] The factors involved in the anesthesia of the newborn are excellently discussed in the article by Spath.[1073]

Operation, on a day-case basis, should always be completed before 3.00 p.m. in order to ensure that the effects of anesthesia are gone before the child is sent home. Children should not be discharged in a sedated or semi-comatose state.[439]

Because of the increased risk of postoperative apnea and bradycardia, low-birthweight and preterm babies are conventionally treated as inpatients with appropriate ICU support and monitoring; however, some benefit from being treated as day cases.[784]

THE OPERATION

Principles

In babies and young children, the inguinal canal has not yet developed its oblique adult anatomy. The superficial ring is directly anterior to the deep ring and the sac is indirect. There is no acquired deformity of the canal. In these cases the fascia transversalis is normal and a simple herniotomy is all that is necessary. Straightforward inguinal herniotomy should give a 100% cure rate.[64,272,1195]

Hemostasis and suture materials

Hemostasis is secured by careful ligating of bleeding points with metric 3 (4-0) braided polyglycolic acid (Dexon) or braided polyglactin 910 (Vicryl). Electrocoagulation with a fine pediatric coagulation probe is also used but great care is needed to prevent propagation and thrombosis of the small vessels in the delicate spermatic cord and cause subsequent testicular damage.

All deep suturing is carried out using Dexon or Vicryl. The skin is closed with metric 4 or metric 6 (4-0 or 5-0) clear* subcuticular Monocryl, Vicryl, PDS or a skin dressing only. If the subcutaneous fat is closed carefully and accurately, no subcuticular suture will be required. Adhesive skin tape skin closure gives very good cosmetic results. The recent introduction of skin adhesives that replace sutures (Dermabond®) allow the surgeon a new choice of skin closure without the need of a dressing.

Position of patient

The child is placed on his back on the operating table. A light cotton blanket (or a warming device) lies over the chest and upper abdomen and a similar blanket over the lower limbs. This precaution prevents heat loss during surgery.

DRAPING

Drapes are applied so that the groin area and scrotum are exposed throughout the operation (Figure 10.8).

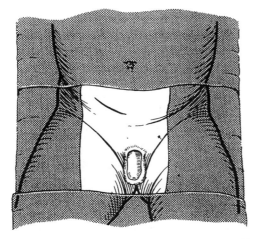

Figure 10.8 *Draping should be so that the scrotum and both groins are visible to the operator.*

The incision

A horizontal transverse incision is made in the transverse skin crease just above and medial to the superficial inguinal ring. The incision should be 1.0–1.5 cm long. The superficial ring and the emerging spermatic cord can be readily palpated under anesthesia. The site for incision and the direction of the subsequent dissection are thus confirmed (Figure 10.9).

---

*Clear PDS is recommended because skin tattooing can occur if a colored polymer is used.

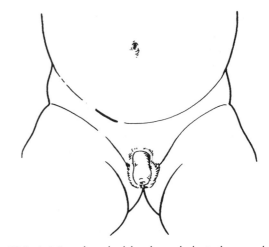

Figure 10.9 *A 1.5 cm long incision is made just above and medial to the external inguinal ring.*

Dissection of the external ring

The superficial ring and cord, which have already been identified by palpation, are approached by gently opening the subcutaneous fat with a blunt hemostat. At this stage the superficial epigastric vessels are encountered and picked up in light hemostats, divided with scissors and ligated. Not all surgeons will divide these vessels unless necessary to complete an adequate dissection.

The superficial inguinal ring and cord are readily identified when the superficial subcutaneous fat has been opened (Figure 10.10).

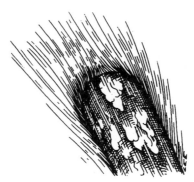

Figure 10.10 *The cord is identified as it emerges from the external inguinal ring.*

Dissection of the cord coverings

Once the cord has been identified its coverings must be opened to give access to the hernial sac. The sac lies on the anterosuperior aspect of the cord as it emerges from the external inguinal ring. One must be especially careful not to injure the minute ilioinguinal nerve during this dissection.

It is covered first by the diaphanous external spermatic fascia, then by the cremasteric fascia, which is readily identified by its neat intertwining pink fascicles of muscle, and more deeply by the very delicate internal spermatic fascia. These structures – the three layers of spermatic fascia – are separated from the enclosed contents of the cord by careful blunt dissection with a fine hemostat.

A 'trick of the trade' is most useful here: a closed hemostat is pushed through the fascial layers into the cord and then opened slowly in the long axis so that a rent is made. If a hernial sac is present it is immediately apparent in the rent. The rent is held open with the hemostat and the sac grasped with a second hemostat placed between the open blades of the first (Figures 10.11–10.13).

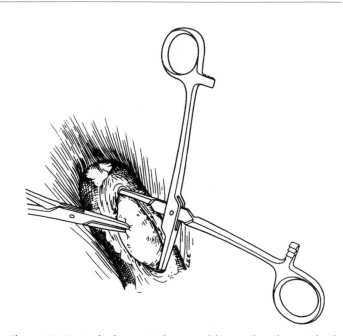

Figure 10.13 *As the hemostat is opened it stretches the rent in the coverings of the cord and the bluish colored indirect sac is immediately visible on the anterior superior aspect of the cord. The sac is grasped in a second hemostat.*

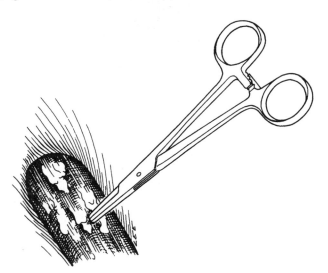

Figure 10.11 *A fine closed hemostat is pushed into the cord between the easily identified interwoven bundles of the cremaster.*

The sac can be identified lying on the anterosuperior aspect of the contents of the cord. It is pale blue and much thicker than the fascial coverings of the cord. The most difficult maneuver in the operation must now be carried out. The components of the cord are in the posterolateral position. Therefore, one should not stray far from this location to minimize the risk of injury to the cord structures.

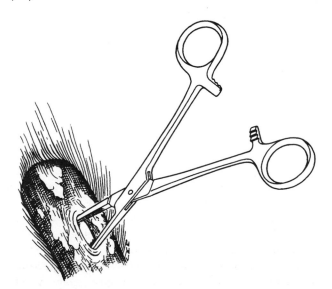

Figure 10.12 *The hemostat is gently opened.*

The sac is either 'complete' (total funicular hernia), that is it extends to the scrotum and encompasses the testicle, or 'incomplete' (partial funicular hernia), that is it extends along only part of the length of the cord.

If the sac is 'complete' its posterior wall must be separated from the other cord contents – the vas deferens, the testicular artery and the pampiniform plexus of veins. This must be done very gently. Above all, the vas or the pampiniform vessels must never be grasped in forceps. Its successful accomplishment is a benchmark by which surgical competence can be measured. First, the internal spermatic fascia fixing the pampiniform plexus to the sac is divided by a scalpel (Figure 10.14).

Then a fine hemostat is gently insinuated between each structure and the thin peritoneal sac wall in turn to push them off the sac (Figure 10.15). When each structure has been pushed off, the proximal sac is held in a hemostat and the sac divided across (Figure 10.16). The distal sac (remainder of the processus vaginalis), testicle and cord can now be manipulated back into place in the scrotum. Gentle traction on the testicle in the scrotum at this time will confirm that it has been returned to its normal site (Figure 10.17).

The proximal divided sac is now dealt with in the same manner as an incomplete sac.[132] The fundus of an incomplete sac (or the proximal remnant of a complete sac) is held in a hemostat and the contents of the cord are gently pushed off its posterior wall using a piece of gauze, while traction is applied to keep the sac taut. The sac must be stripped of cord contents down to its junction with the parietal peritoneum.

DIFFICULTIES DISSECTING THE SAC

If dissection of the proximal sac is difficult or obscured the lateral margin of the superficial inguinal ring should be divided

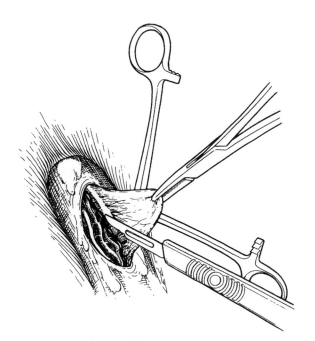

Figure 10.14 *The sac being separated from the cord structures. A gentle stroke with a sharp scalpel will divide the internal spermatic fascia, opening up a plane between the sac and the cord structures.*

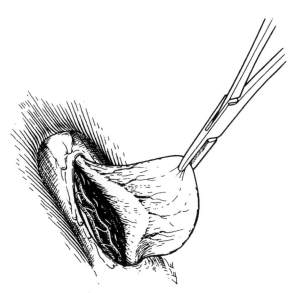

Figure 10.15 *A hemostat holds up the sac and the cord structures are separated from it.*

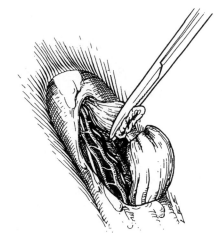

Figure 10.16 *If the sac is complete it must now be clamped and divided across.*

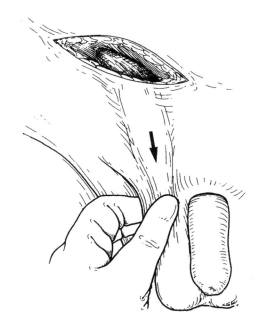

Figure 10.17 *The distal end falls away towards the testicle. The scrotum is manipulated to ensure the testicle is returned to base.*

for 1 cm or so to increase the exposure of the deep ring and the fascia transversalis.

OPENING THE SAC

Once the sac has been completely separated from the cord coverings and contents, many surgeons will open the sac and inspect its contents. This is most important in a female child. If any intra-abdominal contents are in the sac they are pushed back into the greater peritoneal cavity (Figure 10.18). In some instances, many surgeons will simply twist the sac to keep the

contents in the intra-abdominal position. This must be carefully done to ensure that there are no structures in the sac and also to prevent the inadvertent binding of the vas deferens.

The sliding hernia

Bladder, colon or internal genitalia in the female can form part of the wall of a sliding hernia. The hernial sac should be cleaned of cord structures around three-quarters of its circumference, then the sac should be divided on either side away from the sliding organ (along the dotted lines). This is made easier if the superficial ring, external oblique, is divided (as above). The sac can now be closed by a suture picking up the extraperitoneal wall of the bladder (colon, broad ligament), reducing any contents and ligating around the remainder of the sac.

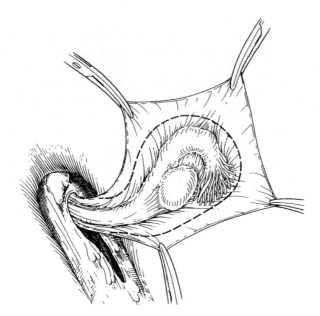

Figure 10.18 *The sac should always be opened. In the female, the ovary and the tube are often sliding components of the sac wall.*

The vascular compromised testicle

If there is recent incarceration the venous return from the testicle will be impeded and there may even be early infarction of the testicle. Such testicles should not be removed; if left undisturbed many will recover, at least partially, and be endocrine-useful in adult life.

Closure

The sac is now ligated circumferentially with a transfixion suture of metric 3 (4-0) absorbable polymer (Figure 10.19). Catgut or catgut derivatives are not advised to suture ligate the sac; catgut loses its strength often capriciously early and precipitates recurrence. There is never any need to dislocate the testicle from the scrotum to deal with the sac, provided the proximal sac is divided across, the distal component of a complete sac can be left alone in situ. Protection of the distal cord and testicle will avoid trauma and vascular damage to the testicle.

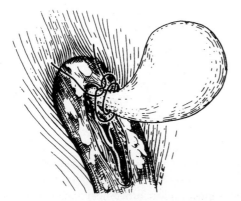

Figure 10.19 *The sac is closed with a transfixion ligature.*

THE EXTERNAL OBLIQUE

If the superficial ring has been extended into the aponeurosis of the external oblique, the divided aponeurosis is now repaired with appropriate polymer sutures.

Subcutaneous tissue

The subcutaneous fat is now closed with two or three metric 3 (4-0) absorbable polymer sutures, carefully placed to close the dead space in the depths of the wound and its immediate subdermal layer. The knots are placed deeply (Figure 10.20).

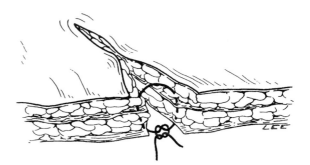

Figure 10.20 *Closure of the subcutaneous fat.*

The skin

The skin is closed with a subcuticular suture of metric 4 or 6 (4-0 or 5-0) polyglycolic acid (Vicryl) or polydioxanone (PDS). Skin tapes or adhesives can also be substituted for the skin closure.

Iatrogenic cryptorchism

At the completion of the operation the position of the testicle in the scrotum should be confirmed. The manipulation of the sac can cause the testicle to be drawn up into the neck of the scrotum or into the inguinal region; if the testicle is not replaced into the scrotum at the conclusion of the surgery, postoperative adhesions will trap it in fibrous tissue and result in cryptorchism. Infection and postoperative cremaster spasm have also been blamed for this unfortunate complication. Vigilance will prevent it. The testicle must be easily palpable in the scrotum at the conclusion of the inguinal herniotomy; if it is not, further exploration and, if necessary, testicular fixation should be accomplished before the anesthetic is terminated[562] (Figure 10.21).

LAPAROSCOPIC REPAIR

The considerations in the preoperative and anesthetic management for the laparoscopic repair of pediatric hernias are similar to that of the open technique. One notable difference is that of the use of abdominal insufflation. The pressures that are used in this setting are generally 5–8 mm Hg. However,

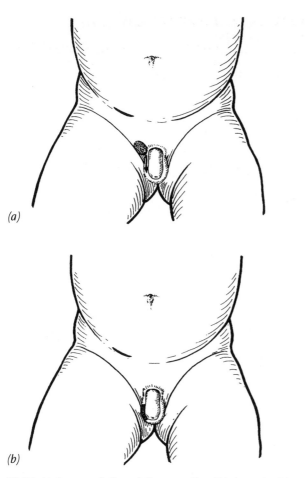

(a)

(b)

Figure 10.21 *At the completion of the operation it is important to check the position of the testicle and ensure that it is in the scrotum.*

pressures as high as 12–15 mmHg have been reported, although these tended to be in older patients.[675]

The use of the laparoscope to view the contralateral side of a hernia differs in that there is no need for a repair of the defect, if found. Therefore, the majority of reported series have repaired the newly diagnosed hernia with one of the open techniques described earlier in the chapter. If the laparoscopic repair is to be performed, the approach must differ.

This repair has been successful in patients as young as 3 weeks of age. The typical approach is similar to that of the adult patient undergoing an intra-abdominal operation. An umbilical incision is used to insert a Veress needle whereupon the abdomen is insufflated to the appropriate pressure. Usually a 5 mm trocar is then inserted followed by a 0° laparoscope. Two additional trocars are then inserted on either side of the abdominal cavity. Depending upon the instruments used, 2 mm, 3 mm or 5 mm trocars will be required. Alternatively, two mm instruments rather than two one mm intruments can be used through 12-gauge venous cannulas. The advantages of the smaller port sizes are the virtual elimination of the risk of trocar site herniation and the improved cosmetic result.

Because these hernias are generally small and the fact that these patients will all experience growth, the use of a prosthetic is rarely indicated. The neck of the sac will be closed with sutures

The use of a non-absorbable 3-0 or 4-0 suture is preferred but the use of absorbable PDS sutures has been reported.[1020] The passage of the suture into the abdominal cavity can be easily done by a direct passage through the abdominal wall into the patient. To accomplish the intracorporeal suturing and tying of the knot, the suture length should be cut to approximately 8 cm. One may close the defect using one to three interrupted sutures or a single purse-string suture[801,1020] (Figures 10.22 and 10.23). It is important to assure that the tissue that is stitched together for the repair includes muscular tissue and not just the peritoneum. If the purse-string closure is performed, the incision into the peritoneum surrounding the orifice is recommended to insure adequate tissue enclosure. The surgeon must,

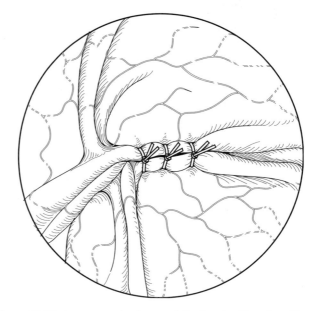

Figure 10.22 *Laparoscopic closure of the inguinal hernia with interrupted 4 0 sutures.*

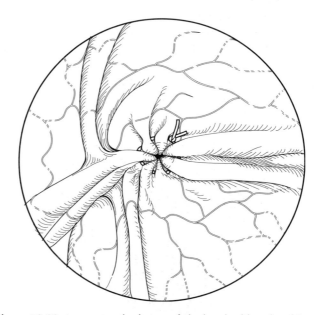

Figure 10.23 *Laparoscopic closure of the inguinal hernia with a purse-string suture.*

of course, be careful not to include any of the cord structures within the sutures.

The sutured closure of the 5 mm port sites is preferred. The 2 or 3 mm sites are too small to close effectively and have not been shown to risk future herniation. Skin closure of the larger incisions can either be with a subcuticular, tape or skin adhesive closure.

POSTOPERATIVE CARE AND FOLLOW-UP

No postoperative care other than normal maternal nursing care is required. The child can be caressed and fed by his mother as soon as he has recovered from the anesthetic. He can be allowed to play and be bathed as soon as necessary.

Most patients recover rapidly from these simple operations and multiple outpatient follow-up visits are probably unnecessary. Probable findings in the postoperative clinic are malposition of the testicle, atrophy of the testicle and the odd transient hydrocele. More importantly, a contralateral hernia may be discovered. Despite the vogue against routine follow-up it is a valuable quality control process for the surgical team and ensures parent happiness. The authors advise it.

COMPLICATIONS

Some children, perhaps 10%, have bruising adjacent to the wound and in the scrotum, which resolves spontaneously. Wound infections are very rare.

Sometimes the testicle may go 'hard' after surgery. An expectant policy should be adopted with this complication. The 'hard' testicle is, in reality, suffering from borderline ischemia and if left alone will likely recover spontaneously. Earlier techniques which involved mobilization of the testicle from the scrotum were accompanied by an incidence of up to 4% of subsequent testicular atrophy.[953] It must be emphasized again that the testicle does not require routine mobilization from the scrotum and delivery into the wound – this maneuver hazards the superficial pudendal anastomotic blood supply and places the testicle at increased risk of ischemia.

Another complication is division of the vas deferens at operation. A specialist unit studying over 7000 cases discovered a 1.6% incidence, or more exactly fragments of vas deferens were found in five of 313 infantile hernial sacs examined histologically after operation.[1078] In other series, the incidence of histologic identification of tissue of the vas varied from 0.13–0.23%.[888] At operation the vas should be fully visualized before the sac is ligated and excised – should prevent this complication. If the vas is damaged, immediate repair is recommended.

Although one may be concerned over the development of a hydrocele following the laparoscopic repair, none have been reported. There have also been no reports of injury to any of the cord structures. The recurrence rate following this repair is 0.78% using interrupted sutures or 4.4% the purse-string closure.[801,1020]

EXTRAPERITONEAL APPROACH TO INGUINAL HERNIA

Introduction

The advantage of an extraperitoneal approach to inguinal hernia was described by Cheatle in 1921.[207] This approach to hernias in children was recommended by Boley and Kleinhams in 1966.[135]

The extraperitoneal approach can be made using a midline vertical incision, a Pfannenstiel incision or a lateral muscle-splitting incision. The midline incision gives good access but is cosmetically unacceptable and not recommended. The Pfannenstiel incision is an extensive approach but does give excellent access to each groin and is recommended if a bilateral pathology must be dealt with.

The lateral muscle-splitting approach is easy to use, gives good exposure and heals well with excellent cosmesis. This approach to strangulated inguinal hernia (and high undescended testicles) has been advocated by Jones of Aberdeen and is recommended for these circumstances.[556] Jones' contribution has significantly improved the quality of surgery available for children needing these difficult operations with potential hazard to the testicle.

This extraperitoneal approach is advised in the following circumstances:

1   For the incarcerated inguinal hernia, which has failed to reduce on gallows traction. In these circumstances the edema and early inflammation around the distended sac can obscure the delicate spermatic vessels and vas. There is no edema proximal to the deep ring and the cord structures can thus be readily identified and preserved using the extraperitoneal approach. Furthermore, strangulated bowel needs inspection and, very rarely, resection. This is easy using this access.
2   When an inguinal hernia is associated with a high (impalpable or within the inguinal canal – so-called 'inguino-emergent') maldescended testicle. This approach facilitates dissection of the sac from the vessels and cord; the sac can be tied off flush with the peritoneum and then the vessels can be mobilized retroperitoneally to the lower pole of the kidney and the vas fully mobilized into the pelvis. After this mobilization the testicle can be placed in the scrotum via the inguinal canal and the abdominal wound closed.
3   The extraperitoneal approach using a Pfannenstiel incision is the technique of choice for the rare instance of bilateral inguinal hernia associated with bilateral maldescent of the testicles, or for bilateral impalpable high maldescended testicles.

A NOTE OF CAUTION

The extraperitoneal approach to inguinal hernia is unusual and the surgeon must gain experience using it in the non-emergency situation. It is not an operation for the inexperienced junior, or for the surgeon who does not have regular experience of operating on small children, to undertake on a newborn with a strangulated inguinal hernia. It must be reiterated – children should be operated on by surgeons who have experience and a special interest and/or training in pediatric surgery.

The operation

PRINCIPLES

In babies the inguinal canal has not developed its adult obliquity; the hernial sac is a peritoneal sac passing through a congenital defect of fascia transversalis at the deep ring, thence through the canal to present at the groin.

When incarceration is present, the constriction is usually caused by the rigid aponeurotic pillars of the superficial inguinal ring. This operation exploits the potential space between the peritoneum and the fascia transversalis. It allows the peritoneal sac to be isolated before it enters the inguinal canal and before it has become edematous and diaphanous in cases of incarceration.

The same patient position, draping, hemostasis and sutures are used as described previously.

THE INCISION

A horizontal transverse incision is made medial to the anterior superior iliac spine across the linea semilunaris to the midpoint of the rectus muscle. This incision is 1.0–2.0 cm cephalad to the incision used for the traditional anterior inguinal herniotomy described on pages 138 and 139. The external oblique muscle is split in the line of its fibers to expose the lateral margin of the rectus muscle that is retracted medially (Figure 10.24).

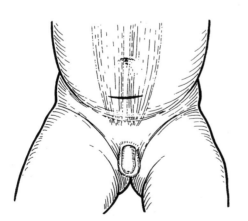

Figure 10.24 *Incision for unilateral extraperitoneal exploration of a child's groin.*

If bilateral hernias are to be explored: (a) a Pfannenstiel incision in the suprapubic skin crease is employed; (b) this incision should extend from the midpoint of one rectus muscle to the midpoint of the second – the rectus muscles are separated in the midline and the extraperitoneal space opened (Figure 10.25)

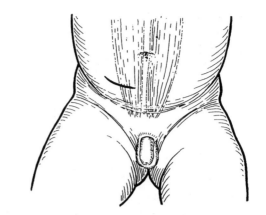

Figure 10.25 *Pfannenstiel incision for bilateral groin exploration. The rectus muscles are separated in the midline.*

EXTRAPERITONEAL ACCESS

Access to the extraperitoneal space is gained to reveal the peritoneum. The whole of the lower edge skin, subcutaneous tissues and the musculo-aponeurotic strata are lifted up with a retractor to reveal the neck of the peritoneal sac and its contents as they plunge into the deep ring (Figure 10.26).

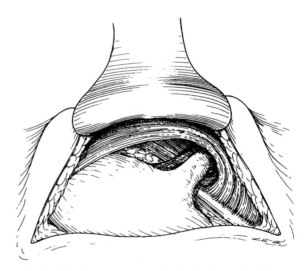

Figure 10.26 *The lower aponeurotic flap is elevated with a retractor to reveal the hernial sac plunging into the inguinal canal.*

DEFINING THE SAC

Gentle taxis and simultaneous external pressure usually reduce the contents of the sac. If the hernia is incarcerated or strangulated the peritoneum of the neck can be opened before the attempted reduction. A soft forceps can be placed on the bowel and used to retrieve the bowel after reduction, enabling assessment of its viability. If there is difficulty reducing the bowel, a curved artery forceps can be passed alongside it through the deep ring and gently opened to dilate rigid structures. If necessary, a superficial dissection of the lower flap will allow the superficial ring to be visualized or split laterally to enlarge it and release a strangulation.

The sac is now empty. It is now a simple matter to lift up the neck of the sac, gently pull away the cord vessels and the vas and clamp across the neck (Figure 10.27).

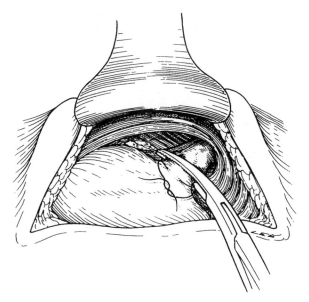

Figure 10.27 *After the sac has been separated from the cord structures, the neck of the sac is clamped and the distal sac divided.*

DIVIDING THE SAC

The neck of the sac is divided and the sac transfixed and tied off flush with the peritoneum. The distal sac (processes vaginalis) is left undisturbed. It is important not to attempt to manipulate the testicle into the abdomen or to attempt to remove the distal sac. If infarction and/or strangulation are present, the vascular supply to the testicle may be compromised; further manipulation and surgical viewing will not improve this! An expectant policy will be rewarded by the recovery of most testicles (Figure 10.28).

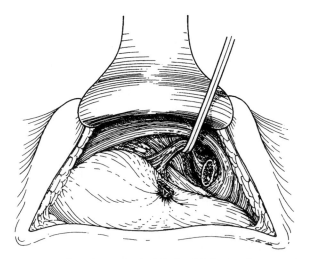

Figure 10.28 *After the sac is tied flush with the peritoneum the cord structures are checked. Do not attempt to disturb the testicle or reduce it into the abdomen.*

CLOSURE

The aponeurotic layers, the anterior rectus sheath and the external oblique are closed with a running metric 3 (3-0) absorbable polymer suture (Figure 10.29).

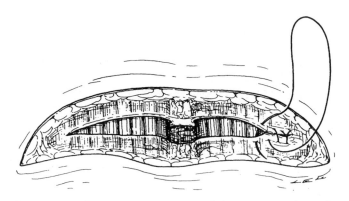

Figure 10.29 *The retractors are removed, the rectus musdes spring back to position, and the anterior rectus sheath is then closed.*

The subcutaneous fat is closed as before and the skin closed with a subcuticular suture of PDS, Vicryl, Monocryl, skin tapes or skin adhesives.

Postoperative care and complications

Postoperative management is exactly the same as for the standard herniotomy (see page 144).

FEMORAL HERNIA IN CHILDREN

Femoral hernia between birth and 14 years of age is uncommon, comprising less than 0.5% of all childhood groin hernias. In the English literature, 44 cases aged under 5 years are recorded. In a small series by Radcliffe and Stringer, the peak age of incidence was 5–10 years of age with equal numbers of boys and girls having a femoral hernia.[932] Strangulation is even rarer, 10 cases being reported in the English literature.[136,1115,1235] The youngest victim of strangulation in a femoral hernia reported is a 5-week-old boy.[1154] Of the 10 cases of strangulation reported, two contained strangulated omentum, which is surprising considering the small size of the omentum in infancy. Other contents of femoral hernia sacs in infancy include female genitalia, ovaries and fallopian tubes, and small intestine.

Femoral hernias are more frequently noticed in girls than boys.[368,532,695] It is suggested that the primary etiology of infantile femoral hernia is a congenitally narrow posterior inguinal wall, fascia transversalis, attachment onto the pectineal ligament (Cooper's ligament) with a low origin of the inferior epigastric vessels; this predisposes to a wide femoral ring with weakened fascia transversalis stretched over it.[533]

Acquired femoral hernia can occur as a complication of an osteotomy for dislocation or subluxation of the hip.[1010]

An acquired prevascular femoral hernia can also complicate a congenital dislocation of the hip.[835]

Diagnosis

Tam and Lister (1984) report 20 cases from Alder Hey Children's Hospital, Liverpool.[1115] The correct diagnosis was made in only three cases by the referring physician and in only 13 cases by the consulting surgeon. This clearly illustrates the difficulty of diagnosis and, perhaps, the low index of suspicion prevailing. That the diagnostic rate improved in the second period of their study would support the argument about the suspicion index. Mistaken diagnoses included: inguinal hernia, four cases; lymphadenitis, two cases; lymphangioma, one case. Attention to the location of the hernia lateral to and below the pubic tubercle on clinical examination should eliminate diagnostic confusion.

In a series of 12 femoral hernias in children in Leicester, nine were misdiagnosed: eight as inguinal hernia and one as a cyst of the cord.[1235] One case was an emergency presentation of a Richter's hernia in a male 6-year-old child. Femoral hernia followed previous inguinal herniotomy in two children.

The differential diagnosis of femoral hernia in a child includes: (a) inguinal adenitis; (b) inguinal hernia; (c) ectopic testis; (d) lipoma; (e) cyst of the canal of Nuck; (f) obturator hernia; (g) cystic lymphoma.

Treatment

There is no uniformly agreed surgical approach to femoral hernias in childhood. The principles would seem to be to remove the sac and close the peritoneum, and then to obliterate the enlarged femoral ring either by suturing the medial inguinal ligament to the pectineal ligament or by closing the defect with pectineus fascia. If the etiological concept of a narrow conjoint tendon attachment to the pubis is supported, it would seem logical to attach the conjoint tendon to the pectineal ligament as in the 'Cooper's ligament repair' of an inguinal hernia.[533] Whichever method of repair is favored, it is crucially important to find and remove the sac. This can be difficult; in two of the 20 cases reported from Alder Hey Children's Hospital, failure to identify and remove the sac at the primary operation resulted in an early recurrence of the hernia.[1115]

The low (crural), the inguinal or the high extraperitoneal approach can be utilized. Because of the difficulties of diagnosis and of identifying the sac, the extraperitoneal approach is probably ideal, as it allows good review of both inguinal and femoral areas at operation. Similarly, the laparoscopic approach allows the surgeon to view all of these areas. The repair can also be affected by this technique.[675] There has been very limited experience with this type of hernia repair in the pediatric population. Lee repaired four hernias using a transabdominal preperitoneal technique and placing a Teflon® (Boston Scientific, Meadox Medical, Inc., Oakland, NJ) plug into the femoral defect. The peritoneum was closed with 5 mm staples or sutures. After a mean follow-up of 16 months (range 6–24), there were no recurrences. These patients ranged in age from 2–17 years of age.[675] This technique can only be considered as 'evolutional' at best. The placement of a prosthetic biomaterial in patients of this age will probably make this operation scarce. It must be stressed, however, that to avoid missing a hernial sac at operation is more important than relying on one particular method of repair.

CONCLUSIONS

- Children with inguinal hernias should be operated on at the earliest opportunity after diagnosis. The operation should be performed by a surgeon experienced and interested in this surgery. There should be no children with inguinal hernias on the waiting list of general surgeons.
- Emergency herniotomy for inguinal hernia in infants is one of the more difficult operations in pediatric surgical practice; this is an operation for an experienced surgeon only. Taxis and sedation will reduce many childhood incarcerated inguinal hernias. Early surgery will reduce the incidence of the condition.
- The extraperitoneal approach can be considered for incarcerated or strangulated inguinal hernias in childhood. Femoral hernias are rare in children, and they will be overlooked unless diagnostic suspicion is maintained.
- Laparoscopy is of benefit to diagnose an unsuspected contralateral hernia and appears to diminish the need for unnecessary groin exploration and its attendant risks. In experienced hands, this technique can also be used to repair both inguinal and femoral hernias. More experience with this modality in the pediatric population is needed to verify its utility in hernia repair.

11

Umbilical hernia: operation in babies and children

INCIDENCE

After birth the normal umbilicus is a relatively simple structure. During the development of the embryo however this region is highly complex. The structures of the umbilical cord can be responsible for umbilical inflammation and drainage, and minor degrees of herniation of the umbilicus are present in many neonates.[858] These tend to regress spontaneously in the majority of cases before the age of 4 years unless the neck of the sac is greater than 2 cm in diameter.[885] However, umbilical hernias are a common source of referral to surgeons. After groin hernias and hydroceles, they are the third most frequent diagnosis pediatric surgeons deal with. Umbilical hernias occur in 4–30% of Caucasian infants, although many resolve spontaneously.[132,637,977,1222]

Umbilical hernias are more common in people of African origin than in white, Indian or Chinese. In the West Indies 58.5% of children of African origin have umbilical hernias compared with 8% of white children, 3.3% of Indian children and 1.3% of Chinese children.[542] In East Africa 60% of African origin children have umbilical hernias, compared with 4% of Indian origin.[726] Other studies confirm that 32%[255] or 42%[339] of Negro children have umbilical hernias. Among the Xhosa tribe in South Africa 61.8% of children have umbilical hernias, some being quite large.[545] Meier and colleagues undertook a prospective evaluation of the umbilical area of 4052 Nigerians living in the vicinity of the Baptist Medical Center in Ogbomoso, Nigeria.[783] The diameter of the fascial defect was measured with the subject supine and the protrusion of the umbilical skin with the subject erect. Protrusion of the umbilical tip past the periumbilical skin was identified in 92% of subjects below the age of 18 years and 49% of those above the age of 18 years. Umbilical hernias defined as protrusion of at least 5 mm and a diameter of at least 10 mm was present in 23% of patients under the age of 18 years and 8% of patients over the age of 18 years. It was concluded that spontaneous closure of umbilical hernias in these African children occurred until the age of 14 years. Because a retrospective analysis of the hospital records revealed very few emergency operations for umbilical hernia related problems, in this group of patients it has been recommended that the low incidence and serious mortality rate associated with management of emergencies does not justify a prophylactic repair. One detailed study from Johannesburg contradicts this evidence; Blumberg found the incidence of umbilical hernia to be the same regardless of race.[132] However, this is the only study that has made such a finding.

Other predisposing causes of umbilical herniation are prematurity and low birth weight, respiratory distress syndrome, rickets and malnutrition.[1170,1222] Umbilical hernias occur in 84% babies weighing 1000–1500 g; 38% in those weighing 1500–2000 g; and 20.5% in those between 2000 and 2500 g.[1170] Prenatal diagnosis of congenital umbilical hernia can be made on the basis of ultrasound and can be differentiated from persistent omphalo-mesenteric duct or omphalocele.[1045] Umbilical hernias often regress spontaneously and do not usually require surgical correction before the age of 4 years, unless the neck of the sac is greater than 2 cm in diameter.[55,885]

INDICATIONS FOR SURGERY

The usual infantile umbilical hernia is a protrusion through the umbilical cicatrix, with a small peritoneal sac and a relatively narrow neck. These hernias become very obvious when the infant cries or strains and are often a source of worry to the parents. The hernia usually is a small cone-like protrusion with the umbilical cicatrix at its apex. A more exuberant hernia with a proboscid protuberance at the center of the belly can lead to great psychological problems and warrant urgent surgery in infancy. Tender distended umbilical hernias occur in and mirror intraperitoneal disease, peritonitis, intestinal obstruction and ascites. Umbilical hernias rarely incarcerate or strangulate. Severe abdominal wall spasm associated with an umbilical hernia incarceration during vigorous swimming has been described in two children. Breathing using the abdominal muscles is critical in competitive swimming – high intra-abdominal pressures can cause umbilical herniation and incarceration in these circumstances, such cases are often dismissed as 'cramp'.[1062]

The abdominal wall around the base of an umbilical hernia should be palpated carefully. It is important to exclude linea alba hernias, interstitial hernias and cystic remnants of the omphalomesenteric duct or allantois.

Infantile umbilical hernias undergo spontaneous regression and cure as the child grows. However, if the hernia is unusually large, with a neck diameter greater than 2 cm, or fails to regress by school age, it should be operated upon. A small aponeurotic defect, diameter less than 1.5 cm, may be prone to incarceration and strangulation; in one large series the incidence of these complications was 5%.[637] A more recent survey of the literature, when reporting three cases of incarcerated umbilical hernia in boys under 4 years old, suggested that the incidence of obstructed umbilical hernia is approximately 1:1500 umbilical hernias. This rare incidence supports a policy of expectant management in the vast majority of children.[885] Although infantile umbilical hernias are remarkably free from complications one very rare complication, spontaneous rupture and evisceration, requires emergency treatment. Spontaneous rupture may be precipitated by local trauma, by umbilical sepsis, by severe coughing or a combination of these factors.[9,72] If spontaneous rupture with evisceration occurs the eviscerated bowel should be covered with warm damp swabs and urgent repair of the hernia performed after resuscitation of the child. Strangulated umbilical hernia in children is very rare. Okada and colleagues reported a case in a 5-month-old girl in whom resection of the ascending colon and 5 cm of terminal ileum was required and the authors suggested that strangulation may have occurred as a result of the fascial defect decreasing in size as the child grew.[866] Complications are absolute indications for surgery. It is important for psychological reasons to preserve the umbilical cicatrix when undertaking surgery.

ARRANGEMENTS FOR SURGERY AND ANESTHESIA

Children with umbilical hernias can be treated on an outpatient day-case basis. The arrangements for this surgery are similar to those described in Chapter 9 (see page 138).

THE OPERATION

Principles

A simple excision of the peritoneal sac and closure of the aponeurotic defect by double breasting in the vertical plane – Mayo's operation – is recommended.[761] This operation has stood the test of time, is easy to perform and is effective. The umbilical cicatrix is carefully preserved and its base sutured to the fascial linea alba to present a cosmetically attractive appearance after surgery. The alternative operation, through a vertical incision, is described by Criado but is not recommended on cosmetic grounds.[253]

For huge umbilical hernias in children the fascial defect may need to be repaired with the use of a cutaneous flap to construct a neoumbilicus.[129]

Hemostasis and suture materials

These details are given on page 139.

Position of patient

The child is placed on his back (supine) on the operating table. A light cotton blanket is placed over the chest and upper abdomen and a similar blanket over the lower limbs. Alternatively, limb stockinets can be used instead of, or in addition to, these blankets. This precaution prevents undue heat loss during surgery. In the smaller infants, heat lamps may be necessary.

DRAPING

Drapes are applied so that the umbilical area is exposed throughout the operation.

The incision

A curved transverse incision is made below the umbilicus: a curvilinear 'smile' incision. There is usually a skin fold skirting the umbilicus and the incision can be placed in it to give the most cosmetically acceptable result (Figure 11.1).

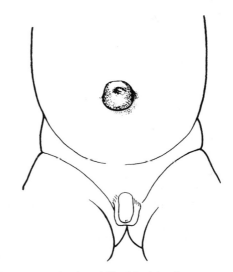

Figure 11.1 *A curved subumbilical incision is recommended.*

Skin flap and exposure of hernial sac

A skin flap, including the umbilical cicatrix, is dissected back to expose the hernial sac, which is dissected free from the surrounding fat. When the neck of the sac is defined, the more rigid outline of the linea alba should now be easily identified (Figure 11.2).

ENLARGEMENT OF OPENING

It is usually possible to reduce the contents of an infantile umbilical hernia without enlarging the opening of the linea

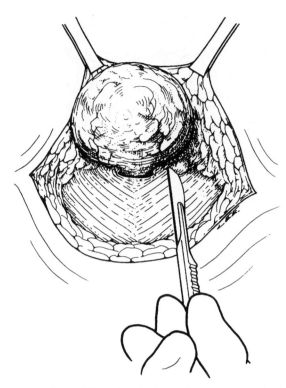

Figure 11.2 *The umbilicus is raised as a flap to expose the hernia.*

alba. However, if the contents cannot be reduced, the opening should be enlarged by small horizontal incisions into the rectus sheath on either side (Figure 11.3).

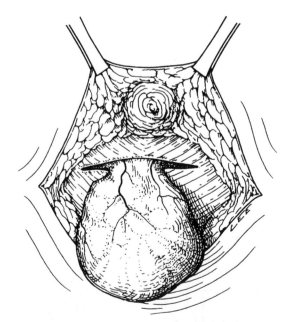

Figure 11.3 *The hernial orifice is enlarged slightly on either side.*

Removal of sac

The sac should be opened and then divided from the parietal peritoneum at its neck. As the sac is divided, its edges are picked up and held in small hemostats (Figure 11.4). If the overlying skin is particularly thin, one must be careful not to carry out excessive dissection if this would predispose the skin to necrosis or ulceration.

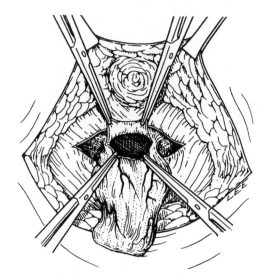

Figure 11.4 *The sac is opened and checked that it is empty. The sac is then excised.*

Repair of linea alba

The linea alba and the peritoneum are sutured as one layer. Hemostasis must first be secured. Often in children there are some substantial vessels running between the peritoneum and the aponeurosis; these should be ligated (Figure 11.5).

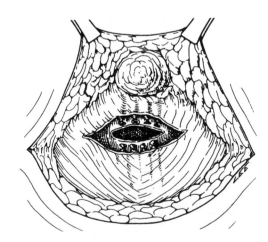

Figure 11.5 *Hemostasis is ensured.*

A double breasting technique (Mayo) is used. The placement of the sutures is facilitated if the lateral extremities of the cut in the linea alba are held up in small hemostats. Three PDS 3-0 sutures are used; they are introduced through the upper flap, then through the lower flap and back through the upper flap. The sutures should traverse the upper flap about 0.5 cm from its margin (the condensation of the aponeurosis at the linea alba aperture). As each suture is introduced it is held, not tied (Figure 11.6).

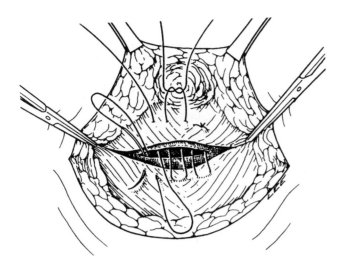

Figure 11.6 *A double breasting, 'vest over pants', Mayo operation is recommended. The first line of sutures is placed and held. Then the sutures are all tied simultaneously, pulling the lower flap up underneath the upper flap.*

When all three sutures have been placed, they are gently tightened and tied. Thus the lower aponeurotic flap is sutured to the undersurface of the upper flap.

The repair is now completed by suturing the edge of the upper flap to the anterior surface of the lower flap. Metric 3-0 PDS is used as continuous sutures (Figure 11.7).

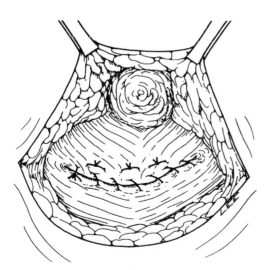

Figure 11.7 *The repair is completed by sewing the edge of the upper flap to the anterior surface of the lower flap.*

Reconstruction of umbilicus and skin closure

The deepest part of the delve of the umbilical cicatrix is now sutured to the linea alba with braided polymer or fine colorless PDS, so preserving the appearance of the umbilicus (Figure 11.8),

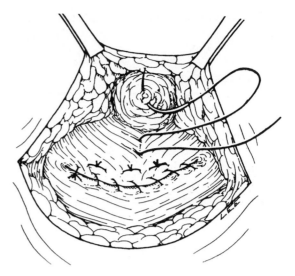

Figure 11.8 *The umbilicus is reconstructed.*

The subcutaneous fat is closed with interrupted sutures of fine absorbable polymer, the knots being tied deeply. Skin closure is with a subcuticular suture of colorless PDS if needed (Figures 11.9 and 11.10). The use of a pressure dressing for

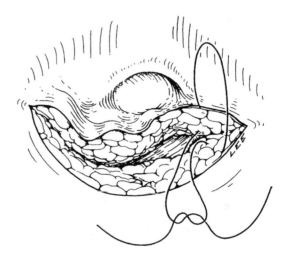

Figure 11.9 *The subcutaneous fat is closed.*

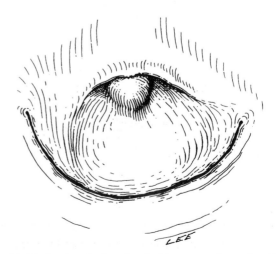

Figure 11.10 *A subcuticular absorbable suture closes the skin.*

48 h may be recommended if there is a substantial amount of dead-space.

POSTOPERATIVE CARE

No postoperative care other than normal maternal nursing care is required. The child can be cuddled and fed by his mother as soon as he is recovered from the anesthetic. He can be allowed to play and be bathed as soon as necessary.

The only postoperative complications are hematoma formation and minor sepsis. With careful hemostasis neither of these should be worrisome. Postoperative hematomas or infection may predispose to recurrence, which is otherwise very rare.[222] Wound healing is usually quick and cosmesis very good.

CONCLUSIONS

- Umbilical hernias in neonates and infants should be treated expectantly.
- Most childhood hernias resolve spontaneously.
- If operation is needed, Mayo's 'vest over pants' technique is recommended.

12

Diagnosis of a lump in the groin in the adult

Knowledge of the anatomy of the groin and a consequently enhanced ability to differentially diagnose groin lumps is somehow projected as part of the image of surgeons. Surgical teachers are apt to regard knowledge of groin lumps as normative for the student and aspirant surgeon. Glassow, certainly an experienced hernia surgeon, reporting his experience of femoral hernia in the female, described 8% of these femoral hernias being misdiagnosed as inguinal hernias.[417] Hardy and Costin have also drawn attention to the difficulties of distinguishing between inguinal and femoral hernias.[475] Although the distinction between femoral and inguinal hernias is difficult enough for practising surgeons, surgical teachers have in the past been obsessed with the diagnosis of groin lumps – the pursuit of the undiagnosable is, after all, an academic trail! Research shows that the differentiation between direct and indirect hernias cannot be sustained clinically.[151] In 180 patients over the age of 20 years with inguinal hernias two clinical tests were applied: the direction of the bulge and pressure on the deep ring to differentiate between direct and indirect hernia.[174] Operative findings indicated that the diagnosis of indirect hernia was correct in 92% of cases, whereas the clinical diagnosis of direct hernia was correct in only 56% of cases. These findings challenge the assumption that direct hernias are more easily diagnosable than indirect. Clinical diagnosis nevertheless remains a test of a medical student's diagnostic skill. However even the position of fixed landmarks such as the midpoint of the inguinal ligament and the mid inguinal point cannot be accurately distinguished.[32] Prior to surgery these two landmarks were used to identify the surface marking of the deep inguinal ring, but at operation the deep ring was found to be 0.25 cm lateral to the mid inguinal point and 0.46 cm medial to the midpoint of the inguinal ligament.

Unfortunate students had better beware; examiners will continue to ask them to distinguish inguinal and femoral, and direct and indirect inguinal hernias!

Every groin lump should be carefully evaluated and hernias must be distinguished from other lesions, but having stated this obvious truth it must be admitted that the distinction between the various types of groin hernia may often be impossible. Multiple groin hernias occur and add further to diagnostic confusion.

The Renaissance and eighteenth-century surgeons responsible for many of the clinico-anatomical descriptions we work to were coping with different clinical problems from those we deal with. We no longer have to diagnose the longstanding inguinoscrotal hernia which is carried in a wicker basket; today's patients frequently present with small lumps of recent origin. The patients are usually well-nourished, not to say obese, and they expect as accurate a diagnosis as possible. But we must recognize that our clinical skills do not deliver a greater than 60% accuracy.[475,916]

As the diagnosis is pursued from 'hernia/no hernia?' to 'hernia/femoral or inguinal?', and from 'inguinal hernia/direct or indirect?', the difficulties increase manifold. Even the experienced worker surgeon, not the academic thinker of the problem, may get the diagnosis wrong. Our differential diagnosis of these lumps demands review. The groin is an area of diagnostic uncertainty. A bizarre example of the diagnosis of a groin lump is reported by Deva et al. from Australia; their patient, a morbidly obese female (weight 182.0 kg, height 152.4 cm, body mass index 78.4) presented with an enlarging groin mass initially thought to be a femoral hernia. Computed tomography (CT) was not possible owing to her weight and ultrasound showed a solid lesion with no bowel demonstrated. The lesion, weighing 1650 g, was resected and found to be fat with no peritoneal sac!?[289]

Only one type of groin hernia can be diagnosed with any certainty; this is the broad neck direct sac in the elderly male, which never strangulates, is often bilateral and rarely causes much discomfort. It is readily apparent when the patient stands and immediately disappears spontaneously when he lies. This patient is happy when told the diagnosis … and the need for no operation.[99] Berliner has observed patients with bilateral hernia who have needed unilateral repair only, for periods of 5–10 years. In the majority, even those doing heavy labor, the asymptomatic side did not require surgery.[120] Small, asymptomatic, direct inguinal hernias that are not enlarging can be managed with judicious neglect and remain stationary in size and continue to be asymptomatic despite heavy labor.[118]

INGUINAL HERNIA – THE ADOLESCENT AND THE ADULT

In the male adolescent or young adult the lump is most likely to be an indirect inguinal hernia. The story then is that when the lump first appeared there was acute, quite severe pain in the groin that passed off and after a day or two went away altogether. The pain may have been related to straining or lifting or playing some violent game. Overall however, it has been estimated that only 7% of patients can attribute the presence of a hernia to a single muscular strain.[1066] This is an important figure in assessing 'cause' in claims for industrial injury in such patients. In 129 patients with a total of 145 hernias, in only nine could a single strenuous event be unequivocally related to the appearance of a lump in the groin. Smith and colleagues have recommended the following guidelines for claims for industrial injury:

1 The incident of muscular strain must be reported officially.
2 There must have been severe groin pain at the time of the strain.
3 The diagnosis by a qualified person should have been made preferably within 3 days of the event and certainly within 30 days.
4 There should be no previous history of inguinal hernia.

At first the lump comes and goes, disappearing when the sufferer goes to bed at night and not being present in the morning until he gets out of bed and stands up. The lump comes in the groin and goes obliquely down into the scrotum. The patient usually describes the sequence well. This is the classic description of an indirect (oblique) inguinal hernia in the young adult (Figure 12.1).

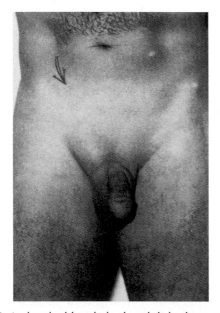

Figure 12.1 *An inguinal hernia in the adult is above and medial to the inguinal ligament and pubic tubercle as the hernia emerges from the superficial inguinal ring.*

In the older man an indirect hernia can occur, but a direct inguinal hernia is more likely. The story here is usually of some associated strain, often at work, the lump then appearing one or two days after the initial pain in the groin has gone away. Such a hernia may not reduce spontaneously. In the older male the lump may be associated with coughing, straining to micturate or disturbances in bowel habit. In these circumstances other predisposing conditions, respiratory disease or urinary tract obstruction or colonic disease that results in constriction of the lumen must be excluded as potentiating factors. As the length of time that the patient has had the hernia increases, the cumulative probability of pain increases to almost 90% at 10 years and the probability of irreducibility increases from 6.5% at 12 months to 30% at 10 years.[460]

Bilateral inguinal hernias in adult males are sometimes manifestations of connective tissue disorder (see page 46), ascites, carcinomatosis peritonei, heart failure or liver disease. The history may give a lead. Indirect inguinal hernias as a complication of CAPD are yet another manifestation of intra-abdominal fluid dilating the adult processus vaginalis.

A varicocele cannot easily be confused with an inguinal hernia in the male. The varicocele is invariably in the left inguinoscrotal line – it is like a mass of worms and disappears spontaneously if the subject lies down. It has no cough impulse.

Inguinal hernias are more common in adult males than adult females in a ratio of 10:1. However, inguinal hernias do occur in women; indeed, indirect inguinal hernias in women are as common as femoral hernias in women, a fact that is often forgotten in the differential diagnosis (see Table 3.2). Direct inguinal hernias are very rare in women.

The closed inguinal canal in the adult female means that small indirect inguinal hernias in women cause much stretching, and hence pain. Indirect inguinal hernias in women present with pain rather than with a lump. Even on the most careful examination a lump may be impossible to find in the suprapubic fat of an adult female. In these situations, the use of sonography and/or CT scanning can be particularly informative.

FEMORAL HERNIA

A femoral hernia accounts for approximately 5–10% of all groin hernias in adults.[459] In an analysis of 379 patients with groin hernia presenting electively at a University Department of Surgery, 16 patients had femoral hernia. The correct diagnosis of femoral hernia was made in only three cases by general practitioners and in only six by surgical staff of all grades indicating a poor rate of diagnosis.

Most femoral hernias occur in women aged over 50 years. Atrophy and weight loss are common in patients with femoral hernias. The incidence of femoral hernias, male to female, is generally reported to be about 1:4 (see Chapter 16). The different pelvic shape and additional fat in women render them more prone to femoral hernias than are men.[417] Women with femoral hernias are usually multiparous – multiple pregnancy is said to predispose to femoral herniation. Femoral hernias are as common in men as in nulliparous women.[120] A wide variety of occupations are likely to be found in any sample of femoral hernia patients, although it is said that nurses are more prone to these hernias than other groups.[915]

Patients complain of a groin lump, groin pain or various obstructive symptoms, nausea, colic, distension or constipation. The symptoms are variable and, particularly in the obese, unless a painstaking clinical examination of the groin is undertaken a small femoral hernia is easily overlooked. Groin pain with a recent onset irreducible groin lump is the presentation in 27%, a painless reducible groin lump occurs in 10%, a painful and reducible groin lump in 7%. Groin pain with no other symptoms and no complaint of a groin lump is the presentation in 3% of patients. Six percent of patients present with recurrent obstructive symptoms (Figure 12.2).[475,916] Missing the diagnosis of femoral hernia has dire consequences.[839] Such patients are often frail and elderly with severe coexisting diseases and late hospitalization is one of the main causes of unfavorable outcome.[627]

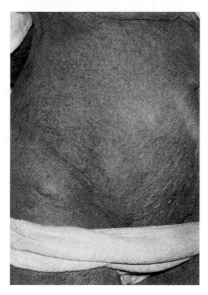

Figure 12.2 *A femoral hernia is below and lateral to the inguinal ligament and pubic tubercle as the hernia emerges into the thigh.*

In diagnosis of a femoral hernia, distension of the saphenous veins is an important confirmatory sign.[392] The accuracy of the diagnosis of femoral hernias in the community varies. In a retrospective review, letters of referral were traceable in 88% of elective patients with an operative diagnosis of femoral hernia. The correct diagnosis is arrived at by the referring general practitioner in less than 40% of cases and the diagnostic rate is only improved by 20% in the hands of surgical staff.[199,459] Patients referred with an inguinal lump or hernia (as opposed to a femoral hernia) were given a later outpatient appointment and consequently a later operation. Therefore all elderly patients referred with an undiagnosed groin lump should receive an early outpatient appointment because femoral hernias presenting with intestinal obstruction as an emergency have a mortality greater than 10%. Kemler and Oostvogel reviewed 111 patients admitted for femoral hernia repair in Tilberg, Netherlands. Those treated electively suffered no mortality and no bowel resection and 10% had significant co-morbid disease. Of the 33 patients treated as an emergency the mean age was 77 years, 20% had significant co-morbid cardiorespiratory disease and following surgery which involved nine bowel resections, three deaths occurred.[579] A conservative policy once diagnosis of femoral hernia has been made is therefore not acceptable.

An even more problematic clinical pitfall is the patient presenting with vague abdominal symptoms, the cause of which is an impalpable Richter's femoral hernia involving a small knuckle of the antimesenteric part of the small intestine.[1168]

OTHER GROIN SWELLINGS

Other structures in the groin each contribute to the harvest of swellings, pains and discomforts patients complain of. These include:

1   *Vascular disease*
    - Arterial – aneurysms of the iliac and femoral vessels; these may be complicated by distal embolization or vascular insufficiency which will make the diagnosis easy. Femoral aneurysm as a complication of cardiac catheterization or transluminal angioplasty is a recent arrival in the diagnostic arena.
    - Venous – a saphenovarix could be confused with a femoral hernia. Its anatomical site is the same, but its characteristic blue color, soft feel, fluid thrill, disappearance when the patient is laid flat and the giveaway associated varicose veins should prevent misdiagnosis.
    - Inguinal venous dilatation secondary to portosystemic shunting can result in a painful inguinal bulge that can even become incarcerated. Preoperative Doppler ultrasound in cirrhotic patients with suspected inguinal hernias is advised.[514]

2   *Lymphadenopathy*
    Chronic painless lymphadenopathy may occur in lymphoma and a spectrum of infective diseases. Acute painful lymphadenitis can be confused with a tiny strangulated femoral hernia. A lesion in the watershed area, the lower abdomen, inguinoscrotal or perineal region, the distal anal canal or the ipsilateral lower limb quickly resolves the argument.

3   *Tumors*
    Lipomas are very common tumors. The common 'lipoma of the cord', which in reality is an extension of preperitoneal fat is frequently associated with an indirect or direct inguinal hernia. Fawcett and Rooney examined 140 inguinal hernias in 129 patients to study the problem of lipoma. A fatty swelling was deemed significant if it was possible to separate it from the fat accompanying the testicular vessels.[346] The fatty swelling was designated as being a lipoma if there was no connection with extraperitoneal fat and was designated as being a preperitoneal protrusion if it was continuous through the deep ring with extra peritoneal fat. Protrusions of extraperitoneal fat were found in 33% of patients and occurred in association with all varieties of hernia. There was a true lipoma of the cord in only one patient. It was concluded that the forces causing the hernia were also responsible for causing the protrusion of extraperitoneal fat. Read has commented that occasionally extraperitoneal

protrusions of fat may be the only herniation and therefore inguinal hernia classifications need to include not only fatty hernias but sac-less, fatty protrusions.[949] Lipomas also occur in the upper thigh to cause confusion with femoral hernias. A lipoma is rarely tender; it is soft with scalloped edges and can be lifted 'free' of the subjacent fat.

4 *Secondary tumors*
A lymph node enlarged with metastatic tumor usually lies in a more superficial layer than a femoral hernia. Such lymph nodes are more mobile in every direction than a femoral hernia and are often multiple. A metastatic deposit of a tumor arising from the abdominal cavity such as adenocarcinoma can present as a rock-hard immobile mass that can be confused as either a primary incarcerated inguinal hernia or a postoperative fibrotic reaction following an inguinal hernia repair.

5 *Genital anomalies*
  • Ectopic testis in the male – there is no testicle in the scrotum on the same side. Torsion of an ectopic testicle can be confused with a strangulated hernia.
  • Cyst of the canal of Nuck – these cysts extend towards, or into, the labium majorum and are transilluminable.

6 *Obturator hernia*
An obturator hernia, especially in a female, lies in the thigh lateral to the adductor longus muscle. Vaginal examination will resolve the diagnosis. Elective diagnosis is rarely entertained.

7 *Rarities*
  • A cystic hygroma is a rare swelling; it is loculated and very soft. Usually the fluid can be pressed from one part of it to another.
  • A psoas abscess is a soft swelling frequently associated with backache. It loses its tension if the patient is laid flat. It is classically lateral to the femoral artery.
  • A hydrocele of the femoral canal is a rarity reported from West Africa. In reality it is the end stage of an untreated strangulated femoral epiplocele. The strangulated portion of omentum is slowly reabsorbed, the neck of the femoral sac remains occluded by viable omentum, while the distal sac becomes progressively more and more distended by protein-rich transudate.

INGUINOSCROTAL PAIN

Inguinoscrotal pain may arise in the groin and radiate to the ipsilateral hemiscrotum, thigh, flank or hypogastrium. Such pain may be neuralgic in type and accentuated by physical exertion. If the cause is a hernia or preperitoneal fat forcing its way out through the deep inguinal ring, these structures are stretched and pain fibers are stimulated. This is thought to cause a local reflex increase of tone in the internal oblique and transversus muscles coupled with neuralgic pain from stretching of the ilioinguinal nerve. The pain due to increase in tone is intermittent, whereas the neuralgic pain leading to hyperalgesia

can be constant and following hernia repair will disappear, indicating that it is neuropraxic in type.[1227]

Numerous other conditions can give rise to acute or chronic pain in the inguinoscrotal and neighboring anatomical regions (Table 12.1). These include gynecological and urological pathology and a variety of musculoskeletal syndromes. An important entity increasingly being characterized is the syndrome of 'broad and deep fossae' or the sportsman's hernia. Thus, patients presenting with pain, as opposed to a painless, reducible swelling in the groin, should undergo very careful clinical evaluation for urological, gynecological and musculoskeletal disorders. In addition to a careful history and examination, a variety of radiological investigations are at the disposal of the clinician.

Table 12.1 *Differential diagnosis of inguinoscrotal pain*

Hernia:	Direct or indirect inguinal hernia, femoral hernia, lipomas of the cord
Scrotal conditions:	Epididymo-orchitis, prostatitis, urinary tract infection, torsion of the testis
Urological conditions:	Tumor or stone disease, urethral extravasation
Gynecological conditions:	Pelvic inflammatory disease, uterine or ovarian tumor
Musculoskeletal disorders:	Adductor tendonitis, adductor avulsion, gracilis syndrome, pubic instability, osteitis pubis, rectus abdominis, tendonopathy, ilio-psoas injury
Spinal abnormalities	
Hip abnormalities	
Enthesopathy	

In many patients presenting with chronic groin pain, a urological disorder is the initial working diagnosis. Chronic prostatitis or seminal vesiculitis is commonly suspected and in many patients may have been treated with multiple courses of antibiotics.

Thorough examination and investigation may reveal no underlying cause; an occult hernia should then be suspected. However, a further increasingly recognized diagnosis should be entertained: 'tennis elbow' of the groin or enthesopathy (inflammation of the insertion – enthesis – of a ligament or tendon).[54] There is frequently a history of sudden onset of pain and then of aggravation by physical exertion. The exact site of tenderness must be ascertained to differentiate the ligamentous or tendinous insertion. Careful palpation using one finger of muscles, ligaments, tendons or scars in the inguinal region will point to the origin of the enthesopathy, which may be in the adductus longus insertion, inguinal ligament insertion, rectus abdominis insertion, or along the inguinal ligament at sites where the transversalis and internal oblique muscles insert. Once the condition has been recognized, symptoms may respond to local injection of lignocaine (lidocaine) and triamcinolone.

Clinical examination of the scrotum must be included in any assessment of inguinoscrotal pain. A small hernia protruding at the deep ring may stimulate the genital branch of the genitofemoral nerve to give scrotal pain in the male or labial pain in the female as its feature. If the patient appears acutely complaining of pain in the groin associated with the lump, the differential examination should include hernias, torsion of the testicles, spasm of the cremaster and trauma to the testicle or cord.

Other causes of inguinoscrotal pain include abdominal aneurysms, degenerative disease of the lower thoracic and lumbar spines and degenerative disease of the hip joint. The genital pelvic viscera, prostate, seminal vesicles and proximal vasa have an autonomic supply from T12 to L2 and from S2, S3 and S4; therefore referred pain from these organs may radiate via the genital branch of the genitofemoral nerve L1 and posterior scrotal nerves S2 and S3 to the groin and external genitalia.

CLINICAL EXAMINATION

The patient should be undressed and the entire abdomen and lower limbs examined.

In the male the first step is to observe where the testicles are. Knowledge of testicle position prevents all the confusions of undescended testicles, etc.

The groin should be examined with the patient standing erect and again with the patient lying flat. Hernias are sometimes only apparent when the patient stands up or only when the patient strains or coughs.

When the patient is examined a rapid decision should be made as to whether the lump is a hernia or not a hernia – this is the crucial initial decision to make. A hernia has a cough impulse, changes in size when the patient strains or lies down and may be reducible. The other lumps in the groin do not change their disposition when the patient stands or lies down.

In the male the differential diagnosis between a direct and an indirect inguinal hernia cannot be made with any certainty, except for the elderly male who has a broad neck direct inguinal hernia that is spontaneously reducible when he lies flat. Similarly, in the female it is very difficult indeed to make the differential diagnosis between an inguinal hernia and a femoral hernia which has emerged from the saphenous opening and its fundus doubled back up over the inguinal ligament. Fortunately both of these differential diagnoses between a direct and an indirect inguinal hernia in the male and between the femoral and the inguinal hernia in the female, although interesting, are not of crucial importance. The operative approach to the groin hernias allows whichever groin hernia is encountered at surgery to be corrected. It is, therefore, better to be able to make the diagnosis of a hernia and be humble enough to acknowledge that having approached the groin the operative strategy may need modifying depending upon the anatomic type of hernia found.

It is difficult to distinguish between an inguinal and a femoral hernia, particularly in an obese person. Femoral hernias may present as 'recurrences' after repair of an inguinal hernia. In these circumstances they are often indistinguishable from inguinal hernias. The diagnostic difficulty is increased by the fact that as a femoral hernia emerges through the cribriform fascia at the fossa ovalis, the fundus comes forwards and then turns upwards to lie over and anterior to the inguinal ligament. Palpation of the external ring and the cord should enable the diagnosis to be made in the male. The difficulty is in the female. If the hernia can be reduced, careful palpation of the hernial aperture should enable the examiner to orientate it relative to the inguinal ligament. If the hernia emerges above the inguinal ligament when the patient coughs, the hernia is inguinal; if below the ligament, it is femoral.

Reducing the hernia and then using one finger to hold it reduced while the patient coughs is a useful test which will enable the inguinal canal or the femoral ring to be identified, almost with certainty. Invagination of the scrotal skin into the inguinal canal, a time hallowed test, is uncomfortable for the patient and does not provide useful information. This maneuver is still useful to identify small hernias at the internal ring. Hernias which extend down into the scrotum are generally indirect inguinal. Scrotal hernias must be separated from other scrotal lumps – hydrocele, varicocele, testicular tumors, epididymal cysts, etc. If the hernia is reducible, the diagnosis is obvious. A cough impulse is a characteristic of hernias, but not of other scrotal masses.

The advent of sophisticated radiological investigation (see below) has enabled small and occult hernias to be more easily diagnosed. The chief utility of ultrasound is to enable scrotal and other swellings to be clearly differentiated.

GROIN DISRUPTION IN ATHLETES

In most athletes with groin pain a musculoskeletal disorder is easily diagnosed and adequately treated. The pectineus muscle, adductors (magnus, brevis and longus) and gracilis muscle should be examined by palpation, passive abduction, adduction against resistance and hip flexion. The rectus abdominis muscle must be examined by active contraction with both legs elevated and by palpation of its origins. Next the hip should be tested using Patrick's test (pressure applied to the knee with the opposite hip stabilized and with the tested hip in a flexed, abducted and externally rotated position with the heel on the opposite knee), observing the full range of movements and by flexion, adduction, internal rotation and compression. A full range of movement should be present in the lower back, including flexion, extension, lateral reflection and rotation, and the thoracolumbar spine should be examined for tenderness. Stretch tests must be performed for the femoral and sciatic nerves, and a full neurological examination carried out of the lower limb and affected groin, with particular reference to ilioinguinal or genitofemoral nerve neuralgias. Finally, the pelvis should be examined by palpation of the pubic arches, crests and tubercles, and the pubic symphysis by compression and direct pressure.[738]

Following this thorough clinical examination, which if necessary is supplemented by plain radiographs of hips and pelvis, including views of the pubic symphysis, there will remain a group of patients who have unexplained groin pain.[447,672] Because the diagnosis and therapy of chronic groin pain in athletes is complex, referral to a specialist sports injury clinic is advisable. Such groin injuries account for only 5% of those attending, but are responsible for a much larger proportion of time lost from competition and work. Herniography has been instrumental in identifying the cause of the sports hernia as the syndrome of 'broad and deep fossae'.[455,1065,1161] In the UK Jeremy A Gilmore has contributed significantly to the understanding of this problem.[415] Gilmore is clear in stating that groin disruption is not a hernia; there is no protrusion of a viscus beyond its normal confines. Groin disruption is a severe musculo-tendinous injury of the groin, which can be successfully treated by the surgical restoration of normal anatomy. Gilmore describes an experience of over 2000 cases referred, 1400 of which required operation, 98% were male with the majority being soccer players. The severity of the pathology found at operation varies, but the main features include: torn external oblique aponeurosis, torn conjoint tendon, conjoint tendon torn from the pubic tubercle, dehiscence between conjoint tendon and inguinal ligament; there being no hernia present either direct or indirect in all cases. Edema and occasionally evidence of hemorrhage is seen in acute cases and the severity of the tears usually correlates with the patient's symptoms.

The history is variable. Some athletes such as runners will tend to describe an insidious onset resulting in a 'groin strain' with a persistent, dull, deep ache in the groin. Athletes involved in contact sports may describe sudden tearing sensations giving rise to continuous aching pain in the inguinoscrotal region. The pain is aggravated by physical exertion and may begin to radiate to the thigh, scrotum or lower abdomen: it is often these symptoms which have led to extensive investigation. The fact that many athletes experience exacerbation of pain with physical exertion or coughing and straining points to an abnormality of the shutter or sphincter mechanism of the inguinal region. It is useful to ask patients to shade in pain areas on an anatomical diagram, to identify the areas in which pain occurs and is developing (Figure 12.3).

The signs found on physical examination are again variable and relate more to the last period of physical exertion than to any other factor. After a period of prolonged rest, physical signs may be minimal. However, following a period of training or sporting activity, the whole inguinoscrotal region may be tender. The key to diagnosis is palpation of the external ring by invagination of the scrotal skin and palpation from inside the inguinal canal. An area of exquisite tenderness is felt, which is aggravated by coughing, and a slight impulse can be detected. A further diagnostic maneuver can be undertaken by asking the patient to adopt a half 'sit-up' and cough while the upper and

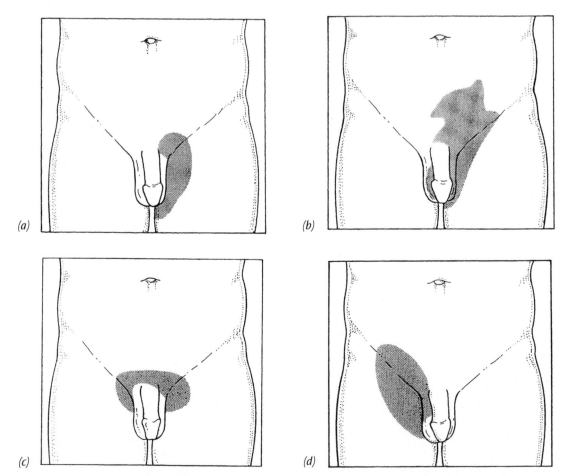

(a)　(b)　(c)　(d)

Figure 12.3 *Pain diagrams, each accompanied by the instruction 'Please shade the areas where you felt pain prior to your operation'.*

lower margins of the superficial ring are examined and the posterior inguinal wall palpated. An enlarged tender ring and posterior pain is evidence of inguinal canal disruption.[729]

The history, exclusion of all other pathologies, and characteristic physical signs as outlined above will enable the diagnosis of groin disruption. However, many clinics will insist on objective evidence, either from a herniogram or supplemented with other radiological investigations (see below). Herniography directed hernia repair has poor specificity and the presence of an occult hernia may not necessarily identify the cause of the pain.[366,1124]

The findings at operation are said to be characteristic: these include a dilated external ring, disruption of the conjoint tendon from the inguinal ligament, absence or attenuation of the transversalis fascia, and a plug of preperitoneal fat at the internal ring. Other explanations are a sheer injury of the common abductor-rectus abdominis anatomical unit[1110] and entrapment by the inguinal ligament of the genital branch of the genitofemoral nerve;[12] however, it must be remembered that the detailed anatomy of the inguinal canal is very variable (see pages 21–31 and an anatomical basis for the 'sportsman's groin syndrome', 'Gilmore's groin', is elusive. Repair of the posterior inguinal wall achieves good results with 87–93% of athletes returning to full sporting activity within 3–6 months. Subsequent follow-up with pain scores in these athletes indicated a marked improvement in the level of pain.[455,738]

Successful treatment depends on an accurate diagnosis, meticulous surgery repairing each element of the disruption and vigorous rehabilitation. Surgery is indicated in patients who fail to respond to a standard rehabilitation programme. Successful operation is achieved by restoration of the normal anatomy by repairing each element: the conjoint tendon, the transversalis fascia, the conjoint tendon which may require re-attachment to the pubic tubercle and the inguinal ligament may also require repair. At operation an open 6-layered suture technique to prevent further disruption has been recommended.[415] Laparoscopic and flat mesh repair have also been reported.[535]

HIDDEN HERNIAS

Hidden hernias are more likely to occur in women than men. This is due to the greater prevalence of femoral hernia in women, linked to the failure to examine or the inaccessibility of the femoral opening, particularly in obese patients. In addition, certain pelvic hernias, such as obturator hernia, occur with a much higher frequency in women and internal hernias such as hernias of the broad ligament of the uterus occur exclusively in women (see Chapter 20).

In a woman, the non-palpable, hidden or occult inguinal and femoral hernia is an infrequent cause of pain.[68,192,1076] Symptoms are likely to be similar to those of the sports hernia: dull inguinal pain is the predominant symptom. There may be tenderness on palpation over the deep inguinal ring, tested either by inversion of the scrotal skin or the skin of the labia majora, and the Valsalva maneuver exacerbates this tenderness. The deep inguinal ring is often abnormally wide and there is hyperalgesia in the distribution of the ilioinguinal or genitofemoral nerves.

Herniography may establish the diagnosis, although a dilated internal ring plugged by preperitoneal fat will obscure radiographic findings. Herniography however is not always accurate. There can be a false-positive rate of up to 20% usually in patients presenting with pain alone, and a false-negative rate of up to 10% usually in patients with pain and a palpable lump but no clinical inguinal hernia in the groin.[469,583,705] More invasive radiological techniques include a combination of herniography and femoral vein phlebography to establish the diagnosis of occult femoral hernia.

Herniography can clinch the diagnosis of obturator hernias; the hernia is seen to protrude downwards anteriorly through the obturator foramen beneath the pubic bone (Figure 12.4). The typical shape is similar to that of a femoral hernia, but the sac is situated more medially. A CT scan with contrast may help in differentiation.[1120]

Hernias of the broad ligament of the uterus can occur through the ligament itself into the mesometrium, through the mesosalpinx, or under the round ligament or suspensory ligament of the ovary. Subacute or acute intestinal obstruction is the mode of presentation of this internal hernia, which can occur in women of all ages.[30] Obstetric trauma may be a causative factor and the diagnosis should be considered in any woman presenting with intestinal obstruction and no obvious cause.

Radiological diagnosis of occult hernia

HERNIOGRAPHY

Herniography can be an excellent and sensitive diagnostic tool, capable of demonstrating hernias in the groin, especially

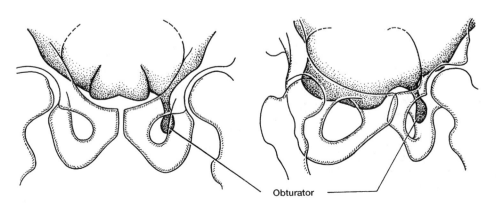

Obturator

Figure 12.4 *Obturator herniogram.*

when physical examination is negative.[68,317,322,451,1161] Indirect herniography by injecting contrast medium into a hollow viscus and observing the position of the contrast-filled viscus has fallen into disuse because of the considerable morbidity. Nevertheless, Allen and Condon found that lateral protrusion of the urinary bladder ('bladder's ears') into the deep inguinal ring developed in 9% of 406 patients undergoing intravenous urography and cystograms.[17]

Direct herniography was first performed in experimental animals by Sternhill and Schwarz[1089] and subsequently performed clinically by Ducharmé in children.[317] Herniography with fluoroscopy and peritoneography, performed by puncture of the abdominal wall and injection of non-ionic contrast medium, is now the preferred method of investigation.[451] Indications are principally symptoms indicative of a hernia but no palpable lump, obscure groin pain (other diagnoses having been excluded by appropriate investigation), and evaluation of patients who remain symptomatic following primary hernia repair.

Technique is important and will be successful only in experienced hands.[451] The patient must be placed on a tilt table with fluoroscopy, enabling tangential views of the pelvic floor and groin. The bladder should be empty at the time of the examination. Through a small skin incision a catheter is inserted through the left lower quadrant of the abdomen into the peritoneal cavity. After screening to confirm the presence of the catheter within the peritoneal cavity, it is advanced towards the pelvic floor. Contrast medium is then introduced, which should be non-ionic in nature, and adequate filling will be obtained with 60–80 ml. The X-ray table is then rotated to the upright position and contrast medium allowed to pool in the various fossae and hernial orifices. The table is then lowered to 25° foot down and the patient is moved to the prone position. The symptomatic side is then turned downward in an oblique position and the patient asked to strain. Hernial sacs should then be screened in several positions to allow full evaluation, including several projections for optimal evaluation of all the fossae. A thorough examination of the entire surgical anatomy of the pelvic and inguinal floor should be performed for exact verification of all potential hernial orifices. A normal herniogram is shown in Figure 12.5.

Classical herniograms for direct inguinal, indirect inguinal and femoral hernia are shown in Figure 12.6. These hernias can be diagnosed from their shape, relation to the pelvic peritoneal

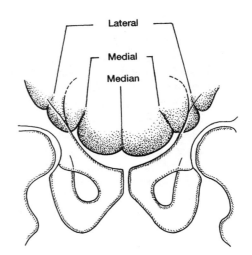

Figure 12.5 *Normal herniogram, showing lateral, medial and median umbilical folds.*

folds and the resulting pelvic fossae. Five pelvic peritoneal folds in the pelvis and groin (lateral umbilical, medial umbilical and median umbilical) divide the pelvic cavity into three fossae: supravesical, medial umbilical and lateral umbilical (see Figure 12.7). An indirect hernia protrudes lateral to the lateral fold through the lateral (inguinal) fossa. A direct inguinal hernia protrudes lateral to the median fold through the medial (inguinal) fossa. A femoral hernia protrudes through the median umbilical fossa in a lateral direction through the femoral canal.

Herniography is also valuable in the postoperative evaluation of patients with persistent symptoms in whom clinically detectable hernias are not evident on physical examination.[468] Hamlin and Kahn performed herniograms in 46 subjects with 54 symptomatic sites.[468] Ten recurrent hernias were found, although only two were symptomatic. In addition, they found 14 hernias in the contralateral, asymptomatic, groin and the herniogram was negative in one patient with a clinical hernia. A herniogram can therefore corroborate clinical findings and eliminate the need for re-exploration. Herniography can also identify patients in whom recurrent hernias have developed that are not detected on physical examination.

Inguinal and femoral hernias are best demonstrated by herniography. Anterior wall defects, ventral, Spigelian and

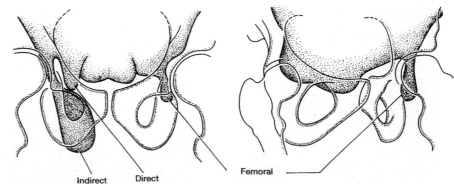

Figure 12.6 *Herniograms; direct, indirect and femoral.*

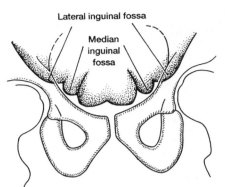

Figure 12.7 *Herniogram showing the lateral and medial inguinal fossae.*

obturator hernias should be evaluated both by herniography and cross-sectional imaging techniques.[478] Herniography should be combined with other imaging techniques to avoid pitfalls caused by contrast not entering and outlining intermittent hernia defects; for this reason post-exercise and oblique and tangential radiographs are essential to enlarge the diagnostic field.

Complications of herniography occur in approximately 6% of patients and are usually minor because it is a minimally invasive procedure. The minor risks include hematoma of the anterior abdominal wall, adverse reaction to the contrast medium, bruising of the pelvic viscera and extraperitoneal extravasation of contrast medium. More serious, infrequent complications include bowel perforation, mesenteric hematoma formation, and pelvic peritonitis. These complications are unusual in experienced hands.

Essentially herniography is a sensitive and reliable investigation, which can be used to diagnose hidden hernias, aid in the diagnosis of the cause of obscure groin pain, and diagnose occult hernias. The investigation can be performed under local anesthesia on an outpatient basis with minimal complications.[723] Visceral perforation is a rare hazard that does not usually require significant intervention, making herniography a safe and useful diagnostic test.[489]

ULTRASONOGRAPHY

Ultrasound examination of the abdominal wall and inguinal region has been used to a lesser degree in the diagnosis of occult hernia and obscure groin pain.[1143] The preferred method is real-time ultrasound for short-focus adjustment, using a linear scanner to clarify surface anatomy. The patient is placed supine with an empty bladder and further examination is performed in the upright position, with the patient passive, or in the Valsalva maneuver, and comparisons made between sides in two vertical planes.

This technique has a sensitivity of 100% and specificity of 97.9% in determining the nature of a lump in the groin. False interpretation is more likely to occur in cases of femoral hernia. The typical findings and interpretation of an inguinal and a femoral hernia are shown in Figures 12.8 and 12.9.

The antenatal diagnosis of abdominal wall defects is now a successful part of obstetric/pediatric surgical practice. Patients born with herniation can then be readily transferred to a pediatric surgical service.[305]

Ultrasound assessment of the contralateral groin accurately diagnosed a patent processus vaginalis in only 15 of 23 infants, with four false-positive and four false-negative cases.[642] Lawrenz and colleagues concluded that ultrasound cannot be used alone to plan the management of the contralateral groin in infants.

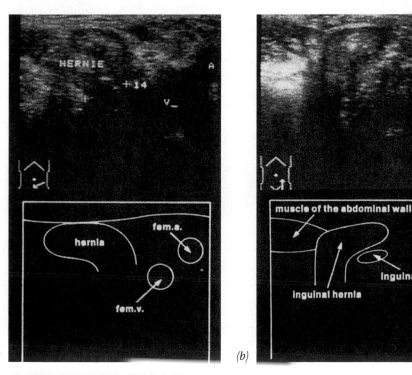

(a)   (b)

Figure 12.8 *Ultrasound examination localizing an inguinal hernia sac in transverse (a) and longitudinal (b) section. (Reproduced with permission from Truong et al., 1995.)*

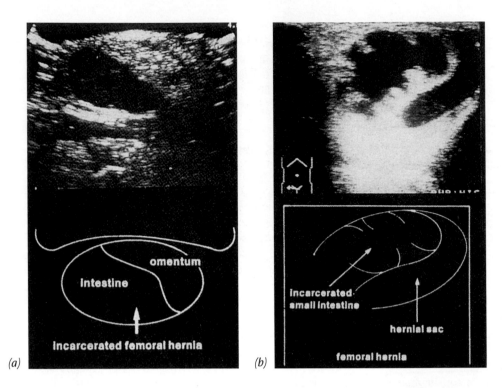

(a) *(b)*

Figure 12.9 *Ultrasound examination showing femoral hernia with incarcerated omentum and small bowel. (Reproduced with permission from Truong et al., 1995.)*

In boys where there is doubt about the diagnosis, ultrasound is a non-invasive and highly accurate diagnostic tool.[210] Using 4 mm as the upper limit of the normal diameter of the internal inguinal ring, occult inguinal hernias can be diagnosed with a 97.9% accuracy. A small study in 19 patients with clinically diagnosed groin hernias assessed the ability of color Doppler and color Doppler sonography to distinguish between different types of groin hernia in adults.[1236] The inferior epigastric artery was used as a landmark to differentiate different types of hernia sac, but was only visualized in 55% of cases making this examination an unreliable method for differentiating hernia types.

COMPUTED TOMOGRAPHY

Cross-sectional imaging by CT scanning has the potential for evaluating disorders of the abdominal wall, including hernias. The diagnosis of hernia is based on the identification of the fascial defect rather than visualization of hernial contents. Preliminary investigations by Hahn-Pedersen and colleagues have shown that examination of the pampiniform plexus during the Valsalva maneuver can differentiate direct from indirect hernias.[456] The practical usefulness of this finding is unknown. The introduction of contrast medium by intubation of the small intestine followed by CT scanning is a very helpful investigation in cases of intestinal obstruction and suspected but occult external hernia.[68,1146] Contrast medium appears in the entrapped loop between the external obturator and pectineal muscles in the case of obturator hernia (Figure 12.10). Inguinal and femoral hernias may not be detected unless they are obstructed because the patient is usually scanned in the supine position.[478] Femoral hernias are distinguished from inguinal hernias because of their location inferior and lateral to the pubic tubercle.[1196] Computed tomography can also clearly

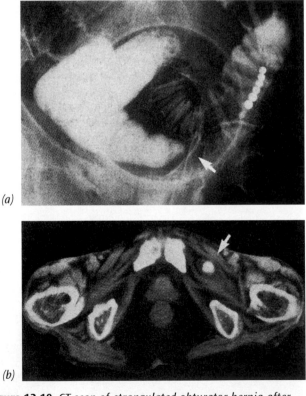

(a)

(b)

Figure 12.10 *CT scan of strangulated obturator hernia after intubation and small bowel infusion of contrast. Obstructed small bowel (a) and contrast in mass between external obturator and pectineal muscles (b). (Reproduced with permission from Tsutsui et al., 1994.)*

demonstrate the anatomical site of a hernia sac, its contents and any occlusive bowel complications due to incarceration or strangulation. Clinical diagnosis of external hernias is particularly difficult in obese patients or in those with laparotomy scars. In these cases CT imaging is essential for a correct preoperative diagnosis and to determine the most effective treatment.[527]

MAGNETIC RESONANCE IMAGING

Magnetic resonance imaging (MRI) and retrograde air insufflation has been used to evaluate bowel obstruction. Using this technique Chung-Kuao Chou clearly demonstrated an internal supravesical hernia.[220] MR imaging is particularly helpful in athletes with groin pain. Osteitic changes particularly in the pubis are detected as areas of low signal intensity on T1-w images of high and homogeneous signal intensity and on T2-w scans without fat suppression. Abnormalities in myotendinous structures are also well-documented by this technique as are involvement of the sacro-iliac joints.[78] Inguinal hernias are easily demonstrated by MRI, which allows the direct visualization of the hernial sac within the inguinal or femoral canal. The disadvantage of MR scanning is that the patient cannot strain in the semi erect or erect position because the procedure is carried out in the prone position.[648]

CONCLUSIONS

- Every effort should be made to distinguish inguinal from femoral hernias before surgery. This is especially important for the open approach but the laparoscopic method will differentiate these definitely.
- Careful identification of the pubic tubercle, the anterior superior iliac spine and, between them, the inguinal ligament is the prerequisite. Inguinal hernias emerge from the fascia transversalis above this line, femoral hernias below it.
- Femoral hernias never pass from the abdomen into the scrotum or labia majora as indirect inguinal hernias do.
- Direct inguinal hernias are almost unknown in women.
- The diagnosis of inguinoscrotal pain can be a challenging clinical problem. A diagnosis can often be achieved with appropriate radiological investigation.

13

Anterior open repair of inguinal hernia in adults

OPERATION OR TRUSS?

Operation must always be advised for incarcerated or strangulated inguinal hernia. A truss is only an option if the hernia can be readily and completely reduced. A large hydrocele encroaching on the external ring, which interferes with fitting a truss, is also a contraindication to management by a truss.

A truss is sometimes advised (ill advised) in the older patient with a reducible hernia, when without real justification, the risks of hernia repair are considered to be excessive. Open repair of a groin hernia does not involve major exploration of a body cavity, manipulation of viscera or hemodynamic hazard. There are no metabolic complications either. Sepsis is rare after groin hernia repair. For these reasons surgery should be advised; a truss is a poor alternative to surgery. Wearing a truss does not guarantee that an indirect inguinal or femoral hernia will remain reduced. A truss increases the patient's chance of developing complications; it may obstruct the venous and lymphatic drainage of intra-hernial viscera and precipitate strangulation. In addition, particularly with the large direct hernia the pressure of the truss leads to atrophy of the muscular and fascial margins of the defect enlarging the hernial orifice promoting enlargement of the hernia and making surgical repair even more difficult.

Sir Geoffrey Keynes in 1927, commented on the complications of a truss:[584]

> 'The tissues underlying such a truss will be found to be matted, thinned out and the muscles almost entirely converted to fibrous tissue. It is impossible to look upon the truss as anything but an antiquated piece of apparatus, the very existence of which is a sorry testimonial to progressive surgery, the use of which generally results in gradual injury to the wearer, and the results of which tax the surgeon's best efforts to undo when the time comes that the truss is no longer able to hold up the protrusion'.

A more recent evaluation by Law and Trapnell assessed 250 consecutive patients referred for surgical repair of a hernia, 52 of whom were fitted with a truss before attending the outpatient clinic. The mean age of these patients was 70 years, the truss had been worn for a median of 35 months (range 2–240); 11 (21%) had been prescribed a truss before referral to a

surgeon, and 23 (44%) had received no instructions, with the result that 35 (77%) fitted the truss while standing. Partial or complete control of the hernia was achieved in only 16 patients (31%) and 33 (64%) had found the truss to be uncomfortable.[641] The authors expressed concern that 40 000 trusses were being sold annually in the UK, mostly through retail outlets, yet advice to patients was incomplete which could result in an increase of complications and morbidity such as atrophy of the spermatic cord and testicle, tissue atrophy and neuritis and a considerably lower quality of life than might be expected from adequate inguinal hernia repair.

Cheek, Williams and Farndon further reviewed the use of trusses in England in 1995, they confirmed that 40 000 trusses were being issued nationally in the UK and that the evaluation of the effectiveness of trusses was inadequate. The rate of truss supply in England, 700 per million, is considerably higher than elsewhere in the developed world. Nowadays with modern anesthesia no patient should be denied surgery, nonetheless there is an urgent need for some research on the value of trusses.[209]

Neuhauser, writing in 1977, has compared the outcome of elective herniorrhaphy in the elderly to management with a truss. His study is important if only because it highlights the difficulties of surgical decision making and points to the value of more sophisticated option appraisal when advising patients. Neuhauser assesses what effect the choice of truss versus elective herniorrhaphy has on the life expectancy of a 65-year-old person.[842]

Reviewing data for (a) the mortality of elective surgery; (b) the mortality of emergency surgery; (c) the probability of recurrence; (d) the yearly probability of strangulation and (e) the life expectancy of the patient, he calculates and compares the effects of using a truss, and thus running the risk of obstruction followed by an emergency operation and its higher mortality, with having an immediate elective operation with its low mortality and the risk that the hernia will recur and need additional elective operations. The most recent data used for these calculations of probabilities are from 1974.

Although these data have been superseded – the mortality rate for elective hernia repair in the elderly is now approaching zero and the mortality rate for emergency hernia operation in the 1960–1969 decade is probably less than the 1% figure used in this study – the conclusion reached is very important. On the data available, elective inguinal herniorrhaphy does not prolong life in the elderly. It may or may not improve the quality of life.

What has changed in the past 30 years is the reduction in the mortality of emergency operation for strangulation. Although much improvement has been gained in the mortality for emergency operation, the need for elective operation to save lives in the elderly has not been eliminated.

Elective inguinal hernia repair in the elderly must be undertaken as a well-planned procedure with full medical support for any co-morbid conditions. An appropriate choice of analgesia between general, local or regional anesthesia must also be taken. Finally the surgery must be undertaken with precision and care to avoid surgical complications, which are poorly tolerated in the elderly.[404] Gilbert reported on 175 patients over the age of 66 years, in whom elective inguinal or femoral hernia repair was performed. Of these patients 50% were ASA grade III (severe systemic disease that limits activity but is not incapacitating), and 22% had undergone coronary artery bypass grafting, indicating that vascular disease is the most common co-morbidity in these elderly patients. Most of the operations were carried out under local or epidural anesthesia; only 17 operations being undertaken under general anesthesia. The preoperative control of symptoms of systemic or medical disease was undertaken in conjunction with a qualified physician. However, exercise tolerance was judged by the simple ability to climb one flight of stairs if local anesthesia was being considered, although more extensive investigations were required if general anesthesia was to be administered. Aspirin and anticoagulants were withdrawn temporarily and heparin cover instituted. In this series there were no deaths and minimal complications. Gilbert emphasizes that there are misconceptions concerning elective inguinal hernia repair in the elderly, based on the premise that the patient has numerous medical complaints and the hernia is a minor, non-life-threatening secondary phenomenon, or that the patient is on multiple medications which would complicate anesthesia, and lastly that the type of anesthesia required is general anesthesia. These myths should be dispelled and all patients assessed and considered for hernia surgery if the hernia itself merits repair. More recently Gianetta from Italy and Gunnarsson from Sweden have reported similar series of elderly patients with equally good results.[401,453] Both studies confirm the safety if concomitant disease is controlled and if domestic arrangements are made in advance so that the patient's need for hospital care can be minimized or, more commonly, eliminated.

A not quite so optimistic overall picture was painted by Gardner and Palasti.[387] In this series of 304 patients over the age of 80 years, the overall mortality for elective hernia repair was 8.9%, with deaths resulting from complications of the primary disease rather than associated medical disorders. The mortality rate, however, was 19.9% when operation was carried out as an emergency, and the authors suggest that health resources should be directed at treating hernias before complications develop. In the USA in 1967 death from the complications of hernia in patients over the age of 60 years was one of the ten leading causes of death.[504] This represents a 20-fold

increased risk of dying from attempted inguinal hernia repair when complications develop compared with patients who undergo surgery on an elective basis.

So the argument about whether to recommend an elective operation for an inguinal hernia, or to recommend a truss, must take into account the patient's assessment of his own quality of life. In the period 1982–1994 there was an increase in men undergoing inguinal hernia repair in Scotland in the over 65 age group indicating that age alone is no longer a barrier to successful treatment of inguinal hernia.[1040]

The operation will not prolong his life, but it may make it more comfortable. However, will a truss prove 'dirty, tight, uncomfortable, hot and smelly'? Will it represent a horrible affront to a man's self-image? Will wearing a truss have strong negative sexual overtones? Confronted by a male with a hernia, should we allow the patient to choose between truss or operation?

The incidence of strangulation of inguinal hernia is not known with any accuracy; the usual cited rate is 4% over the entire time the patient has the hernia;[615] rates from 1.7% to 6% are quoted, but are unhelpful because they are not based on a time period.[735,1238]

In a retrospective study Gallegos and colleagues studied the cumulative probability of strangulation in relation to the length of history calculated independently for inguinal and femoral hernias at the Middlesex Hospital over a 3-year period.[380] Of 476 hernias (439 inguinal, 37 femoral) there were 34 strangulations (22 inguinal, 12 femoral). After 3 months the cumulative probability of strangulation for inguinal hernias was 2.8%, rising to 4.5% after 2 years. For femoral hernias the cumulative probability for strangulation was 22% at three months and 45% at 21 months. They concluded that the rate at which the cumulative probability of strangulation increased was in both cases greatest in the first 3 months. For femoral hernia there is no question that the risk of strangulation is greater, 40% being admitted as an emergency with strangulation or incarceration.[1214] The age-standardized rate of incidence for strangulation is 13/10 000 population.

The delay in treatment of patients with groin hernia is multifactorial.[769] In patients presenting with strangulation more than half had noted the presence of a hernia for a month, a quarter had not reported it to their family doctor, and a further quarter were known by family practitioners or non-surgical medical personnel to have a hernia but had not been referred to a specialist. Although 10% had been previously assessed with a view to elective repair, half of these were considered unfit to undergo operation. There remains, however, a group of patients representing approximately 40% of the whole, who present primarily with strangulation within days of developing a hernia.

The only data available on untreated hernia relate to Paris in the 1890s and to contemporary Latin America. In both these series very low incidence rates are recorded for strangulation.[115,843] The yearly probability of incarceration and strangulation for all ages was 0.0037 in the 1890s French series and 0.002[116] for all ages and 0.100[343] for those over 65 in Colombia. Although these low probabilities and the relatively high frequency with which inguinal hernia occurs in the adult population (5–8% of the elderly male population) would seem to make hernia repair an unattractive option to the elderly male with a symptomless rupture, today lives could be saved.

In a district general hospital, doing more elective operations for primary inguinal hernias did not alter either the incidence of emergency operation for strangulated inguinal hernia[930] or the mortality of strangulated hernia.[1128]

Allen, Zager and Goldman attempted to investigate the reasons why elective surgery is not being undertaken to prevent emergency admissions.[16] A questionnaire was sent to 406 senior physicians, general practitioners, geriatricians and general surgeons. Although 71–90% would not advocate elective surgery for a small, painless, reducible inguinal hernia in a 79-year-old male; only 49% (physicians) to 78% (surgeons) would advocate elective surgery for an asymptomatic femoral hernia in a frail 80-year-old woman. Elective surgery in the latter case can be carried out with virtually no morbidity or mortality, yet a strangulated femoral hernia in an elderly patient carries a mortality in excess of 25%. This study concluded that general practitioners, physicians and surgeons are wrongly exercising a selective policy at the expense of the elderly.

Statistical data from the National Center For Health Statistics in the USA from the decades ending 1968, 1978 and 1988 investigated mortality from hernia.[790] In 1971 Medicare discharges for inguinal hernia without intestinal obstruction showed that 94% of patients had surgery with a probability of death of 0.005 (5/100 000). However, for inguinal hernia with obstruction, 88% underwent surgery with a mortality rate of 0.05, which represents a ten-fold increased risk of death. Encouragingly, the death rate from hernia with obstruction fell from 5/100 000 (1968) to 3/100 000 (1988), indicating that elective surgery had contributed to a reduction in the mortality rate of complicated hernia.

The mortality of strangulated inguinal hernia remains significant because of late diagnosis and referral, and increasing co-morbidity in elderly patients.[33,155] The low probability of strangulation with the low mortality of early emergency operation has offset the need to advise elective operation for all patients with inguinal hernia to save lives in the elderly. Elective operation may or may not improve the patient's quality of life. The patient must make an informed decision, aided by the surgeon.

A truss is very rarely a useful short-term option; for instance, the patient with an inguinal hernia of recent onset when there is severe cardiovascular or respiratory disease which is not yet controlled by physic, or a recent onset groin hernia in a woman with a third trimester pregnancy.

TRUSS DESIGN

The adder-headed spring truss is the standard for an inguinal hernia (Figure 13.1). If the hernia is large, or if it extends to the scrotum, a rat-tailed truss with a perineal band to prevent the truss slipping is used. Sir Astley Cooper comments that if the customer has a 'very protuberant abdomen' the perineal band may not be necessary. The head of the truss should rest

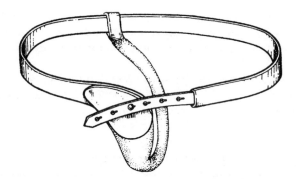

Figure 13.1 *The spring truss is the standard truss for an inguinal hernia. A truss with a perineal band is used in inguinoscrotal hernia or in persons whose physique predisposes to slipping of the head of the truss.*

over the inguinal canal, not over the external ring; it should exert its pressure inwards and upwards. When the truss is worn it should control the hernia easily when the patient stands with the legs apart and coughs violently.

Different gauges of spring are needed, depending on the physique and occupation of the patient. Lightweight trusses to wear in bed – 'evening' or 'French' trusses – used to be popular. The head of the truss will need designing for individual needs, too (Figure 13.2). The hernia must be completely and easily reducible by the patient if a truss is to be worn. A truss will predispose to strangulation if the hernia is not fully reduced. Another problem with a truss is the difficulty of controlling a large direct hernial opening close to the pubis, the proximity of the bone making occlusion of the opening by the truss difficult.

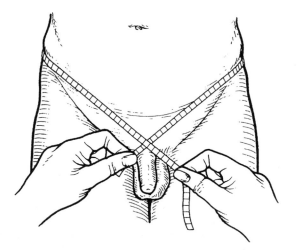

Figure 13.2 *Measuring for a truss. The head of the truss should be centered over the midpoint of the inguinal canal; the circumferential spring should be worn about 3 cm below the iliac crest.*

The adult patient should only remove his truss after he is in bed, and he should put the truss on again before he stands. It is most important that habitual truss-wearers keep their hernias permanently reduced and controlled by the truss. There is said to be an increased risk of strangulation if the hernia normally controlled by a truss prolapses. The skin beneath the truss head needs great care. Local tissue atrophy, cremaster atrophy leading to pendulous testicles, ilioinguinal neuritis causing pain, varicocele and testicular atrophy are complications of a truss.

Older textbooks credit 'cures' to prolonged treatment – the London Truss Society recorded that of 96 886 patients treated with a truss 4387 (4.53%) were 'cured'.[584]

INDIVIDUALIZED HERNIA SURGERY

Faced with many uncertainties regarding the optimal treatment of groin hernias and the requirement to develop operative strategies that are generalizable and applicable to every case, the surgical community has attempted to define the requirements in each scenario. The concept that an operation, which may give ideal results in experienced hands – the Shouldice operation for instance – may be difficult to learn and will give indifferent results in non-expert hands, while at the same time damaging normal tissue (for example dividing all the posterior inguinal canal wall in every case), has encouraged surgeons to define the different anatomic types of inguinal hernia and then match the repair to the defect found.

Nyhus classification

The first attempt at classification was made by Nyhus in 1991.[855] Nyhus defined the status of the fascia transversalis in the posterior wall of the inguinal and femoral canal. He recommended minimalist repair of the medial side of the inguinal ring only when this was necessary and he warned against extensive posterior wall repair at the expense of disrupting a normal inguinal posterior wall. He railed against surgery that resulted in overtreatment of many comparatively simple hernias. Nyhus classified groin hernias into four types, which enabled individualization of surgery to be recommended.

TYPE I

Type I hernias are indirect inguinal hernias in which the internal abdominal ring is of normal size, configuration and structure. They usually occur in infants, children or young adults. The boundaries are well delineated and Hesselbach's triangle is normal. An indirect hernial sac extends variably from just distal to the internal abdominal ring to the middle of the inguinal canal.

TYPE II

Type II hernias are indirect inguinal hernias in which the internal ring is enlarged and distorted without impinging on the posterior wall (floor in American surgical anatomy) of the inguinal canal. Hesselbach's triangle (the posterior wall of the canal) is normal when palpated through the opened peritoneal sac. The hernial sac is not in the scrotum, but it may occupy the entire inguinal canal.

TYPE III

Type III hernias are of three subtypes: direct, indirect, and femoral.

1 *Type IIIA* hernias are direct inguinal hernias in which the protrusion does not herniate through the internal abdominal (inguinal) ring. The weakened transversalis fascia (posterior inguinal wall medial to the inferior epigastric vessels) bulges outward in front of the hernial mass. All direct hernias, small or large, are type IIIA.
2 *Type IIIB* hernias are indirect inguinal hernias with a large dilated ring that has expanded medially and encroaches on the posterior inguinal wall (floor) to a greater or lesser degree. The hernial sac frequently is in the scrotum. Occasionally the cecum on the right or the sigmoid colon on the left makes up a portion of the wall of the sac. These sliding hernias always destroy a portion of the posterior wall of the inguinal canal. (The internal abdominal ring may be dilated without displacement of the inferior epigastric vessels. Direct and indirect components of the hernial sac may straddle those vessels to form a pantaloon hernia.)
3 *Type IIIC* hernias are femoral hernias, a specialized form of posterior wall defect.

TYPE IV

Type IV hernias are recurrent hernias. They can be direct (type IVA), indirect (type IVB), femoral (type IVC), or a combination of these types (type IVD). They cause intricate management problems and carry a higher morbidity than do other hernias.

Gilbert classification

Gilbert, another American expert, proposed another classification system based on anatomic and functional defects described at operation. Gilbert classified groin hernias into five classes: types 1, 2 and 3 are indirect and types 4 and 5 direct.[405] Type 1 has a tight internal ring through which passes a peritoneal sac of any size. When this sac is surgically reduced, it will be held within the abdominal cavity by the intact internal ring. Type 2 has a moderately enlarged internal ring which measures no greater than 4 cm. Type 3 has a patulous internal ring, greater than 4 cm, with the sac frequently having a sliding or scrotal component which usually impinges on the direct space. In type 4 hernias essentially the entire posterior wall (floor) of the inguinal canal is defective. Type 5 consists of a direct diverticular defect in a suprapubic position. Rutkow and Robbins added a sixth type to encompass those groin hernias which consist of both indirect and direct components and a seventh for femoral hernias.[993] As in any classification system, there can be numerous variations and combinations which are difficult to account for, and these variables (i.e. primary/recurrent, sliding component, reducible/incarcerated, lipoma) must be noted.

Bendavid classification

Bendavid of the Shouldice Hospital has proposed an even more elaborate system, the TSD (type, staging, and dimension) classification scheme (personal communication, 1992). Five types of groin hernias are described: type 1 or anterolateral (formerly indirect): type 2 or anteromedial (formerly direct); type 3 or posteromedial (formerly femoral); type 4 or posterolateral (formerly prevascular); and type 5 or anteroposterior (formerly inguinofemoral). Each type is characterized by three stages which denote the extent of the herniation anatomically.

TYPE 1

Stage 1: Extends from the deep inguinal ring to the superficial inguinal ring.

Stage 2: Goes beyond the superficial inguinal ring but not into the scrotum.

Stage 3: Reaches into the scrotum.

TYPE 2

Stage 1: Remains within the confines of the inguinal canal.

Stage 2: Goes beyond the superficial inguinal ring but not into the scrotum.

Stage 3: Reaches into the scrotum.

TYPE 3

Stage 1: Occupies a portion of the distance between the femoral vein and the lacunar ligament.

Stage 2: Goes the entire distance between the femoral vein and the lacunar ligament.

Stage 3: Extends from the femoral vein to the pubic tubercle (recurrences, destruction of lacunar ligament).

TYPE 4

Stage 1: Located medial to the femoral vein: Cloquet and Laugier hernias.

Stage 2: Located at the level of the femoral vessels: Velpeau and Serafini hernias.

Stage 3: Located lateral to the femoral vessels: Hesselbach and Partridge hernias. (In type 4 hernias the stage does not imply the severity of the lesion.)

TYPE 5

Stage 1: Has lifted or destroyed a portion of the inguinal ligament between the pubic crest and the femoral vein.

Stage 2: Has lifted or destroyed the inguinal ligament from the pubic crest to the femoral vein.

Stage 3: Has destroyed the inguinal ligament from the pubic crest to a point lateral to the femoral vein.

In the TSD scheme the 'D' refers to the diameter (in centimeters) of the hernial defect at the level of the abdominal wall. Where a defect is not circular but ovoid or elliptical, the widest laterolateral measurement is recorded. There is also a series of subclassifications for type 2 hernias: the letters 'm, l, c, e' denoting whether a defect is located through the medial, lateral, central or entire portion of the posterior wall of the inguinal canal.

Examples of Bendavid's TSD scheme are as follows. An anteromedial hernia, near the pubis, 2 cm in diameter is labelled type 2, stage 1 (m), D2. An anterolateral hernia with a deep inguinal ring measuring 4 cm and extending into the scrotum is classified type 1, stage 3, D4. Where a hernia repair has failed twice, this is indicated as 2R and noted after the type; e.g. a twice-recurrent anterolateral hernia extending to the superficial inguinal ring with an internal ring measuring 5 cm would be labelled type 1 (2R), stage 1, D5. When a portion of a viscus contributes to a sliding hernia, the letter 'S' is noted after the type, as are the letters 'I' for incarceration and 'N' for necrosis. When the herniating component consists simply of adipose tissue, the letter 'L' is noted after the type and all the other characteristics of the TSD classification scheme are provided.

Aachen classification

Schumpelick from Aachen has simplified these systems on the basis of the more traditional European anatomic classification.[1027] On the basis of this typing, he added a grading system of measurement of the hernial orifice. Grade I represents the normal diameter of the internal ring of up to 1.5 cm. He chose 1.5 as the measure because that is the average diameter of a surgeon's index fingertip or the length of the branches of laparoscopic scissors, simplifying the practical measurement. Indirect and direct hernias with an orifice of 1.5–3.0 cm are graded as category II. Grade III hernias are those with an orifice of greater than 3 cm. In combined hernias, the total diameter of the two defects is calculated and 'c' (for combined) is added.

The different localizations of the defect are indicated by the abbreviations L (lateral or indirect), M (medial or direct), and F (femoral).

A Unified System of Classification proposed by Zollinger

This system builds upon the traditional indirect, direct, and femoral anatomic locations using (i) the defect sizing of the Aachen system and Gilbert; and more importantly (ii) the competence of the internal ring and integrity of the direct floor as emphasized by Nyhus. Zollinger derived his classification from a survey of 50 North American and 25 European hernia surgeons which revealed that four systems were in active use: Traditional, Nyhus, Gilbert and the Aachen system.[1241] In the Unified System:

1 Small indirect hernias (Type I) have an intact internal ring, while small direct ones (Type III) have an intact rim of functioning direct floor. Large indirect hernias (Type II) have loss of internal ring function, while large direct ones (Type IV) have lost the integrity of the entire direct floor. Although the designations small and large correlate with abdominal wall defect sizes, the preservation or loss of

function, rather than a precise defect measurement in cm, is the dominant factor in this classification.

2 A combined inguinal hernia (Type V) is defined as one with loss of internal ring competence (Type VA), direct floor integrity (Type VC) or both (Type VB).

3 In addition to femoral hernia (Type VI) an additional category of inguinal–femoral hernia 'Other' (Type O) is included for those not defined with a category number such as the femoral plus inguinal combinations, the very rare prevascular, and the special circumstances such as massive inguinal hernias.

RECOMMENDATIONS

On the basis of these systems of classification some principles, long since adhered to, can be appreciated:

- If the deep ring is of normal diameter and the fascia transversalis is of normal strength it does not need to be disrupted; a simple excision of the indirect sac will suffice to cure the condition.
- If the deep ring is stretched but the remainder of the posterior wall is normal a simple plastic operation to tighten the deep ring and resection of the indirect hernia sac will suffice; the Lytle operation only is needed.
- If the posterior wall is deficient (i.e. there is a direct hernia) a repair of the defect with reinforcement either by the Lichtenstein operation with mesh – or the Shouldice operation – is needed.
- With recurrent hernias, especially with complex recurrent hernias, an extraperitoneal mesh replacement will be necessary. Against this background of surgical requirements for individualized hernia repair the reports from personal case studies, cohort studies and randomized trials must be assessed. A key discriminant must be the generalizability of any operative recommendation. A systematic review of the literature concerning the choice of operation for groin hernia; has recently been published and confirms the recommendations in Chapters 13, 14 and 15.[208]

The Unified classification is a sound basis to classify groin hernias and the individualization of the operation to repair the defects, along the lines indicated, should be applied. The operations recommended are all described in detail in Chapters 13, 14 and 15.

THE OPERATION

The surgical literature abounds with descriptions of operations for inguinal hernia (Table 13.1). However, few of these essays describe new or original principles. The foundations underlying the modern approach to inguinal hernia were laid by Marcy, who observed the anatomy and physiology of the deep inguinal ring and correctly inferred the importance of the obliquity of the canal.[742] Bassini, who had heard Marcy's lecture in 1881, grasped the significance of this anatomic arrangement

Table 13.1 *Techniques for inguinal hernia repair*

Single-layered closure
Halsted I (1890)[461]
Madden (1971)[730]

Multi-layered closure
Bassini–Halsted principle
Bassini (1887)[90]
Ferguson (1899)[352]
Andrews (1895)[35]
Halsted II (1903)[462]
Fallis (1938)[343]
Zimmerman (1938, 1952)[1239]
Rienhoff (1940)[954]
Tanner (1942)[1116]
Shouldice repair
Glassow (1943)[353]
Griffith (1958)[436]
Lichtenstein (1964, 1966)[689]
Palumbo (1967)[880]

Cooper's ligament repair
Lotheissen–McVay principle
Narath (cited by Lotheissen, 1898)[711]
Lotheissen (1898)[711]
McVay (1942, 1958)[779]

Preperitoneal approach
Cheatle (1920)[206]
Henry (1936)[491]
Musgrove and McGready (1940)[830]
Mikkelson and Berne (1954)[788]
Stoppa (1972)[1098]
Condon (1960)[235]
Nyhus (1959)[854]
Read (1976)[943]
Rignault (1986)[959]
Paillier (1992)[875]

Primary repair with prosthetic materials
Koontz (1956)[615]
Usher (1960)[1155]
Lichtenstein (1972)[689]
Trabucco (1989)[1138]
Valenti (1992)[1159]
Corcione (1992)[246]

Plug repair
Lichtenstein (1970)[689]
Bendavid (1989)[109]
Gilbert (1992)[407]
Robbins and Rutkow (1993)[960]
Gilbert (1998)[409]

Laparoscopic repair
Ger (1990)[399]
Corbitt (1991)[245]
Ferzli (1992)[353]

and, in particular, the role of the fascia transversalis and transversus abdominis tendon.[90]

Many surgeons have contributed to the recognition of the essential role of the transversalis fascia in the pathology of groin hernia, resulting from degeneration and a change in structure and function.[946,989]

Bassini stressed the importance of dividing the fascia transversalis and reconstructing the posterior wall of the canal by suturing the fascia transversalis and transversus muscle to the upturned, deep edge of the inguinal ligament. In his repair, Bassini included the lower arching fibers of the internal oblique muscle where they form the conjoint tendon with the transversus muscle. He called the upper leaf of his repair the 'triple layer' that is, fascia transversalis, transversus abdominis and internal oblique.

Bassini's original observations about the fascia transversalis and 'triple layer' have somehow been lost from the later literature. Many of the failures of 'Bassini's operation' occur in cases where the fleshy conjoint tendon only has been sutured to the inguinal ligament.

Division of the cremaster muscle and the posterior wall of the inguinal canal are essential components of the original Bassini hernia operation. Many surgeons, however, still perform the Bassini operation, dividing neither the cremaster muscle nor the posterior wall of the inguinal canal, possibly because Bassini did not actually describe these steps in his original papers.[946] Attilio Catterina, a colleague of Bassini's, later described and depicted the operation in a book illustrated with numerous watercolors. This atlas, although it was published in many languages in the early 1930s in Europe, was never published in North America, nor disseminated widely to European surgeons, possibly accounting for the inaccurate dissemination of Bassini's technique.

Wantz has accurately traced the history of the relationship between Bassini and Catterina, which resulted in the enthusiastic promulgation of Bassini's technique through his atlas, illustrated by the surgeon artist O. Gaigher, and numerous lectures across the European continent.[1186] Catterina, a protégé and colleague, and latterly Professor of Surgery at Genoa, recognized the importance of Bassini's quantum leap in surgical technique and the fact that Bassini had failed to get the technical points across to his surgical audience. Bassini specifically described dividing the cremaster muscle and the posterior wall of the inguinal canal (Figure 13.3).

The Bassini operation without these two essential steps gives poor results; hence in America this corrupt Bassini operation was abandoned in favor of the McVay–Cooper's ligament repair, Marcy's simple ring closure, or Nyhus preperitoneal approach. Bassini was also the first surgeon to insist on the use of non-absorbable suture material to repair his triple layer.

The third person in seminal herniology is Halsted. Halsted's original input was to advise drawing the external oblique down behind the cord in order to strengthen the repair.[461] He later abandoned this. His major contribution is really 2-fold: he insisted on scrupulous atraumatic technique and he emphasized, as Bassini had, the importance of adequate follow-up. In a more general sense, Bassini and Halsted are epoch persons because they introduced quality control and audit to surgeons. Florence Nightingale's exhortation that 'to understand God's will we must study statistics' was translated into surgical science by Bassini and Halsted![462]

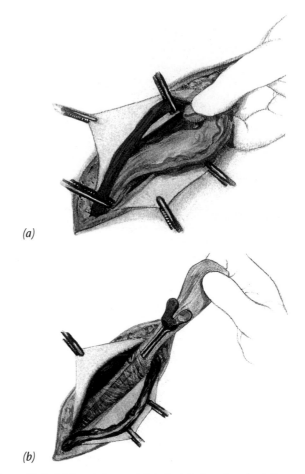

(a)

(b)

Figure 13.3 *(a) Bassini completely isolated and excised the cremaster muscle and its fascia from the cord. He thus ensured complete exposure of the deep ring and all the posterior wall of the inguinal canal, an essential pre-requisite to evaluate all the potential hernial sites. (b) Bassini stressed the complete exposure and incision of the fascia transversalis of the posterior wall of the inguinal canal. To complete the repair he sutured the divided fascia transversalis, together with the transversus muscle, and the internal oblique muscle, 'the threefold layer' to the upturned inner free margin of the inguinal ligament. (From Catterina, The Bassini Procedure, published by H.K. Lewis, 1934.)*

OPERATIVE TECHNIQUE

The choice of technique will reflect the surgeon's training, the type of hernia and the age of the patient.

THE SHOULDICE OPERATION[424,1042]

The main principles are:

- The normal anatomy should be reconstituted as far as possible. The deepest layer to be defective, in either indirect or direct hernias, is the fascia transversalis. This should, therefore, be repaired first.

- All the potential hernia sites must be assessed and repaired if necessary. The 'missed' hernia is a cardinal mistake.
- Only tendinous/aponeurotic/fascial structures should be sutured together. Suturing red fleshy muscle to tendon or fascia will not contribute to permanent fibrous union of these structures; nor will it result in anything resembling the normal anatomy.
- The suture material must retain its strength for long enough to maintain tissue apposition and allow sound union of tissues to occur. A non-absorbable or very slowly absorbable suture material must therefore be employed.[120,1042]

The tension in the Shouldice operation continuous suturing is low – initial suture tension is 100 g on spring balance, which falls to 50 g with the next suture – falling to 25 g. Even in large direct hernias it is only 25 g distributed.[1042] The suture tension similarly is low in bilateral hernias repaired asynchronously 48 h apart.[1182] This low tension maintains tissue apposition throughout healing and promotes sound repair.

Suture materials

The suture material of choice for the repair is metric 3 polypropylene. In the original Shouldice series from Toronto, monofilament stainless steel wire was used. Myers and Shearburn,[832,1042] and Devlin and Barwell,[86,294,298] originally used stainless steel wire, but have subsequently used polymers. Stainless steel wire is a most effective suture material, but it is difficult to use, whereas polypropylene is as effective and is much easier to handle.

Indications and contraindications to surgery

Elective surgical repair is the treatment of choice for inguinal hernias in adults. Operation is recommended for all hernia patients from pubescence to retirement. Surgery is advised because inguinal hernias: (a) cause discomfort; (b) are at risk of obstruction and strangulation; (c) cause disfigurement; and (d) give rise to scrotal skin problems.

With the elderly male aged over 75 years a less definite policy must be adopted; if the hernia is direct and spontaneously reducible the patient often has few if any symptoms attributable to it and surgery is perhaps not always mandatory. Indeed, the risks of anesthesia and surgery in this age group may be greater than the chances of developing complications necessitating urgent surgery.

Administrative and management arrangements for inguinal hernia – surgery

A careful administrative policy is necessary if the greatest benefits (for the patients and the community) are to be obtained from a policy of elective surgery for inguinal hernia. This is discussed on pages 51–60. Three regimens are mainly used:

1 Day-case – 8 h stay – applicable to all healthy males who have good home circumstances. This is the most common approach in the United States. In fact, the majority of patients, old and young, are discharged within a few hours of surgery.
2 Overnight – less than 24 h stay – applicable to healthy males with less appropriate social status. This is typically reserved for the patients with medical problems that necessitate closer observation. Age is a relative consideration. The advent of home healthcare has made, even this length of stay less common.
3 Five-day stay – most suitable for older patients, patients with contemporaneous medical conditions or patients who are socially disadvantaged. One should question the need for surgery if this becomes predicated preoperatively. The risks with or without surgical intervention should be carefully considered.

Anesthesia

Local, regional or general anesthesia may be employed (see pages 105–114)

Position of patient

The patient is placed on his back on the operating table. Access is improved if the head of the table is tilted downward by about 15 degrees; the head-down tilt is an important method of improving access (Figure 13.4). This is particularly beneficial if the hernia is incarcerated.

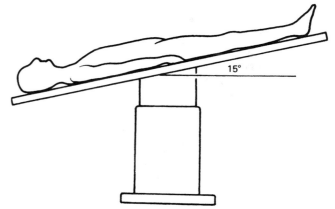

Figure 13.4 *The patient is placed on the operating table with a head-down tilt of 15°. The head-down tilt improves access by emptying the lower abdomen of contents so that the upper wound edge does not continuously overhang the operating field.*

The incision

The incision is placed 1 cm above and parallel to the inguinal ligament. Laterally the incision begins over the deep inguinal ring, runs to the pubic tubercle, then curves caudally (vertically) and runs down over the pubic tubercle. It is important to keep the knife at right angles to the patient's skin on this curve if the incision is to avoid undercutting the flap on its lower outer side. More importantly, the extension provides good access to the cord as it emerges from the superficial inguinal ring.

A skin crease incision gives a cosmetically more sound scar and is preferred by some surgeons, but to expose the pubic tubercle and Cooper's ligament the lower end of the incision needs under running, with the attendant additional dissection, hematoma formation, etc. For these reasons the uncosmetic but surgically more acceptable incision described is preferred by many surgeons. However, many other surgeons find that this operation can be performed quite well with such an incision. It is important not to dissect in the subcutaneous fat superficial and medial to the pubic tubercle. Dissection in this area hazards the cord to pudendal anastomosis and may predispose to testicular ischemia (see Chapter 24) (Figure 13.5).

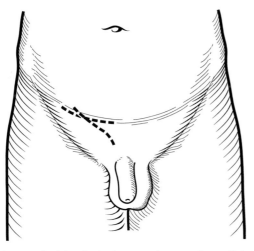

Figure 13.5 *An incision is made 1 cm above and parallel to the inguinal ligament; the incision should expose the superficial inguinal ring. Incision and dissection medial to the pubic tubercle is unnecessary and harmful.*

Exposure

After the skin has been divided the subcutaneous fat is opened in the length of the incision down to the external oblique aponeurosis. Careful hemostasis must be attained. The superficial pudendal and superficial epigastric vessels are tied and the smaller vessels dealt with by diathermy. A self-retaining retractor is now introduced and opened. This retractor serves two purposes: it opens the wound to facilitate access, and the slight traction it exerts on the skin ensures hemostasis in the small vessels in the immediate subdermal tissues.

After the subcutaneous fat has been opened down to the external oblique aponeurosis, the deep fascia of the thigh is opened to allow access to the femoral canal. The femoral sheath is exposed below the inguinal ligament and checked to make sure it is intact. It is important not to overlook a concomitant femoral hernia, which may present in the postoperative period (Figure 13.6).

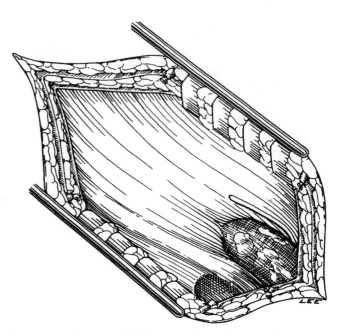

Figure 13.6 *The external oblique aponeurosis exposed.*

Dissection of the canal

The external oblique aponeurosis is next opened in the long axis of the inguinal canal. This incision extends down to the superficial inguinal ring, the margin of which is divided. With the ring opened, the upper medial flap of the external oblique is grasped in a hemostat and lifted up off the underlying cremaster fascia. The incision in the external oblique should commence at the most superior point of the superficial ring. The optimum site is to divide the external oblique about 2–3 cm cranial to the inguinal ligament; this 'high' incision allows maximal tissue for final closure and reconstitution of the inguinal canal (Figure 13.7).

The aponeurosis is gently freed from underlying structures by careful dissection up to its fusion into the lateral anterior rectus sheath.

Similarly, the lower lateral leaf of the external oblique is mobilized and freed of the underlying cord coverings down to the up-turned deep edge of the inguinal ligament, which is exposed (Figure 13.8).

Thus the whole of the cord is exposed.

Dissection of the cord

The cremaster muscle/fascia is now divided in its long axis from its proximal origin down to the level of the pubic tubercle.

The cremaster is made into two flaps – an upper medial and a lower lateral flap. These flaps are raised off the pampiniform plexus of veins, the other contents of the cord and the vas deferens. The flaps of the cremaster are each traced proximally to their origin from the internal oblique and the adjacent fascia, and distally to the pubic tubercle. The cremaster is clamped, divided and ligated at its origin and similarly dealt with distally at the level of the pubic tubercle (Figure 13.9). The genital branch of the

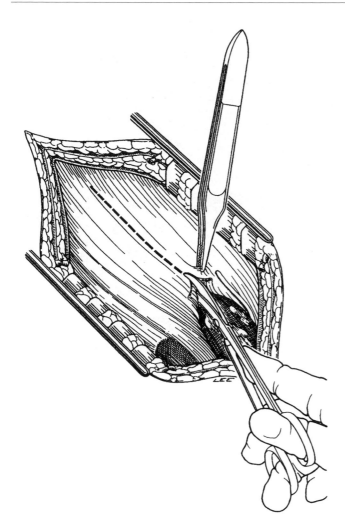

Figure 13.7 *Opening the inguinal canal.*

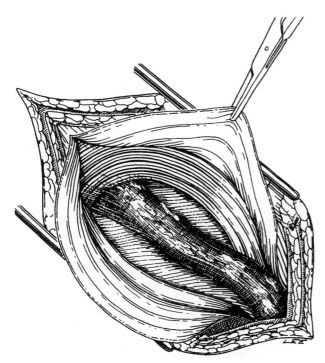

Figure 13.8 *Dissection of the canal.*

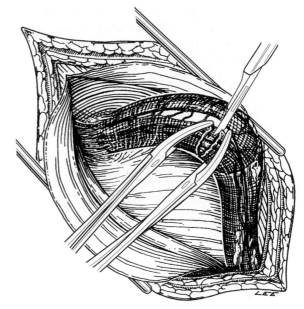

Figure 13.9 *Division and removal of the cremaster.*

genitofemoral nerve should be carefully sought, routinely separated from the cremaster muscle and cleanly divided. This maneuver reduces the incidence of chronic genitofemoral nerve neuralgia.[1189] The removal of the cremaster muscle from the cord structures is not considered necessary by all surgeons. Many, in fact, such as the authors feel that it is preferable to leave the cremaster muscle in situ.

After the cremaster has been removed, the contents of the cord and any hernia contained therein should be visualized. If there is a 'lipoma' – extraperitoneal fat around the fundus of an indirect sac[346] – in the cord, it is usually excised at this stage. Removal of a lipoma must not be used as an excuse to strip out all the fat and areolar tissue in the cord; if this is done the patient will suffer considerable postoperative testicular edema and may develop a hydrocele. Caution and prudence are necessary when dealing with an extensive lipoma; too extensive a dissection can hazard the testicular blood supply, particularly the veins.

Identification of the fascia transversalis

After the contents of the cord have been adequately visualized, they are lifted up and the continuation of the fascia transversalis onto the cord at the deep ring is identified. The condensation of the fascia transversalis about the emerging cord is the deep ring and it must be dissected accurately. The correct identification and dissection of the deep ring is crucial to the subsequent repair operation – a technical detail emphasized by Bassini[90,425] and more recently by Lytle.[718]

The internal spermatic fascia must be dissected off the deep ring all around the cord. Only when the cord is fully dissected like this can the deep ring be assessed.

The medial superior margin of the cord needs careful inspection now to identify any indirect sac. However small – even a tiny crescent of peritoneum entering the cord between the vas and medial margin of the deep ring – such a sac must be dissected cleanly and removed, otherwise it will enlarge postoperatively and appear later as a fully developed indirect hernia. A peritoneal crescent is the herald of an early recurrence if it is not treated adequately[933] (Figure 13.10).

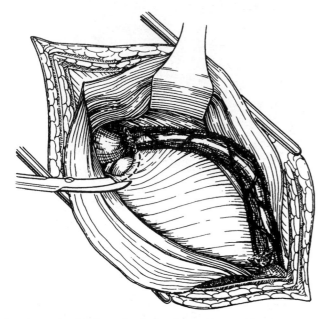

Figure 13.10 *The deep ring is freed from the cord by sharp dissection.*

It is important to check all the hernial sites at operation. A femoral or a direct inguinal hernia may easily be overlooked if exposure is inadequate. If a hernia is missed it will either appear postoperatively or later as 'a recurrence'. Whether the recurrent hernia is through a repaired portion of the inguinal region or not is immaterial to the patient; it is 'a recurrence' from the patient's perspective and most importantly necessitates another operation. Careful inspection of all hernial areas must be carried out at each operation.

HERNIAL SACS

Indirect

If an indirect hernial sac is present it should easily be found now. It lies on the anterosuperior aspect of the cord structures and should be ligated before amputation because omission of ligation (with the Shouldice operation) increases the recurrence 4-fold.[1190] To minimize the risk of postoperative ischemic orchitis, scrotal sacs are transected at the midpoint of the canal, leaving the distal part undisturbed (see Chapter 25). The anterior wall of the distal sac can be incised to prevent postoperative hydrocele formation. Further management depends on the presence and nature of the contents of the indirect hernial sac (Figure 13.11).

NO CONTENTS

If the sac is empty and does not extend beyond the pubic tubercle, it is lifted and freed from the adjacent structures by careful

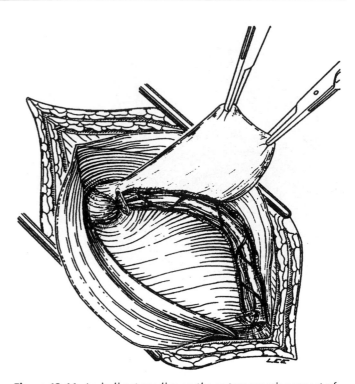

Figure 13.11 *An indirect sac lies on the anterosuperior aspect of the cord and is easily found after removal of the cremaster. If the sac is only in the canal and does not emerge beyond the superficial inguinal ring it is removed completely.*

dissection. It is traced back to its junction with the parietal peritoneum, transfixed with an absorbable polymer suture, which is tied around it securely, and the redundant sac excised (Figure 13.12). If an indirect hernia sac extends beyond the pubic tubercle the sac is transected and the distal sac left in situ (Figure 13.13).

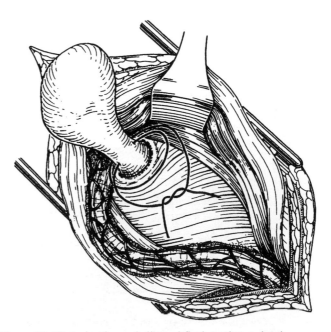

Figure 13.12 *A simple sac is ligated flush to the parietal peritoneum.*

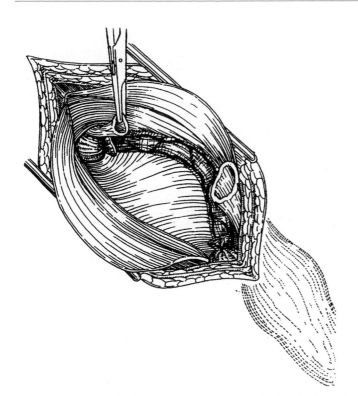

Figure 13.13 *If the indirect sac extends beyond the inguinal canal it must never be dissected beyond the pubic tubercle, instead the proximal sac is identified across and ligated flush with the peritoneum at its neck. The distal sac is left in situ to preserve the rich anastomosis of vessels that occur in the cord and prevent ischemia of the testicle.*

SMALL BOWEL AND/OR OMENTUM, WITH OR WITHOUT ADHESIONS

Unless the hernia is strangulated and the small bowel non-viable, any adhesions are divided and the small bowel is returned to the abdominal cavity. Strangulated omentum or small bowel can be resected at this stage. The diagnostic decision as to what should be done about very adherent and frequently partially ischemic omentum is difficult. If there is any doubt about omentum it is best excised, because to return omentum of doubtful viability to the peritoneal cavity invites the formation of adhesions.

SLIDING HERNIA

Such a hernia may contain the cecum and appendix (on the right side) in its wall, the sigmoid colon (on the left side) or the bladder (in the medial wall on either side). The following guidelines apply in these circumstances:

- No attempt should be made to separate cecum or sigmoid colon from the sac wall. This may compromise their blood supply and lead to further unnecessary problems.
- The appendix must not be removed, as this could introduce sepsis.
- Appendices epiploicae must never be removed from the sigmoid colon – they may harbor small colonic diverticula, excision of which will precipitate sepsis.

- On the medial side of a sac there should be no attempt to dissect the bladder clean. If the bladder is inadvertently opened, a two-layer closure with absorbable polymer and urethral drainage are required for 7 days at a minimum. Recovery will obviously be delayed.

A sliding hernia is dealt with by excising as much peritoneal hernial sac as possible and then closing it using an 'inside out' pursestring suture. When it is closed it is pushed back behind the fascia transversalis (Figure 13.14).

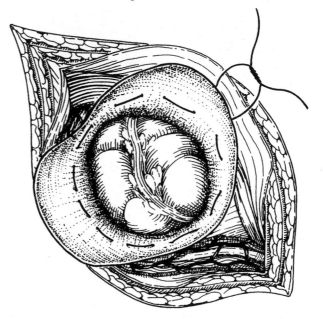

Figure 13.14 *Closing the sac of a sliding hernia.*

Direct

The direct sac may be either a broad-based bulge behind and through the fascia transversalis or, less commonly, it may have a narrow neck. In the first type, interference with the peritoneum is not needed – the sac should be pushed behind the fascia transversalis, which will subsequently be repaired (Figure 13.15). In the second, which is usually at the medial end of the canal, extraperitoneal fat is removed, the sac carefully cleared, redundant peritoneum excised and the defect closed with a polymer transfixion suture. Care must be taken to avoid the bladder, which is often in the wall of such a sac (Figure 13.16).

Combined direct and indirect

Lastly, a combined direct and indirect 'pantaloon' sac straddling the deep epigastric vessels may be found. In such a case the sac should be delivered to the lateral side of the deep epigastric vessels and dealt with as described for an indirect hernia (Hoguet's maneuver).[508,931]

The indirect sac is completely freed from the vas, spermatic vessels and the adjacent fascia transversalis at the deep ring. It is best then to mobilize the fascia transversalis medially so

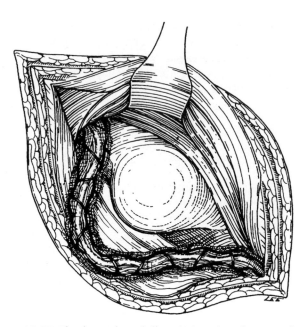

Figure 13.15 *The dome-shaped direct bulge; there is no need to open this sac.*

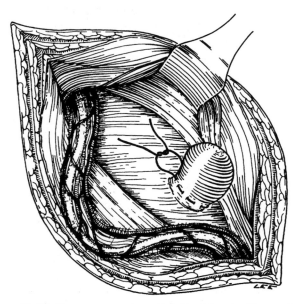

Figure 13.16 *The narrow neck medial direct hernia. The sac is isolated, closed and excised.*

that the whole of the sac can be drawn laterally. Whether or not the direct sac should be opened at this stage is a question of judgement. The hazard of wounding the bladder must be acknowledged. Any opening into a direct sac must be commenced laterally; care must be taken to identify the bladder margin medially and any peritoneal incision must stop short of this. Alternatively the direct sac can be opened – a finger inserted into the peritoneal cavity through the indirect sac will identify the dimensions of the direct sac and facilitate dissection and mobilization.

Once the indirect and direct sacs are mobilized redundant peritoneum is excised and the peritoneal defect closed. Repair of the fascia transversalis is then undertaken (Figure 13.17).

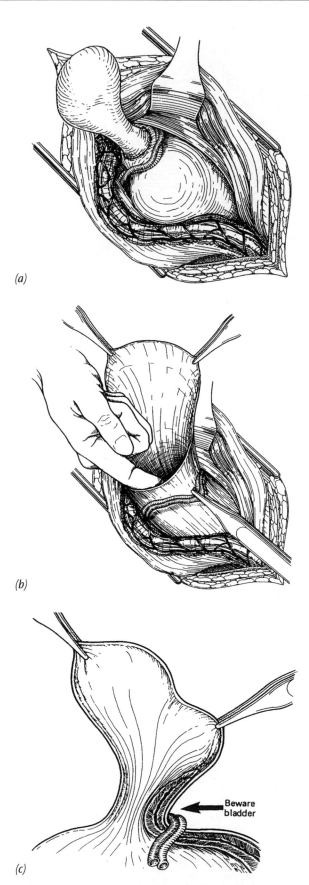

(a)

(b)

(c)

Beware bladder

Figure 13.17 *Hoguet maneuver. The combined direct/indirect sac (pantaloon hernia) is delivered lateral to the deep epigastric vessels. Any redundant peritoneum is excised and the sac closed.*

Dissection of fascia transversalis

The most essential part of the Shouldice operation is the repair of the fascia transversalis. This structure should already have been identified at its condensation around the cord forming the deep inguinal ring. The condensed medial margin of the deep inguinal ring is freed from the emerging cord by sharp dissection. When this is completed the medial margin of the ring is grasped in a dissecting forceps or a hemostat and lifted up off the underlying extraperitoneal fat. Dissecting scissors are now passed through the ring between the fascia and the underlying fat. By this maneuver the fascia is separated from the underlying structures, particularly the deep epigastric vessels. If there is no direct herniation and no gross distortion of the deep ring only the margin of the deep ring, the 'sling' of the deep ring, needs dividing, if there is a direct hernia and attenuation of the fascia transversalis, the fascia transversalis is now divided along the length of the canal, beginning at the deep inguinal ring and continuing down to the pubic tubercle. The upper medial flap is lifted up away from the underlying fat.

Attention is now turned to the lower flap. If it is penetrated by cremasteric vessels arising from the deep epigastric vessels these should now be divided and ligated close to their origin. If care is not taken with the cremasteric vessels they may be torn off the deep epigastric vessels and troublesome hemorrhage will follow. If a direct hernia is present it will bulge forward at this time and must be pushed back in order to free the lower lateral flap of the fascia transversalis. This flap must be freed down to its continuation as the anterior femoral sheath deep to the inguinal ligament. The lower, condensed fascia transversalis as it merges to the anterior femoral sheath is the iliopubic band (see page 33). Any grossly attenuated fascia transversalis about a direct sac is excised. With the fascia transversalis opened and developed the femoral canal should be checked again (Figure 13.18).

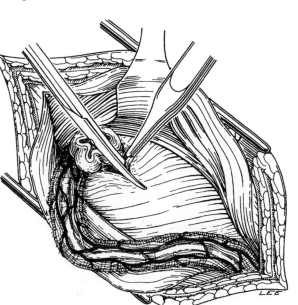

Figure 13.18 *Dissection of the fascia transversalis.*

Repair of fascia transversalis

If the previous dissection has been carried out carefully, and if hemostasis is now complete, the remainder of the operation should be easy. First, the fascia transversalis is repaired and the deep ring is carefully reconstituted using a 'double breasting' technique. The posterior wall of the canal must be reconstituted so that all of the peritoneum and the stump of a hernial sac are retained behind it. To do this, the lower lateral flap of the fascia transversalis is sutured to the deep surface of the upper medial flap. The repair is begun towards the medial end of the canal. Where the medial margin of the deep ring only has been divided and the more medial aspect of the posterior wall of the canal shown to be sound, no direct herniation, only the divided fascia transversalis at the medial margin of the deep ring, the 'sling', will need careful two layered reconstruction with a non-absorbable suture, Lytle operation[720] (Figure 13.19). If there is a direct hernia the whole of the posterior wall of the canal will have been divided and will need repair, the first suture being placed in fascia transversalis where that structure becomes condensed into the aponeurosis and periosteum on the pubic tubercle. The lower lateral flap of the fascia transversalis is then sutured to the undersurface of the upper flap at the point where the upper flap is just deep to the tendon of the transversus abdominus (conjoint tendon). At this point there is a thickening or condensation of the fascia transversalis (the 'white line' or 'arch'), which holds sutures easily.

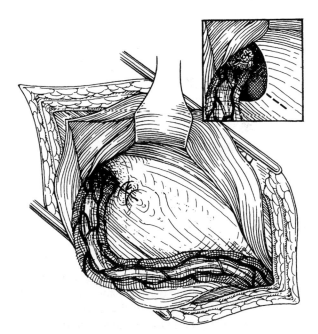

Figure 13.19 *After the neck of the sac has been divided at the deep inguinal ring the fascia transversalis of the deep opening is identified and assessed. If ring is normal sized the stump of the sac is reduced and no more need be done. If the ring is marginally dilated (stretched) it should be carefully dissected and possibly divided slightly (inset) and then sutured tightly around the medial side of the cord with polypropylene to reconstitute a competent deep inguinal ring.*

Care must be taken with the closure of the fascia transversalis as it approaches the lateral rectus sheath, which must be adequately repaired to the fascia transversalis and the pubic tubercle. The anatomy here is variable and the falx inguinalis (see page 30) should be included in the repair.

The fascia is sutured laterally until the stump of an indirect hernia lies behind it and it has been snugly fitted around the spermatic cord (Figure 13.20).

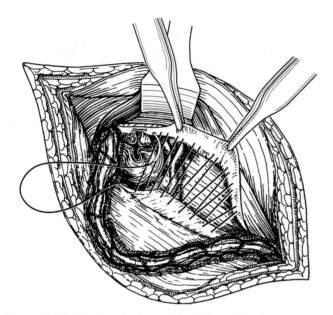

Figure 13.20 *Suturing the lower lateral flap of fascia transversalis to the undersurface of the upper medial flap along the 'white line' or 'arch'.*

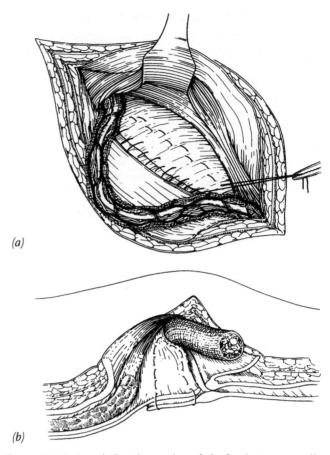

(a)

(b)

Figure 13.21 *Completing the overlap of the fascia transversalis repair. The margin of the upper medial flap is sutured to the anterior surface of the lower lateral flap (a). A neat closure up to the cord makes a new deep ring (b).*

The direction of suturing is then reversed. The free margin of the upper medial flap is brought down over the lower lateral flap and sutured to the fascia transversalis at its condensation (the iliopubic tract), just above the upturned deep edge of the inguinal ligament in the floor of the canal. Suturing is continued back to the pubic tubercle, where the suture is tied. By this maneuver the fascia transversalis is 'double breasted' on itself, the 'direct area' of the canal is reinforced and the internal ring carefully reconstituted and tightened.

It is important not to split the fascial fibers. Sutures should be placed about 2–4 mm apart and bites of different depth taken with each so that an irregular 'broken saw tooth' effect is produced.

The repair of the fascia transversalis is the crucial part of the operation. The fascia must be dissected and handled with care if its structure is to be maintained (Figure 13.21).

A 'trick of the trade' sometimes facilitates this suturing of the fascia transversalis: after the upper medial and lower lateral leaflets of fascia transversalis have been developed to clearly show the 'white line' of the transversus tendon through the fascia above and the iliopubic tract below, a loose swab (sponge) is pushed into the dissection to keep the extraperitoneal fat out of the way when the first sutures are introduced (Figure 13.22). When these sutures are loosely in place the swab is removed and the suture tension adjusted to give tissue closure.

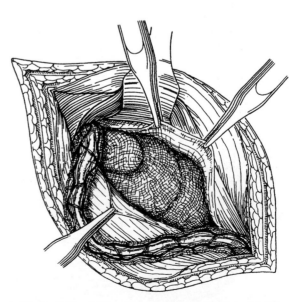

Figure 13.22 *If the subjacent extraperitoneal fat and peritoneum is bulging, a 'trick of the trade' is to pack it down with a gauze swab. This must be removed before the sutures are snugged tight.*

REINFORCEMENT WITH THE CONJOINT TENDON

The conjoint tendon is now used to reinforce the repair of the fascia transversalis medially. A suture is started laterally through the upturned deep edge of the inguinal ligament medial to the margin of the reconstituted deep inguinal ring and continued to the deep tendinous surface of the conjoint tendon, which is directly to the medial side of the deep ring. Sometimes, particularly if the cord is bulky, it is easier to proceed in reverse by passing the needle first through the undersurface of the conjoint tendon and then under the cord and through the upturned edge of the inguinal ligament.

At the point where this suture is inserted, the deep surface of the conjoint tendon is just beginning to become aponeurotic (the tendon of the transversus muscle) and it should hold sutures easily. The suture is continued in a medial direction, picking up the upturned edge of the inguinal ligament and the undersurface – the aponeurotic part – of the conjoint tendon down to the pubic tubercle (Figure 13.23). The direction is then reversed, suturing the aponeurotic part of the conjoint tendon, the internal oblique tendon now, loosely to the external oblique aponeurosis about 0.5 cm above the inguinal ligament. The 'broken saw tooth' technique previously mentioned is again used, and as it is done the suture is gently pulled snug, not tight, so that the conjoint tendon and rectus sheath are rolled down onto the deep surface of the external oblique aponeurosis. Suturing is continued laterally until the conjoint tendon ceases to be aponeurotic at the medial edge of the emergent spermatic cord. The suture is then tied.

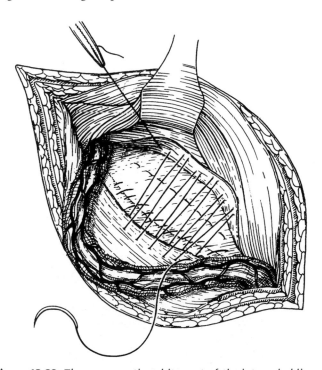

Figure 13.23 *The aponeurotic, white part of the internal oblique tendon and the conjoint tendon are used to reinforce the repair.*

The reconstruction of the posterior wall and the floor of the inguinal canal are now complete. The cord is now placed back in the canal (Figure 13.24)

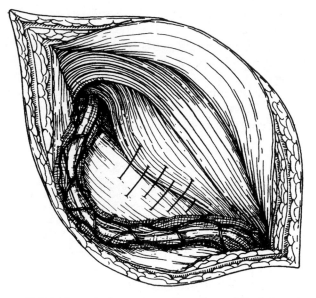

Figure 13.24 *The anterior aponeurotic surface of the internal oblique aponeurosis is loosely sutured to the aponeurosis of the external oblique medially.*

Closure

EXTERNAL OBLIQUE APONEUROSIS

Now that the cord has been replaced the external oblique aponeurosis can be closed over it. Again a 'double breasting' technique is used. Remembering that aponeurotic wounds are slow to regain strength, polypropylene sutures are used for this layer. The suturing is commenced medially, the lower lateral flap being sutured to the undersurface of the upper medial flap. Suturing is from medial to lateral and back again, so that the upper flap is brought down over the lower flap and a new superficial inguinal ring is constructed at the medial end of the canal. Care should be taken to close any secondary clefts in the external oblique (see page 23).

The repair is now complete, and if all the layers have been sutured exactly as described the loads on the suture lines should be well distributed; there should be no undue tension and no splitting of fiber bundles. Indeed, the structures should have just 'rolled together' (Figure 13.25).

SUBCUTANEOUS TISSUE

The subcutaneous tissue is carefully closed with interrupted sutures. No 'dead spaces' should be left and the fat should be closed so that the skin is closely approximated. If there is much tissue trauma or dead space, a closed drain is useful in this layer but seldom necessary[98] (Figure 13.26). The skin is closed with a subcuticular absorbable suture (Figure 13.27).

SUTURE TECHNIQUE IF MONOFILAMENT STAINLESS STEEL WIRE IS USED

As an alternative to polypropylene, 34-gauge stainless steel wire can be used. This is the original material used by Shouldice

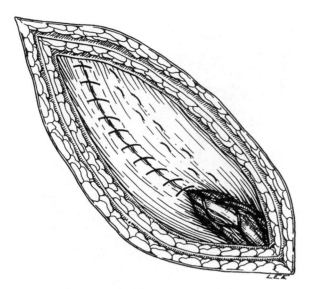

Figure 13.25 *The external oblique aponeurosis is closed, double breasted, anterior to the cord. Thus the inguinal canal is reconstituted with the cord obliquely traversing it.*

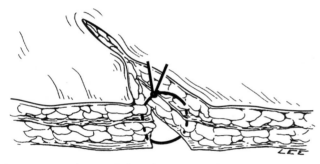

Figure 13.26 *Closure of the subcutaneous tissue.*

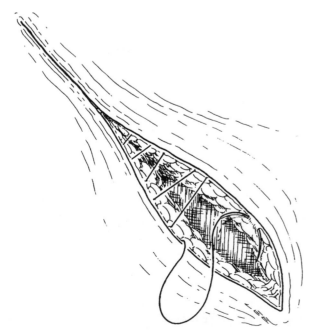

Figure 13.27 *The skin is closed with a subcuticular continuous absorbable polymer suture.*

himself. Stainless steel is an excellent suture material as it is strong, and causes little tissue reaction. However, special attention must be given to the technique if it is not to be broken or kinked in use. It is best to carry the wire as a loop on a long hook between each suture. The assistant must wield the hook carefully while at the same time keeping out of the operating surgeon's way and simultaneously maintaining the tension in the loop constant (Figure 13.28).

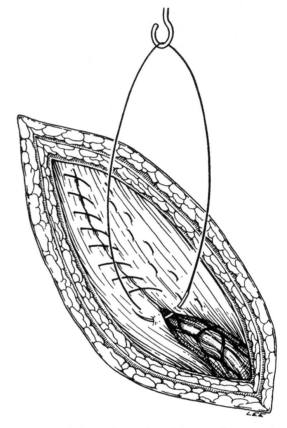

Figure 13.28 *Technique of suturing with monofilament wire.*

McVAY/COOPER'S LIGAMENT OPERATION

The McVay/Cooper's ligament repair is most useful in the management of concomitant femoral and inguinal hernias.[778] In this operation the anterior femoral fascia (sheath) is carefully dissected to clear the anterior wall of the femoral artery and vein, and all fat and lymph nodes are removed from the femoral canal to eliminate any potential femoral hernia (Figure 13.29). If a femoral sac is found it is converted to an inguinal sac and then dealt with.

The incision, exposure, dissection of the canal and cord are identical to the two other approaches (Shouldice and Lichtenstein) described. The cord is dissected free, but no dissection is necessary medial to the pubic tubercle. The transversalis fascia is incised and the posterior wall of the canal is resected. The dissection is then taken deeper to expose and free the iliopectineal (Cooper's) ligament. Next, the anterior femoral fascia is exposed, beginning the dissection lateral to the femoral

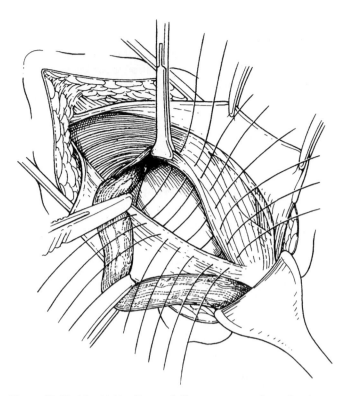

Figure 13.29 *The McVay/Cooper's ligament operation: clearing the anterior femoral sheath.*

artery, progressing medially across the anterior surface of the artery and vein. The femoral canal is then cleared of fat and lymphatics, taking care to identify any abnormal obturator circulation, and to carefully ligate any collaterals. After the inferior dissection is completed the tendinous portion of the transversus arch is developed. Any attenuated fascia transversalis and internal oblique is cleared from the transversus aponeurosis. A generous relaxing incision (see page 182) is made as medial as possible in the internal oblique aponeurosis – anterior rectus sheath – deep to the external oblique aponeurosis before the two aponeuroses fuse (see below). In obese females this dissection will involve the placement of deep Deaver retractors, with the patient placed in the Trendelenburg position.

The cord is opened and any indirect sac dissected free, ligated high and excised. If no indirect sac is immediately apparent the anterior medial part of the canal is dissected further to identify any small peritoneal tab that is present to ensure that an indirect sac is not overlooked.

The sacs are then opened, excised and closed, or if there is a direct bulge it is inverted and the extraperitoneal fat closed over it. Anyway, the extraperitoneal tissue is 'tidied up' by inverting it all with an absorbable polymer suture.

The repair is now initiated by bringing the transverse abdominis arch down to the inguinal ligament. This is best achieved with a layer of interrupted sutures, beginning at the pubic tubercle and continued laterally to the medial edge of the femoral vein. Each is placed carefully under direct vision and held before serial knotting (Figure 13.30) and are placed between the transversus arch the 'white line' and the iliopectineal (Cooper's) ligament. The femoral vein is retracted and protected by a retractor.

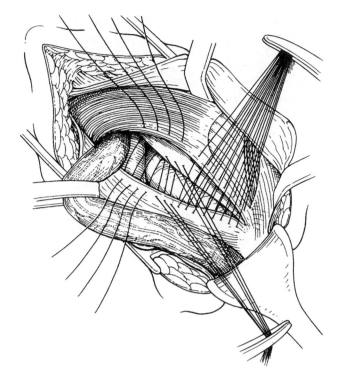

Figure 13.30 *Sutures are placed between the transversalis abdominis arch and Cooper's ligament as far as the femoral vein.*

The femoral canal is then closed by placement of two or three transition sutures of non-absorbable sutures between Cooper's ligament and the anterior femoral fascia (sheath). The lateral suture is placed just lateral to the last suture in Cooper's ligament; the medial two or three are medial to this and go between the Cooper's ligament sutures (Figure 13.31).

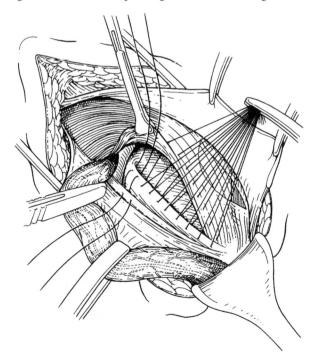

Figure 13.31 *The femoral canal is closed with two or three transition sutures between Cooper's ligament and the anterior femoral fascia.*

The repair is now continued laterally between the transversus abdominis arch and the anterior femoral fascia with the line of sutures just displacing the internal ring laterally, but not placing any sutures lateral to the cord. These sutures are of monofilament, non-absorbable material. The sutures are now tied beginning medially and a new internal ring created such that a hemostat can be inserted between the last tied suture and the cord (Figure 13.32).

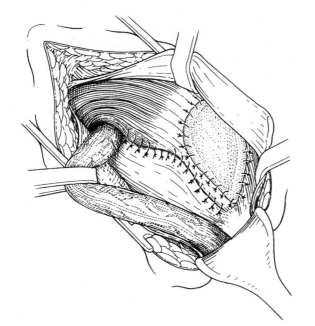

Figure 13.32 *The sutures are tied, medial to lateral. The defect of a relaxing incision can be filled with polypropylene mesh.*

Attention is now turned to the relaxing incision. This may be secured with sutures of monofilament, non-absorbable sutures or a polypropylene mesh patch can be used to repair the defect (Figure 13.33). Rutledge states that he reinforces the

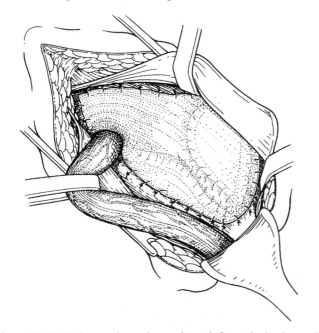

Figure 13.33 *Onlay mesh can be used to reinforce the basic repair.*

basic repair with an onlay graft polypropylene mesh in approximately 10% of patients.

The cord is replaced and the external oblique aponeurosis closed anterior to the cord. The operation is completed by closure of the subcutaneous fat and skin (see pages 178–179).

Relaxing incision

The employment of a relaxing incision to avoid tension at the suture line in inguinal hernioplasty is an old concept (Figure 13.34). Many surgeons do not use this technique either

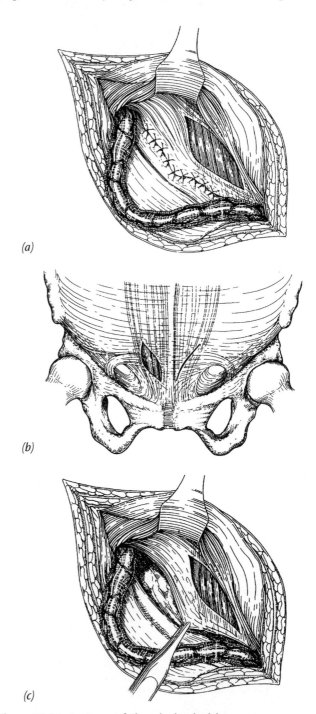

(a)

(b)

(c)

Figure 13.34 *Anatomy of the relaxing incision.*

because they do not understand the concept or because they extensively mobilize the fascia transversalis/transversus tendon for their primary repair (as in the Shouldice operation). If this mobilization is adequate and if sutures are placed closely and at even tension, the repair can be effected without a relaxing incision. However, a relaxing incision is useful; Halsted recommended its use for the more difficult ruptures and Halsted's former resident Bloodgood recommended it when the conjoint tendon had been obliterated. Even earlier, Wolfler and Bloodgood had separately recommended incision of the rectus sheath so that a flap of its aponeurosis could be turned down and sutured to the inguinal ligament to reinforce the direct area.[131,1220] Fallis (1938),[343] Reinhoff (1940)[954] and Tanner (1942)[1116] also emphasized the usefulness of this maneuver. Although in the UK the operation is known as 'Tanner's slide', it does have a long international pedigree to recommend it. Mattson (1946) has stressed the importance of rectus sheath in repair of large and recurrent direct hernias[758] and more recently McVay (1971) has emphasized that a relaxing incision is mandatory if a 'Cooper's ligament' repair is to be secure.[777]

McVay prefers the 'slide' technique to the flap method of utilization of the rectus sheath; not only does the slide technique allow fixation of the strong musculo-aponeurotic rectus sheath to Cooper's ligament, but in doing so it replaces the posterior wall of the inguinal canal with a strong viable aponeurosis exactly where the fascia transversalis is weak. The slide down transversus tendon is fixed inferiorly to Cooper's ligament as the virgin fascia transversalis would be. It must be re-emphasized that the relaxing incision is used to allow an adequate repair in the transversus abdominis/transversalis layer.

In McVay's experience of the Cooper's ligament repair, a recurrence rate of under 1% in 1000 cases over 16 years is recorded. In part these excellent results are due to the securing of an adequate viable posterior wall for the inguinal canal (the intact rectus sheath with its blood supply) to the firm anchorage of Cooper's ligament. This tissue is superior to any transplanted fascia or prosthetic material.

Concern is expressed by some surgeons that an adequate slide, that is an incision adequate enough to allow easy apposition of the transversus aponeurosis to Cooper's ligament, leaves a triangular defect lateral to the rectus through which a hypogastric hernia could develop.[744] This is not a complication reported by exponents of the Cooper's ligament repair. Moreover further consideration of the anatomy will remind surgeons that the lateral margin of the rectus sheath is strong below the semilunar line of Douglas. This is the area where the fascia transversalis is most dense. Fears of herniation at this site can be discounted; both McVay and Ponka, who regularly employ this technique, recall no instances of pararectal herniation after using a relaxing incision.[913]

The technique for the relaxing incision is important. The upper medial flap of the external oblique is raised and then dissected medially where it overlies the anterior rectus sheath. At this site the anterior rectus sheath consists of the interdigitated aponeurotic fibers of the internal oblique and transversus

muscles. They form one continuous lamina in the lower abdomen caudal to the semilunar line of Douglas and they are loosely attached to the more superficial external oblique aponeurosis. This loose attachment allows the two laminas, the superficial external oblique and the deep rectus sheath, to move independently in axis at right angles to each other – a mechanism of importance in closing the inguinal canal shutter.

In any event, a few deft scalpel strokes and blunt dissection will separate the external oblique aponeurosis from the internal oblique rectus sheath almost as far as the midline. The external oblique lamina is firmly retracted medially, the relaxing incision is then made in the deep lamina of the rectus sheath, which is the continuation aponeurosis of the internal oblique and transversus muscles after they have merged to become the conjoint tendon. The relaxing incision should be about 1.5 cm from the midline: it should commence about 0.5 cm cephalad to the pubic crest and extend upward and very slightly lateralward for 7–8 cm. Care must be taken to avoid the iliohypogastric nerve. The conjoint tendon and the underlying fascia transversalis can now be slid down to make the repair. Hemostasis must be secured: failure to gain first-class hemostasis can lead to bleeding into the rectus sheath which can fill with much blood before spontaneous clotting and compartment hematoma pressure will arrest the surgeon's carelessness.[945]

The hernia repair is now made. This will draw the conjoint tendon and adjacent tissues downwards and laterally, causing the relaxing incision to gape and expose the red belly of the rectus muscle. Do not be alarmed – when the external oblique is closed, the 'gap' in the rectus sheath is adequately closed and no rectus herniation will result.

There are mistakes to be avoided; no incision must ever be made medial to the red muscle belly of the rectus. This area is the linea alba, where all the layers fuse and no slide of one layer or another can occur. An incision in this most medial area will lead to iatrogenic herniation in the lower midline. Similarly, dissection and exploration of the lateral margin of the rectus, the Spigelian fascia, where the internal oblique and transversus muscles are banding together and, most importantly, where the fascia transversalis fuses with the aponeuroses, will lead to weakness here and be prone to a postoperative pararectus hernia. It is the continuity of the fascia transversalis posterior to the rectus muscle, the rectus muscle itself and the intact external oblique aponeurosis anteriorly which prevents herniation after the relaxing incision has created a defect in the deep lamina (internal oblique) of the anterior rectus sheath.

The employment of a 'slide' does not exonerate the surgeon from an adequate repair of the inguinal canal. All the authors who employ a slide also stress it is no alternative to a full-scale inguinal repair. McVay and Ponka use a Cooper's ligament repair, whereas Tanner repairs the fascia transversalis as a separate layer before reinforcement by conjoint tendon. The 'slide' or relaxing incision permits approximation of the fused portions of the fascia transversalis, the transversus abdominis aponeurosis and the internal oblique aponeurosis (the transversus arch, the conjoint tendon or the 'triple layer of Bassini' – principles repeating themselves under different definitions!).

OUTCOMES OF OPEN SUTURED TECHNIQUES

To the present day there has been a continuous and inventive search for the ultimate inguinal hernia repair. Surgeons become the evangelical protagonist of one technique, whereas the more pragmatic suggest that a number of different operations must be in the armamentarium of a hernia surgeon. Nevertheless, a surgeon should adopt a single technique for primary inguinal hernia, direct or indirect, in the adult male, because there is no doubt that results improve with standardization of technique and continued practice and application.

For more than 25 years, McVay has concerned himself with the anatomy and technique of inguinal hernia repair and with evaluating his methods.[778] With Halverson his review of 1211 hernioplasties performed and followed up over a 22-year period is a notable contribution.[464] This report highlights the continuing attrition of excellent early results when follow-up is purposeful and complete: in 1958 McVay reported a recurrence rate of 2.24%, but by 1969 this had increased to 3.5% – this projects to 4.2% at the end of 25 years. A humbling experience, but also a tribute to the enthusiasm of the team and to their pursuit of excellence.

From the statistical studies two important conclusions can be drawn – most (62%) of recurrences have occurred by 5 years, but there is a continued new recurrence rate for up to 25 years. To project the final recurrence rate to 25 years the following tabulation can be used:

All patients followed up	Multiply rate by
1 year	5.0
2 years	2.5
5 years	1.5
10 years	1.2

It is suggested that in a group of hernioplasties with mixed durations of follow-up it is more realistic to break the series up into one-year, two-year and five-year groups and then use this tabulation to derive conclusive recurrence rates. Unless a report contains the number of hernias followed up for each given time, it is misleading. Short-term studies are so misleading that most of them can be ignored. Unless the surgeon re-examines the patient, any estimate of recurrence rates is guesswork.

The McVay/Cooper's ligament operation is a standard technique with much to recommend it. It repairs the fascia transversalis and is particularly applicable to the medial end direct hernia and to the femoral hernia in the female. Rutledge records 906 consecutive primary Cooper's ligament repairs with a recurrence rate of 1.9% overall: 3.5% for direct and 1.1% for indirect inguinal hernia.[1000] The patient follow-up was 97%, 80% of patients being examined, and average follow-up was nine years. The operative technique, however, is extensive, requiring deep retraction with Deaver's retractors, Trendelenburg position, and in 13% of patients a Marlex mesh overlay was used. With a 5% testicular atrophy rate in skilled hands, this operation might have medicolegal consequences.[1001] Rutledge comments that the recurrence rate rises to 5.5% if the cord is brought out straight

through the external oblique and transplanted subcutaneously. Testicular atrophy occurred in 7.9% of recurrent hernia repairs. In the series there were two instances of pulmonary embolism. In a further patient, femoral vein compression was demonstrated phlebographically. An alternative, less invasive, technique is to use Duplex scanning.[851]

Marsden defines a recurrence as 'a weakness of the operation area necessitating a further operation or the provision of a truss'.[747–749] Thus defined a recurrence is an operative failure; this is superior to descriptions of a 'bulge' or 'thrill' at the operative site. It also allows of a follow-up question: 'Do you wear a truss?' or 'Have you had a second operation?' These are questions any patient can respond to. Non-progressive asymptomatic bulges are not defined as recurrences.

The Shouldice Hospital in Toronto was established in 1945 and by the end of 1952 Shouldice was able to record 8401 groin hernia repairs. With experience his recurrence rate had dropped considerably, from 6.5% in his first 461 cases followed up from 1943, 1944 and 1945–1952, to 0.1% in the most recent cases followed up to 2½ years from 1952.[1046] Glasgow, in 1984, reviewed 10 353 cases with a 10-year recurrence rate of 1.1%[425] (Figure 13.35).

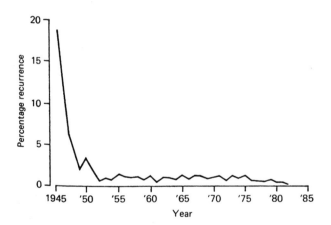

Figure 13.35 *Recurrence rates of all hernias repaired at the Shouldice Clinic, Toronto, 1945–1982. Each year's group of surviving patients was followed up for life and results were updated yearly. (From Alexandra 1986, with permission.)*

The Shouldice surgeons stress meticulous anatomic repair of the fascia transversalis, the use of non-absorbable sutures and early ambulation. Results in different specialist clinics yield uniformly excellent outcomes compared with other operations and with a recurrence rate of under 1%, justifies the adoption of this operation by those surgeons adequately trained in the technique.[120,301]

However results suggest from non-specialist units has shown that the Shouldice operation may not be the gold standard operation that it has been heralded to be for the last 20 years.[850] A retrospective review of 1936 operations performed during 1992 in eight hospitals in Sweden (catchment 761 000) revealed a 17% recurrence rate in a setting where 25% of surgeons were using the Shouldice operation.[850] The Shouldice Hospital has never performed a prospective randomized trial comparing its technique against any other. It has taken more than 40 years after the inception of this technique for the publication of the first such studies to materialize (Table 13.1).

Kingsnorth and colleagues, in a trial designed to rule out surgeon-dependent variables, prospectively randomized 322 patients with primary inguinal hernias to Shouldice repair or plication darn. Surgery was undertaken by 15 operators of whom 14 were surgeons in training who received a preliminary period of training until they were proficient with the operative techniques. After a mean follow-up of 30 months (range 24–48) there were seven recurrences in the Shouldice group (4.3%) and four in the plication darn group (2.5%). This recurrence rate is approximately five times higher than that recorded by the Shouldice Hospital, and the authors suggest that the failures were caused by collapse of the posterior wall within 6 months of repair, indicating that this is the area of technical difficulty in reproducing the Shouldice Hospital results.[603] More trials have reproduced these results. Panos and colleagues achieved a 6.6% recurrence rate for the Shouldice operation in a residency training program.[882] Fingerhut, reporting for the French Association for Surgical Research in a controlled trial of 1593 patients, found a recurrence rate of 6% using polypropylene for the Shouldice repair and 3% for stainless steel at 5 years.[355] Tran and colleagues from Cologne reported a dismal 10% recurrence rate for the Shouldice repair at 2 years in 142 patients with primary hernias operated on by both consultant surgeons and surgeons in training.[1139] Kux and colleagues tested the standard Shouldice operation with four rows of polypropylene, and a modified Shouldice operation with two rows of polypropylene sutures against the Bassini operation using absorbable or non-absorbable sutures.[628] With an impressive personal clinical follow-up of 93.6% in surviving patients, the recurrence rate in the standard Shouldice operation group was 3.6% between 3 and 4 years, with a 2.3% recurrence rate in the modified Shouldice operation. Three board-certified surgeons and six residents performed the operations and the failure rate for recurrent hernias was 7.6%. An important observation long known to hernia surgeons was that of the 27 patients found to have a clinical recurrence, almost half were not aware of it.

The conclusion that must be drawn from these studies is the need for adequate training of surgeons undertaking the Shouldice operation, and meticulous reconstruction of the posterior inguinal wall as the cornerstone of this technique. With this caveat good long-term results can be obtained in a non-specialist setting.

THE LICHTENSTEIN TECHNIQUE

The true tension-free hernioplasty using mesh and no suture closure of the hernial defect was introduced in 1984 by Irving Lichtenstein and colleagues.[1049] Lichtenstein's experience with the use of polypropylene mesh in inguinal herniorrhaphy, however, began much earlier.[689] In a personal experience of 6321 cases reported in 1987 with a 91% follow-up over a period of 2–14 years, a recurrence rate of 0.7% was achieved. At this time apart from the innovation of polypropylene mesh, Lichtenstein

had abandoned high ligation and excision of indirect sacs, but continued to use single-layer approximation of the transversus abdominis and the inguinal ligament with a relaxing incision. After a period of evolution the perfected tension-free hernioplasty was reported by Lichtenstein, Shulman, Amid, and Montelier in 1989.[694]

Repair of the posterior abdominal layer with a suture line was abandoned, except for a simple imbrication suture for large sacs that aided flattening of the posterior wall before placement of the mesh. The recurrence rate in over 1000 cases was 0% at 1–5-year follow-up, with no mesh infections and the authors stated that the technique was simple, rapid, relatively pain-free allowing prompt resumption of unrestricted physical activity. This report prompted a campaign of popularization of the tension-free hernioplasty.[891]

Like the Shouldice Hospital the Lichtenstein Institute surgeons have written multiple publications in the surgical literature, repeating their experiences with a gradually enlarging number of patients.[25,1049,1051] The authors emphasize that the hernial defect edges are not co-apted and the sole strength of the repair is based on blocking the defect with a tension-free patch. Many thousands of patients have now undergone repair with this operation at the Lichtenstein Institute; the operation being performed under local anesthesia and patients discharged within a few hours of operation with minimal discomfort, for which mild analgesics are prescribed. Unrestricted activity is encouraged and patients discharged from the Unit are able to resume normal activity in 2–10 days. A postal survey performed by Shulman of 70 surgeons utilizing this technique who did not have a special interest in inguinal hernia surgery indicated similar results in 22 300 repairs.[25]

The use of prophylactic antibiotic cover in the form of powder instillation or a single perioperative intravenous bolus is a vexed question. The Lichtenstein Institute has used both methods, but has not made a firm recommendation. However, Gilbert and Felton in a co-operative multicenter prospective study of 2493 inguinal hernia repairs by 65 surgeons found a wound infection rate of less than 1% whether or not biomaterials or antibiotics were used.[408] Moreover, the removal of polypropylene biomaterials from infected wounds was not necessary to eliminate infection and indeed is not recommended because of technical difficulty and inevitable recurrence. The authors conclude that the expense incurred for routine prophylactic antibiotic cover in inguinal hernia operation when biomaterials are used could not be reconciled by any benefits obtained.

In the UK the Lichtenstein technique was first reported by Kingsnorth and colleagues, and subsequently by a private hernia clinic, The British Hernia Centre.[270,567]

Kark and colleagues, reporting on 1098 tension-free hernia repairs, reported only one recurrence after primary repair and an overall sepsis rate of 0.9%.[567] This report emphasized the cost savings associated with the operation and the rapid return to activity: with 50% of office workers returning to work in one week or less, and 60% of manual workers in two weeks or less. Nevertheless, the operation can present technical difficulties to the novice, as illustrated by a report from Brussels in which

139 primary inguinal hernias were repaired by tension-free hernioplasty and a 4.6% recurrence rate was reported during a mean follow-up of 12.7 months. The probable technical fault was failure to overlap the pubic tubercle and the entire posterior inguinal wall by a wide margin of mesh.[1003] These authors reported a 50% saving of resources by utilization of the tension-free hernioplasty.

The first randomized trial reporting a comparison between the tension-free hernioplasty and the Shouldice operation was reported by Kux and colleagues, verifying the low recurrence rate (one recurrence in the Lichtenstein group over a 30-month period), and a reduced requirement for postoperative pain relief. Patients under the age of 60 years were excluded from this study.[628]

The EU Hernia Trialists Collaboration examined all randomized and quasi-randomized trials comparing open mesh with open non-mesh methods for repair of groin hernia.[338] Fifteen eligible trials, which included 4005 participants, were identified. Return to usual activities was quicker in the mesh group for seven of the 10 trials (P value not significant). There were fewer reported recurrences in the mesh groups (1.4% compared with 4.4%). Therefore using the powerful statistical methods followed by the Cochrane Collaboration the currently available literature indicates that mesh repair is associated with three times fewer recurrences than non-mesh, in the repair of inguinal hernia.

The Lichtenstein tension-free hernioplasty

The incision, exposure, dissection of the canal and cord and the dealing with indirect hernial sacs is identical for that described for the Shouldice operation (see pages 170–176). In the case of large direct sacs, in order to flatten the posterior inguinal wall to facilitate placement of the mesh, a running, inverting, absorbable suture is applied to the transversalis fascia (see video clip 'Lichtenstein repair').

The external oblique aponeurosis needs to be lifted up and dissected from the underlying internal oblique muscle high enough to accommodate a 6–8 cm wide patch. Because a considerable degree of overlap is required of Hesselbach's triangle, the pubic tubercle and laterally beyond the internal ring. Medially this dissection should be taken beyond the pubic tubercle to the midline (Figure 13.36).

Polypropylene mesh precut to 8 cm × 16 cm is now tailored to the individual patient's requirements. This will involve trimming 1–2 cm of the patch's width and the upper medial corner so that it will tuck itself between the external oblique and internal oblique muscles without wrinkles (Figure 13.37).

The cord is now retracted downward and the mesh aligned into the inguinal canal such that its inferior border lies parallel with the inguinal ligament, and its medial border overlaps the pubic tubercle by 1–2 cm. Using a non-absorbable monofilament running suture beginning at the upper, medial, rounded border of the mesh, the suture is placed into the tough aponeurotic tissue of the midline and secured with a knot. This suture then continues around the edge of the mesh taking bites of firm connective tissue under direct vision, but avoiding the periosteum of the bone.

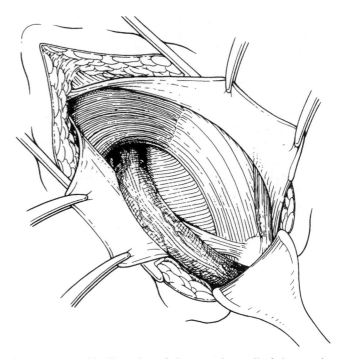

Figure 13.36 *Wide dissection of the posterior wall of the canal.*

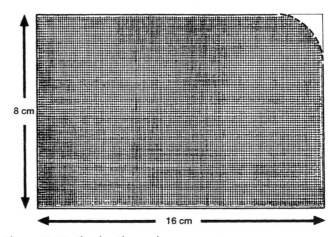

Figure 13.37 *Shaping the mesh.*

As the suture continues it picks up the lower edge of the shelving margin of the inguinal ligament. Having secured the mesh medially and also secured it to 1–2 cm of inguinal ligament, this suturing is temporarily halted (Figure 13.38). A slit is now made at the lateral end of the mesh creating two tails, a wider one (two-thirds above) and a narrow one (one-third below) (Figure 13.39). The lower, narrower tail together with the needle and its running suture are now passed behind the cord, which is then retracted upwards (Figure 13.40). The wider upper tail and the narrow lower tail are overlapped and grasped in a hemostat to retract the mesh and prevent unnecessary wrinkles.

The running suture between the lower edge of the mesh and the shelving margin of the inguinal ligament is now completed to a point just lateral to the internal ring (Figure 13.41). The upper leaf of the external oblique aponeurosis is now retracted strongly upward and the upper edge of the mesh is sutured

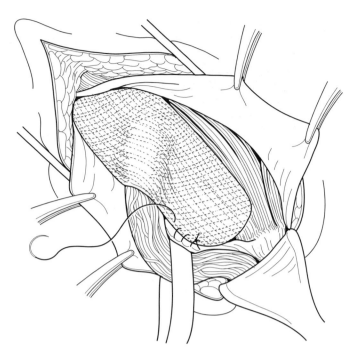

Figure 13.38 *Initial half of continuous suture to allow mesh to overlap pubic tubercle and appose to inguinal ligament.*

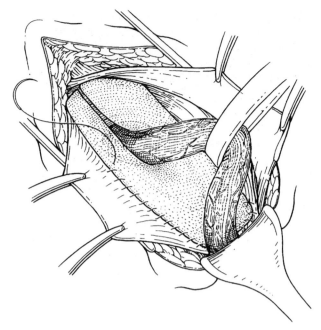

Figure 13.40 *The lower 'tail' of the mesh is flipped behind the cord, followed by the continuous suture with needle, and the cord is retracted upwards.*

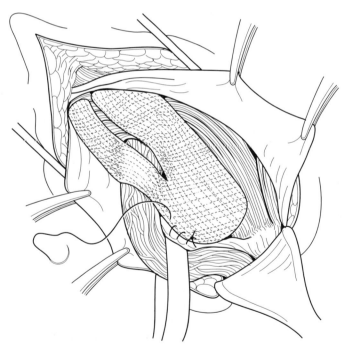

Figure 13.39 *The mesh is slit (one-third below; two-thirds above), up to the medial margin of the internal ring.*

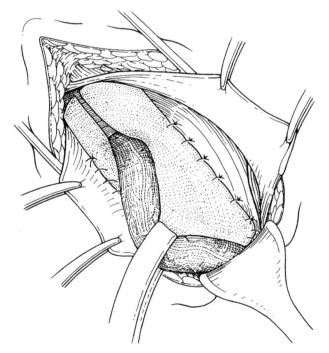

Figure 13.41 *The continuous suture line along the inguinal ligament is now continued to the lateral border of the internal ring.*

to the underlying internal oblique aponeurosis or muscle with a series of interrupted sutures approximately 2–3 cm apart. Care is taken to avoid underlying blood vessels and sensory nerves, such as the ilioinguinal and iliohypogastric nerves (Figure 13.42). The mesh should not be completely flattened, but should be seen to have some degree of anterior convexity in

order to remain tension-free. The last fixation suture is placed laterally at approximately the same level as the internal ring.

The lower edges of each of the two tails are now fixed to the inguinal ligament at a point just lateral to the completion knot of the lower running suture. A point is chosen in the lower edge of the upper tail approximately 1 cm beyond the lateral margin of the internal ring to avoid unnecessary buckling of the mesh

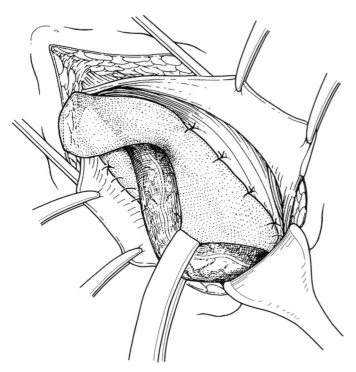

Figure 13.42 *Three or four sutures tack the mesh cranially.*

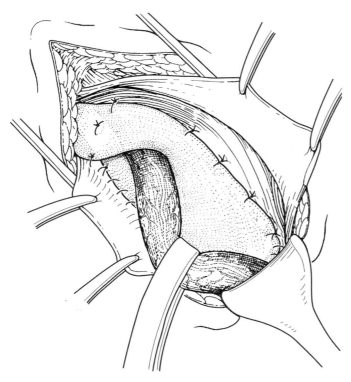

Figure 13.43 *'Tails' are overlapped and crossed and a single suture placed to create a new 'internal' ring.*

(Figure 13.43). Having created a new internal ring with cross-over and overlap of the two tails, excess patch on the lateral side is now trimmed in order to leave approximately 3–4 cm of mesh beyond the internal ring. This lateral tail is now tucked underneath the external oblique aponeurosis and may be prevented

from movement, curling up or wrinkling by placing sutures between it and the underlying muscle (Figure 13.44). The size of the new internal ring is now tested with a hemostat, which should pass easily between the cord and the mesh. If this gap is too wide it may be closed loosely with a non-absorbable suture (Figure 13.44).

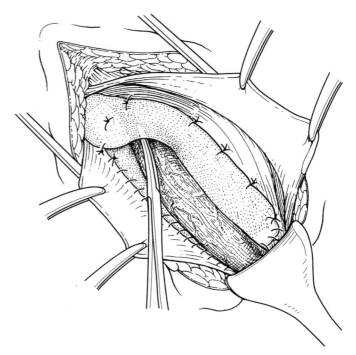

Figure 13.44 *Sutures may now be placed lateral to the ring to prevent shifting and curling. An artery clip is run down between the mesh and new internal ring to ensure an adequate aperture.*

Having completed repair of the posterior inguinal wall with the polypropylene mesh, the cord is placed back into the canal, and wound closure is identical to that described for the Shouldice operation (see page 170).

POSTOPERATIVE CARE

Immediate active mobilization is the key to rapid convalescence. The 'client with a hernia' must not be allowed to become institutionalized into the 'postoperative patient'. If the operation has been performed under local anesthesia, the patient should be helped to walk as soon as he is returned to the ward. If general anesthesia has been used, the patient must be made to get up and walk as soon as he is conscious. There may be slight pain after surgery and a suitable mild analgesic should be prescribed. Analgesics with narcotic properties are not always needed.

If social circumstances allow, patients should be discharged within a few hours of operation with minimal discomfort for which mild analgesics are prescribed. Unrestricted activity is encouraged, and indeed most patients should resume normal activity in 2–10 days. 'Take it easy' is the wrong advice.[1049]

Integrity of the hernia repair depends on good surgical technique, rather than any supposedly deleterious, premature physical activity undertaken by the patient. Return to full activity does not increase recurrences and indeed caution will engender anxiety and perhaps justify the patient's decision to remain off work for up to 6 weeks.[443] It is contradictory and counterproductive to warn against strenuous activity and is a recipe for long-term disability. Troublesome wound soreness is rare 7–10 days after the operation.

The wound dressing can be removed by the patient on the first through the fifth postoperative day based upon the surgeon's experience and recommendation. After the dressing is removed the patient can shower or bath normally.

Light office or professional work can be resumed after about one week and most other heavier jobs after about 2–4 weeks. Patients are told that they may undertake any work which does not cause pain to their wounds.[791,996,1052]

INGUINAL HERNIA IN WOMEN

During the 26-year period 1945–1971, more than 75 000 hernia repairs were performed in the Shouldice clinic, Toronto; of these 1672 (2.2%) were primary inguinal hernias in women and 414 (0.05%) primary femoral hernias in women. Of the inguinal hernias, 1548 were indirect and only 124 were direct. Thus primary indirect inguinal hernia is 13 times more common than direct hernias. Direct inguinal hernias in women are very rare, and when they do occur they present usually in the lateral part of the posterior wall close to the deep epigastric vessels rather than in the medial canal as they do in men.[417,422] In contrast to femoral hernia, pregnancy and vaginal delivery are not risk factors and obesity appears to be protective.[495] Recurrent inguinal hernias in women are more frequently indirect than direct – medial direct recurrences are a complication of previous groin surgery, Pfannensteil incisions, or of

the high repair of femoral hernia. Occasionally, this is the result of an overlooked hernia that is missed at the prior operation.

In women, the round ligament should be excised and the inguinal canal closed.[417] The fascia transversalis is sutured down to the iliopubic tract and medially onto the iliopectineal line as in the McVay/Cooper's ligament operation, thus reducing the risk of subsequent femoral herniation (Figure 13.45).

BILATERAL HERNIA

Bilateral hernias should not usually be repaired simultaneously by the Shouldice technique, for three reasons.

1   If sepsis occurs it may be bilateral if introduced at the same operation.
2   After simultaneous bilateral herniorrhaphy there is often much edema and swelling of the penis and scrotum, which can make voiding tiresome and will delay convalescence.
3   There is evidence that simultaneous bilateral herniorrhaphy using the Shouldice technique may stretch the fascia transversalis unduly and predispose the patient to subsequent femoral hernia[420,421] (see Chapter 25).

A small study by Serpell and colleagues investigated 31 patients undergoing bilateral simultaneous inguinal hernia repair, and five patients undergoing bilateral sequential repair, and compared these two groups against 75 patients having unilateral inguinal hernia repair. There were no differences in wound complications, postoperative respiratory complications or other adverse effects between the three groups.[1039] However, operating time and hospital stay was reduced by two days in those patients undergoing simultaneous repair.

A larger but retrospective study from the Mayo Clinic, of patients undergoing hernia repair, compared 333 patients who

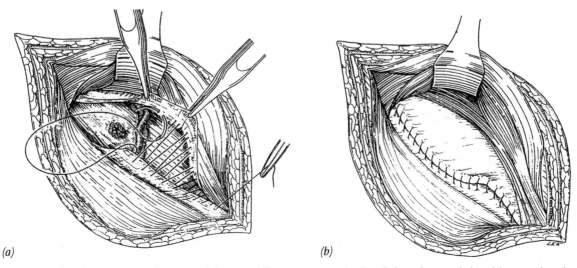

(a)   *(b)*

Figure 13.45 *Inguinal hernia in women: the sac and the round ligament are excised and then the canal closed by suturing the fascia transversalis to the iliopectineal ligament.*

underwent sequential unilateral repair against 329 who underwent simultaneous bilateral repair. Although there was greater morbidity in the bilateral group, these complications for specific events were not significantly different between the two groups, except for urinary retention, which occurred in 6.1% of the unilateral group, and 15% for the bilateral group. These results have a cautionary note: bilateral synchronous inguinal hernia repair in the elderly has a relatively high incidence of urinary retention; moreover the recurrence rate reported from the Mayo Clinic was 8.5%.[792]

The Lichtenstein operation and laparoscopic inguinal hernia repair both lend themselves more easily to simultaneous repair of bilateral inguinal hernias.[27,1014] With the Lichtenstein operation the simultaneous repairs can be carried out under local anesthesia and with the laparoscopic repair there is less pain after operation and a faster return to activity and work. In 2001 the National Institute for Clinical Excellence in the UK published guidance on the use of laparoscopic surgery for inguinal hernia. Laparoscopic surgery was recommended as an option for the repair of bilateral inguinal hernia (and recurrent inguinal hernia see below).[838]

There is ever-growing volume of data that verifies the usefulness of the laparoscopic approach for bilateral hernias. It is important to use a large piece of mesh in these cases to cover the myopectineal orifice adequately. Some suggest the use of a very large single piece of mesh.[200] Compared to unilateral repair of inguinal hernias, the bilateral repair appears to be safer and more cost effective and without increased risk of morbidity or recurrence.[1023]

Another advantage of laparoscopy is the ability to diagnose (and repair) unsuspected bilateral hernias. The incorrect diagnosis of unilateral rather than bilateral inguinal hernias has been found in 13% to 58% of patients that were evaluated in this manner.[252,610]

RECURRENT INGUINAL HERNIA

Recurrent inguinal hernias are always difficult and operation should only be undertaken by an experienced surgeon who is interested in this problem. If there is sepsis or sinus formation, operation should not be undertaken until it has settled. It may be necessary to remove all foreign suture material from the wound at a first operation and then wait some months before attempting the repair. For a first-time recurrent hernia there are several options. Where the first operation was complicated by hematoma, sepsis, sinus formation or a complex hernia, the anterior open approach is not recommended because ischemic orchitis and testicular atrophy is a significant risk. In the absence of these factors an anterior approach with which the operator is familiar such as the Shouldice operation or the Lichtenstein technique can be recommended. Generally, tissue planes can be identified if a slow and gentle dissection is made. If the hernia is multiple recurrent or if there has been much sepsis or scarring, or a major tissue deficit exists, the extraperitoneal open approach or laparoscopic repair (pages 194–206) is

advised. The laparosocopic approach is very effective in this situation.[100,126,349,1162] It should never be necessary to divide the cord in order to repair a recurrent hernia.

STRANGULATED HERNIA

The use of mesh is not absolutely contraindicated if the amount of contamination is kept to a minimum and broad-spectrum antibiotics are used during and after the operation for several days.[883,1225] In 35 patients, nine of whom required intestinal resection for necrosis there were two postoperative wound infections in the series of 35 patients studied by Pans: neither of these patients had had an intestinal resection. Wysocki and colleagues studied 16 patients in whom one had a bowel resection with no septic complications.

The Shouldice operative technique is recommended to treat a strangulated inguinal hernia, where there is gross contamination following bowel perforation due to necrosis. The additional risk of infection in this situation militates against the use of mesh, infection of which may cause morbidity. If additional access is required to deal with gangrenous gut, the deep ring can be enlarged medially by dividing the deep epigastric vessels between ligatures, taking care to avoid the bladder. It is, however, preferable to perform an additional standard paramedian or midline incision for access to the main peritoneal cavity rather than to have to do an awkward resection of gangrenous tissue through the groin incision.

OTHER MESH HERNIOPLASTY PROCEDURES

A modification of the tension-free hernioplasty using a plug to block the defect in the posterior inguinal wall supplemented by a sutureless swatch or patch as an overlay on the posterior inguinal wall has been described.[443,996,1052] Robbins and Rutkow reported the mesh-plug hernioplasty in 1993, which is a cone-shaped polypropylene structure, supplemented with a small flat mesh. They report a very low recurrence rate with low postoperative discomfort and rapid return to normal activities.[960,995] The essential feature of the mesh plug hernioplasty is minimal dissection. For indirect hernias the sac is approached by separating the cremaster fibers longitudinally along the spermatic cord so as not to destroy the cremaster reflex. The sac is dissected free, down to the preperitoneal fat pad at the level of the internal ring and a pocket created for positioning of the mesh plug (Figure 13.46). For direct hernias the attenuated transversalis fascia is elevated with an Alice clamp and the neck of the sac is completely circumscribed with sharp dissection to allow the preperitoneal fat space to be entered (Figure 13.47). For both indirect and direct hernias the mesh plug can now be inserted, tapered end first into either the internal ring (Figure 13.48) or the defect in the posterior wall (Figure 13.49). The mesh plug is then secured either to the crura of the ring or to surrounding intact tissue of the posterior wall by several interrupted sutures. This mesh plug repair is then reinforced with an onlay flat patch

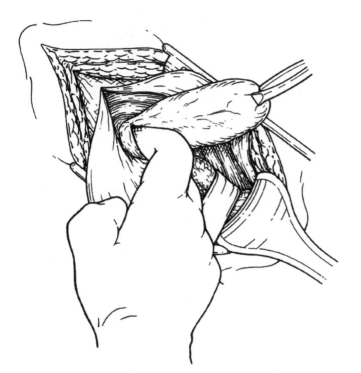

Figure 13.46 *A pocket is created for positioning of the mesh in the preperitoneal space.*

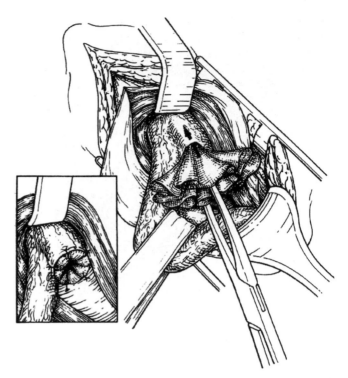

Figure 13.48 *The plug is inserted into the perperitoneal space via the internal ring.*

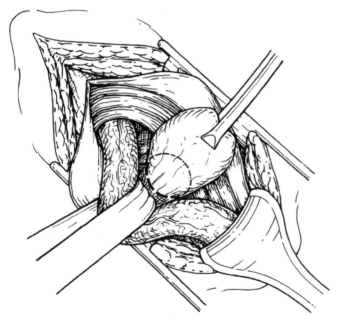

Figure 13.47 *The preperitoneal space is entered via an incision in the transversalis fascia at the neck of the sac.*

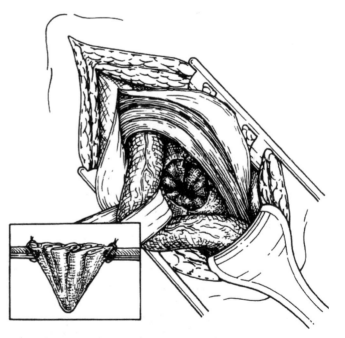

Figure 13.49 *The plug is inserted into the preperitoneal space through the direct hernia defect.*

based on the anterior surface of the posterior wall of the inguinal canal from the pubic tubercle to above the internal ring (Figure 13.50). A slit in the mesh to accommodate the cord, and the two ends are sutured back together around the cord, and this suture represents the only fixation. The authors have extended the technique to treat all inguinal hernias, femoral hernias, recurrent groin hernias, and small incisional hernias. In 1563 cases two recurrences were recorded with an average

follow-up of 82% at 2.4 years. Because of its simplicity this operation is gaining popularity. The plug utilized however is a 3-dimensional semi-rigid structure, which occludes only part of the posterior wall, combined with an onlay (sutureless) swatch. The recurrence rate will only become apparent by long-term follow-up, but there is some indication that unacceptable rates of postoperative pain occur in up to 5% of patients treated with

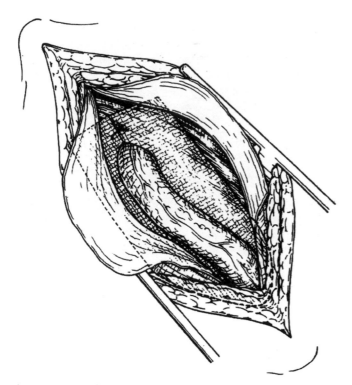

Figure 13.50 *Onlay mesh reinforces the plug repair.*

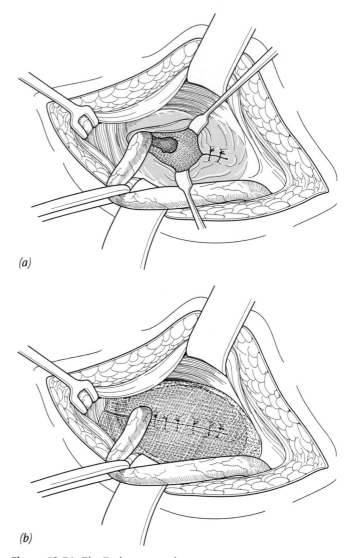

(a)

(b)

Figure 13.51 *The Trabucco repair.*

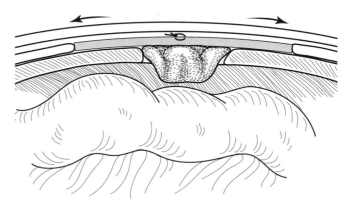

Figure 13.52 *The corcione repair.*

the plug from studies by several authors.[594,656,878,898] Other plug devices are also available but there are few clinical reports with large series of patients with any substantial follow-up (see Chapter 7).

Trabucco working from the Trabucco Hernia Institute in New York has spent several years in the search for a single layer mesh with the ideal rigidity and desired characteristics. Having experimented with 12 different models made of pre-shaped, single layer polypropylene varying in weight, thickness and porosity. Trabucco concluded that the single layer rigid polypropylene mesh was the most favorable.[1137] Trabucco has designed a pre-shaped mesh which can be used in all primary inguinal hernia repairs and fits into the sub-aponeurotic inguinal space and which does not have a tendency to wrinkle, curl or shift (Figure 13.51).

Corcione has adopted a personal modification of the suture-less mesh repair, which is called the 'held-in mesh repair'. A 5 × 5 cm umbrella folded plug is placed through the deep ring in direct and indirect hernias and after continuous plication of the transversalis fascia, the internal ring is narrowed and the plug is locked in. A second suture layer is placed in the transversalis fascia ending at the pubic tubercle where the two ends are passed through the medial part of the mesh and tied above it. The flat mesh is then placed over the posterior wall of the inguinal canal and a perpendicular slit made in it for passage of the cord, which is then closed with a single suture.[246] (Figure 13.52) In 930 inguinal hernias repaired in 798 patients there was only one recurrence after 2 years: outpatient surgery was performed in 61% and local anesthesia in 95% of patients.

Valenti has described the protesi autoregolantesi dinamica – PAD, which consists of two superimposed layers of surgical mesh, placed in the interaponeurotic layers (Figure 13.53). Each moves independently where they are superimposed: where the lower layer medially and the upper layer laterally overlap. More than 500 patients have been repaired with a recurrence free follow-up after 5 years and little postoperative discomfort.[1159]

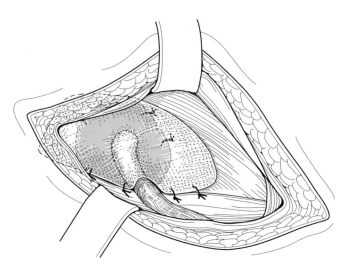

Figure 13.53 *Protesi autoregolantesi dinamica – PAD repair.*

CONCLUSIONS

- For primary inguinal hernia in adults the method of repair will reflect the surgeon's training, the type of hernia and the age of the patient.
- The Shouldice operation and the Lichtenstein repair conform to the principles of good repair surgery, namely careful and accurate identification of anatomic planes and the use of appositional suture material or implanted mesh to repair the defect. When combined with good management policies, both techniques are cost-effective.
- The Shouldice operation gives excellent results in the hands of well-trained surgeons. However, the operation is technically demanding.
- The Lichtenstein repair has gained popularity because of its simplicity and equally good results in the hands of experts and trainee surgeons. Variants in the placement or configuration of mesh have their protagonists but have not been popularized except for the mesh-plug repair, which may be associated with an increased incidence of chronic groin pain.
- The recurrence rate after inguinal hernia repair is operator dependent: the choice of operator is as important as the choice of operation.[599] One should not, however, overlook the potential applications of the laparoscopic approach.

14

Extraperitoneal or preperitoneal open repair of groin hernias using prosthetic reinforcement

The technique outlined in this chapter extends the extraperitoneal approach of Annandale, Cheatle and Henry to access all the hernial sites in both groins simultaneously and then repair the defect(s) in the fascia transversalis by inserting a sheet of prosthetic mesh between the peritoneum and the parietes to replace any deficiencies in the fascial layer. The technique was originally described by the Amiens herniology team of Stoppa and colleagues in 1972. Read has described a similar technique using Marlex mesh to repair large direct and recurrent inguinal hernias. Rives and colleagues have been the early protagonists of the unilateral preperitoneal approach. They described using two or three stitches to approximate the transversus abdominis arch to Cooper's ligament in order to close the myopectineal orifice. The mesh is not sutured in place and only intra-abdominal pressure maintains its place over the hernial defect(s). This approach has been further championed by Wantz for both recurrent complex and primary groin hernia. A further variant has been described by Nyhus, exclusively for a recurrent inguinal hernia in which anatomical repair of the defect by approximation of the transversalis fascia to the iliopubic tract or Cooper's ligament is performed before reinforcement of the defect with polypropylene mesh placed in the preperitoneal space with suture fixation. Recently, variations of these techniques have been described by Ugahary and Kugel.[622,1150]

As originally described, the French do not attempt any repair of any of the hernial orifices; the prosthesis is placed in position and held there by the intra-abdominal pressure of the peritoneum against the parietes, like ham in a sandwich. There are two objections to this sublime technique: first, if hernial orifices, particularly large direct inguinal defects, are left open they bulge postoperatively and although they are not true hernias patients do complain of the unsightly 'rupture'; secondly, it is technically difficult to introduce the mesh into the pelvis over the femoral vessels on each side adequately if it is not fixed down as the operator retreats upward to close the parietal wound. For these reasons, suturing, and then quilting the prosthesis into position is recommended. However, currently there are proponents of both suturing or not suturing the prosthesis, based upon the surgeon's experience.

INDICATIONS

The prosthetic reinforcement technique via the extraperitoneal route is indicated in:

- Intricate (combination) groin hernias where there are multiple defects either unilateral or bilateral; for instance, combinations of prevascular, femoral, indirect and direct inguinal and low Spigelian hernias.
- Giant inguinoscrotal hernias, either unilateral or bilateral, where replacement of abdominal contents through a groin incision only would be technically difficult.
- Recurrent or multiple recurrent groin hernias. Incision through the virgin extraperitoneal plane makes these operations simpler.
- Incisional herniation after Pfannenstiel incisions and incisional hernias through the lateral rectus sheath (acquired Spigelian hernia). Repair is difficult because the posterior rectus sheath is absent, but placement of prosthetic mesh in the extraperitoneal layer resolves this.
- Primary or recurrent unilateral hernia using the Kugel® patch, which is perhaps the most common usage of this technique today.

The disadvantages of the extraperitoneal prosthetic operation include the need for general anesthesia with good relaxation to enable access to the lower pelvis. It requires a more extensive dissection making the presence of a skilled assistant who can handle a retractor deftly important.

A potential problem with this technique is sepsis, which will prejudice the outcome; sepsis with polypropylene mesh will nearly always resolve without removal of the prosthesis. Attention to aseptic technique and absolute hemostasis are critical factors in the success of this operation. The French, and the late George Wantz in the USA, championed the use of Mersilene mesh, which is more supple than Marlex. The polyester meshes are a multistrand material and may be more prone to sepsis and also carries a risk of fistulization (see Chapter 7).

A common postoperative complication is edema and/or ecchymosis of the lower flap and genitalia. This edema is sometimes quite considerable; it does, however, always settle. It is advised to inform the patients of this possibility preoperatively.

Calne (1967)[173] has described an alternative strategy to cope with bilateral inguinal or femoral hernias without resorting to the extraperitoneal approach via a Pfannenstiel incision. Both inguinal canals are opened by incising the external oblique aponeurosis. Oblique and narrow neck direct sacs are excised and their necks closed. Large direct sacs are left undisturbed. Femoral sacs can be dealt with at the same time. Bilateral orchiectomy will facilitate the operation but is not essential. The extraperitoneal space is opened behind each rectus and the internal oblique and transversus muscles displaced cephalad. Polyester mesh (Mersilene) is then threaded behind the rectus. The mesh is then fixed by four strong sutures to the periosteum of the anterosuperior iliac spines and pubic tubercles on either side. The mesh is stretched out and fixed under some tension. Excess mesh is trimmed. The edges of the mesh are sutured to the inguinal ligament inferiorly, allowing a small space to transmit the cord if it is to be left intact, and to Cooper's ligament, when there is femoral herniation, to close the femoral canal. The mesh is also sutured to the posterior layer of the anterior rectus sheath and the inferior borders of the internal oblique and conjoint tendons.

Ten operations were recorded; one patient who had a bladder diverticulum excised at operation developed a wound infection and persistent sinus. There was one unilateral recurrence at 16 months postoperatively. The longest follow-up was 4 years in a woman with bilateral recurrent femoral hernias; the other follow-up periods are short, the maximum being 11 months. This open operation is seldom seen in the current era of hernia surgery but its principles are followed in the laparoscopic totally extraperitoneal hernioplasty. (See Chapter 15.)

THE BILATERAL OPERATION

Preoperatively

The patient must void urine immediately prior to operation; the urinary bladder must be empty to allow adequate exposure of the anterior pelvis. If the anatomic situation is complex and compromised by much scarring, the operation may be slow and take a long time. An indwelling catheter is advisable in these circumstances.

Position of patient

The patient is laid on his back on the operating table. The table is tilted to 15 degrees, head down; this empties the pelvis of intestine to allow the operator to work on the anterior pelvic parietes. Draping should allow a lower midline or Pfannenstiel incision.

The traditional incision

Access must be gained to the entire groin regions on both sides. A skin crease horizontal Pfannenstiel incision gives the best cosmetic result and should be used preferentially. Where there are scars from previous operations on groin hernias it is best to avoid these and the delayed healing that may occur in reopened skin scars. In these circumstances, a midline skin incision with midline incision of the linea alba and separation of the rectus muscles is recommended (Figure 14.1).

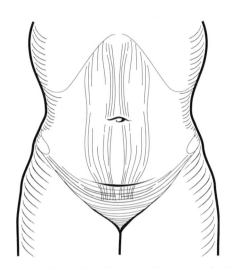

Figure 14.1 *Access through a Pfannenstiel or a vertical incision separating the rectus muscles.*

Development of extraperitoneal space

The red bellies of the rectus muscles are separated from the underlying peritoneum by finger dissection. A self-retaining retractor is inserted to hold the wound open. With a combination of sharp scissor dissection and blunt dissection the plane between the peritoneum and the parietes is opened behind the pubis down to the anterior prostatic capsule. This plane is extended laterally behind the pubis and obturator internus muscles. Hernial sacs may now be encountered entering the various potential defects in the parietes (Figure 14.2). This is usually a rapid and easy part of the operation if these tissues have not previously been operated on.

Mobilization of indirect inguinal hernial sacs

The necks of indirect sacs are identified as they spring from the main peritoneal sac. Dissection is made around them – a pledget in a curved artery forceps is a useful implement here. Once the sac is identified contents should be reduced, if possible before the sac is opened. The sac should then be dissected back from the internal hernial orifice (deep ring). In the usual

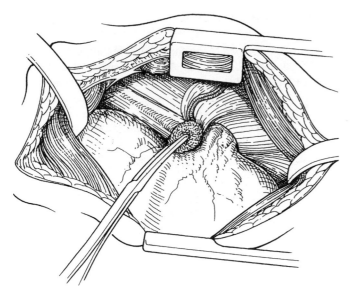

Figure 14.2 *Developing the extraperitoneal plane.*

hernia the whole sac can easily be milked back from the canal. The sac is then opened and any remaining contents reduced. The sac is now transfixed and ligated so that the stump is closed off flush with the peritoneum (Figure 14.3).

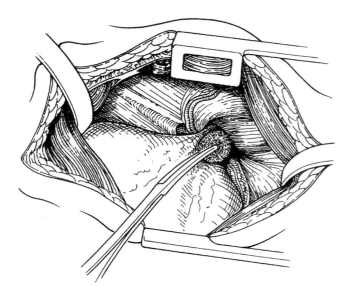

Figure 14.3 *Mobilizing indirect sacs. These sacs are 'milked' out of the cord at the deep inguinal ring.*

Discarding distal indirect sacs

When a scrotal hernia is present, the proximal 2 or 3 cm of the sac should be milked back as before. The neck can now be divided across and closed flush to the parietal peritoneum with a transfixion suture. Before the distal sac springs away into the canal, its anterior wall should be slit for several centimeters, to prevent fluid accumulation within it and formation of a scrotal hydrocele. It can then be left in the scrotum with impunity.

Attempts to milk all of a scrotal sac back into the abdomen and then peel it out of the scrotum will result in damage to testicular vessels, bleeding and an unpleasant and troublesome scrotal hematoma (Figure 14.4).

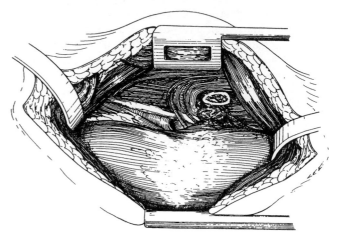

Figure 14.4 *Distal sacs, which extend into the scrotum, should not be forcibly pulled up; if they are there will be excessive bruising and hematoma in the scrotum. The neck of the sac is isolated, cleaned of tissue and cord structures, and divided across. The distal end is left open to fall back into the undamaged scrotum. Not all surgeons feel it is necessary to ligate the sac.*

Mobilization of direct inguinal and femoral sacs

Direct inguinal and femoral sacs are usually easily reduced, although if they are recurrent sacs some easement with careful scissors dissection may be required (Figure 14.5).

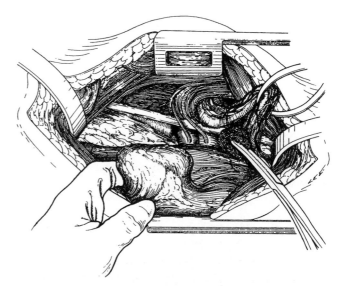

Figure 14.5 *Direct inguinal and femoral hernias are dealt with; they are reduced out of their parietal defect. Direct sacs are broad necked and do not require formal amputation.*

Parietalization of cord structures

After the hernial sacs have been dissected, the stump of the indirect sac is grasped in a long hemostat. Traction upwards on the stump will display the testicular vessels and vas running on the peritoneum posteriorly. These structures should now be mobilized away from the peritoneum for 4 or 5 cm (parietalization). This will allow the cord structures to be placed against the parietes and the prosthesis to be placed between them and the peritoneum so that the mesh closes the deep ring. Great care must be taken during this dissection to avoid the femoral nerve, which lies lateral to the deep ring. Ordinarily the femoral nerve is buried in and protected by the dense iliac fascia and is easily avoided, but if there has been previous surgery the dissection will be through much fibrous tissue and the nerve is at risk. Similarly, after vascular operations the nerve may be displaced and at risk (Figure 14.6).

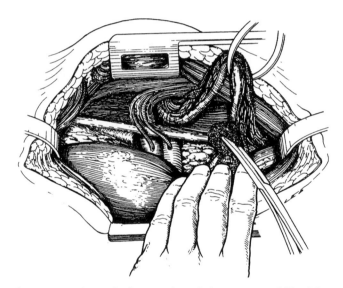

Figure 14.6 *The testicular vessels and the vas are mobilized for 4 or 5 cm from the deep ring. These structures are then spread out, 'parietalized', before insertion of the mesh.*

Closure of direct orifices

If large direct defects are present these may now be closed with continuous metric 2 (0 or 00) polypropylene sutures, picking up the iliopubic tract inferiorly and the white condensation of fascia transversalis superiorly (Figure 14.7). Because of the use of large prosthetic reinforcement, this maneuver is not considered necessary and is seldom performed today.

Measuring and cutting out the prosthesis

The prosthesis should reach from the anterior superior iliac spine to the same point contralaterally. Vertically it should reach down behind the pubis and behind the pubic rami on either side. Cephalad it must extend 3.0 cm above the lower margin of the conjoint tendon (the transverse arch). It will

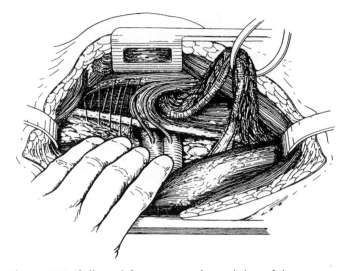

Figure 14.7 *If direct defects are prominent, it is useful to suture them loosely across before inserting the mesh. A suture to approximate the conjoint tendon to the pectineal ligament medially will prevent bulging immediately postoperatively.*

need to extend higher if a Spigelian hernia or incisional hernia is to be repaired. If a Pfannenstiel incisional hernia is present the mesh should extend up almost to the umbilicus. In practice, the transverse size of the prosthesis usually measures the distance between the anterosuperior iliac spines, and the height should be equal to the distance from umbilicus to the pubis. The lower lateral corners of the prosthesis are trimmed back about 2.0 cm on each side and rounded to accommodate the basin-like shape of the pelvis (Figure 14.8).

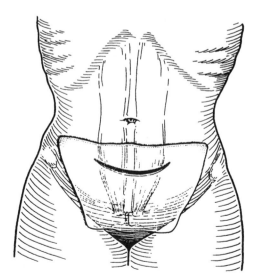

Figure 14.8 *Measuring out the prosthesis.*

Stoppa recommends that the prosthesis be shaped into a chevron (Figure 14.9). The measurement of the width of this mesh is the distance between the two anterior iliac spines minus 1–2 cm. The height is the measurement of the distance from the umbilicus to the pubis.[1095]

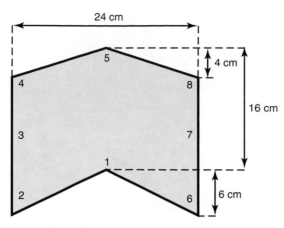

Figure 14.9 *The cardinal points of positioning of the clamps onto the prosthesis to aid in its insertion are shown.*

Placement of prosthesis

The prosthesis is grasped along its lower margin in four long artery forceps. Using these forceps, the prosthesis is placed on the peritoneum in the pelvis. The chevron prosthesis is more easily placed by grasping the mesh with eight long curved tonsil clamps at the points indicated in Figure 14.9. These are placed sequentially in numerical order from one to eight. Number one is placed at the pubis and number five is toward the umbilicus.

SUTURE TO PECTINEAL (COOPER'S) LIGAMENT

Laterally the pectineal ligament is identified close to the femoral vein; the prosthesis is fixed to the pectineal ligament at this point with a single interrupted polypropylene suture, which is held untied in a hemostat. Further untied sutures are placed medially. When a series, at least three on each side, of sutures have been placed they are tied. After these sutures have been tied, the prosthesis should overlap the bony pelvis by 2 or 3 cm, extending down into the pelvis to the prostatic capsule (Figure 14.10).

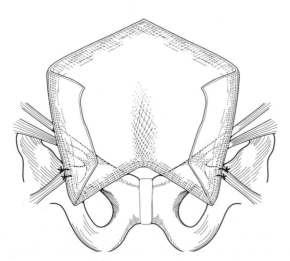

Figure 14.10 *Suturing the prosthesis to the pectineal ligament.*

SUTURE TO LATERAL INGUINAL LIGAMENT

The lateral extremity of the prosthesis is now fixed to the deep surface of the inguinal ligament lateral to the deep ring and adjacent to its attachment to the anterior superior iliac spine. Care must be taken to avoid the cord structures and the femoral nerve that lies on the iliopsoas muscle beneath. There is a hazard to the lateral cutaneous nerve of the thigh, which must be avoided. This maneuver completes the closure of the deep ring and the parietalization of the cord (Figure 14.11).

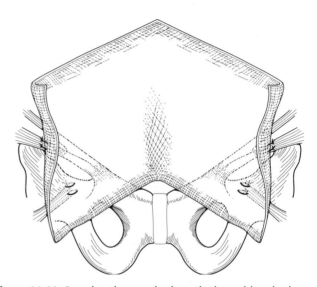

Figure 14.11 *Suturing the prosthesis to the lateral inguinal ligament.*

SUTURE TO CONJOINT TENDON AND RECTUS SHEATH

The prosthesis is next sutured to the arch of the conjoint tendon – two interrupted sutures of polypropylene are sufficient (Figure 14.12). It is possible to achieve this fixation to the parietes cephalad to the deep ring and the direct area by a quilting suture from one lateral margin of the prosthesis to another.

With experience and careful placement technique a single polypropylene suture to the pectineal (Cooper's) ligament may suffice, thus avoiding any danger to the nerves.

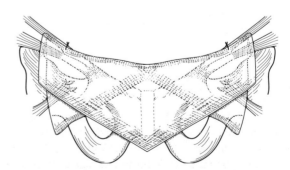

Figure 14.12 *Suturing the prosthesis to the conjoint tendon.*

SUTURE-FREE METHOD

The need for the use of any sutures at all has been questioned. In the current teachings of René Stoppa, he states that there is a need for only one suture that is placed at the umbilical site (Figure 14.13). The intra-abdominal pressure will maintain the proper positioning of the mesh as he designs it to fit into the pelvis based upon Pascal's hydrostatic principle.[1095]

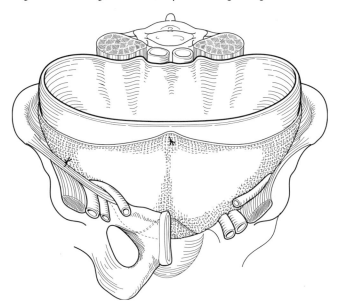

Figure 14.13 *Current recommended placement of the single suture to fixate the giant prosthesis.*

Closure

SUTURE TO ANTERIOR RECTUS SHEATH

The linea alba is reconstituted, starting at the pubis and picking up the prosthesis in the midline. A continuous polypropylene metric 2 suture is used for this (Figure 14.14).

CLOSURE OF MIDLINE

The midline linea alba is closed in front of the prosthesis so that the linea alba closure is reinforced (Figures 14.15 and 14.16).

Closed suction drains can be placed into the pelvic extraperitoneal space but are seldom necessary.

Subcutaneous tissue and skin closure should be secure as to the preference of the surgeon.

Postoperative care

The patient is mobilized as early as possible after the operation. Edema of the lower flap of the Pfannenstiel incision is common; it resolves slowly but spontaneously. The drains, if used, are removed at between 24 and 48 h. Convalescence is smooth, but care must be taken to identify any signs of sepsis, which must be treated vigorously with appropriate antibiotics. If the

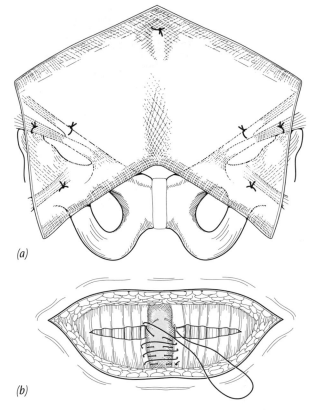

(a)

(b)

Figure 14.14 *Closure: the prosthesis is sutured to the linea alba.*

patient shows a temperature above 38.5°C (101°) blood cultures should be taken and antibiotics started immediately. The antibiotic regimen will need adjusting if positive blood cultures are obtained.

The extraperitoneal, or preperitoneal, approach to groin hernias children is described in Chapter 10, page 144.

THE UNILATERAL OPERATION

Preoperative preparation and positioning of the patient is the same as for the bilateral operation. There are differences in the newer techniques that have been developed recently which are described below. The 'traditional' method is presented first.

The incision

A half-Pfannenstiel incision placed 2–3 cm below the level of the anterior iliac spine and extending from the midline laterally for 8–10 cm, is positioned well above the deep inguinal ring (see video clip 'Open preperitoneal inguinal hernia repair'). Next, the rectus sheath is incised to expose the red belly of the underlying rectus abdominus muscle and the incision carried laterally into the aponeurosis of the internal oblique/transversus abdominus muscles for 1–2 cm (Figure 14.17).

An assistant then retracts the rectus muscle medially and it is dissected from the underlying filmy transversalis fascia. It may be necessary to divide and ligate the inferior epigastric

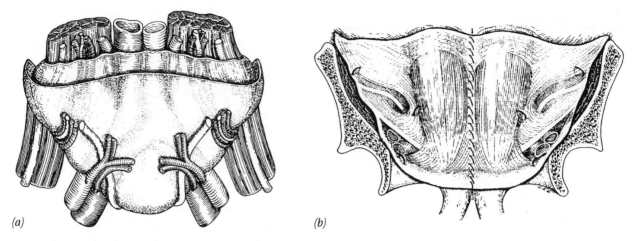

(a)   *(b)*

Figure 14.15 *The completed operation: the mesh lies in the extraperitoneal layer and completely encloses the anterior pelvic peritoneum.*

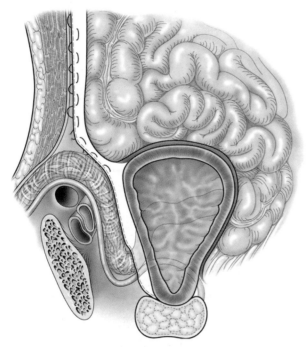

Figure 14.16 *Parasagittal section to demonstrate the mesh in the extraperitoneal layer and lining the pelvis down to the prostatic capsule.*

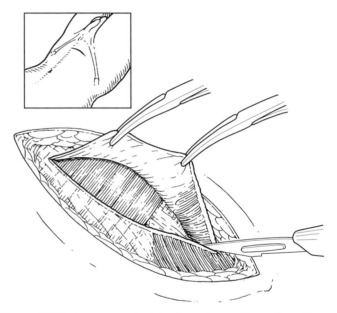

Figure 14.17 *A transverse incision is made two fingers-breadth above the pubic symphysis from the midline, deepened to incise the rectus sheath and laterally into the aponeurosis of the oblique abdominal muscles.*

vessels which cross the operative field but these can usually be preserved (Figure. 14.18).

Development of extraperitoneal space

Following incision of the transversalis fascia the preperitoneal space is entered. The underlying viscera are retracted manually with the non-dominant hand and the preperitoneal space is developed by blunt dissection using a pledget mounted on a deep hemostat (Figure 14.19). The exposure should bring into view the oblique muscles of the abdominal wall, the superior pubic ramus, the posterior wall of the inguinal canal, and the structures of the cord entering and leaving it, the femoral opening, and the pectineal (Cooper's) ligament.

Indirect inguinal hernia sacs, direct inguinal and femoral sacs are mobilized and managed surgically as for the bilateral operation.

Parietalization of cord structures

Wantz emphasizes this maneuver in order that the spermatic cord is dissected away from the peritoneum to permit these structures to be placed against the pelvic wall so that the

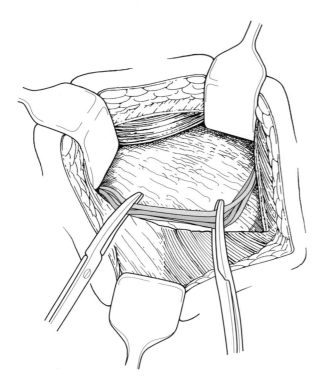

Figure 14.18 *The rectus muscles retracted medially. The transversalis fascia is incised and the inferior epigastric vessels ligated and divided.*

prosthesis can be laid between them and the peritoneum.[1186] This step, however, is not performed by Rignault,[959] nor does he carry out any approximation of the margins of the defect with sutures. Nyhus[857] closes the defect, but does not parietalize the cord before placement of a supplementary polypropylene mesh

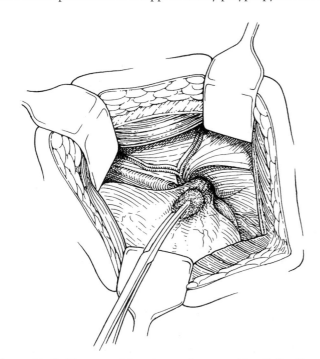

Figure 14.19 *The prepositioned space is exposed in all directions, in preparation for the mesh.*

prosthesis. Ugahary and Kugel both attempt to parietalize the cord structures.[622,1150]

The Nyhus technique of closure of the defect without parietalization is illustrated in Figures 14.20 and 14.21. The upper margin of the defect is thickened transversalis fascia and the

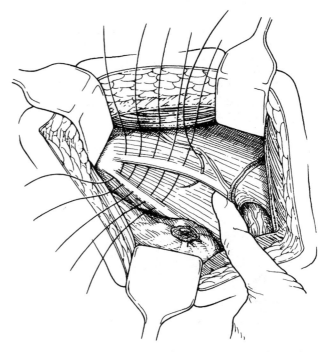

Figure 14.20 *Redundant peritoneal sac has been excised. The fused transversalis fascia–transversus abdominis layer is approximated to the iliopubic tract (below).*

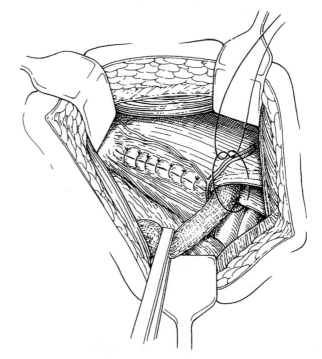

Figure 14.21 *The transversalis fascia sling lateral to the cord is closed to reconstruct the internal ring.*

arch of the aponeurosis of the transversus abdominus muscle; the lower margin is iliopubic tract. The more medial sutures also pick up Cooper's ligament inferiorly and lateral sutures can be placed lateral to the internal ring.

Measuring and cutting out the prosthesis

As for the bilateral operation, wide coverage of the myopectineal orifice is necessary. The optimal shape is trapezoid (Figure 14.22). The final position of the prosthesis is shown in Figure 14.23. The essential points of fixation by sutures are:

1 Medially to the pectineal (Cooper's) ligament by two or three interrupted sutures.
2 Laterally to the fascia over iliacus.
3 Behind the abdominal wound with two or three tacking sutures (Figure. 14.24).

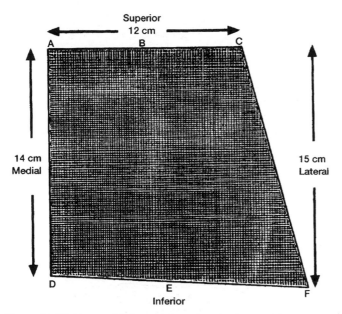

Figure 14.22 *Trapezoid shapes of mesh to be inserted in preperitoneal space. The letters A–F illustrate the position of the mesh after placement (Figures 13.23 and 13.24).*

Closure

It is essential to close the anterior rectus sheath with a continuous, non-absorbable monofilament suture which also repairs the lateral extension into the internal oblique/transversus abdominus muscle; failure to do this could result in an incisional hernia or acquired Spigelian hernia lateral to the rectus sheath.

Minimal access preperitoneal placement of the prosthesis

The introduction of the laparoscopic techniques for the repair of inguinal hernias has caused some surgeons to re-evaluate the need for large incisions to position biomaterial to repair the hernia. Currently the two biggest proponents of these concepts

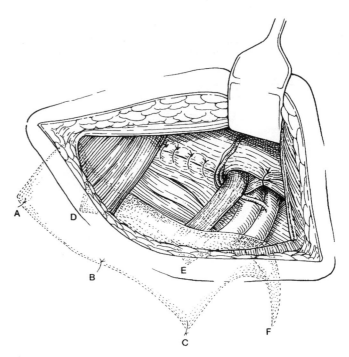

Figure 14.23 *Positioning the mesh. The lower corner of the mesh (D) lies behind the symphysis pubis, the lower central part (E) is sutured to the pectineal (Cooper's) ligament and the lower lateral corner of the mesh lies on the iliacus, where it may be sutured to the pelvic fascia.*

are Kugel and Ugahary.[622,1150] Either operation can be performed with local, regional or general anesthesia. Unlike the procedures above, these operations require two separate incisions to repair bilateral hernias. Both of these techniques utilize an incision 3–4 cm in length. The procedure is aided by placing the patient in the reverse Trendelenberg position to move the intestines away from the pelvis.

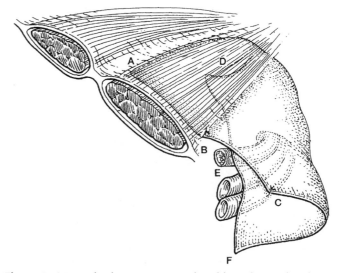

Figure 14.24 *Anchoring sutures are placed into the pectineal (Cooper's) ligament and sometimes to the iliacus fascia. Superiorly the mesh is tacked to the abdominal wall above the incision (A, B and C), thus reinforcing the abdominal incision.*

The location of these incisions differs, however. The incision for the Kugel repair is placed at the midpoint from the anterior iliac spine and the pubic tubercle (Figure 14.25). The incision

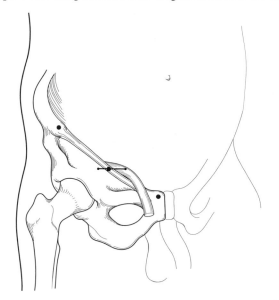

Figure 14.25 *Location of the incision for the Kugel repair of inguinal hernias. The left and right dots denote the pubic tubercle and the anterior iliac spine. The incision is positioned between these two structures and can be made in either the transverse or vertical plane.*

for Ugahary's operation is made approximately 3 cm above and lateral to the internal ring (Figure 14.26). The location of that incision leads this procedure to be also known as the gridiron hernioplasty. With either repair, the location of the incision is

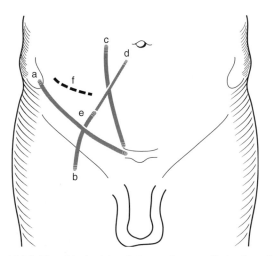

Figure 14.26 *The skin incision is located normally in the softest part of the affected lower abdomen. Markings of the surface anatomy: (a) inguinal ligament, (b) femoral artery, (c) lateral border of the rectus muscle, (d) line perpendicular to the inguinal ligament from the femoral artery before it becomes the iliac artery (indicates the surface projection of the interior epigastric vessels), (e) the internal ring should be lateral to the epigastrics and above the inguinal ligament, (f) placement of the skin incision will be about two fingers laterocranial from the internal ring.*

critical to the performance of the procedure in an easy fashion. Once the incision is made, the entrance to the preperitoneal space is accomplished by a muscle splitting dissection of the flat muscles of the abdomen.

The preperitoneal space is entered by incision of the transversalis fascia. Ugahary incises the fascia in the transverse plane while Kugel places the incision in the vertical direction. The dissection of the space then is performed so that there will be enough free space that is slightly larger than that of the prosthetic biomaterial that is to be placed for the repair of the hernia. This space is developed with the use of either forceps and other instruments[622] or with the use of long thin retractors.[1150]

The plane of dissection will be posterior to the epigastric vessels and will extend approximately 2–3 cm above the incision in the transversalis fascia. The cord structures should be separated from the peritoneum 3 cm[622] or 7–10 cm[1150] above the internal ring. Typically this will expose Cooper's ligament and the pubic bone medially. Care must be taken not to injure the vessels to the testes during this dissection. If the visualization is difficult, a laparoscope can be inserted into the preperitoneal space to assist in the identification of the structures.

Ugahary uses a polypropylene mesh that is 10×15 cm in size. The center is marked with a colored suture to assist in the orientation of the prosthesis. This is then tightly rolled around a 300 mm forceps with the side that will be facing the inguinal floor on the outside of the roll (Figure 14.27). This facilitates the

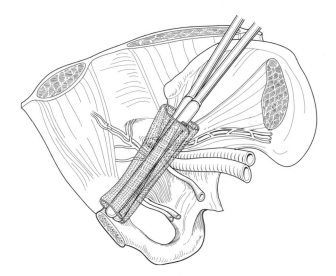

Figure 14.27 *The preparation of the prosthesis. With an anatomical forceps the prosthesis is rolled up, the visceral site with the colored stitch being inside the coil.*

unrolling of the mesh. The mesh is then inserted into the space with the very distal end placed behind the pubis. The suture will be near the epigastric vessels while the very lateral end of the mesh will be at the level of the wound. The retractors are removed. One is then re-inserted into the roll of the mesh. A second retractor is then used to unroll the mesh by a sweeping and rotating motion. In sequential fashion, the two retractors are used to hold the mesh in place while the other completes the flattening of the mesh. A short depressor is used to flatten out the distal ends of the mesh rather than a retractor. One absorbable suture is used to fix the lateral corner of the mesh to the transversus muscle (Figure 14.28). The polypropylene mesh will then have assumed the shape of the myopectineal orifice quite similar to that of the laparoscopic approach or the GPRVS repair of Wantz (Figure 14.29).

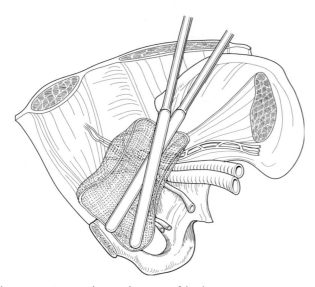

Figure 14.28 *Drawing to show use of both retractors, one to hold the mesh and the other to spread the mesh flat, smoothing out folds.*

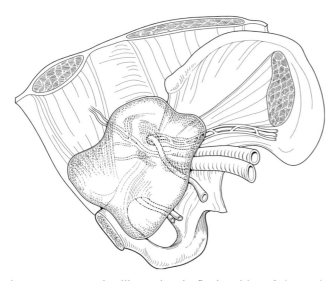

Figure 14.29 *Drawing illustrating the final position of the mesh in the preperitoneal space behind the myopectineal orifice.*

Kugel uses a Kugel Patch™ to repair these hernias (see Chapter 7). Briefly, this consists of two layers of an oval shaped polypropylene mesh that is welded with an integrated polyester ring. This ring allows the mesh to open up upon insertion while the design of the flat portion allows sutureless placement of the prosthesis. He recommends the use of an 8 × 12 cm patch for the repair of unilateral inguinal hernias.

Malleable retractors are used to maintain the space created by the preperitoneal dissection.

The index finger is inserted into the slit that is placed on one of the meshes whereupon the patch is rolled onto the finger. Usually it is easier to use the right index finger for a left hernia and the left finger for a right hernia (Figure 14.30). The

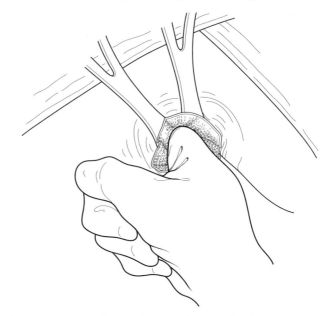

Figure 14.30 *Insertion of the patch is simplified by using a malleable retractor as a shoehorn.*

finger is directed toward the pubic bone by sliding along Cooper's ligament. The finger is removed and the retractor is eased out of the space. This retractor can then be used to further flatten the patch if necessary. When properly placed, the patch is completely open and lies parallel to the inguinal ligament with 60% of the patch above the inguinal ligament. The lateral edge of the patch should lie 2–3 cm beyond the incision in the transversalis fascia. In this position this will cover the inguinal floor and the femoral space as do the other preperitoneal repairs (Figure 14.31). A single absorbable suture to fix the lateral edge of the patch to the transversalis is recommended.

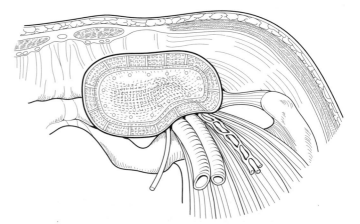

Figure 14.31 *Preperitoneal view showing proper placement of the patch. (Reprinted from Am J Surg 1999; 178: 298–302 with permission.)*

Closure of the muscle layers is with absorbable 2-0 or 3-0 sutures or a simple running stitch. Scarpa's layer may be closed, if desired. The skin is closed with a 3-0 or 4-0 absorbable subcuticular stitch.

These patients are sent home the day of surgery. Postoperative analgesia is either non-steroidal anti-inflammatories or codeine-based formularies. There are no specific restrictions other than that which is limited by pain. Most resume activities in 5–7 days.

Results

The Stoppa bilateral operation, termed the 'Giant Prosthesis for Reinforcement of the Visceral Sac' (GPRVS), was reported by the Amiens group in 1984.[1098] Of 255 operated patients[265] (84.2%) had an uncomplicated postoperative course. The hematoma rate was 7.9% and the local sepsis rate was 5.8%. Many of these patients were elderly or poor risk and had undergone multiple previous operations. Late results, with a follow-up rate of 91.3% at 2–10 years, revealed a recurrence rate of 2.5%. All the recurrences occurred during the first postoperative year, indicating that the pattern of recurrence does not follow the same course as anterior repairs. Few of the infections were deep and related to the prosthesis, and antibiotics or a combination of antibiotics and drainage, with eventual healing, treated superficial suppuration. The merits of Dacron mesh (Mersilene) used by the French surgeons are discussed in Chapter 7. Rignault, utilizing large sheets of mesh without closure of hernial defects, reports similar results; during a 14-year period 767 patients underwent preperitoneal prosthetic inguinal hernioplasty with a 2% sepsis rate and a 1.2% recurrence rate for recurrent hernias, of which there were 239 operations.[959] Once again, most recurrences were seen within the first postoperative year and were related either to sepsis or to technical mistakes made by inexperienced surgeons.

Nyhus, reporting his preperitoneal approach and prosthetic buttress repair for recurrent hernia, assessed 203 operations in 195 patients.[857] Regional anesthesia was used in most patients, no perioperative antibiotics were given and long-term follow-up was available for 115 hernias (56%) in 102 patients (52%) over a period of 6 months to 10 years. Eight patients had repeat recurrences at a mean of 30 months after repair but only two of these (1.7% of those followed up) have recurred after sutured repair supplemented with mesh buttress. The other six recurrences occurred in an earlier experience when no mesh buttress was being used. The authors state that the preperitoneal approach for recurrent groin hernia with reinforcing mesh buttress should be the procedure of choice for all recurrent groin hernias.

Other groups have reported similar results. Mozingo and colleagues treated 100 recurrent hernias in 84 men, with three re-recurrences occurring within 6 months of surgery at a follow-up of 6 months to 5 years. They reported few complications and no testicular complications.[820] Hoffman and Traverso used the technique in 175 patients with 152 primary and 52 recurrent inguinal hernias. They had one recurrence and wound complications occurred in 12 patients (5.9%).[507] Like Nyhus, these authors do not employ parietalization of the cord

and close the defect with interrupted sutures before a large rectangle of polypropylene mesh is sutured to cover the entire myopectineal orifice, with fixation to Cooper's ligament, transversus abdominus medially and rectus muscle superiorly and laterally.[507] Finally, Horton and Florence[516] have described a preperitoneal approach, entering directly through the posterior inguinal wall under local anesthesia, allowing the patient to go home within one or two hours of surgery. Because wide visualization of the preperitoneal space cannot be achieved with this approach it is likely that the mesh may shift, uncovering areas of the myopectineal orifice and causing the potential for recurrence. Additionally, suture fixation is blind resulting in a risk to vascular and neural structures in the preperitoneal space.

A further study from the Netherlands has confirmed the excellent results of the preperitoneal mesh repair in 75 patients with 150 hernias (24 primary and 126 recurrent) using Marlex mesh. The technique used placing the cord structures in a vertical slit in the mesh, is identical to that often used when there are difficulties mobilizing and parietalizing the cord in recurrent hernias.[101]

Neither the gridiron nor the Kugel hernioplasty are supported by more than a few publications of the results. Ugahary has reported the results of 427 hernia repairs in 364 patients from September 1995 to December 1998. Of these, 369 were primary and 58 were recurrent hernia repairs. There were seven recurrences (1.7%). The most common causes of these recurrences were displacement of the mesh. Additionally, the initial meshes were smaller (8×10 cm) and had a slit placed for the exit of the cord structures. The larger mesh is used today without a slit whereupon the cord is parietalized. Most of the recurrences were noted within the first ten patients of the surgeon's operative experience and were seen within the first week postoperatively. Unfortunately, the length of follow-up was not provided.[1149] Longer periods of follow-up with at least a 3-year median interval are necessary to verify the effectiveness of this technique.

As originally reported, Kugel had a recurrence rate of 0.62%. There were five recurrences in 808 patients operated upon from January 1994 to July 1998.[622] In all cases, this was due to the lower edge of the patch that had lifted off the parietal surface allowing the hernia to recur underneath the patch. These occurred in the first 6 months. Because of this, the patch was placed in a more posterior position. There were two wound infections that required drainage but not removal of the patch. By May 1999 he had performed 882 repairs with the same number of recurrences for a rate of 0.57%. A total of 785 repairs were for primary hernias (89%) and 97 were for recurrent hernias (11%). There were no more infections.[623] As with the gridiron repair more data with longer follow-up is needed to confirm his success and the durability of the repair as they become more widely adopted.

ADVANTAGES AND DISADVANTAGES OF THE EXTRAPERITONEAL OPERATION

It is important to have a sense of proportion regarding the advantages and disadvantages of this approach to groin hernias.

The advantages of the extraperitoneal (preperitoneal) approach are:

- It can allow the bilateral exploration through a single incision (excluding the Ugahary and Kugel methods).
- All hernial orifices are visible and easily explored.
- Multiple sacs can be dealt with.
- It is always easy to isolate sacs and divide and close them flush with the peritoneal cavity.
- The anatomy of sliding hernias is more completely visualized.
- If necessary, the peritoneal sac can be opened, e.g. if strangulation is present.
- The layer of dissection is an unscarred virgin layer.
- The repair is placed in the essential transversalis fascial plane.
- In recurrent hernias there is no dissection of the cord vasculature and hence no risk of testicular ischemia.

Some disadvantages of the extraperitoneal approach are:

- It is impossible under local anesthesia and without muscle relaxation (excluding the Ugahary and Kugel methods).
- More assistance, retraction and illumination are required than using the conventional anterior exposure of groin hernias.

- The retraction of the rectus muscles laterally makes it difficult to identify the medial margins of direct inguinal defects. This is overcome with the minimal access procedures to a large extent.

CONCLUSIONS

- The open extraperitoneal mesh operation is very valuable in the surgery of complex, or recurrent, groin hernias.
- The approach exploits the extraperitoneal plane, which is usually unscarred and easy to dissect. There need be no opening into the peritoneal cavity and no manipulation of viscera. Postoperative ileus is not encountered. With care, bleeding is minimal and a rapid convalescence the rule.
- The more extensive procedures should not necessarily be the first choice routine operation for primary, uncomplicated groin hernias.
- However, the minimal access operations seem to be successful in these cases in experienced hands. Currently, in some areas these are used primarily. Longer follow-up is needed.

15

Laparoscopic groin hernia repair

INTRODUCTION

The first report of a hernia repair using laparoscopy was made by Ralph Ger in 1982.[398] In a patient with right indirect inguinal hernia the neck of the sac was closed with a series of staples using an operating laparoscope and a cannula placed in the right iliac fossa. Although this procedure was carried out in November 1979, Ger states that the first patient to be treated by laparoscopic closure of the neck of the sac was under the care of Dr Fletcher of the University of West Indies, Jamaica.

The use of prosthetic material for laparoscopic repair of an inguinal hernia was introduced by Corbitt[245] and Schultz[1026] in 1991. These repairs involved the use of a polypropylene plug, patch, or both to close the inguinal canal in a tension-free manner. Because of unacceptably high early recurrence rates these approaches were abandoned in favor of laparoscopic placement of a preperitoneal prosthetic biomaterial. This repair follows the same principles as the open Stoppa repair.[1099] After reducing the hernia sac a large piece of mesh is placed in the preperitoneal space covering all potential hernia sites in the inguinal region. The mesh becomes sandwiched between the preperitoneal tissues and the abdominal wall and, provided it is large enough, is held there by intra-abdominal pressure until such time as it becomes incorporated by fibrous tissue.

The intraperitoneal placement of mesh was introduced by Fitzgibbons and colleagues[359] as a method of laparoscopic hernia repair. This operation is performed using minimal dissection by leaving the hernia sac in situ and covering the defect with mesh, which is stapled to the surrounding peritoneum. The major concerns with this repair are the risk of injury to underlying structures from staples and of obstruction or fistula formation as a result of adhesions between bowel and exposed mesh. These concerns had resulted in this repair being performed in only a few centers. Other materials, such as expanded polytetrafluoroethylene, are thought less likely to cause adhesions and were also being investigated with this repair.

Currently, the laparoscopic approach for the repair of inguinal hernias is achieving success and there are many areas of the world where this is the preferred method of repair. However, it does not seem that this methodology will become the standard of care for all inguinal hernias. In skilled hands the laparoscopic approach is also effective for incarcerated inguinal hernias[680] and recurrent inguinal hernias after a prior laparoscopic repair.[349] There seems to be a trend to limit the use of this technique in those inguinal hernias that are either bilateral and/or recurrent. This trend however does not take into account patient preference, surgical training and the need to maintain a good level of skill or performance for those already undertaking the operation. Conversely, the laparoscopic herniorrhaphy for incisional and ventral hernias is increasing in popularity. It might possibly become the standard of care for this problem given the results that have been seen thus far.

EXTRAPERITONEAL OPERATION

(CD)

Anesthesia

Although totally extraperitoneal hernia repair can be performed using either local or epidural anesthesia, it is our preference to use general anesthesia with complete muscle relaxation and mechanical ventilation. This ensures that the respiratory and cardiovascular changes that occur with extraperitoneal CO_2 insufflation are minimized. These changes are similar to or less than those observed with intraperitoneal CO_2 insufflation, and may be related to the size of the space created during the preperitoneal dissections.[1202] All patients undergoing totally extraperitoneal hernia repair receive DVT prophylaxis. Use of antibiotic prophylaxis is controversial in this situation with little evidence for or against their use.

Position of the patient on the table

Before attempting totally extraperitoneal hernia repair it is important to ensure that the patient's bladder is empty. This can be achieved by asking the patient to micturate before entering the operating suite. Alternatively, a urinary catheter could be inserted but this is generally unnecessary. The patient should be placed on the operating table in the supine position with a 15° Trendelenburg tilt. Ideally both hands should be placed by the patient's side to allow the operator and the assistant to stand opposite each other at the patient's epigastric level. The operator stands on the side opposite to the hernia being repaired.

When bilateral repairs are to be done, the operation can be started by standing on the side of the patient opposite the larger hernia defect. The television monitor should be placed at the foot of the table (Figure 15.1). If two monitors are being used one should be placed at either side of the lower end of the operating table.

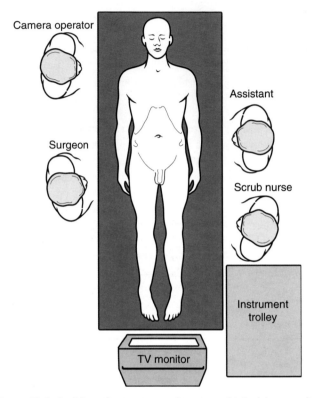

Figure 15.1 *Position of operator, assistants and television monitor at the operating table for repair of a left inguinal hernia.*

Trocars and trocar position

One 10 mm cannula and two 5 mm cannulas are generally used for this operation. The 10 mm cannula should have a blunt-nosed trocar as it is inserted using an open technique. The 5 mm cannulas should have built-in fixation threads to prevent them from moving in and out of the extraperitoneal space as instruments are passed through. In addition, because of the confined operating space, the 5 mm cannulas should be short (60 mm). All the cannulas can be placed in the lower midline. In this instance, the 10 mm cannula is placed in a sub-umbilical position; one of the two 5 mm cannulas is placed one-third of the way between the symphysis pubis and the umbilicus and the other half way between the symphysis pubis and the umbilicus (Figure 15.2).

Alternatively, many physicians prefer for the two smaller trocars to be placed laterally near the anterior axillary line above the iliac crest on either side of the patient. These latter trocars will usually be positioned after the dissection is nearly completed through the larger midline trocar. This will frequently be accomplished with the use of the laparoscope itself.

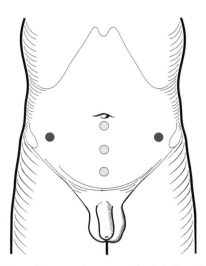

Figure 15.2 *Sites of trocar placements for totally extraperitoneal hernia repair. The mark on either side of the abdomen indicates the alternate location for the 5 mm trocars.*

Laparoscope

Some surgeons substitute the 0° laparoscope for a 30 or 45° laparoscope after developing the extraperitoneal space. We find that this is not necessary and that the operation can be completed satisfactorily with a 0° laparoscope. Currently either the 5 or 10 mm laparoscope can be used for the entire procedure. In particularly difficult cases, the 5 mm laparoscope is preferred as this can be placed in the lateral ports to visualize the anatomy from the contralateral aspect.

Developing the extraperitoneal space

A transverse incision of 1–1.5 cm below the umbilicus is made. The tissues are then separated with scissors or hemostat and retracted with two retractors to expose the anterior rectus sheath on the side of the hernia to be repaired. The sheath is opened with a no. 11 bladed scalpel through a small transverse incision. The midline and rectus muscle are identified and the space between the rectus muscle and the posterior rectus sheath developed using the hemostat. A large right-angled retractor (to retract the rectus muscle anteriorly to allow the insertion of a blunt-nosed 10 mm trocar and cannula) is then inserted into this space and moved medially, laterally and posteriorly to develop the preperitoneal space. The skin around the cannula can be sealed with a figure-of-eight stitch and at this stage insufflation with CO_2 can commence, insufflation pressure being kept to 10–12 mmHg. There are balloon-tipped trocars that allow the surgeon to insert them into this space. These need not be secured to the skin, but the balloon will be inflated which will maintain its position as well as seal off the preperitoneal space so that the CO_2 will be contained.

A 0° laparoscope is then inserted through the 10 mm cannula and can be gently used as a blunt dissector to further enlarge the space. It is important to feel the pubic symphysis, and stay in the midline and immediately posterior to the rectus muscle with the laparoscope during this dissection. Once the pubic arch is visible, two 5 mm cannulas are inserted under direct vision in the positions previously described.

The preperitoneal space may also be developed using balloon dissection. A deflated balloon on the end of a cannula, of which many different types are available (Figure 15.3), is placed

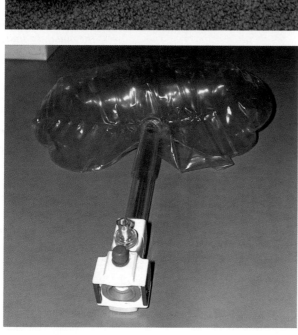

(a)

(b)

Figure 15.3 *(a) The deflated PBD2 balloon for dissection of the preperitoneal space. (b) The inflated PBD2 balloon for dissection of the preperitoneal space.*

in the preperitoneal space using the access described. The balloon is then filled with air and the space developed under direct vision using a 0° laparoscope. This method is helpful in the learning period when surgeons are still unfamiliar with the preperitoneal anatomy. While balloon dissection is slightly more rapid, it has the disadvantage of adding additional expense to the operation. In addition, it is associated with bladder and bowel injury in patients who have had previous lower abdominal surgery.[484] In those patients who have had prior lower abdominal surgery or prostatectomy, it is preferred to either perform the entire operation without the use of a balloon dissector, or to perform a transabdominal preperitoneal operation. Some surgeons will occasionally merge the two techniques. In these cases, the surgeon will enter the abdomen above the umbilicus with a 5 mm port and inspect the lower abdominal contents. If there are no adhesions, which is frequently the case, the dissection can

be converted to the totally extraperitoneal operation either with or without the use of the balloon dissection.

Dissection

Two dissectors, which will grasp but not tear the peritoneum, are important for this part of the procedure. A sharp pair of scissors will sometimes be used but is seldom necessary. It is important to identify the anatomical landmarks in an ordered fashion. The pectineal (Cooper's) ligament on the same side as the hernia should be exposed first. At this stage in thin patients you may see the external iliac vein laterally and accessory obturator vessels, if present, will be found crossing the pectineal ligament. Separation of the perivascular and extraperitoneal fat is performed in the avascular plane between both using gentle blunt dissection, and is aided by the CO_2 insufflation. Characteristic filamentous tissue, which breaks down easily, will be observed between the two planes (see video clip).

The retropubic space can now be developed in the midline and on the side of the hernia to above the level of the obturator nerve and vessels. The inferior epigastric vessels should next be identified and the space between them and the extraperitoneal fat developed. During this part of the dissection it is important to keep the epigastric vessels up against the rectus muscle using one dissector while the other is used to separate the tissues. If this is not done the epigastric vessels will come down into the operating field and small branches between them and the rectus muscles will be torn, giving rise to troublesome bleeding. Between the inferior epigastric vessels and extraperitoneal fat a fascial layer is encountered. This represents the deep layer of the fascia transversalis (Figure 15.4; see color insert) and should be divided using a combination of blunt and sharp dissection to open up the space lateral to it. This may not always be necessary if the dissection allows the complete separation of these structures.

Much of this will be accomplished with the dissection balloon if this is the chosen technique. The choice of the use of the balloon or blunt dissection has been shown to be equally effective in creating the space necessary to perform this operation. The attention to the epigastric vessels is limited when this is used because the unfurling of the balloon will sometimes pull these vessels down rather than leaving them in situ. This may limit the insufflation of the balloon whereupon the surgeon must complete the dissection manually. Also, for those surgeons that prefer the lateral location of the 5 mm trocars, some of the dissection will usually be necessary with the laparoscope and/or one of the dissection graspers that would be inserted through one of the lateral or midline trocars.

Indirect inguinal hernias

At this stage it should be possible to identify the sac of an indirect inguinal hernia (Figure 15.5; see color insert). The sac will be found immediately lateral to the inferior epigastric vessels as it enters the internal ring. The sac should be grasped at the

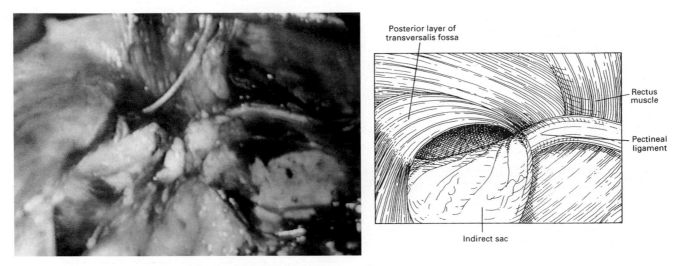

Figure 15.4 *Endoscopic appearance of the deep layer of fascia transversalis.*

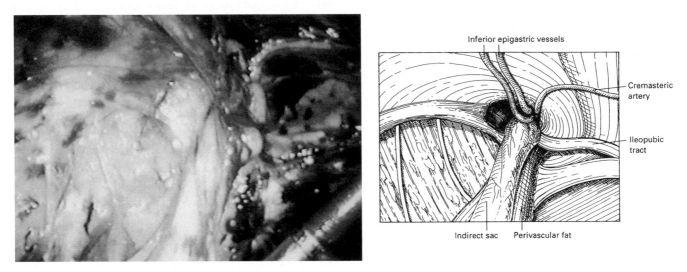

Figure 15.5 *Endoscopic appearance of an indirect sac.*

internal ring and reduced by retracting and dissecting the adhesions between it and the inguinal canal. Tension needs to be kept on the sac during this part of the dissection by using both dissectors in a stepwise fashion; otherwise as the sac is released to regrip it, it will return to the inguinal canal because of its elasticity and inguinal attachments. It is important to dissect all the tissues around the sac down to the peritoneum. These tissues represent attenuated transversalis fascia (see Chapter 2) which invests the cord and indirect sac as it enters the internal ring. Once this has been achieved the sac can be lifted up and the vas deferens will be visible at its posterior border and may be dissected off it along with the testicular vessels. The vas runs medially and crosses over the iliac vessels as it descends into the pelvis, while the testicular vessels take a course slightly lateral to the iliac vessels. In small to moderately sized indirect inguinal hernias, the apex of the sac can be identified and the sac completely reduced into the extraperitoneal space. If the sac is large and entering the scrotum, it may be wise to divide and ligate it at a convenient point as one would do with open hernia repair. The testicular vessels and vas deferens should be completely

skeletonized of any lipomatous material that may be in the inguinal canal. Not infrequently, a small hole may be made in the sac during its reduction. This should not impair the ability to complete the dissection and such defects can usually be ignored. However, it should be noted that great care must be exercised to avoid a large tear of the peritoneal sac during these maneuvers. This will result in the insufflation of the intra-abdominal space, which will limit the available preperitoneal space and subsequent 'working room' for the operation to continue. Additionally, this could expose the patch material to the intestinal contents of the abdomen with resulting adhesions. Posteriorly the peritoneal dissection should be taken back until the vas can be seen descending into the pelvis. Laterally it should go at least to the level of the anterior superior iliac spine while medially dissection should cross the midline and go well below the pectineal ligament (Figure 15.6). This is to ensure complete exposure of the myopectineal orifice and that there is adequate space for insertion of the mesh.

Lateral to the testicular vessels the femoral branch of the genitofemoral nerve and the lateral cutaneous nerve of the

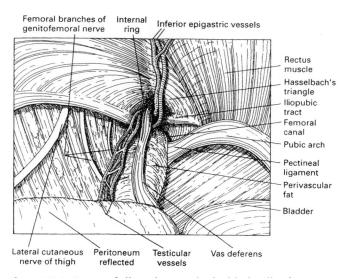

Figure 15.6 *Extent of dissection required with details of anatomy observed at endoscopy.*

thigh can be identified in patients with little adipose tissue (Figure 15.7). Care should be taken not to damage these or a small branch of the deep circumflex iliac artery, which lies lateral to the cutaneous nerve of thigh. These structures all lie beneath the iliopubic tract. Therefore, any fixation of the meshes must be placed above this line to assure that these nerves are not in harm's way. Also in thin patients the external iliac vessels will be easily identified, the artery appearing between the testicular vessels and the vas and the vein lying medial to the artery. In all patients the characteristic pulsation from the external iliac vessels will be observed in this position. Small peritoneal branches arising from the iliac artery may also be noted during the dissection and as these are usually at the posterior limit of the dissection they can be preserved. As all dissection is carried out in an avascular plane there should be only a limited need to use electrocautery during the operation. Most dissection is performed by gentle separation of tissues

using atraumatic-dissecting forceps. If there is an injury to larger vessels such as the epigastric artery or vein, then the use of hemostatic clips or suture ligation will be necessary. If this fails then one could place transfascial absorbable sutures to maintain hemostasis of these vessels.

Indirect inguinal hernias in females

The approach to these hernias is similar to that of the indirect inguinal hernias in the male patient. Once the sac is reduced the round ligament can be left in situ or divided and ligated at the internal ring depending on the surgeon's preference.

Direct inguinal hernias

A direct inguinal hernia will be encountered during the dissection to expose the pectineal ligament. The defect lies laterally to the border of the rectus muscle and is medial to the inferior epigastric vessels except when a combined direct and indirect hernia is present. Sometimes a direct defect can appear to encroach on the femoral canal and in this circumstance may be confused with a femoral hernia. Patients with a direct hernia will also occasionally be found to have a femoral hernia. The direct hernia sac and preperitoneal fat are usually easy to reduce by grasping the sac with atraumatic forceps and simple pulling. While the hernia is being reduced the characteristic appearance of a pseudosac, which is attenuated transversalis fascia, will be displayed. This should be allowed to retract into the defect. As with indirect hernias, the sac is reduced into the extraperitoneal space and no attempt is made to open or ligate it. The vas deferens and testicular vessels need to be exposed to exclude a synchronous indirect hernia. The extent of the dissection should be identical to that of the indirect hernia repair. It is important to be careful during this part of the operation as the peritoneum is easily torn at the internal ring in patients with a direct hernia. It is generally best if the peritoneum is

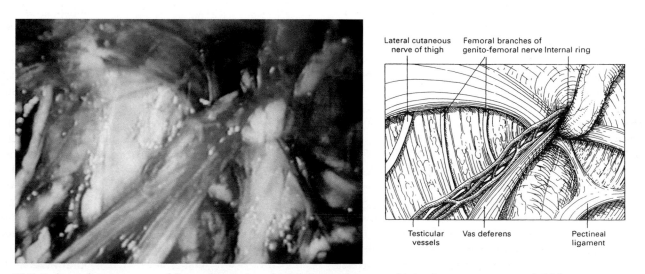

Figure 15.7 *Endoscopic appearance of femoral branches of genitofemoral nerve and lateral cutaneous nerve of thigh.*

pushed with the laparoscopic forceps rather than pulled at this location so that this tear will not occur.

Femoral hernias

As the pectineal ligament is exposed as far lateral as the external iliac vein in all patients, a femoral hernia should not be missed during totally extraperitoneal hernia repair. This can be reduced in the same manner as for direct hernias. One should be attentive to the possibility of the inclusion of an organ such as the bladder or ovary into the hernia contents. When found these structures should be carefully reduced to avoid injury. Once this has been done dissection should proceed as for other groin hernias.

Recurrent hernias

A reasonable amount of experience with totally extraperitoneal hernia repair is required before dealing with recurrent hernias following an open repair. This is because the anatomical landmarks are often distorted due to the previous repairs. The inferior epigastric vessels may have been divided and thus be in part absent or visible as a much smaller vessel. Dense adhesions form between the neck of the recurrent sac and the previous repair and because of this it is wise to use careful sharp dissection to free it from these adhesions. Elsewhere the peritoneum is often very thin and easily torn, as stitches may have gone through it from the previous repair. Because of the frequent use of a prosthetic biomaterial in the prior repair, the occurrence of a tear in the peritoneum should be expected during the dissection. This is especially frequent in the patient that has had a prior plug-and-patch repair. In this latter situation, it is probably best to use a transabdominal approach so that the peritoneum can be repaired at the completion of the procedure.

If the laparoscopic technique is selected for the repair of a recurrent hernia after a laparoscopic repair, it is usually best accomplished with a transabdominal preperitoneal (TAPP) technique. This will allow the surgeon the ability to dissect the peritoneum under direct vision and allows the assurance that there are no adhesions from an intra-abdominal organ. This is particularly recommended when the patient has had a previous repair that utilized a polypropylene biomaterial (which is invariably the case).

Bilateral hernias

Bilateral hernias can be repaired using the same access as for unilateral hernias and additional trocars are not required. Once dissection has been completed on one side the operator simply switches to the other side and reduces the contralateral hernia. Although one large piece of mesh can be used for bilateral hernia repair, it is our preference to use two pieces of 15 cm by 10 cm. In this circumstance it is helpful to staple one to the pectineal ligament before the contralateral mesh is placed into position.

For all indirect hernias and most direct hernias the mesh does not need to be tacked, stapled or sutured in place. If, however, a large direct defect encroaches upon the femoral canal or there is a femoral hernia the mesh should be stapled or sutured to the pectineal ligament to prevent the inferior border of the mesh from slipping upwards and into the defect. The mesh does not need to be divided to fit around the cord or, indeed, sutured or tacked around the cord.

On desufflating the extraperitoneal space it is important to ensure that the inferior fold of the mesh does not roll up with the peritoneum. If an adequate dissection has been carried out this will not occur. After desufflation all cannulas are removed and the rectus sheath at the sub-umbilical incision is closed with 2/0 or 0 Vicryl, while skin is closed with interrupted 4/0 nylon or absorbable subcuticular stitches and/or adhesive tapes.

Fixation of the mesh

To secure the mesh a spiral tacking device is generally used, however, there is some evidence that fixation may not be necessary.[585] A newer device allows the placement of a 'construct' that is similar to a key ring to fixate the mesh (see Chapter 7). In either instance, two or three tacks or constructs are placed only in the pectineal ligament in the situations previously mentioned. Some surgeons secure the mesh to rectus muscle medially and the transversus abdominis laterally. Fixation at this position provides no additional support for properly positioned mesh and can be avoided in all but the large inguinal or femoral hernia repairs. Alternatively the mesh can be sutured to the pectineal ligament with a 2/0 Prolene stitch.

When placing these fixations devices, it is often easier to insert them into the pectineal ligament if the instrument is inserted via an ipsilateral trocar. The angle of the ligament is such that a firm grasp of the ligament is best afforded if this approach is used. This will prevent the slippage off the ligament that is common as the instrument is fired. The contralateral trocar is used for placement of the additional fixators along the muscle above the iliopubic tract.

Experimental studies have shown that it may be efficacious to use a fibrin sealant to secure the mesh rather than metal devices.[571] This has the obvious advantage that the risk of injury to vascular or neural structures is virtually eliminated while resulting in less pain to the patient. More studies in such products will become important to the field of herniology in the future.

CONVERSION TO OPEN REPAIR

It is necessary in approximately 1% (or as few as 0.23%) of cases to convert open preperitoneal repair.[564] This usually occurs as a result of a large tear in the peritoneum or, when a very large (estimated defect of 5 cm or greater) direct hernia is encountered. In the latter circumstance a 15 cm × 15 cm piece of mesh is required and is more easily placed at open surgery. If the hernia is unilateral, a small transverse incision is placed over the ipsilateral rectus muscle at the level of the lower 5 mm cannula and the preperitoneal space entered lateral to the rectus muscle. If there are bilateral hernias, a Pfannenstiel incision is made at the same level to gain access to the preperitoneal space.

In the majority of instances when the prospect of conversion becomes a reality, one may convert instead to the transabdominal preperitoneal repair. With this approach the entire abdominal cavity will allow a much larger working space and usually obviates the need for conversion to the open approach. The larger piece of mesh can be inserted and placed. The remainder of the procedure will proceed as the traditional TAPP repair.

CONTRAINDICATIONS TO TOTALLY EXTRAPERITONEAL HERNIA REPAIR

Although there are no absolute contraindications to totally extraperitoneal hernia repair in the elective setting, large inguinoscrotal or irreducible hernias are relative contraindications. Previous lower midline or ipsilateral paramedian incisions also come into this category. Extraperitoneal endoscopic repair is difficult and time-consuming in these circumstances such that it is difficult to justify attempting it in the first place. In these instances, one may elect to attempt a TAPP repair and convert to the open operation if it is obvious that this, too, is not feasible. If there is a concern in regards to the possibility of adhesions that may make the extraperitoneal approach risky, a small laparoscope is inserted into the abdominal cavity and the areas of suspicion are inspected. This is done through an infra-umbilical skin incision with the abdominal entry moved to above the potential site for the fascial incisional for placement of the 10 mm trocar. If there are no adhesions in the area or none that involve the bowel, the 5 mm port can be removed after the abdomen is evacuated of the carbon dioxide. The larger 10 mm port is then inserted via the infra-umbilical incision whereupon the extraperitoneal procedure will be performed with assurance that there is no risk of injury to the bowel during the creation of this space.

TRANSABDOMINAL HERNIA REPAIR

This differs from the totally extraperitoneal approach in that the preperitoneal space is entered through a transverse peritoneal incision made above the hernia defect. The abdomen is entered using either closed or open laparoscopy and two additional cannulas are placed lateral to either rectus muscle at the level of the umbilicus. These can be two 5 mm cannulas or a 5 mm and 12 mm cannula if staples are to be used. Typically, however, the use of all 5 mm ports is possible. The peritoneal incision should extend from the medial umbilical ligament medially to the level of the anterior superior iliac spine laterally. If the patient has a direct hernia it is wise to divide the medial umbilical ligament, which carries the obliterated umbilical artery (see Chapter 2) to ensure adequate exposure of the pectineal ligament and retropubic space beyond the midline.

Once the preperitoneal space has been entered, dissection is as for totally extraperitoneal hernia repair. One of the important aspects of transabdominal hernia repair is adequate closure of the peritoneum after the repair. Suturing or stapling the peritoneum can accomplish this closure effectively. Care must be used if the peritoneum is closed with the helical tacks. These devices are of such a size that it can be difficult to affect an adequate closure of the peritoneum especially if there is a paucity of preperitoneal fat. A defect left between tacks, staples or sutures forms a potential source for internal herniation of the small bowel. Any port site larger than 5 mm should be closed to prevent the development of port site hernias.

As with the totally extraperitoneal approach there are no absolute contraindications to this repair; indeed, it can be easier to perform for patients with large inguinoscrotal hernias or with extensive lower abdominal adhesions.

RESULTS

There have been many studies that have examined the efficacy of laparoscopic inguinal hernia repair compared with the various open methods that are available today. A few of these are listed in Table 15.1. In several of these papers, the methodology of data collection and patient selection make firm and accurate comparisons difficult between the series. In fact, in many cases the data cannot be compared directly. Nevertheless, as shown in these series, it appears that the rate of complications in the laparoscopic patients does not exceed that of the open patients. Additionally, the rate of recurrence is not statistically different. What is not shown in this table is the indisputable fact that the laparoscopic repair requires a general anesthetic in most cases, takes more operative time to complete and the hospital costs are more expensive. Most of these series are consistent in finding that laparoscopic patients return to normal activities and work sooner. This saving in costs to the community makes the overall costs of the laparoscopic operation less than the open operation.

While the majority of information in the literature reveals that the laparoscopic repair is associated with less pain, Picchio found that the tension-free open hernia repair is superior to the TAPP in terms of postoperative pain with no important differences in recovery.[910] This finding is in the minority, however, as most studies consistently show that pain is less with the minimally invasive approach, particularly if an objective analysis such as measured treadmill walking is used as a measure of return-to-physical-work comparing open hernia repair to laparoscopic repair. Rosen found that the laparoscopic repair offered an early advantage to the open repair by this measure.[971] This study reaffirms the clinical setting regarding the laparoscopic repair. Other reports have found similar findings regarding the lessening of postoperative pain with this repair.[709,821]

The trend in most centers around the world is for the laparoscopic repair to be limited to bilateral and recurrent inguinal hernias. The results for this indication are excellent. No recurrences were seen in one study comparing open versus laparoscopic.[1014] Another study found that the incidence of recurrence after bilateral repair was 0.6%.[1023] Felix recommends this repair for recurrent hernias following laparoscopic repair.[349]

Table 15.1 *Randomized trials of inguinal herniorrhaphy*

Author and year	Method	Median follow-up (years)	Number of hernias	Rate of complications (%)	Rate of recurrence (%)
Payne (1994)	TAPP	N/A	48	12	N/A
	Lichtenstein	–	52	18	N/A
Stoker (1994)	TAPP	0.6	75	–	0
	Lichtenstein	–	75	–	0
Maddern (1994)	TAPP	N/A	44	40	N/A
	Double darn	–	42	47	N/A
Barkun (1995)	TAPP	1.2	43	22	2.0
	Darn/Lichtenstein	–	49	12	0
Liebl (1995)	TAPP	1.3	54	N/A	0
	Shouldice	–	48	N/A	0
Lawrence (1995)	TAPP	N/A	58	12	N/A
	Darn	–	66	2	N/A
Vogt (1995)	IPOM	0.7	30	–	0
	Multiple types	–	31	–	0
Schrenk (1996)	TAPP	N/A	28	–	5.0
	TEP	–	24	–	16.7
	Shouldice	–	34	–	2.9
Liem (1997)	Open	2.0	509	–	6
	TEP	–	493	–	3
Johansson (1997)	TEP	1.7	179	–	1.0
	Open mesh	–	168	–	3.0
	Anterior repair	–	177	–	0
Champault (1997)	TEP	3.0	51	4.0	6.0
	Stoppa	–	49	29.5	2.0
Beets (1998)	TAPP	1.75	42	67	12.5
	GPRVS	–	37	62	1.9
Wellwood (1998)	TAPP	N/A	200	–	N/A
	Tension-free	–	200	–	N/A
Cohen (1998)	TAPP	N/A	78	–	1.85
	TEP	–	67	–	0
Khoury (1998)	TEP	3.0	150	–	2.5
	Plug and Patch	–	142	–	3.0
Johansson (1999)	TAPP	1.0	604	–	⎫
	Open preperitoneal mesh	–	–	–	⎬ No statistical significance
	Tissue repair	–	–	–	⎭
MRC Laparoscopic Hernia Trial Group (1999)	Laparoscopic	1.0	468	29.9	1.9
	Open	–	433	43.5	0
Lorenz (2000)	TAPP	2.0	86	11	2.3
	Shouldice	–	90	9	1.1
Sarli (2001)	TAPP	–	20	34.7	0
	Tension-free	–	23	35	4.3
Wright (2002)	TEP	5.0	149	N/A	2.0
	Tension-free	–	107	–	0
	Stoppa	–	32	–	9.4
	Sutured	–	12	–	0

IPOM, intraperitoneal onlay mesh repair (laparoscopic); TAPP, transabdominal preperitoneal repair (laparoscopic); TEP, totally extraperitoneal repair (laparoscopic).

Nevertheless, the results for primary repair are impressive. Kapris reported a 0.62% recurrence rate over a 7-year period. Past the learning curve the recurrence rate was 0.16% after 45 months. The total complication rate exclusive of recurrence was 3.68% (2% were due to urinary retention).[564]

There is little question that the laparoscopic method is more expensive in terms of operative time and equipment costs.[288] There are reports that have found that the hospital costs were less with the TAPP repair,[709] but the total of hospital and non-hospital costs were slightly less with the Shouldice operation. Beets *et al.* found that the costs associated with the giant prosthetic reinforcement of the visceral sac (GPRVS) repair were similar to that of the laparoscopic TAPP repair (US$1150 vs. US$1179).[100] Other considerations that are seldom explored are the costs to the patient and the employer. Heikkinnen *et al.* revealed that the total expenses for employed patients were lower when compared with the open repair.[488] Few similar studies have been done and, in fact, most insurers do not consider the societal costs as a benefit to any operative procedure. In Beets' report, the TAPP patients returned to work 10 days sooner than those with the GPRVS. As shown in Table 15.1, however, there were approximately six times as many recurrences with the laparoscopic procedure, but these operations were performed with relatively inexperienced surgeons.

A summary of all of these comments can be found in the follow-up report by Fingerhut at a European consensus conference.[356] This conference convened in 1994 and again in 2000. At that time, there were more than 60 clinical trials and more than 12 500 patients entered into them. The members of this conference concluded that laparoscopic inguinal repair was associated with less postoperative pain, more rapid return to normal activities but took longer to perform, was more costly and might increase the risk of rare complications. A meta-analysis of all randomized trials by the EU Hernia Trialists Collaboration Group found, in addition to the above, that laparoscopic patients had less chronic pain and numbness, while hernia recurrence was similar to that observed with open mesh repair. While some of these findings could be disputed in experienced centers, they are consistent with the current literature.

The choice between the TAPP and the TEP is merely a matter of personal preference, however. There is no clinical difference between the conversions to open, the complications seen, or the recurrence rates between these two operations in experienced hands[1163] (Table 15.2). The only difference noted in this study was that the TAPP took 32 min longer to complete than did the TEP. This was due to the need to close the peritoneal flap. This would indicate, then, that the TEP may be the more expeditious and less costly procedure based upon the operating room expenses. The MRC Trial Group did not find any clinical difference between the use of the TAPP versus the TEP operation.[821]

DISADVANTAGES OF LAPAROSCOPIC HERNIA REPAIR

One of the drawbacks of laparoscopic surgery has been the steep learning curve associated with its use. This was particularly evident in the early stages of development of the operative procedure. In large part, the surgeons that were attempting to perform this operative procedure had limited experience with the laparoscopic methodology, the laparoscopic anatomy or an adequate understanding of the need to cover the entire myopectineal orifice. As with other forms of hernia repair, recurrence rates and complications were notably higher in this learning period. Such recurrences are often not true recurrences but failure to repair the hernia in the first instance; for example, an indirect sac may be missed or inadequately reduced, mesh size may be too small or incorrectly placed. If any of these circumstances arise a persistent hernia will usually be apparent within days or weeks of the attempted repair. In a study by Liem *et al.*,[696] evaluating the learning curve for four laparoscopic surgeons inexperienced in totally extraperitoneal repair, the actuarial recurrence rate was 10% at 6 months postoperatively. Over 50% of recurrences were due to overlooking or insufficiently reducing an indirect hernia sac.

We estimate that it may take as many as 100 laparoscopic hernia repairs before an inexperienced laparoscopic surgeon can bring the operating time for laparoscopic hernia repair into a range similar to that for open hernia repair. On the other hand, the surgeon that is experienced with other advanced laparoscopic operations will take approximately 30–50 cases to build an adequate experience and a decreased operative time.[288] Since operating time is expensive this has significant cost implications. Added to this, laparoscopic hernia repair is already more costly than open repair, principally because of the use of disposable instruments. These costs, however, can be brought into a range similar to that of open repair by using reusable rather than disposable instruments and by suturing rather than stapling or tacking when indicated. A hidden cost, often not considered, is use of the laparoscopic equipment itself, which is currently less durable and more expensive than conventional instruments. These costs can be minimized by frequent use and extra care by nursing and medical staff during their use.

The relative difficulty in performing laparoscopic hernia repair using local anesthesia is often cited as a drawback of this operation. This only applies, however, when safe general anesthesia is not available at an institution. Despite its many

Table 15.2 *Complications following endoscopic hernia repair*[879]

Procedure	Number	Recurrence	Neuralgias	Testicular pain	Chronic wound pain
Transabdominal preperitoneal	1944	1%	2%	0.5%	0.3%
Totally extraperitoneal	578	0%	1%	1.5%	0.3%

proponents there is no evidence that use of local anesthetic is safer than general anesthesia for hernia repair. Edelman, however, has reported satisfactory results using local anesthesia with a laryngeal mask for the TEP compared with the open repair of inguinal hernias. Perhaps such a method may become more popular in the future.[324]

CONCLUSIONS

- Laparoscopic hernia repair is technically more demanding than open anterior approaches. This, combined with a poor knowledge of the preperitoneal anatomy by many, will limit its use to surgeons with a special interest in laparoscopic or hernia surgery.
- It has advantages in terms of reduced postoperative pain, lower wound morbidity, a more rapid return to normal activity and less chronic pain and numbness than open repair. The benefits that are realized to the individual patients can be expanded into the societal advantages because these patients are returned to the work force more rapidly.
- Many surgeons are finding this technique more beneficial for the patients with bilateral and/or recurrent hernias. These advantages need to be balanced against increased costs and a high recurrence rate in the learning curve period.
- Results from large randomized clinical trials evaluating laparoscopic hernia repair have shown it to be an effective method for the repair of the inguinal hernias.

Acknowledgement

The authors wish to acknowledge the assistance of P.J. O'Dwyer in the preparation of this chapter.

16

Femoral hernia

A femoral hernia is a protrusion of a peritoneal sac, covered with extraperitoneal fat, into the femoral sheath. The most common femoral hernia enters the femoral canal, which is that 'space' in the sheath medial to the femoral vessels as they proceed from the abdomen into the thigh. A femoral hernia sac may contain all or part of an abdominal viscus, including the ureter.[234]

Femoral hernias occur much less frequently than inguinal hernias and are more frequent in females than males. The ratio of femoral to inguinal hernias varies: figures from 1:18 to 1:8 are recorded. A round figure of 1:10 is generally accepted. The female to male ratio of femoral hernias is 4:1.[291] Male patients with femoral hernias have frequently undergone an inguinal hernia repair.[420] Femoral hernias are more frequent on the right than left side in a ratio of 2:1 and are bilateral in 1 in 15 persons. The incidence of femoral hernias in children is very low but it appears that this is twice as common in females than males.[867] In females the incidence increases with age as 42% of femoral hernias are in women aged over 65 years.[993] Femoral hernias are operated on up to eight times more frequently than inguinal hernias in female patients in the Shouldice Hospital.[108,291] In the patients that are 75 years of age or older, the incidence of femoral hernias is more than twice that of the general hernia repair population. In the elderly, emergency herniorrhaphy is necessary in 44% of the patients with femoral hernias.[453] Inguinal hernia is thus an important and difficult to make differential diagnosis of a groin swelling in a woman. In tropical Africa, femoral hernias are very rare; it is postulated that the frequency of inguinal lymphadenitis involving Cloquet's node in the femoral canal protects tropical Africans from femoral hernia.[230]

One study that evaluated the value of diagnostic laparoscopy during the repair of hernias found that the diagnosis of a femoral hernia that was present at the time of operation was unsuspected preoperatively in 11% of the 253 patients that were studied.[252] This raises several questions regarding the actual incidence of these hernias in the hernia patient population. However, even the authors felt that this high rate of a femoral component may have reflected a bias in patient selection because of the predominance of bilateral hernias in this series. Seventy-two percent of the patients with unsuspected femoral hernias had bilateral hernias, which may signify a diffuse fascial weakness as the etiology of these newly discovered hernias. The use of diagnostic laparoscopy in the pediatric patient population appears to offer benefits as well.[675] Similarly, the use of diagnostic laparoscopy for undiagnosed chronic pain can reveal unsuspected femoral hernias.[498]

The etiology of femoral hernia is poorly defined. In contrast to inguinal hernia, there is no easy embryological explanation. The fact that femoral hernias are most frequently found in middle-aged and elderly females and the disparity in incidence between parous and nulliparous women suggests that intra-abdominal pressure and the stretching of aponeurotic tissue consequent on pregnancy are important factors. Chronic cough, intestinal obstruction, constipation and excessive physical labor may also contribute to raised intra-abdominal pressure. Weight loss in the elderly female is also associated with femoral hernia. Nurses are said to be more prone to femoral hernia. Ten percent of femoral hernias follow a previous operation for an inguinal hernia; indeed, femoral hernias in men almost always occur after an operation for an inguinal hernia.[420,915]

A very rare congenital femoral hernia in males is associated with descent of the testicle through the femoral canal into the thigh. Four well-documented cases are recorded in the literature. Absence of the ipsilateral testicle from the scrotum and an incompletely reducible femoral hernia should arouse suspicion.[1091]

ANATOMY

Femoral hernia has a sinister reputation because of the unyielding anatomy of the femoral canal. The whole canal (i.e. the space between the pubis and the iliopsoas muscle) is bounded anteriorly by the inguinal ligament, posteriorly by the pectineal (Cooper's) ligament at its attachment to the iliopectineal line of the pubic bone, medially by the sharp lateral margin of the lacunar ligament and laterally by the iliopsoas muscle with its overlying fascia (Figure 16.1).

The canal is divided into two compartments, the lateral being occupied by the femoral artery and femoral vein, and the smaller medial by areolar tissue, some lymphatics and a lymph node. The femoral vessels are encased in the femoral sheath of fascia transversalis. Anteriorly the sheath is continuous with

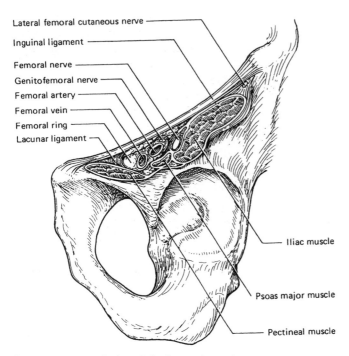

Figure 16.1 *Boundaries of the femoral canal.*

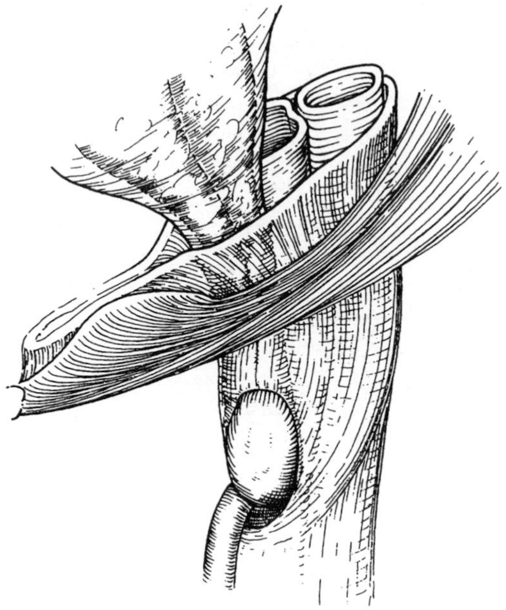

Figure 16.2 *Anatomy of a femoral hernia. The hernial sac progresses down the femoral sheath 'funnel' to present in the thigh. In the thigh the fundus of the hernia carries the attenuated cribiform fascia before it.*

the fascia transversalis deep to the inguinal ligament; posteriorly the femoral sheath fuses with the pectineal ligament. The sheath extends into the thigh. From the abdomen the sheath resembles a funnel extending down to the fossa ovalis where the saphenous vein penetrates the cribriform fascia (anteroinferior femoral sheath). It is through this small medial compartment or funnel that the usual femoral hernia penetrates into the thigh.[376,719,1238]

Once in the thigh the sac pushes anteriorly onto the relatively weak cribriform fascia – the anterior femoral sheath that surrounds the fossa ovalis opening for the saphenous vein. It carries the stretched cribriform fascia before it and bulges into the thigh. The fundus is then forced upwards to lie over the inguinal ligament. Two factors combine to make it turn superiorly: these are fusion of the femoral sheath with the deep fascia of the thigh and the repeated flexion of the hip joint (Figure 16.2).[719] Because of the upward turn towards the inguinal ligament the femoral hernia can be misdiagnosed as an inguinal hernia.

In its advancement into the thigh the hernial sac carries with it some extraperitoneal fat about its fundus and it may draw the extraperitoneal anterolateral wall of the bladder down with it on its medial aspect. Once the sac is entrenched in the thigh, the medial wall of the hernia, consisting of peritoneal sac, extraperitoneal fat and fascia transversalis, is pressed up against the sharp margin of the lacunar ligament medially, the unyielding pectineal fascia and pubic bone posteriorly, the inguinal ligament anteriorly and the femoral vein laterally. As the hernia emerges from the saphenous opening the sharp upper margin of the cribriform fascia also contributes to the structuring of the sac.[11,1238]

The compression of the sac leads to fibrosis in it at its neck so that it constricts any contents, omentum or intestine. This

stricturing of the sac neck is an important factor in the mechanism of strangulation. Very often, the strictured sac neck is the confining structure in a strangulated hernia rather than the lacunar or pectineal ligaments.

Compression of the femoral vein and the saphenous vein by a femoral hernia may occur; indeed, visible distension of these veins is a diagnostic sign in the differential diagnosis of a femoral hernia from other groin swellings. Saphenous vein distension is particularly pronounced in cases when the femoral hernia has progressed through the cribriform fascia into the thigh and in doing so has compromised the saphenous vein at its termination into the femoral vein.[392]

DIFFERENTIAL DIAGNOSIS

This subject is discussed in Chapter 11.

MANAGEMENT OF FEMORAL HERNIAS

Operation should always be advised, for two reasons:

1 It is impossible to make and fit an adequate truss to control such a hernia.
2 The incidence of strangulation in these hernias is high. Many femoral hernias occur in elderly women, and a strangulated femoral hernia in the elderly woman carries a considerable morbidity.

Many femoral hernias present with incarceration or strangulation. The ratio of elective to emergent operations for these hernias varies anywhere from 1.3:1 or 1.5:1 to 5:1.[294,495,391] In some other reports, the emergent cases outnumbered the elective ones by 10:1.[1128] The ratio of elective to emergent femoral hernias compared to that of inguinal hernias is approximately 6.4:1.[401] In other words, the need for an emergent operation for a femoral hernia is over six times greater than that of an inguinal hernia. The female patients incur 76.7% of the incidence of strangulated femoral hernias than the male patients.[495] In this latter series, the frequency of strangulation of femoral hernias was 43% (versus only 5% of inguinal hernias) but others have reported an incidence of 50%.[879] This demonstrates the need to repair all of these hernias when the diagnosis is made. Additionally, there is an increased frequency of co-morbidities in the elderly patients thereby making the non-elective operations more risky.[847]

When a patient presents with intestinal obstruction and a femoral hernia, if the hernia is not tender and therefore not strangulated, reduction by taxis may be employed in the short term. But if there is any local tenderness, suggesting that strangulation has occurred, taxis should not be employed. A partial enterocele (Richter's hernia) is common in femoral hernias. These patients may have confusing symptoms and signs; a high index of diagnostic suspicion should always be maintained. Urgent operation after adequate resuscitation and cardiorespiratory management in elderly shocked patients needs emphasizing.

Tingwald and Cooperman (1982) have emphasized the problems presented by the elderly with groin hernias.[1128] Due to the increased risk of postoperative complications, some surgeons are becoming increasingly reluctant to perform elective procedures on these patients.[264] However, with femoral hernias delay only increases the likelihood of incarceration, and then emergency surgery in a more ill patient will be required. Elective repair of a femoral hernia is an urgency; these patients are at considerable hazard of strangulation if they have to wait for surgery. The National Confidential Enquiry in England has repeatedly warned of the high mortality of emergency surgery for strangulated femoral hernias in the female.[155,837] All these facts are confirmed by the most recent series from North Tees; the coexisting medical morbidities in the emergency cases included respiratory disease, chronic obstructive airways disease (19%), coronary artery disease (40%), neurological disease (10%) and diabetes mellitus in 8%. The morbidity following emergency operation was also higher than elective operation, with pulmonary embolism occurring only in the emergency cases.[847]

OPERATIVE APPROACHES TO FEMORAL HERNIA

A femoral hernia is a variety of groin hernia – a defect in the fascia transversalis which is exploited by a peritoneal sac traversing the muscular weakness of the myopectineal orifice of Fruchaud – exactly similar to a patent processus vaginalis in an indirect inguinal hernia exploiting the deep ring in the fascia transversalis posterior wall of the inguinal canal, or a direct hernia peritoneal sac expanding into an acquired defect of the fascia transversalis. This being so, repair of a femoral hernia inexorably follows the same canons of repair as an inguinal hernia repair. Isolate and excise the peritoneal sac, repair the fascia transversalis defect and then reinforce this repair by adjusting the local aponeurotic attachments.

In sequence, a femoral hernia occurs when the femoral sheath, a funnel of fascia transversalis enclosing the femoral vessels beneath the inguinal ligament, becomes dilated. A peritoneal sac enters the femoral funnel and then, as a plunger, causes it to dilate. As the fascia transversalis pushes onto the ligament it becomes scarred and often strictured around its neck, and in doing so pushes the attachment of the transversus abdominis aponeurosis medially along the pectineal line until the medial margin of the femoral sheath abuts on the inguinal ligament anteriorly, the lacunar ligament medially and the pectineal ligament posteriorly. After excision of the peritoneal sac, the femoral sheath must be repaired medially and the hernioplasty must prevent further herniation; to do this, the attachment of the fascia transversalis to the pectineal ligament must be broadened. This reconstruction of the medial femoral sheath can be reinforced by suturing the tendon of transversus abdominis to the pectineal line (McVay/Cooper's ligament repair) or from below by turning up a flap of pectineus fascia to close the medial femoral canal or finally by plugging it with a mesh prosthesis.[82,778]

As an alternative, the entire operation can be conducted in the extraperitoneal (preperitoneal layer) and a mesh repair of the canal constructed in this layer.[1098,1188]

Eponyms really confuse the surgeon here and are best discarded temporarily. Three approaches that apply a tissue repair to femoral hernioplasty are described; because none of these is universally applicable, the surgeon must be acquainted with all three:

1 The abdominal,[1114] suprapubic,[615] retropubic,[1180] preperitoneal[854] or extraperitoneal[207,494,1098] operation. This approach, developed by Henry, is often known as the McEvedy approach, although Henry used a midline incision and McEvedy a para-rectus incision.[770] A Pfannenstiel incision enables bilateral hernias to be operated simultaneously by this approach. (Eponyms: Cheatle,[207] Henry,[494] McEvedy.[770])
2 The inguinal or 'high' operation. (Eponyms: Annandale,[37] Lotheissen,[711] Moschowitz.[816])
3 The crural or 'low' operation. (Eponyms: Bassini,[89] Lockwood.[702])

The open extraperitoneal approach gives excellent access to the femoral canal and to the general peritoneal cavity should that be necessary to deal with a strangulated viscus. However, this approach to the pelvis is unfamiliar to most surgeons and, therefore, not to be recommended to the inexperienced surgeon operating on his first strangulated femoral hernia at the dead of night.[856]

The open inguinal approach is familiar, but has the twin drawbacks of disrupting the inguinal canal mechanism and not providing adequate access to a strangulated viscus. If this approach is used, an excellent repair of the fascia transversalis (Shouldice technique) must be employed to avoid the complicating inguinal hernia. This is particularly so in women, in whom direct inguinal hernia is almost unknown … except as a complication of this operation.

The open crural approach to the femoral sac is good and bloodless, and repair of the hernia is easy by this method. Its most significant disadvantage is that access to a strangulated viscus is often very inadequate. The crural approach is recommended for elective operation and to the occasional or novice surgeon. This is the quickest and least traumatic operation to perform.[321,847,1123] If a visceral strangulation is present it is best to perform either a lower midline or Pfannenstiel incision and deal with the crisis through an incision which is familiar to most abdominal operators. With an emergency situation, or for the inexperienced surgeon, this is no place for an anatomical extravaganza.

THE 'LOW' OR CRURAL OPERATION

Preoperative management

In the uncomplicated case no special preoperative management is required. The bladder is frequently a sliding component of the medial wall of a femoral hernia, and preoperative catheterization is a sensible precaution, which will lessen the likelihood of bladder injury.

If the hernia is strangulated or obstructed, preoperative nasogastric aspiration and adequate fluid replacement is mandatory. The patient must be fully resuscitated and co-morbidities, especially in the elderly, adequately managed.

Anesthesia

General anesthesia is preferred, but local anesthesia can be employed. Local infiltration with extra injection around the sac neck will suffice.

THE OPERATION

Position of the patient

The patient is placed supine on the operating table, which is tilted head down 15°.

DRAPING

If the hernia is not strangulated, draping to allow access to the groin only is required. If strangulation or obstruction is present or suspected, towels should be placed to enable easy access to the lower abdomen if a laparotomy becomes necessary. A sterile adhesive drape can be used.

The incision

A skin incision is made over the hernia. The incision is about 6 cm long and parallel to the inguinal ligament.

After the skin is divided, it is easy to separate the subcutaneous fat down to the coverings of the hernia sac. Hemostasis should be secured before the sac is mobilized.

Mobilization of sac

The sac, having emerged from the femoral canal, carries before it fascia transversalis and extraperitoneal fat in front of which is the attenuated cribriform fascia and the femoral fascial layer of the thigh. Because of these fascial layers, the sac usually makes a forward upward turn in its path at the fossa ovalis; thus its fundus will be found lying over the inguinal ligament. It is important to appreciate this before mobilization is attempted. Once the sac is identified, the fascial layers are cleaned from it by blunt dissection, which is best achieved by breaking up the adherent scar tissue and fat with a hemostat and then wiping the fascia off with a gauze swab. These extraperitoneal coverings of the sac are frequently quite thick and fibrosed and are most often the real constricting layer when strangulation has occurred (Figure 16.3).

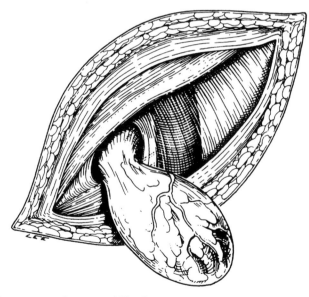

Figure 16.3 *The sac mobilized.*

Identification of femoral opening

The neck of the sac is now cleared of fat and fascia so that the boundaries of the femoral canal can be identified. It is best to identify the medial and anterior margins of the canal first. The medial margin is the lacunar ligament and is easily seen as it sweeps around from the inguinal ligament to the subjacent pubic bone. Anteriorly, the rolled-over edge of the inguinal ligament can readily be separated from the sac underneath it. The sac should next be lifted up. The fascia on the pectineus muscle is easily recognizable and if this is traced back to the ramus of the pubis, the posterior margin of the canal – the pectineal ligament – can be recognized.

Attention is now turned to the lateral boundary of the canal – the femoral vein. This is the most vulnerable structure in this area and is difficult to identify because it is covered with a quite opaque fascial sheath. One maneuver is to identify the femoral artery by touch; the artery lies immediately lateral to the vein so the vein must be in any space between the sac and the palpable artery. A careful dissection is made on the lateral side of the sac, preferably using Metzenbaum scissors and keeping close to the sac. The dissection of the sac is only complete when the entire circumference of its neck has been clearly defined (Figure 16.4).

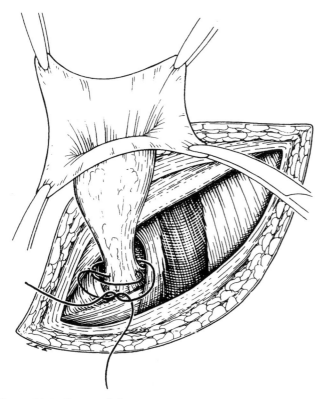

Figure 16.4 *Closure of the sac.*

Inspection of contents of sac

The lateral side of the fundus of the sac should now be opened. The medial side should be avoided, as it may be partly formed by the bladder. There is always much adherent extraperitoneal fat on the fundus which generally contains many distended veins. If these bleed they can confuse the anatomy, so the fat should be gently broken through with a hemostat point and the bleeding carefully controlled.

Inside the extraperitoneal fat the true peritoneal hernia sac will be found. It is grasped in a hemostat and then opened.

Any contents of the sac can now be gently freed, adhesions divided and the contents reduced back into the general peritoneal cavity. If strangulation is present, an alternative approach to the remainder of the operation may be necessary. Often a small nubbin of strangulated dead omentum may be

discovered; this should be isolated, its blood supply ligated, and then excised.

Closure and excision of sac

When it is certain that the neck of the sac is isolated and that the sac is empty, it can be closed and excised. Traction is applied to the open sac and, using metric 3.5 braided absorbable polymer on a 40 mm round needle (0 or 00 suture on a soft-tissue needle), a transfixion suture should be securely tied around the neck. The redundant sac is cut off, leaving a generous cuff beyond the transfixion suture. The stump of the sac will now recede through the femoral canal and out of sight (Figure 16.5).

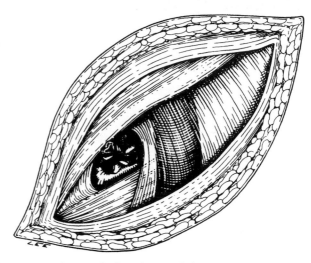

Figure 16.5 *The canal after closure of the sac.*

Repair of canal

The canal is repaired using a single figure-of-eight suture of metric 3 (0 or 00) polypropylene (or other non-absorbable suture) on a J-shaped (or round) needle.

The femoral vein is retracted laterally and the pectineal ligament clearly identified on the superior ramus of the pubic bone. The first suture is placed through this ligament from its deep aspect at the point where the medial margin of the femoral vein would lie if it were not retracted. It is necessary to experiment with the retractor and identify this point correctly. If the suture is placed too far laterally the vein will be compromised, and if placed too far medially the repair will be unsound (Figure 16.6).

The next bite must pick up the inguinal ligament and iliopubic tract of fascia transversalis at a corresponding distance from its pubic attachment, so that the suture forms the base of an isosceles triangle. Next, the pectineal ligament is picked up, again from deep to superficial, halfway between the first pectineal suture and the lacunar ligament and finally the inguinal ligament is picked up, again halfway between the first suture and the attachment of the ligament to the pubis.

Now the free end of the suture is passed deep to the two loops and the two ends are tied securely. When the suture is

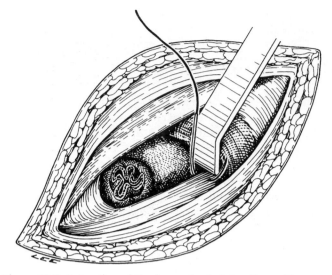

Figure 16.6 *Retraction of the femoral vein laterally enables visualization of the pectineal (Cooper's) ligament. The first suture is not introduced.*

pulled tight, the medial 0.75 cm or so of the inguinal ligament will be approximated to the pectineal line and the femoral canal closed. Furthermore, if the knot is placed at the medial side, it will be away from the femoral vein which will not be damaged by it (Figure 16.7).

Comment on crural operation

Although the primary defect is in the fascia transversalis at the wide part of the femoral canal (the open funnel), this operation does not primarily address itself to this defect. This is the major negative feature of the operation. The fascia transversalis is, inevitably, tangled up when the sac is originally closed, the stump of sac and extraperitoneal fat blocks the medial part of the funnel, the attachment of the inguinal ligament to the pectineal ligament reduces the potential size of the femoral canal.

The skin and subcutaneous tissues are closed as before. If the dissection has been difficult, or if there is much 'dead space', a drain should be used. Disadvantages of the 'low' approach, which are important in obstructed patients, are as follows:

- Difficulty in delivering obstructed bowel for review. This is most relevant in Richter's hernia (partial enterocele) where the involved loop is especially liable to slip back into the abdomen and be irretrievable.
- It is impossible to put an anastomosis, which is bulky, back into the abdomen through the femoral canal. A separate laparotomy is needed if bowel resection is necessary. This may lead to contamination of the main peritoneal cavity unless great care is taken.
- The crural operation provides inadequate exposure if there is difficulty reducing and mobilizing the contents of a hernial sac.
- It can be difficult to excise a thickened fibrous sac down to flush with the parietal peritoneum.

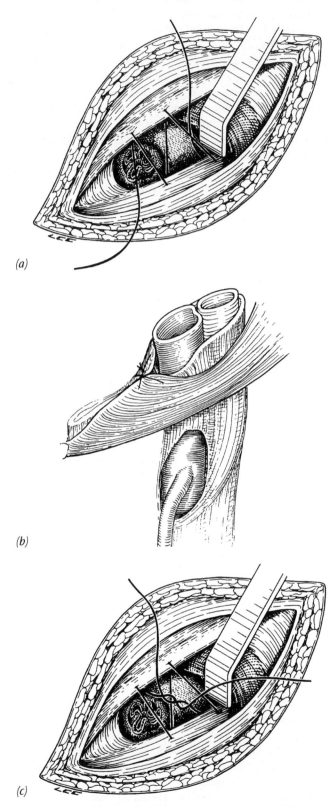

(a)

(b)

(c)

Figure 16.7 *(a, b) The next suture picks up the inguinal ligament and subjacent iliopubic tract of fascia transversalis. Care must be taken to avoid the cord structures in the wall. The suture is placed to form the base of an isosceles triangle with the apex at the pubic tubercle. (c) The knot is tied deeply at the medial side away from the femoral vein.*

- In longstanding hernias, access for an adequate repair is limited.

INGUINAL OPERATION

This operation achieves the same objective of closing the medial portion of the femoral canal which has been described using the crural approach. However, in the inguinal approach the femoral canal is exposed by opening the posterior wall – the fascia transversalis – of the inguinal canal and achieving initial closure, using the fascia transversalis, of the femoral cone. Approximating the inguinal to the pectineal ligaments, if the inguinal ligament is grossly stretched, can reinforce this repair.

The incision and dissection for this operation are exactly the same as those employed in the Shouldice operation for inguinal hernia. After the fascia transversalis in the posterior wall of the inguinal canal has been opened, the extraperitoneal fat on the neck of the femoral hernia can be identified and removed by blunt dissection (Figure 16.8).

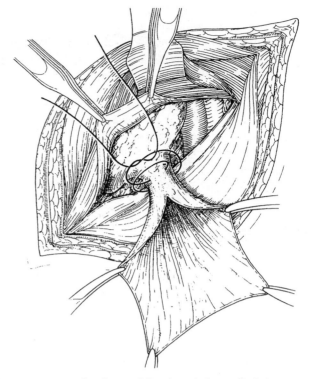

Figure 16.9 *Transfixation and ligation of the neck of the sac.*

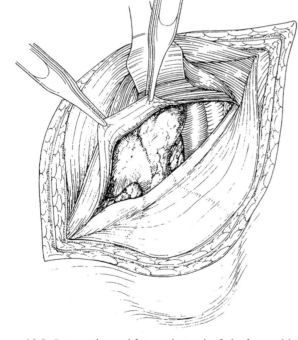

Figure 16.8 *Extraperitoneal fat on the neck of the femoral hernia can be identified and removed by blunt dissection.*

The sac can now either be delivered above the inguinal ligament or opened below the ligament and its contents reduced. The neck of the sac is then transfixed and ligated (Figure 16.9).

The medial extremity of the inguinal ligament is now sutured to the pectineal ligament by figure-of-eight non-absorbable sutures. In this instance, care must be taken to insure that the deep closure does not impinge upon the femoral vein. In this operation these are inserted from above, that is through the incision in the posterior wall of the inguinal canal.

The inguinal canal is then repaired using the Shouldice (or Bassini) technique, care being taken to reinforce the femoral repair with the overlapped fascia transversalis at the medial part of the canal. It is advisable, particularly in women with a broad pelvis, to reinforce the medial repair by suturing the insertion of the transversus muscle tendon (conjoint tendon) to the pectineal ligament (Cooper's ligament repair).

Comment on inguinal operation

The inguinal approach for the repair of femoral hernia is not recommended as the operation of choice because it is technically more difficult and more time consuming than the crural operation and because it disrupts an otherwise normal inguinal canal.

However, some experts, notably Tanner in Britain[1116] and Glasgow in Canada,[419] recommend this operation strongly. If this approach is used, the repair of the transversalis/transversus layer to the pectineal ligament must be adequate and must extend the tendinous attachment of the transversus muscle laterally along the pectineal ligament as far as the femoral vein. Often, to do this without tension, a generous 'medial slide' of the lateral rectus sheath/conjoint tendon must be made.

EXTRAPERITONEAL (PREPERITONEAL) OPERATION

This operation illustrates the genius of an expert surgical anatomist exploiting fascial plane dissection at its most elegant.

Henry's extraperitoneal approach to the anterior pelvis gives an excellent exposure of both femoral canals simultaneously, but it is not an operation for the novice. In the hands of an expert it is a fine operation enabling bilateral femoral hernia to be dealt with simultaneously through one incision.[34,494]

The patient is placed on the operating table and the bladder emptied by catheterization. A vertical midline suprapubic incision is made, the aponeurotic layer is opened vertically in the midline and the peritoneum exposed.

Alternatively, a Pfannenstiel incision, with a supra-pubic side-to-side opening of the anterior rectus sheath and separation of the rectus muscles, gives good access and a much more acceptable skin scar.

The recti are retracted to either side and the space between the peritoneum and the abdominal wall muscles is opened by gentle blunt dissection in order to approach the femoral canal on either side. If only a unilateral hernia is present a pararectal vertical (McEvedy)[770] or skin crease (Ogilvie)[864] incision can be used.

Femoral sacs are dealt with by reduction of their contents, transfixion of their necks and resection of redundant sac (Figure 16.10). If strangulation is present, the subjacent peritoneum can easily be opened, the contents of the sac inspected, and so forth (Figure 16.11).

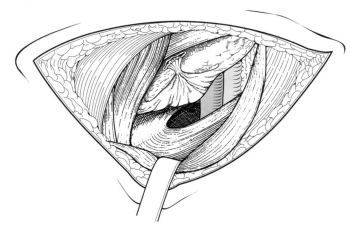

Figure 16.10 *An adequate approach to a unilateral hernia can be made through an oblique or vertical pararectus incision.*

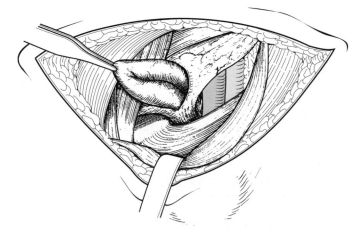

Figure 16.11 *Opening a femoral hernial sac.*

The femoral canal is repaired using a non-absorbable suture, as described in the inguinal operation. The anterior abdominal wall is closed layer by layer.

Comment on extraperitoneal operation

The extraperitoneal operation has advantages, but also disadvantages:

- An extensive mobilization of the lower abdominal wall is required.
- It cannot easily be performed using local anesthesia.
- With mobilization there is a risk of bleeding and hematoma formation between the peritoneum and the endopelvic fascia.
- Unless an adequate repair of the abdominal wall is made, an abdominal incisional hernia can ensue.

THE THREE OPEN APPROACHES

The femoral hernia surgeon should ideally be familiar with all three approaches:

1 The low approach is recommended for the easily reducible uncomplicated femoral hernia especially in the thin patient, and in the frail ASA class 3 or 4 patient, when it can be undertaken electively using local anesthesia.
2 The inguinal approach is best used when there is a concomitant primary inguinal hernia on the same side which can be repaired simultaneously.
3 The extraperitoneal approach is used when obstruction or strangulation are present, in patients who have undergone previous groin surgery, when inguinal and femoral hernias occur together, and in bilateral cases where both sides can be repaired simultaneously.[34,1180]

OPEN PROSTHETIC REPAIR

The above tissue repairs are becoming much less common in the developed nations of the world. The use of prosthetic biomaterials is becoming the preferred method. This is especially true for recurrent repairs in which the recurrence rate is 22% as reported by the Shouldice Clinic in Toronto, Canada. Approximately 20% of primary and 50% of recurrent femoral hernias are repaired with mesh at that institution.[201] Other retrospective studies have identified a reduction in the rate of recurrence from 2–10% to 0–1.1% with the use of prosthetic biomaterials.[108,111] The choice of the mesh prosthetic is somewhat limited when compared to those available for the repair of inguinal hernias (see Chapter 7). The choice of the Shouldice Clinic is the use of a flat mesh that extends from Cooper's ligament to under the internal oblique muscle.

The use of the Kugel patch for the repair of femoral hernias is known to the authors. There are no reports in the literature that provide any information that verify its usefulness for this hernia operation. Long-term follow-up data is also lacking.

Plug-and-patch

The concept of the plug-and-patch repair is based upon the prior 'umbrella plug' and 'dart' repairs of the inguinal hernia. The development of the preformed plug for the inguinal hernia repair has resulted in its use for the femoral hernia. The open approach to the femoral hernia is similar to that of the inguinal approach above or one can use the femoral approach directly. The inguinal incision does have the advantage of an easier inspection of the entire inguinofemoral area should the preoperative diagnosis be anatomically incorrect.

The sac will be identified and the neck dissected accordingly. In this repair, unlike the tissue repairs described above, the sac is not ligated. The dissection is carried into the preperitoneal space so that the neck of the sac is also dissected. This is necessary so that the sac can be fully imbricated into the preperitoneal space. If this is not carried out satisfactorily, there will be a higher risk of recurrence. After this dissection is completed the defect is then filled with the plug. It is important that the inner petals of the plug are removed so that the plug will fill this area with ease, as it is usually too firm to be placed into this site as manufactured. This can result in a permanently palpable mass effect at the site of the former femoral hernia site. Additionally, there is a risk of causing a relative area of venous obstruction as the plug may occupy too much space and impinge upon the femoral vein.

It is important to fixate the plug after it is positioned in the defect. Several absorbable sutures are required such as polyglactin[104] (Figure 16.12). This will prevent the migration

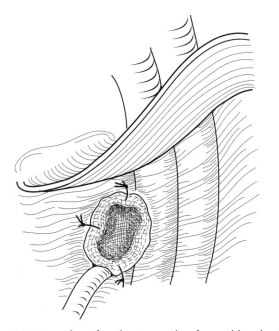

Figure 16.12 *Insertion of a plug to repair a femoral hernia. Note that all the internal petals of the plug have been removed to allow its insertion.*

that has been reported with the use of the plug. The scarification that will eventuate will secure the plug and repair the hernia defect. The closure of the subcutaneous tissue and skin will usually be performed with an absorbable suture.

There have been few reports in the published literature regarding the use of the plug and patch in the repair of femoral hernias. Because of the very nature of the infrequency of the femoral hernia, the numbers of patients have always been small. One of these early reports included only 24 cases and represented less than 1% of the patients in that series. There were no apparent complications or recurrences in these few patients.[994] Other reports have shown similar results.[401,997]

Laparoscopic femoral hernia repair

The repair of the femoral hernia with the laparoscopic placement of a preperitoneal mesh is identical to the transabdominal preperitoneal or the totally extraperitoneal inguinal operations. These are described in Chapter 15. There is no difference in technique because the exposure of the myopectineal orifice by these two procedures will provide an excellent visualization of the femoral hernia. The identified sac and the frequently encountered prevascular fat will easily be reduced by the laparoscopic approach. It is important to carefully inspect the femoral hernia so that any incarcerated fat will be identified and removed. These defects can be quite small and this could sometimes be overlooked. Any associated inguinal hernias could also be identified at that time.

The repair would proceed as would the chosen inguinal repair but one should ensure that the prosthetic mesh is of sufficient size to provide an adequate coverage of the entire inguinal and femoral areas. It is critical that this mesh provides enough overlap to prevent the presentation of an inguinal hernia in the future postoperative period.

Unfortunately, because the repair of femoral hernias with the laparoscopic method is identical to that of the inguinal hernia repair, most series do not differentiate between the two herniorrhaphies. The actual incidence of isolated femoral hernia repair with the laparoscope may be 1.5% but the identification of an additional 13.7% of unsuspected femoral hernias in this series suggests that there may be a significant number of 'missed' hernias during the anterior approach to inguinal herniorrhaphy.[574]

The postoperative care of the patient will be similar to that of the inguinal hernia repair patients. As can occur with the latter group, the site of the prior herniation can frequently fill with seromatous fluid and continue to present as a mass at the site of the former hernia. This is so common that this should be explained to the patient preoperatively to avert the concern that will be forthcoming if this had not been addressed in the office.

STRANGULATION

Strangulation is very uncommon in patients aged under 40 years old. Strangulation is more frequent in females than males and reaches its highest incidence and greatest morbidity in women in their seventh and eighth decades.

If strangulation is suspected, it is more prudent to avoid the laparoscopic repair. The surgeon does have the option to initiate the procedure with the TEP method to inspect the bowel if the suspicion is that of incarceration without strangulation. Should bowel infarction become manifest; the surgeon could then perform a midline incision to resect the non-viable bowel. The TEP approach would have prevented entry into the abdominal cavity so that contamination would be avoided. In the majority of patients, however, the laparoscopic approach will not ever be a reasonable possibility so that the sac should be approached as described below. Once the sac is identified it will be seen to contain bloodstained fluid if strangulation has occurred.

The sac should be opened on the lateral aspect of its fundus and the contents inspected. A variety of intra-abdominal viscera may be found in the femoral hernia sac. Waddington, in 1971, reviewed 128 patients with strangulated femoral hernia; the most frequently strangulated viscera were, in rank order, small bowel, then small bowel and omentum, then omentum alone, then appendix, colon, bladder and lastly fallopian tube.[1174] No viscus should be returned to the peritoneal cavity unless it is definitely viable. Viability of any viscus can only be assessed after its blood supply has been normalized by removing the constriction at the neck of the sac.

Any bloodstained fluid in the sac is sampled for microbiological culture and the remainder sucked out. The contents of the sac are gently manipulated so that the neck of the sac is revealed clearly. It is very important to be careful with a strangulated loop of gut, as operative perforation can seriously hazard the patient's recovery. Quite frequently, careful dissection of the neck of the sac and removal of edematous extraperitoneal fat about it are all that is required to release the strangulation. The constricting agent is usually the thickened transversalis fascia and peritoneal neck of the sac and the edematous extraperitoneal fat about it, rather than the ligamentous structures which form the anterior, posterior and medial margins of the sac. The femoral vein is very rarely involved in the strangulation process, which confirms that the neck of the sac itself is most usually the constricting agent.

When the sac has been opened, the inguinal ligament can generally be retracted upwards and the femoral vein laterally so that the neck of the sac can be divided.

After the strangulation has been released, any contained viscera are wrapped in warm saline packs and left alone for a full 5 min before being inspected. Omentum of doubtful viability is best excised. Small intestine must only be returned to the peritoneal cavity if it has all been inspected and shown to be vital. Often there is a linear necrosis of the bowel where it has been compressed by the neck of the sac; this should be oversewn.

If a considerable segment of gangrenous small bowel needs resection, more gut is prolapsed into the wound. Alternatively, if there is technical difficulty, a lower midline incision can be made and bowel resected through the groin wound (to avoid contamination of the peritoneal cavity). Anastomosis is then carried out through the main peritoneal cavity. It is worth stressing the importance of not contaminating the main

peritoneal cavity and not returning non-viable bowel into it. The use of a lower midline incision for all cases of difficulty is strongly recommended.

Waddington recommends the low, crural, approach and this was used in 119 of his 128 cases. In only one out of 14 patients needing a bowel resection and anastomosis was a paramedian incision needed for supplementing peritoneal cavity access.[1174]

Wheeler (1975) reports typical results for the UK from the University Hospital, Cardiff. In an 11-year study period (1963–1973), 78 patients underwent a total of 80 operations for femoral hernia. In 44 instances the operations were for acute strangulation; the remaining 36 operations were elective.[1207]

In the Cardiff series, three approaches were used – the low approach gave the least recurrences, whereas the inguinal (high) and the extraperitoneal (preperitoneal) using a midline incision approaches were the least satisfactory (Table 16.1). The choice of the high approach in strangulation is interesting; this choice confirms 'traditional' British teaching that the high approach offers advantages if resection is necessary. On the other hand, the poor results with the inguinal approach demand unfavorable comparison with other series in which this approach has given excellent results.

Table 16.1 *Femoral hernia operations undertaken at Cardiff, 1963–1973* (after Wheeler, 1975)*

Procedure	No. operations	No. recurrences	Percentage recurrence
Abdominal pararectal incision (McEvedy)	32 (20)	4	12.5
Midline (Cheatle)	3 (2)	1	33.3
Inguinal (Lotheissen)	7 (3)	3	43.0
Crural (Bassini)	23 (7)	1	4.4

* Figures in parentheses indicate emergency procedures for strangulation.

The more recent series from Stockton-on-Tees represents English district surgical practice in the 11 years 1976–1987; during this period 145 patients (38 male, 107 female) with 146 hernias (99 right, 47 left) underwent femoral hernia repair. In the elective group all but one patient had been aware of the lump for over a month before surgery, in contrast to the emergency group in which 27 (43%) had been aware of the lump for over one month. The most significant difference between the emergency and elective groups was age: 43 (68%) of patients in the emergency group were aged over 65 years compared with only 25 (30%) of those having an elective operation ($P < 0.0001$). Both groups had similar incidences of coexisting medical pathology. The preferred operation technique was the low crural (Bassini–Lockwood) operation. There were no deaths in the elective group but five in the emergency group – an overall death rate of 3.4% (8% in the emergency group). The morbidity was also significantly higher in the emergency group. The most common cause of death was pulmonary embolism. At a median follow-up of 5 years, five patients had a recurrence (3.4%). Three of the recurrences were direct inguinal hernias after the use of the inguinal operation.[848]

This study highlighted the problems of patients who delay in seeking medical advice and the difficulties general practitioners have in making a correct diagnosis of femoral hernia, only 35% of femoral hernias were correctly diagnosed by general practitioners in this series.[847]

Ponka and Brush report that the crural low repair gives the fewest recurrences in their experience.[916] Likewise, Duvie from West Africa reports that the low approach gives a low recurrence rate (0%), a shorter operation time and postoperative stay – although it must be commented that this report was of a very small study with no recurrences in either the 'high' or the 'low' group.[321]

UNUSUAL VARIANTS OF FEMORAL HERNIA

So far we have considered the commonest variety of femoral hernia; there are, however, six rare variants, all of which pass from the abdomen into the thigh through the space bounded anteriorly by the inguinal ligament, posteriorly by the pectineal ligament and the origin of the pectineus muscle, medially by the lacunar ligament and laterally by the fusion of the femoral sheath (fascia transversalis) with the iliac investing fascia. These variants are:

- The hernia associated with maldescent of the testis through the femoral canal (cruroscrotal hernia). This is discussed on page 217.
- The prevascular hernia (Narath's hernia), in which the sac emerges from the abdomen within the femoral sheath but lies anteriorly to the femoral vein and artery. This hernia can be either medial or lateral to the deep epigastric vessels. Narath described this condition associated with congenital dislocation of the hip. He reported six hernias in four patients, each hernia appearing on the same side as the dislocated hip (there were two bilateral cases). Importantly, the hernias did not appear until after the dislocations were reduced by manipulation. The same condition has been described as a complication of an innominate osteotomy for congenital dislocation of the hip.[1010] Similar hernias develop in adults after previous

groin surgery or after vascular operations on the external iliac vessels. Repair by an extraperitoneal approach is recommended.[249,835]

- When the neck of the sac lies lateral to the femoral vessels – the external femoral hernia of Hesselbach and Cloquet.[225,502]
- The transpectineal ligament femoral hernia when the sac traverses the pectineal part of the inguinal ligament and lacunar ligament (Laugier's hernia).[639]
- When the sac descends deep to the femoral vessels and pectineal fascia (Callisen's or Cloquet's hernia).[172]
- When the sac, instead of progressing anteriorly and superiorly through the cribriform fascia, proceeds into the thigh deep to the investing fascia – this hernia is always multilocular and may be mistaken for an obturator hernia. A variant described by Astley Cooper in 1804 and sometimes referred to as Cooper's hernia.[238]

All these variants are best managed using either the extraperitoneal mesh prosthetic operation described in Chapter 14 or the laparoscopic methods described in Chapter 15.

CONCLUSIONS

- Femoral hernia is a common clinical problem, which warrants urgent elective repair to avoid the complication of strangulation. Strangulated femoral hernia carries a high morbidity and mortality in the elderly.
- The mechanism of femoral herniation, a distension and failure of the fascia transversalis in the femoral sheath, is described.
- Methods of repair are outlined – the low, crural, operation is the least traumatic open operation and gives the lower recurrence rate. The laparoscopic method has proven to be a viable alternative to the surgeon that is proficient with that technique.
- The crural operation is not suitable in multiple hernias or when resection of gut is required.
- In these circumstances, the surgeon must have the ability to perform the appropriate operation for the patient. The options include a formal laparotomy, or either the extraperitoneal or inguinal operations as described above. Laparoscopy is well-suited for the patient with multiple hernias, bilateral hernias or a recurrent femoral herniation.

17

Umbilical hernia in adults

EPIDEMIOLOGY AND PATHOLOGY

Umbilical hernias in adults can be a cause of considerable morbidity and if complications supervene they can lead to death. Umbilical hernias are much less frequent in the adult population than inguinal hernias (see Table 3.2). Umbilical hernias account for 0.03% of the hernia operations performed in the UK. Of the patients with umbilical hernias, 90% are women, invariably women who are overweight and multiparous. There is no racial predisposition to adult umbilical hernias.[542] Umbilical hernias have a high risk of incarceration.[533] When these hernias incarcerate and strangulate, they frequently contain transverse colon and/or stomach. Strangulated umbilical hernias have a considerable morbidity,[533] a morbidity dictated by the age of the patient and concomitant disease, atherosclerosis, obesity and diabetes mellitus. Umbilical herniation can complicate abdominal distension, pregnancy and cirrhosis.[202] After pregnancy these hernias can regress spontaneously. In cirrhosis the ascites must be controlled before repair is attempted. Adventitious portosystemic shunts about the umbilicus may complicate operative repair,[81] although a recent study suggests that excessive blood loss in these patients can be avoided.[904]

In a retrospective review only 11% of patients with adult umbilical hernias recalled persistence of a childhood umbilical hernia: this and other observations suggests that the adult umbilical hernia is not through the original umbilical scar but is 'para' umbilical in anatomy.[542] This view is supported by Askar, who postulates that the adult hernia is through the decussation of the fibers of the linea alba adjacent to the umbilical cicatrix.[58]

Acquired umbilical hernia following laparoscopic cholecystectomy has recently been reported from Turin.[278] Forced dilation of the aponeurotic layer is proposed as the etiology despite primary suture of the trocar site. Such dilation should be avoided in removal of the gallbladder. At the initiation of the adoption of the laparoscopic technique for cholecystectomy, this was the site at which the gallbladder was removed. In many cases, forceful dilatation was required. With the introduction of smaller laparoscopes, the gallbladder is commonly removed from the epigastric port. While this will diminish the incidence of the umbilical herniation following the operation, there may be an increased occurrence of the port site herniation at that site in the future.

MAYO OPERATION – HISTORICAL NOTE

William Mayo first used an overlapping technique to repair an umbilical hernia in 1895. In a paper read to the American Academy of Railway Surgeons on 4 October 1898 he publicly called attention to the impracticality of covering the defect left by excision of large umbilical hernia with muscle. He advocated overlapping the adjacent aponeurotic structures which were at hand and securing a wide area of adhesion rather than edge-to-edge union. He experimented with a side-to-side overlap and abandoned this because of technical difficulties. Mayo recommended the vertical overlap because 'on assuming the recumbent posture the stretched tissues allow of great mobility and one can often grasp the abdominal wall and overlap a number of inches without difficulty.'[761,762]

When reporting his results and technique in 1903, he had performed the vertical overlapping operation 25 times; there were no deaths and so far he had had no recurrences. He encountered the problem of 'loss of habitation' in large hernias filled with viscera. He stressed a few operative details worthy of repetition today: he cleared the aponeurosis of fat for 'one or two inches' around the neck of the sac; he opened the sac; he extended the hernia aperture on either side to allow a better overlap, he used non-absorbable sutures (silk on this occasion, but previously kangaroo tendon) and 'railroaded' the upper flap down to the overlap with the lower flap. Interestingly, at this time, Mayo recommended initial closure of the peritoneum with chromic catgut prior to aponeurotic closure.

Mayo's definitive paper was given to the 54th Annual Session of the American Medical Association in 1903 – the discussants were Ochsner, Murphy and Ferguson. All three commended the operation; Ferguson went further and embarrassed Mayo by referring to it as the 'Mayo operation'.[761]

INDICATIONS FOR OPERATION

Most patients with umbilical hernias complain of a painful protrusion at the umbilicus. This discomfort is indication enough for operation. In many patients, this protrusion may be asymptomatic but will be discovered by the primary physician or general practitioner on routine physical examination.

Frequently, it is found in association of an inguinal hernia by the surgeon. Absolute indications for surgery include obstruction and strangulation. Irreducibility is not an absolute indication for surgery: many longstanding umbilical hernias have many adhesions in a loculated hernia and are thus irreducible. In larger hernias the overlying skin may become damaged and ulcerated. Skin complications may dictate the need for operation after the skin sepsis has been controlled. Surgery is advised for all umbilical hernias unless there are strong contraindications, which include obesity, chronic cardiovascular or respiratory disease, or ascites (umbilical hernias can be manifestations of cirrhotic or malignant peritoneal effusions). In even these situations, however, the need for surgery may dictate that the procedure be performed after adequate preoperative preparation of the patient.

Spontaneous rupture of umbilical hernias is rare but is recorded especially in patients with ascites and cirrhosis. Cheselden's 1721 patient who developed a 'preternatural anus' is an example of the spontaneous cure of an umbilical hernia.[211] The English Queen Caroline succumbed to an incarcerated umbilical hernia in 1737 because of the surgical delay in lancing her hernia to allow drainage.[331]

Umbilical hernias are an important complication of cirrhosis and ascites; the ascites should be controlled either medically or with a shunt before hernia repair is undertaken. Umbilical herniation is sometimes a consequence of chronic ambulatory peritoneal dialysis (CAPD).[333] In all patients that are to initiate CAPD, any hernia that is found prior to the insertion of the catheter must be repaired.

SUTURE MATERIALS

For details see Chapter 6. Suffice to say that in nearly all circumstances, the use of a permanent suture is required.

Anesthesia

General anesthesia with full muscle relaxation should be employed. The use of either spinal or epidural anesthesia can also be considered in some patients. In the very ill patients, intravenous sedation can be employed with local anesthesia. This is usually only appropriate in the hernias that are smaller rather than the larger, incarcerated hernias.

Patients who require an extensive intraperitoneal dissection often have considerable adynamic ileus after surgery and need postoperative nasogastric suction and fluid and nutritional support.

A further note of caution is indicated; if the patient has portal hypertension, an extensive portosystemic anastomosis will be present at the umbilicus. Careful dissection and ligation of vessels is important if massive hemorrhage is to be avoided.[904] If this is diagnosed preoperatively, the best course of action would be to control the portosystemic hypertension prior to surgery. Many techniques are available to accomplish this, which is beyond the scope of this text.

THE OPEN OPERATION

Position of patient

The patient is laid on his back on the operating table. Drapes are applied to allow good access to the umbilical area and the abdomen if extended access is required.

The incision

The smaller umbilical hernias can be approached quite satisfactorily with an upper or lower circumlinear incision (see video clip 'Umbilical hernia'). Hernias that are less than 2–3 cm are frequently done in this manner. In the case of the larger hernias, especially those that contain a significant amount of intestinal contents that may or may not be incarcerated. In these cases, it may be best to employ an extended semilunar incision beyond the lateral limits of the curved incision. The ellipse of stretched skin and the enclosed umbilical cicatrix are excised. It is important to discuss this with the patient preoperatively as some may not desire to have the umbilicus resected.

Care must be taken not to excise too much tissue when deciding the dimensions of these incisions. Although the umbilical cicatrix is best excised, removal of too much skin will place the final wound under tension and jeopardize its healing. It is better to aim on the side of caution and take little skin away at the commencement of the operation; more skin can always be excised later (Figure 17.1).

Removal of redundant skin and fat

If there is a significant excess of skin and subcutaneous fat, it can be removed through these semilunar incisions. The incisions are deepened down to the muscular aponeurosis, care being taken to ensure that the incisions are vertical and at right angles to the fascia so that the skin is not undermined and its blood supply compromised (Figure 17.2). This part of the dissection can be very bloody, and a cautious approach and careful sequential hemostasis are recommended. The judicious use of electrocautery will significantly decrease the amount of bleeding. One must be careful not to cause a burn that is full-thickness so that there will not be a slough of skin at that site (Figure 17.3).

More often than not there is no need to resect the skin. The hernia can be repaired and the redundant skin will contract into the appropriate shape and size after a few weeks to several months. It is important to place a suture between the base of the umbilicus and the repair, at the completion of the operation so that the umbilicus will resume its natural shape.

Identification of neck of sac

When the incisions have been deepened to the aponeurosis, the margins of the aponeurosis about the peritoneal neck of the sac can be sought and dissected (Figure 17.4). It is important that the fascial edges be clearly visible to allow for an effective repair of the hernia.

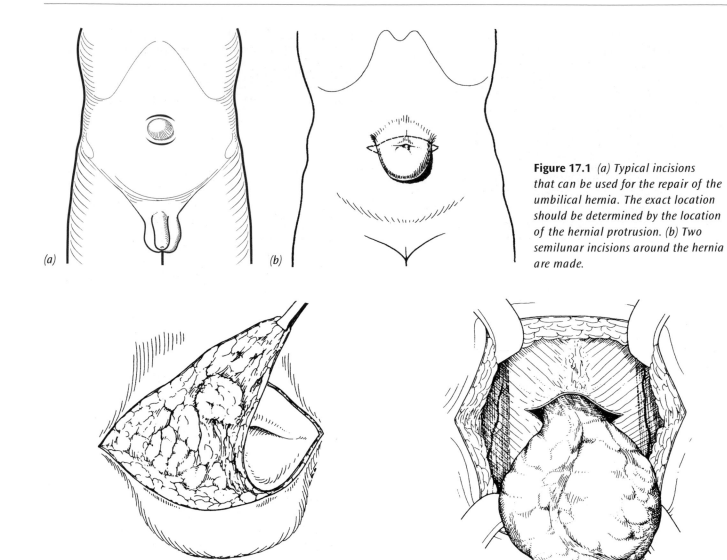

Figure 17.1 *(a) Typical incisions that can be used for the repair of the umbilical hernia. The exact location should be determined by the location of the hernial protrusion. (b) Two semilunar incisions around the hernia are made.*

Figure 17.2 *The redundant skin and scar tissue are excised.*

Figure 17.4 *The neck of the sac is identified. The aponeuroses on either side of the neck are opened laterally for 1 or 2 cm to allow the neck of the sac to be isolated.*

Management of sac – I

Having isolated the neck of the sac, all the overlying fat and skin can be dissected off leaving the peritoneum of the sac protruding bare through the defect in the abdominal wall. The sac can now be opened and its contents inspected (Figure 17.5). Often the contents are densely adherent to the lining of the sac, particularly at the fundus. Adhesions must be divided and ligated where necessary to control bleeding. Again, the admonition about the avoidance of blood loss should be remembered. Densely adherent omentum, particularly if it is partly ischemic, is best excised. All dissection should be made under direct vision. The bowel must be carefully preserved intact. Bowel puncture can lead to fistula formation postoperatively. Postoperative fistula and sepsis may precipitate death.

After the contents have been freed from the sac they are ready to be returned to the main peritoneal cavity (Figure 17.6). Prior to the re-introduction of the contents into the abdominal

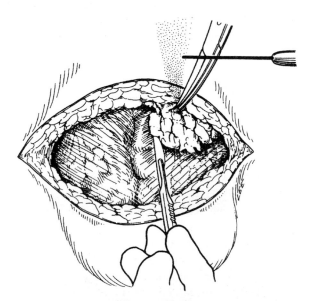

Figure 17.3 *Careful hemostasis will avoid blood loss and its consequences. Absolute hemostasis is critical to optimum wound healing.*

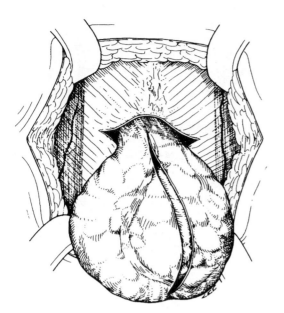

Figure 17.5 *Having cleared the sac of redundant fat and fibrous tissue it is opened carefully. The incision into the sac should commence at the neck, not the fundus. Adhesions are less dense at the neck of a hernial sac; they are most dense at the fundus.*

cavity, it is critical that there is absolute certainty that hemostasis is gained. A considerable amount of intra-abdominal hemorrhage can occur before clinical signs become obvious in the patient. This can lead to adverse outcomes.

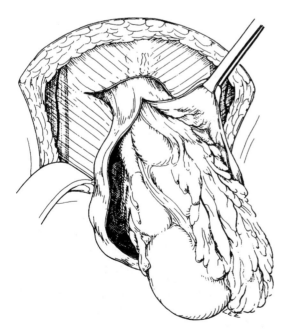

Figure 17.6 *The incision is extended to the fundus; adherent omentum and transverse colon are mobilized before reduction.*

Management of sac – II

If the sac is vast and multiloculated, an alternative can often usefully be employed. Once the peritoneum of the neck at any one point has been identified, it should be opened and a finger

inserted. There are fewer adhesions at the neck of the sac than at the fundus, where recurrently ischemic bowel is frequently densely adherent. A 'trick of the trade' is always to start the dissection at the neck; only the inexperienced operator would attempt to commence dissection at the fundus (Figure 17.7).

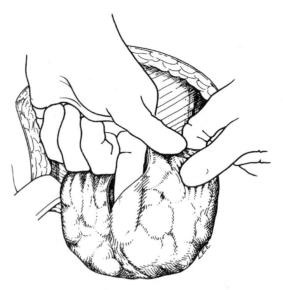

Figure 17.7 *If the sac is multiloculated, a finger is inserted through the initial opening in the neck of the sac.*

Assistants then hold up the whole mass of sac, contents and overlying fat and skin while the neck is dissected around, using the finger in the sac to direct the angle of dissection. This dissection can be tedious if the sac is multiloculated and the contents very adherent. When necessary, the operator may need to change from side to side of the operating table to facilitate this maneuver. Once the neck has been divided, attention can be turned to the contents of the sac. Adhesions are divided and doubtfully viable omentum excised (Figure 17.8). Here again, careful attention to hemostasis is paramount.

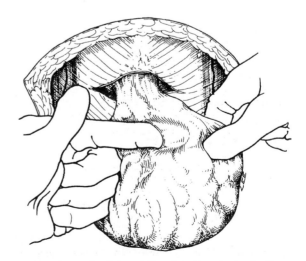

Figure 17.8 *The neck of a multiloculated sac is slowly dissected and divided.*

Enlargement of aponeurotic aperture

The defect is then more clearly defined by enlarging the opening in the abdominal wall laterally for 1 or 2 cm on either side, the rectus muscle being retracted as the posterior rectus sheath is divided, taking care not to injure the epigastric vessels (Figure 17.9). This technique is also used for placement of preperitoneal prosthetic biomaterial, when it is indicated.

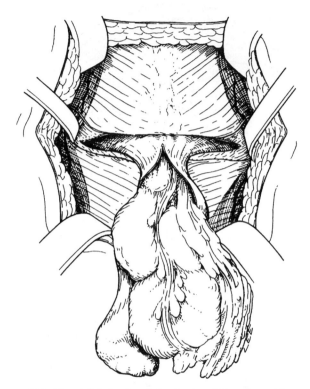

Figure 17.9 *The deficit in the abdominal wall is enlarged laterally for 4 cm on either side; the rectus muscles are retracted to make this possible.*

Frequently, however, the fibrous ring of the neck must be divided, to allow for the reduction of the contents of the sac back into the abdomen. The redundant sac is excised (Figure 17.10). If the sac is not large, as in the case of the smaller hernias, this can merely be either reduced or imbricated into the preperitoneal space without ligation or excision.

Open tissue repair of the defect

MAYO TECHNIQUE

The margins of the opening – aponeurosis, posterior rectus sheath and peritoneum – are now grasped in large hemostats and held up by assistants (Figure 17.11). The deep sutures are next placed. Strong non-absorbable material are used on a round-bodied needle.

The suture enters the upper (cephalad) flap from without, between 2 and 3 cm from its margin. The needle is then grasped on the deep surface of the upper flap, passed across the defect and then from the outside through the lower flap. Then the

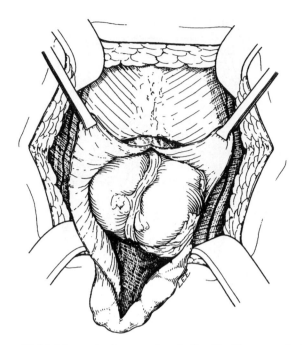

Figure 17.10 *The contents are reduced after the fibrous neck of the sac has been cleared.*

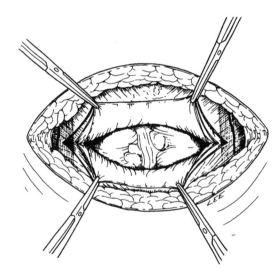

Figure 17.11 *The margins of the parietal defect are now picked up in large hemostats.*

needle is pulled back through the lower flap, across the defect and through the deep surface of the upper flap. The suture thus placed is held in a clip. Many more such sutures are now inserted and held untied until all are in place. Once all have been placed, they are tied.

There are four useful technical points:

1 In the upper flap the sutures must all be placed further than 2 cm from the margin – up to 4 cm is permissible.
2 In the lower flap the sutures must all be at a distance greater than 1 cm from the margin.
3 It adds to the stability of the suture lines if the sutures are staggered, not all at the same interval from the margins of the defect.

4 The more sutures that are put in, the easier they are to close and tie, and the strain is more evenly distributed (Figure 17.12).

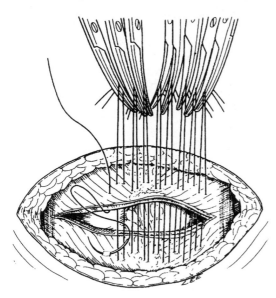

Figure 17.12 *The first layer of deep sutures is now placed. The sutures enter the upper flap 3 cm from its margin. They go through both aponeurotic layers (anterior and posterior rectus sheaths) on either side and through the full thickness of the linea alba in the midline. The sutures are then carried down to and then through the lower flap 1 cm from the margin. The sutures are left lax and held in hemostats.*

After the sutures have all been placed the flaps are brought together, the upper being 'railroaded' down the sutures until it lies overlapping the lower flap (Figure 17.13).

The sutures are now tied, fixing the tissues firmly (but not too tightly) together. A triple layer, double throw knot is used. When all the knots are complete the ends are cut short.

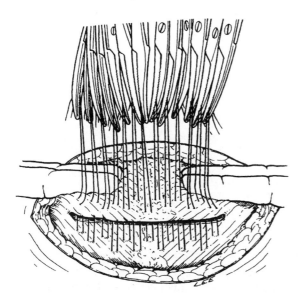

Figure 17.13 *The sutures in the upper flap are all placed. The upper flap is now 'railroaded' down onto the lower flap.*

A fine suction drain is now placed in between the two flaps of the aponeurosis. The edge of the upper flap is sutured to the anterior surface of the lower flap using the same non-absorbable material as previously. Suture bites of over 1 cm into both upper and lower flaps are used (Figure 17.14).

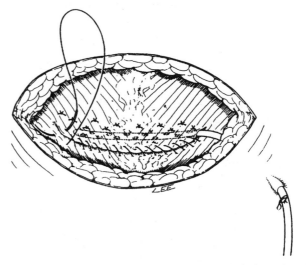

Figure 17.14 *The sutures are tied and a suction drain introduced. The upper flap is sutured to the anterior surface of the lower flap. This gives the classic Mayo or 'vest over pants' overlap.*

OTHER TECHNIQUES

The other methods of the open tissue repair of umbilical hernias are generally that of a fascia to fascial re-approximation with either continuous or interrupted non-absorbable sutures. The fascia will typically be closed in a transverse fashion although the use of a small midline incision may be preferred if the intestine is incarcerated and viability is questioned. The disadvantage of the tissue repairs is the recurrence rate that has been reported to be as high as 42%.[300]

Open prosthetic repair of the defect

FLAT MESH

Because of the high rate of failure with the Mayo repair and the other efforts at primary tissue closure, the use of a prosthetic biomaterial has been employed, particularly in high-risk patients. In a randomized clinical trial of 200 patients, Arroyo and colleagues compared suture with mesh repair and 98% of patients had local anesthesia.[51] A mesh-plug was used if the defect was <3 cm and a flat mesh if the defect was >3 cm. After a mean postoperative follow-up of 64 months the hernia recurrence rate was 11% for sutured repair and only 1% for mesh repair. In contrast, Bowley and Kingsnorth reviewed 473 primary adult and 18 recurrent umbilical hernias repaired in one institution over a 5-year period. There were 18 recurrences (3.8%) at a follow-up range of 12–60 months: 16 of these were sutured repairs, 11 of which were in high-risk patients i.e. obesity, ascites or chronic renal failure.[140] The results of this study do not support the routine use of mesh in primary adult umbilical hernia.

The method of placement will vary according to the preference of the surgeon. The common methods of insertion and fixation are those that place the mesh over the abdominal defect and suture the mesh along the side of the defect with either a continuous or interrupted suture (Figure 17.15).

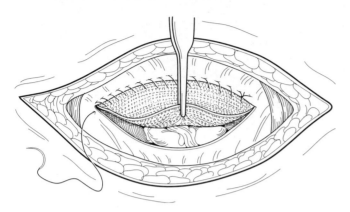

Figure 17.15 *Continuous running suture will affix the fascial edge of the hernia defect to the prosthetic border. Alternatively, interrupted sutures can be used.*

Another common method will utilize the techniques that have been described by Rives–Stoppa or that of Devlin (see Chapter 22). In this placement the mesh is placed in the preperitoneal space and secured to the fascia with transfascial sutures. The benefits of this method are the larger overlap of the prosthetic material and the security that is provided by the mesh itself. Excellent outcomes have been reported with this technique[299] (Figure 17.16).

PLUG AND PATCH

The use of plug and patch in the repair of inguinal hernia is well established. There have been only a few reports of the use of this prosthetic in the repair of umbilical hernias.[300] The placement of the mesh is similar to that of the inguinal approach in that the plug is inserted into the fascial defect and the overlay is applied. As with the inguinal repair, the

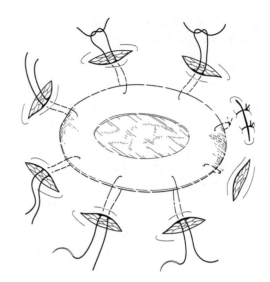

Figure 17.16 *Repair of the umbilical hernia using a preperitoneal prosthetic that is secured similarly to the Rives-Stoppa technique of ventral hernia repapir.*

preperitoneal space must be entered and the fascial edges should be clear of tissue so that the fixation with sutures can be done effectively. There is no need, of course, for a slit in the prosthetic mesh for the exit of any structures, if this is also utilized in the repair. The need to remove any internal petals of the plug would be made at the operating table (Figure 17.17).

The short-term results of this method of repair appears to be acceptable but there are no reports of long-term follow-up in these patients. There has been one report of a 5-year experience with a follow-up period of 6–60 months.[827] Using local anesthesia, this repair placed a plug into the defect and sutured the fascia over the plug with a second suture line in 94 patients. There were no recurrences noted in this presentation and only a few cases of seroma were found. There must be concern over the possibility of similar complications that have been reported with the use of the plug in inguinal hernia repair, however.[656] This would include chronic pain, migration, and erosion into the contents of the abdomen. It is critical to provide secure

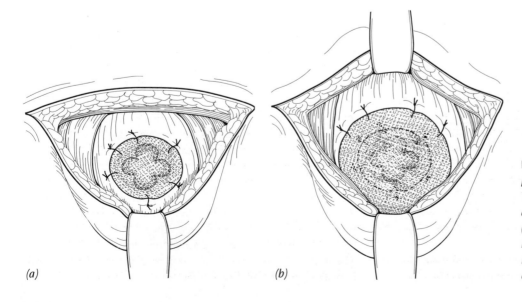

(a)   *(b)*

Figure 17.17 *(a) Placement of the plug into the umbilical hernia defect. This must be fixed with several sutures along the periphery of the device. (b) The overlay of the prosthetic mesh has been placed over the plug shown in (a). Note the overlap of the patch of the hernial defect.*

fixation of the plug device. The subcutaneous tissue and skin will be closed by whatever method the surgeon chooses.

PROLENE HERNIA SYSTEM® (PHS)

The PHS has been used in the repair of umbilical hernias. This has not been reported in the literature but the authors are aware of several individual surgeons that have placed this into the umbilical hernia defect. This can be done with either local or general anesthesia depending upon the size and contents of the hernia. The size of the PHS chosen will be dictated by the size of the defect but generally the use of a medium or large device is adequate in most cases. The preperitoneal space must be dissected more than that needed for the plug so that the underlay will lay open and flat. It is best to ensure that that portion of the product is flat because any wrinkle of any flat mesh can incite the development of adhesions in that area (despite the fact that the mesh is in the extraperitoneal space (Figure 17.18).

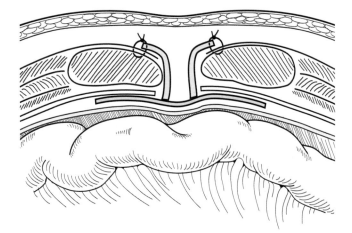

Figure 17.18 *Overhead view of the PHS repair of an umbilical hernia. The round underlay portion is placed in the preperitoneal space. The overlay portion has been modified to confirm to the needs of the defect itself as it is no longer elliptical in shape.*

Once this is placed the overlay will lie over the linea alba and the anterior rectus sheath. It can then be fixed with interrupted absorbable sutures (0 or 00) (Figure 17.19). The subcutaneous fat should be closed to cover the mesh and the skin can be closed by the method of the surgeon's preference.

KUGEL® PATCH

The Kugel patch was designed for the repair of inguinal hernias as a non-laparoscopic approach to the posterior aspect of the inguinal floor. Since the initial product that was developed there are now modifications of the device so that it may be used for other hernias of the abdominal wall (see Chapter 7). Whichever one is used the approach to the umbilical hernia is similar to the use of this product for the repair of ventral hernias and the PHS described above. One must choose a device that is oval or elliptical in shape and that may or may not have another layer of ePTFE on one surface.

The smaller defects can be repaired with local anesthesia as is those noted above. The preperitoneal space must be dissected

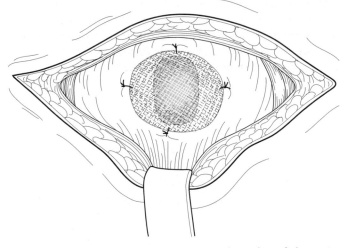

Figure 17.19 *Sagittal view of the correct orientation of the PHS prosthesis. The rectus muscle and sheath is 'sandwiched' between the layers of the device. Note that the underlay portion is in the extraperitoneal plane.*

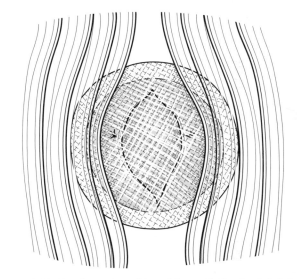

Figure 17.20 *Kugel patch positioned beneath the fascial defect to repair an umbilical hernia. Only a few sutures are required to fixate this product.*

away from the posterior rectus sheath so that the mesh and ring will have enough area to open adequately (Figure 17.20). Upon insertion of the device and appropriate positioning, it must be sutured to the fascia. Absorbable, interrupted sutures (0 or 00) are usually employed. It is recommended that only the anterior layer of the patch be sutured to the fascia. The overlying fascial defect can sometimes be re-approximated but this is not necessary and will frequently be impossible because of the extent of the defect size. The subcutaneous tissue and skin are then closed as with the other devices. Few series have been reported but in Kugel's own series of 246 patients in which this was used for both umbilical and ventral hernias, the recurrence rate was 0.82%.[624] This report did not segregate the patients but one did require removal of the patch due to a chronic draining sinus. As of 2001, there were a total of 90 umbilical hernias, both primary and recurrent, had been repaired without a recurrence.[625]

Laparoscopic repair of the defect

The laparoscopic repair of umbilical hernias is still evolving. Many of the reports in the literature that describe the use of this technology for incisional and ventral hernia have included at least a few umbilical hernias in the series. The methodology is identical to that of the laparoscopic incisional hernia repair as described in Chapter 23. As such, this requires the use of a general anesthetic. In the majority of instances, however, there is little need to dissect adhesions from the abdominal wall. Not uncommonly it will be necessary to remove incarcerated contents of the hernia. Because of the frequent small size of the fascial defect, it is sometimes necessary to enlarge the fascial opening to allow for the reduction of the herniated contents.

It is important to inspect the posterior rectus sheath and the peritoneum at the sites adjacent to the hernia defect. A common finding in these patients is the presence of a significant amount of preperitoneal fat that will inhibit the firm attachment of the prosthetic to the fascia, as this will be interposed between the patch and the native tissue. In these cases, it will be necessary to dissect away this excess of adipose tissue before the insertion and fixation of the prosthesis.

In LeBlanc's series of patients there has not been a recurrence with the use of this technique for any primary umbilical hernia. In the initial 100 patients, there was only one primary umbilical hernia repaired with this method.[663] In the second 100 cases there were only two but subsequent to that the indications have been increased for this repair due to the unacceptable rate of recurrence in our patients, many of which are significantly obese (LeBlanc, personal series). Franklin reported a 0.6% recurrence rate after laparoscopic repair of 62 umbilical hernias using polypropylene mesh. The lone recurrence was in a patient that did not have a mesh used and was closed with sutures alone.[374] In one prospective study, the recurrence rate in 144 patients was only 4% in a series that included 23 umbilical hernias. The number, if any, of these recurrences that were of the umbilical repairs was not stated.[1134] There have been other reports that have also included the use of the laparoscope for the repair of umbilical hernias successfully.[74,345,612] These reports, like the others, did not separate the use of the umbilical hernia and were also small series but reinforce the fact that the laparoscopic technique can be used successfully to repair these defects.

As the laparoscopic repair of ventral hernias of the abdomen expands, so will its use for the repair of hernias of the umbilicus. The ultimate use of the method and indications has yet to be finalized at this time.

Closure

When repairing the defect by the open or laparoscopic methodology, one must assure meticulous hemostasis. Suction drainage may be necessary in some of the patients but generally is not necessary if obliteration of any dead space can be accomplished with the dressings and/or a binder, if required.

The subcutaneous fat is closed in layers using fine absorbable suture such as a 3-0.

The skin is most commonly closed using a slowly absorbable subcuticular suture. Other methods of closure could be the staple or suture skin closure. This is usually not preferred because of the difficulty of the extraction of these devices from the skin. Additionally, they will elicit a significant inflammatory response that can be uncomfortable to the patient and worrisome to the surgeon.

The laparoscopic repair does not obliterate the dead space and may frequently result in seroma formation. In these patients one may employ the use of an abdominal binder to affect the closure of the dead space quite effectively. If trocars are used that are larger than 5 mm it will be necessary to close the fascia at those sites to minimize the risk of port-site herniation. The easiest method to accomplish this will be with one of the laparoscopic fascial closure devices designed for that purpose. The skin incisions are closed with subcuticular sutures or skin tapes.

Postoperative care

If there has been extensive handling and dissection of the small gut and omentum during the operation, postoperative nasogastric suction and parenteral metabolic support may be needed until normal peristalsis is re-established. However, this is seldom required in the usual case.

Early ambulation and breathing exercises are essential. The postoperative problem, which most frequently arises, is respiratory embarrassment caused by the wound pain and the newly raised intra-abdominal pressure.

The laparoscopic technique appears to allow the patient the ability to return earlier to normal activities. In both methods, a significant problem is constipation that commonly develops postoperatively. Early ambulation and use of laxatives or suppositories may be of benefit.

CONCLUSIONS

- Umbilical hernias in the adult are unsightly and painful, especially the larger defects with a fair amount of contents. Incarceration, obstruction and strangulation are common. Operation should always be recommended.
- The vertical overlapping operation as described by Mayo can be used successfully in patients where there are no risk factors.
- The use of a prosthetic biomaterial for the repair of the larger defects has been associated with a lowered rate of recurrence. There are few reports in the literature of the results of the repair of this type of hernia.
- The use of the laparoscopic repair of these hernias has been reported with acceptable results and may become a viable alternative to the repair of this hernia.

18

Epigastric hernia and laparoscopic 'port site' hernia

An epigastric hernia is a protrusion of extraperitoneal fat between the decussating fibers of the linea alba. These hernias usually occur in the midline of the epigastrium between the xiphisternum and the umbilicus, but small hernias can occur away from the midline and may protrude into the rectus muscle sheath. If these hernias enlarge considerably they may develop a peritoneal sac, which may be subcutaneous in midline hernia or interstitial, within the rectus sheath, in more lateral hernias.[57]

INCIDENCE

The population incidence of epigastric hernia is undetermined. These hernias are infrequent in infants and young children, occurring in teenagers or young adults. They are more frequent in males than females in the ratio 3:1.[963] They account for 3.4% of external hernias in a series from Nigeria,[330] in the US Armed Forces they account for 5.0% of external abdominal hernias but this figure may be an underestimate because these small fatty hernias are often not classified separately in official data.[502] Other authors record a similar low incidence. They are frequently found in young men taking up physical exercise such as athletes or those in military service.

SYMPTOMATOLOGY

Epigastric hernias cause symptoms quite out of proportion to their size. The very narrow sharp-edged opening in the linea alba predisposes to attacks of strangulation of the extraperitoneal fat which then becomes swollen, edematous and tender. During attacks the patient will suffer severe abdominal pain.

The occurrence of such attacks is an adequate indication for operative treatment. It is, however, important to investigate the patient fully; a small innocent epigastric hernia is sometimes blamed for symptoms which are in fact due to some intra-abdominal condition, such as a peptic ulcer, cholelithiasis or hydronephrosis. At the same time it is true to say that an epigastric hernia may sometimes produce symptoms which closely resemble those due to a peptic ulcer. Pemberton and Curry, in a 1936 classic paper, reviewed 296 patients with epigastric hernia treated at the Mayo Clinic from 1910 to 1936.[900] They concluded that no group of visceral symptoms could be said to be typical of epigastric hernia and great care must be taken to exclude intra-abdominal disease before operation is undertaken on a patient with an epigastric hernia associated with visceral symptoms. This caution needs emphasizing. The most frequently occurring intercurrent disorders causing visceral symptoms are peptic ulcer and cholelithiasis. The intermittent nature of their symptoms can be confused with other intermittent abdominal pathologies such as idiopathic hydronephroses and congenital obstructions of the small gut.

Small epigastric hernias that entrap the ligamentum teres or the adjacent extraperitoneal fat of the falciform ligament can cause symptoms similar to foregut disease. This is due to visceral afferent stimuli from the falciform ligament being transmitted via the coeliac plexus.[818] The exclusion of these diagnoses by endoscopy and ultrasound gallbladder scan should be routine before epigastric hernia repair.

Epigastric hernias are not uncommon in older children. Often, they are first noticed when the child complains of pain in them, caused by nipping of the fat in the hernia by the tight margins of the aponeurosis. In children, many epigastric hernias resolve spontaneously.

PATHOLOGICAL ANATOMY

The linea alba is an area of decussation of the three tendinous aponeurotic muscle strata of the anterior abdominal wall. At the midline these three aponeuroses, the external oblique, the internal oblique and the transverse abdominis are formed of fine tendinous fibers invested in loose areolar tissue.

The fibers of the external oblique have a downward, forward and medial inclination and additionally, especially around the umbilicus, describe a gentle upward curve (Figure 18.1). Above the umbilicus most aponeurotic fibers cross the midline and

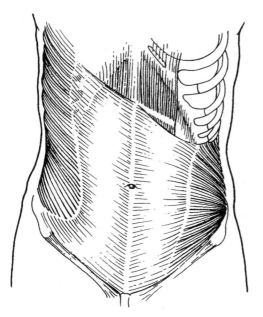

Figure 18.1 *The fibers of the external oblique have a downward and medial direction. They run around the umbilicus and are almost horizontal there. (After Askar, 1984.)*

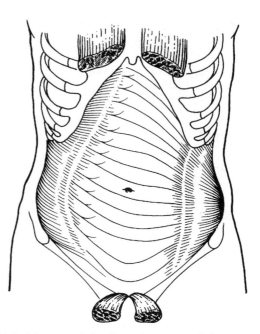

Figure 18.2 *Diagram of the digastric pattern of the transversus (right) and the posterior lamina of the internal oblique (left). (After Askar, 1984.)*

appear as the superficial fibers of the opposite side; they thus form the superficial layer of a double strata external oblique aponeurosis. When they make the cross over from one side to the other they decussate with the fibers of the opposite side; in 40% the fibers decussate only once at the midline – 'single decussation' – whereas in 60% of abdominal walls they decussate twice additionally to give three decussations, 'triple decussation'. This triple decussation is seen only above the umbilicus and never below (see Figure 18.4). In single decussation the fibers of the deep strata of one side emerge to gain the superficial status of the other side. In triple decussation the deep fibers appear superficial at the midline and then deep again after crossing the midline and decussating again. Below the umbilicus, except for a small area immediately adjacent to the umbilicus, this pattern of triple decussation is not seen; all the fibers of the external oblique invariably pass downwards and medially in a single stratum, then all the fibers cross the midline in a single decussation to give the external oblique a clearly defined pattern. This pattern of single or triple decussation with interlocking fibers gives the external oblique a very fine reinforced mesh structure about and above the umbilicus.

The internal oblique muscle consists of fan-shaped muscle bundles laterally. The upper fibers are directed upwards and medially, the middle horizontally and the lower arch downwards and medially. The aponeurotic bundles in both the superficial and the deep strata follow the same direction. At the midline (the linea alba) the anterior lamina fibers fuse with and are continuous with the fibers of the contralateral external oblique (Figure 18.2).

The fleshy bundles of the transverse abdominal muscle, the deepest layer of abdominal musculature, are not strictly transverse, the upper bundles go horizontal and upwards and the lowermost ones are horizontal. In 5% of specimens all the fibers go medially towards each other. The lowermost fibers of the transverse muscle are directed downwards and medially and are often parallel to the inguinal ligament (Figure 18.3).

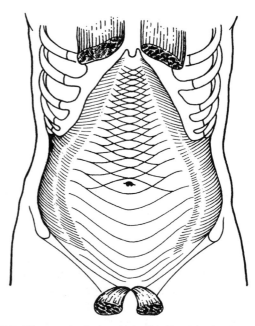

Figure 18.3 *Diagram to demonstrate the digastric structure of the two contralateral transverse abdominal muscles. (After Askar, 1984.)*

The various muscle bundle and aponeurotic fiber directions give the anterior abdominal wall a reinforced criss-cross 'plywood' structure particularly in the upper abdomen. The anterior abdominal wall can be divided into two structural–functional zones, an upper 'parachute area' aiding respiratory movement and a lower 'belly support' area. The anatomy of the midline aponeurosis is related to epigastric hernia formation. Epigastric herniation is found exclusively in patients with a single anterior and single posterior lines of decussion, this is found in only 30% of cadaver specimens examined (Figure 18.4); unco-ordinated tearing strains on the aponeurotic fibers of the linea alba, for instance in vigorous sports, coughing or vomiting, will stretch the decussations and allow the development of fatty protrusions between their bundles.[56]

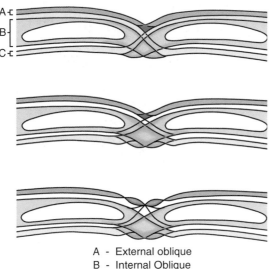

A - External oblique
B - Internal Oblique
C - Transversus

Figure 18.4 *Diagram of the decussation of the middle fibers of the aponeuroses. Single anterior and posterior decussation 30%. Single anterior and triple posterior decussation 10%. Triple anterior and triple posterior decussation 60%. (After Askar, 1984.)*

REPAIR TECHNIQUES

All epigastric hernias should be repaired surgically. For the most part, the repair of these hernias is nearly identical to that of the incisional and ventral hernias that are described in detail in Chapters 23. The only cure for the sometimes disabling and troublesome symptoms is surgical and exploration should always be advised.

Most surgeons recommend simple techniques to repair the defect. Simple suturing may be appropriate for the smaller defects (e.g. <3–4 cm) if the closure can be accomplished without tension. Askar, whose contributions to an understanding of the anatomy of this lesion are seminal, in 1978 recommended fascial darning[56,58] of layer defects. However, the introduction of inert polypropylene mesh to repair such defects using the extraperitoneal plane has rendered fascial darning obsolete. The preoperative evaluation of the patient by physical examination and possibly with ultrasound scanning should center upon the identification of multiple defects so these can be repaired at the time of surgical intervention.

Anesthesia

A general anesthetic is usually employed, but repair can be quite satisfactorily performed under local infiltration with lidocaine or bupivacaine. The use of a spinal or epidural anesthetic technique can also be employed in the open method in those patients that this may be appropriate, such as those with severe cardiac abnormalities.

THE OPEN OPERATION

Suture materials

For the sutured repair, non-absorbable sutures are preferred. The size should be of sufficient strength so an 0 or 00 suture would be appropriate in the adult patient. There are many available in monofilament or braided polypropylene, polyester or expanded polytetrafluoroethylene. In children, PDS is advised.

Prosthesis selection

The choices of a prosthetic biomaterial are many (see Chapter 7). The most common device that is used when this is applied is that of the flat meshes although there are many unpublished verbal reports of the use of the plugs or the Prolene Hernia System for this herniorrhaphy.

Draping

Drapes are arranged so that the whole of the epigastric area from the costal margin to just below the umbilicus is exposed for surgery. Not infrequently the hernia is found to be larger than anticipated and placing the drapes widely facilitates an extended incision.

The incision

A vertical incision has the advantage that the abdomen can easily be opened if this is deemed necessary. On the other hand, if the diagnosis is certain and preoperative investigations have excluded multiple defects and the hernia small, a transverse skin crease incision gives better cosmesis (Figure 18.5).

The fatty hernia, which is enclosed within a fine capsule, is dissected out from the surrounding abdominal fat. The opening in the linea alba, which is usually tiny, should be enlarged by incisions from opposite sides running laterally into the linea alba (Figure 18.6). If it is anticipated that there may be additional defects or intra-abdominal pathology, the use of a vertical incision in the linea alba is more appropriate.

The hernia is incised at its neck to determine whether there is a peritoneal sac and to reduce contents if present into the abdomen (Figure 18.7).

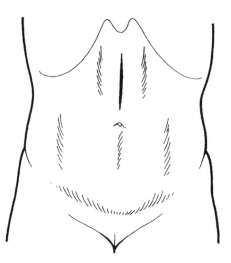

Figure 18.5 *A vertical incision is made over the hernia.*

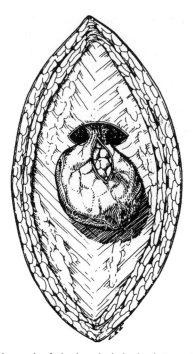

Figure 18.7 *The neck of the hernia is incised. Sometimes these hernias contain small sacs with omentum in them.*

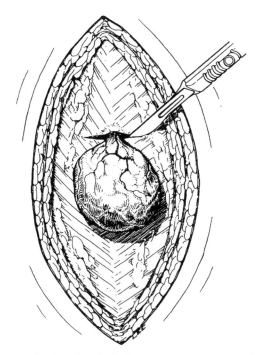

Figure 18.6 *The fatty hernia is dissected out carefully.*

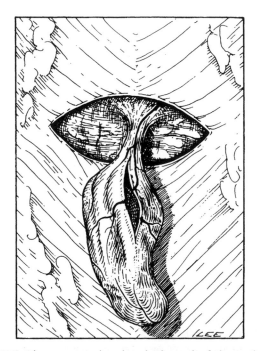

Figure 18.8 *The omentum is reduced. The neck of the sac is closed with a transfixion suture. The redundant sac is then excised.*

The neck of the hernia can then be ligated with a transfixion suture of absorbable polymer and the hernia excised (Figure 18.8). This is seldom done in the current era, however. The contents and the sac are returned to the abdomen and/or the preperitoneal space instead. When this is done the preperitoneal space must be dissected adequately to allow the complete reduction of these structures to prevent recurrence of the hernia.

At this stage the linea alba should be carefully examined for other defects. If necessary, palpation extraperitoneally may reveal other nearby aponeurotic defects that must be repaired. A small aponeurotic defect can usually be closed with a polypropylene or PDS continuous suture without tension.

Alternatively the opening in the linea alba is closed by overlapping its edge with two rows of interrupted polypropylene or PDS – the first row inserted as mattress sutures and the second as simple sutures (Figures 18.9 and 18.10).

As mentioned above, a prosthetic biomaterial could be placed after the reduction of the hernia and its contents. At this point the repair is nearly identical to that of the

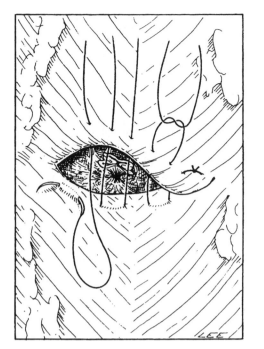

Figure 18.9 *The upper flap of aponeurosis is sutured to the lower flap – the 'Mayo operation'.*

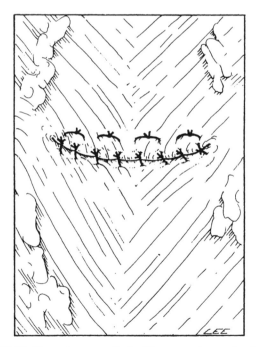

Figure 18.10 *The sutures are tied with an overlap and a further line of sutures placed between the margin of the upper flap and the anterior surface of the lower flap.*

ventral/incisional and umbilical hernia repairs that are described in Chapters 17 and 23.

The subcutaneous fat can be closed with an absorbable suture if this is the surgeon's preference. Many, however, do not feel that this is necessary. The skin is now closed with interrupted sutures, staples or a subcuticular suture.

THE LAPAROSCOPIC OPERATION

Position of patient

The patient is placed supine on the operating table. The laparoscopic approach will require the monitors to be placed at the head of the table on either side of the patient. The arms of the patient may or may not be tucked at the side for this procedure.

Laparoscopic repair

The repair of the epigastric hernia is identical to that of the ventral/incisional hernia repair described in Chapter 23. The one difficulty that will be encountered more frequently with this hernia is that which occurs when the hernia is high in the midline and near the xiphoid. In these hernias, there may be insufficient soft tissue beyond the hernia defect to allow the placement of transfascial sutures.

In some patients, these sutures may be placed on either side of the xiphoid or above the ribs. It is not recommended to place sutures around the ribs as this may result in significant and permanent pain to the patient. In those patients that the patch overlap lies behind the sternum, several additional fixation devices should be applied. Additionally, it is advised that the patch overlap be beyond the 3 cm minimum that is described for the 'usual' ventral hernia, such as 4–5 cm. It is also recommended that deep non-absorbable sutures be placed laparoscopically to firmly attach the biomaterial as the penetration of the metal fixation devices may be inadequate at this site (Figure 18.11).

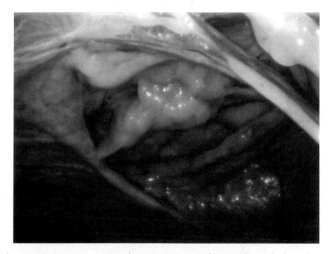

Figure 18.11 *Laparoscopic appearance of an epigastric hernia. Note the falciform ligament to the left of the hernia.*

LAPAROSCOPIC 'PORT SITE' HERNIAS

'Port site' hernia following gynecological laparoscopy was first recorded in 1968[347] and following the introduction of CAPD catheters in 1984.[328] The early case reports were of incarceration or Richter's type strangulation of bowel occurring within days of the laparoscopy or sometimes not for years after the initial laparoscopic intervention. The incidence of such herniation is estimated at 1 in 550 cases of laparoscopy, so it is no longer a rarity.[613] The herniation occurs most frequently after the use of the larger diameter laparoscopes (10 mm and 12 mm) although two cases following the use of 5 mm laparoscopes in gynecological practice are recorded.[895] Most cases are recorded when the port site is through the midline, but the umbilicus, transrectal port sites and flank port sites can all give rise to herniation. While most of the literature on this topic is from the gynecological literature, the occurrence of this in the general surgical community is well known.[951] Most patients present with localized pain and a lump but vomiting may occur if intestinal obstruction occurs. The importance of not dilating port sites and thus stretching the aponeurotic boundaries must be emphasized.[272] Direct suture of trocar sites avoids the hazard.[477] A comprehensive review of the subject by Krug identifies all these points.[613]

It may be difficult to directly suture the fascial defect of the larger trocars in the obese patients. In these patients, it is best to use one of the fascial closure instruments made specifically for that purpose. The newer dilating tipped trocars that do not cut into the fascia but rather dilate it may diminish the risk of post-laparoscopic hernias at the port sites. The increasing usage of the 5 mm and smaller trocars will also decrease the incidence of this occurrence. Technical and instrumentation innovations will enhance this improvement further.

CONCLUSIONS

- Epigastric hernias usually contain extraperitoneal fat only.
- These hernias cause symptoms disproportionate to the hernia size. The symptoms of peptic ulcer disease or biliary disease may be confused with those of an incidental epigastric hernia.
- Epigastric hernias are repaired by excising the protruding extraperitoneal fat or the rare peritoneal sac; the defect in the aponeurosis is then closed with a non-absorbable suture. Laparoscopy provides the ability to affect an excellent repair also.
- 'Port site' hernia following laparoscopy is no longer a rarity.
- The herniation occurs most frequently after the use of the larger diameter laparoscopes (10 mm and 12 mm).
- Direct suture of trocar sites decreases the incidence of this hernia. It is best to use a fascial closure instrument. The newer dilating tipped trocars and the increasing usage of the 5 mm and smaller trocars will also decrease the incidence of this occurrence.

19

Lumbar hernia

ANATOMY

The lumbar area is bounded above by the twelfth rib, below by the iliac crest, behind by the erector spinae (sacrospinalis) and in front by the posterior border of the external oblique (a line passing from the tip of the twelfth rib to the iliac crest). Within this area two triangles are described: the superior lumbar triangle (of Grynfelt) and the inferior lumbar triangle (of Petit). The superior lumbar triangle is an inverted triangle, its base is the twelfth rib, its posterior border is the erector spinae and its anterior border the posterior margin of the external oblique, its apex is at the iliac crest inferiorly. The base of the inferior lumbar triangle is the iliac crest, its anterior border is the posterior margin of the external oblique muscle, its posterior border is the anterior edge of the latissimus dorsi muscle and its apex is superior.

Both the superior and the inferior lumbar triangles vary in size depending on the attachments of muscles to the iliac crest (Figure 19.1). The floor of both triangles is the thoracolumbar fascia incorporating the internal oblique and the transversus abdominis to a variable degree. The T12 and L1 nerves both cross the superior lumbar triangle.

CLINICAL FEATURES

Congenital lumbar hernia does occur and can be bilateral.[5] Such congenital hernias present as a bulge in the loin and may be associated with intestinal symptoms. Lumbar hernias may be acquired, following sepsis in the retroperitoneal tissues[832] as a result of osteomyelitis or tuberculosis of the vertebral bodies or iliac crest which disrupts the lumbodorsal fascia,[1194] or following surgical operations on the kidneys.[396] Traumatic lumbar hernias occur following direct blunt trauma[617] and seat-belt injuries in vehicle accidents.[336,766]

This type of hernia is also described following the anterior approach to the lumbar spine for vertebral interbody fusion for lumbar disc disease. These are usually not true hernias as there is no true fascial defect. In some cases a fascial defect may be demonstrable but, in the majority, this is not the case. These abdominal wall deformities result from the injury to the nerves that innervate the upper portions of the external oblique, internal oblique, transverses abdominus and rectus muscles. The path of the T11 and T12 nerves can be traversed during the dissection of open space for the above operation as well as during the exposure for a nephrectomy. The deformity can be progressive as the protrusion of the upper portions of the paralyzed muscles will cause an outward protrusion of the normal portions of these muscles (Figure 19.2).

Lumbar hernias may contain a variety of intra-abdominal organs; hernias of the colon are most frequent but small intestine, stomach and spleen are also likely candidates for herniation. A particular curiosity is the sliding hernia of the colon, which causes intermittent obstructive symptoms.

Differential diagnosis must include tumors of the muscles, lipoma, hematoma associated with blunt trauma, abscess and

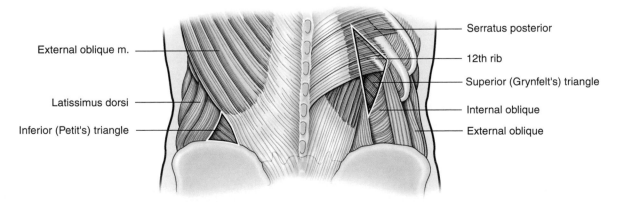

Figure 19.1 *Dissection of the lumbar region to illustrate the anatomy of the inferior lumbar triangle (left) and the superior lumbar triangle (right)*

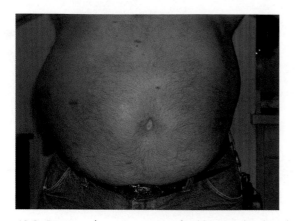

Figure 19.2 *Preoperative appearance of a 'denervation hernia' after a right nephrectomy.*

renal tumors. Small fatty protrusions of retroperitoneal fat through the lumbodorsal fascia have been implicated as a cause of low back pain.[243,341]

Backache radiating to the groin, presumably due to irritation of lateral cutaneous branches of the tenth, eleventh and twelfth intercostal nerves, has been recorded. Tiny fatty hernias along the tracks of cutaneous nerves through the lumbar fascia give rise to severe low back pain with radiation to the buttocks and thigh. These hernias are palpable and tender. They are similar to the fatty hernias that occur through the linea alba and anterior aponeurosis. Local anesthetic infiltration abolishes the pain and confirms the diagnosis. Local excision and closure of the defect cures the condition. The diagnosis is made/confirmed by CT scan, which will delineate the defect.[336,765]

The patients that have the 'denervation' injury that leads to the protrusion of the flank will frequently complain of back pain that is related to the defect. It is difficult to explain the source of this complaint as many of these patients will have had a long pre-existing complaint of back pain requiring the disk surgery. The most common presentation is the acknowledgement of the significant cosmetic deformity that is caused by the musculature paralysis. This will cause asymmetry to the contour of the abdomen.

THE OPERATION

In the acute traumatic situation, where full laparotomy to exclude intraperitoneal bleeding is mandatory, the abdomen should be explored through a midline abdominal incision.

Extensively damaged, ischemic colon in the hernia will need resection with the formation of a stoma appropriately. The defect in the lumbodorsal fascia should be sutured with non-absorbable sutures. The defect in the fascia is best repaired with a prosthetic biomaterial to act as a reinforcement.

When the hernia is being dealt with electively an oblique loin incision (in the line of the intercostal nerves) is made over it. Any sac is identified and the contents reduced. The peritoneum is closed and an extraperitoneal repair prosthetic mesh repair effected.

In the situation of the denervation injury, the repair is more problematic. Because no fascial defect is present many surgeons are reluctant to repair what is reasonably believed to be a cosmetic problem. Nevertheless, we have seen several patients that have a strong desire to undergo a reparative operation. The difficulty lies not only in the decision to operate but also in the type of repair that can be done in these patients. The data on any of these choices is sparse. There are three basic options in which to approach this problem.

The first is seemingly a very simple procedure. The involved flank muscles can be exposed and sutured in the form of a plication. Several layers of these sutures can be applied which will result in a very appreciable improvement in the appearance of the contour of the abdomen at the time of surgery and shortly thereafter. Unfortunately, the denervated muscle cannot be cured nor does the plication provide a final solution. The muscle adjacent to the plication is still paralyzed and will bulge as before within several months to a few years.

Because of this failure, the use of a prosthetic biomaterial is recommended. The surgeon must provide for a very wide overlap of the prosthetic to effect a long-term result. The prosthetic can be placed in the extraperitoneal or the prefascial position. In the latter position, the preperitoneal space must be entered through a flank incision that will probably be placed in the site of the prior incision. The muscles are divided and the extraperitoneal space is dissected. A large piece of biomaterial is placed in that location. It is important to ensure that the mesh extends from above the ribs to the level of the iliac crest. Only in this manner will all of the denervated muscle be covered. The difficulties lie in the dissection of the preperitoneal space, as this area will be densely scarred. This will result in violation of the abdominal cavity in almost all patients. Because of this fact, the use of an expanded polytetrafluoroethylene biomaterial is favored. The next problem is one of fixation of the patch. The easiest and surest approach is the placement of transfascial permanent sutures in the manner of the incisional repairs of Devlin, Rives-Stoppa and the laparoscopic repair of incisional hernias (Chapter 23). At the locations of the bony structures such as the ribs and the iliac crest, it may be necessary to hand-suture these sutures and/or place one of the metal fixation devices such as the tacks or the Salute™ constructs.

Another, less favored, method, is the prefascial method. In this case, the denervated muscles are plicated. A large piece of a prosthetic biomaterial is then placed from above the ribs to below the iliac crest. This can be sutured with permanent sutures in an interrupted or continuous fashion. The disadvantage of this approach is that the denervated muscle is supported from above rather than behind the fascia. This will not provide the long-term cosmetic result that can be seen with the preperitoneal approach.

A more favored method that has been done in a few patients is that of the laparoscopic method. In this method the approach and technique is similar to that of the incisional hernia repair described in Chapter 22. A significant difference is that the patient must be turned in the lateral decubitus position (Figure 19.3). A 'bean-bag' greatly assists in this position. The use of

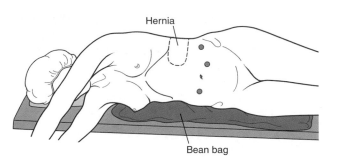

Figure 19.3 *Position of patient to repair a lumbar hernia of the left side. This position is also used for the repair of the "denervation hernia". The three dark cirlces connote the approximate location of the trocar sites.*

transfascial sutures and metal fixation devices is identical to the incisional hernia operation and that of the extraperitoneal method described above. The cosmetic result with this method has been excellent in some patients and acceptable to all (Figure 19.4).

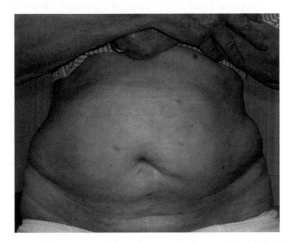

Figure 19.4 *Postoperative appearance of a repaired left-sided 'denervation hernia' that developed after an anterior operative approach to the lumbar spine.*

CONCLUSIONS

- The incidence of lumbar hernias is low.
- The problem of the denervation "hernias" may become more prevalent in the future. Repair of these deformities can be difficult and fraught with failure if not approached in a reasoned manner.
- The use of prosthetic reinforcement is felt to be best and the laparoscopic approach may be of benefit, although more study and follow-up would be helpful.

20

Pelvic wall hernias, obturator hernia, sciatic hernia, perineal hernia, supravesical hernia

PELVIC WALL HERNIAS

Clinical features and diagnosis

Hernias through the walls of the pelvis are rare. The confines of the pelvis are compact and complex. The pelvis consists of bones and ligaments and muscles, penetrated by different nerves which supply the lower limb. Those which are sometimes accompanied by peritoneal protrusions are the obturator nerve, the sciatic nerve, the posterior cutaneous nerve of the thigh and the pudendal nerves. All the foramina which transmit these nerves can form hernial sites. Urogenital and rectal prolapse, which are examples of herniation through the floor of the pelvis, are not included in this section; neither are the iatrogenic incisional hernias which sometimes complicate operations for pelvic malignancy.

All pelvic wall hernias have similar clinical features. A peritoneal sac, closely allied to an important nerve, may contain pelvic or other abdominal organs. The hernia sac will protrude into the adductor muscles if it is an obturator hernia and into the buttock if it is a sciatic hernia. Perineal hernias present in the perineum of both sexes and in the labia in the female. Supravesical hernias present in the lower abdominal wall or into the anterior pelvis retropubically. Sciatic and perineal hernias are more prominent when the patient stands and often disappear altogether when the patient is recumbent.

These hernias can be a source of chronic pelvic pain in women. This is an often overlooked source of this type of syndrome. Pelvic pain in these women can be caused by a variety of entities which can include myofascial abnormalities in approximately 7% of the patients.[191]

These hernias may incarcerate or strangulate and are readily demonstrated on herniography[1063] or CT scanning. Nowadays CT is the diagnostic modality of choice.[116] Finally all these hernias can be treated by excision of the peritoneal sac and extraperitoneal reinforcement of the defect using a mesh prosthesis.[212] A diagnostic (and therapeutic) option is laparoscopy, which can easily confirm the diagnosis if not confirmed preoperatively. In this case, excision of the sac is unnecessary.

OBTURATOR HERNIA

Obturator hernia was first described by Arnaud de Ronsil in 1724. Hilton performed a laparotomy for the condition in 1848.[505] Sir Cecil Wakeley described the anatomy of this hernia in 1939; he comprehensively reviewed the literature and described two cases of his own.[1177] A further excellent review of the topic was by Craig in 1962.[250]

Obturator hernias are rare and few surgeons have seen many cases. They represent 0.073% of all hernias.[127] They may contain preperitoneal tissue, colon, small intestine, the appendix, uterus, ovarian tube or ovary. These are rarely visualized clinically nor are they demonstrable by palpation except in an occasional case. However, the condition is curable by operation and although the clinical features are elusive, contrast herniography and CT scanning have transformed the diagnosis.[116,256,529]

Anatomy

Obturator hernia occurs through the obturator canal which is situated at the upper lateral part of the obturator membrane covering the obturator foramen and which transmits the obturator vessels and nerve. The obturator (adductor) region is the medial upper third of the thigh between the extensor and flexor muscle groups. The nerve is a mixed motor and sensory nerve supply to the adductor muscles of the thigh and the skin overlying them. The obturator nerve arises from the ventral rami of L2, L3 and L4. At the obturator foramen the nerve divides into anterior and posterior branches separated by a few fibers of the obturator externus muscle. The posterior branch gives a slender articular branch, which penetrates the posterior capsule of the knee joint and is distributed to the anterior knee joint[432] (Figure 20.1).

The hernial sac may follow the path of the anterior or that of the posterior division of the nerve. Rarely the hernia has been found to descend beneath the superficial part of the obturator membrane. The path of the hernia is of little clinical importance; it is important to remember that the obturator nerve is posterolateral and it should be visualized and avoided if the

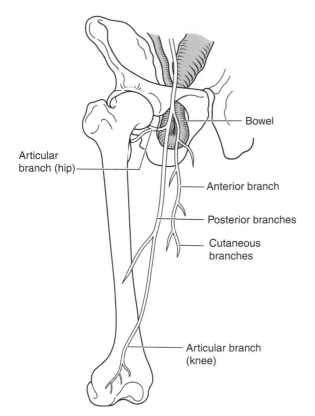

Figure 20.1 *An obturator hernia develops in the obturator foramen where it is alongside the obturator nerve. A strangulated or obstructed hernia may cause groin discomfort and pain in the knee and an absent adductor reflex in the thigh.*

obturator membrane requires division to release the hernial sac (Figure 20.2).

Most authorities cite anatomic variation as an etiological factor. Obturator hernia is six times more common in females than males; the more marked inclination of the broader female pelvis, together with multiple pregnancy, are factors in the sex incidence. Obturator hernia usually occurs after the 50th birthday, and is sometimes preceded by weight loss. The largest series recorded is 20 cases from the University of Chang Mai, Thailand – all the

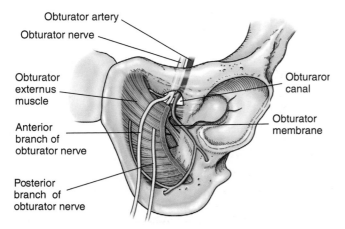

Figure 20.2 *The obturator canal transmits the obturator vessels and nerve.*

patients were female.[751] In another series from the Orient all five patients were women aged over 55 years.[629] Watson, in his series collected from the literature, found one case, a female aged 12 years old.[1194] Obturator hernia is more common in Oriental (Chinese and Japanese) than Caucasian women.

Obturator hernia is a rare condition and can present with no obvious external signs. It should be particularly suspected in elderly women with a history of recurrent small bowel obstruction. Obturator hernia has a considerable incidence of potentially lethal complications.

Clinical features

Obturator hernia nearly always becomes manifest only when acute symptoms of strangulation supervene.[40,471,550] The rigid margins of the obturator foramen cannot stretch, so strangulation is inevitable if a hernia develops and gut or genitalia (the broad ligament and ovary) then enter the sac.[703,1229,1057,1146]

Fifty percent of obturator hernias present with groin discomfort and with pain or parasthesia radiating to the knee, caused by pressure on the adjacent nerve: the Howship–Romberg sign.[250,1057,1070] This sign can be made more specific by noting whether coughing and thigh movements, especially extension, abduction and external rotation, make the pain or parasthesia worse. The sign may be difficult to elucidate in the elderly dehydrated patient. Another test is an absent adductor reflex in the thigh: the Hannington–Kiff sign.[472] The adductor reflex is a stretch reflex and is elicited by placing the index finger at right angles across the adductor muscles, 5.0 cm above the knee, and percussing onto the extended finger with a patella hammer. The contraction of the adductor muscle will be seen and felt. The reflex is absent in cases of strangulated obturator hernia. Comparison with the opposite side, which is often hyperactive in cases of obturator hernia strangulation, will confirm the diagnosis. The absence of the adductor reflex in a patient with a normal patellar reflex is a strong indicator of compression of the obturator nerve from whatever cause.

If infarction of bowel occurs in thin, emaciated, elderly females who present with strangulated obturator hernia, blood-stained fluid is exuded into the upper thigh and presents as a faint bruise in the femoral triangle just below the medial part of the inguinal ligament (Figure 20.3). If the infarction progresses to perforation subcutaneous emphysema develops in the upper thigh.[565] A fistula into the rectosigmoid has been described following the development and drainage of such emphysema.

Vaginal examination confirms the diagnosis, a tender mass being felt in the obturator region. Rectal examination is unhelpful because the obturator foramen is not palpable per rectum (Figure 20.4).

A partial enterocele (Richter's hernia) is often found in obturator hernial sacs. The rigid margins of the obturator membrane make early strangulation inevitable. A partial enterocele will make the clinical features more ambiguous, and the diagnosis will be missed if a careful physical examination is not done.

Rheumatoid-like pains in the groin and in the lower back can be caused by the bladder in an obturator hernia;[765] similar

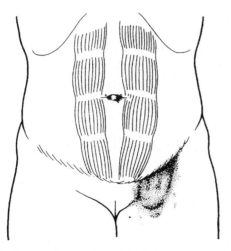

Figure 20.3 *The hernia may be palpable in the upper thigh lying in the femoral triangle between the adductor longus and pectineus muscles. If the hernia is strangulated there may be a telltale area of bruising over the hernial sac in the thigh.*[28]

groin pains following a hip prosthesis have been described as causing confusing differential diagnoses with concomitant obturator hernia.[391] We can only re-emphasize the diagnostic difficulties of obturator hernia. Appendicitis in a strangulated obturator hernia sac in a Ghanaian male has been described from Accra.[41]

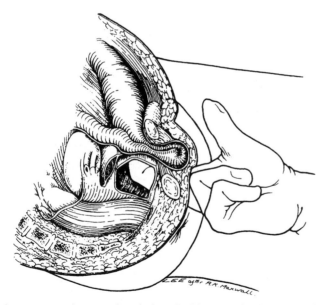

Figure 20.4 *Obturator hernia is palpable on vaginal examination.*

Modern radiographic techniques can readily demonstrate and diagnose obturator hernia. Plain abdominal radiographs will demonstrate the characteristic intestinal gas patterns if there is obstruction. Herniography using an intraperitoneal water-soluble contrast will sometimes delineate an obturator hernia sac as a small localized diverticulum in the upper lateral corner of the obturator foramen. These hernias protrude beneath the superior ramus of the pubis.[451] In cases of obscure groin pain herniography can be particularly helpful.[190,322,1064]

The radiological diagnosis of obturator hernia has been revolutionized by CT scanning which does not require the potentially hazardous puncture of the peritoneal cavity to instill the contrast medium in herniography.[256] This is nowadays the diagnostic modality of choice.[116,529,1231]

One must not overlook the benefit of laparoscopy for diagnosis. This may not be necessary with the use of the CT which also provides the surgeon with preoperative knowledge of the anatomic defect. It is, however, a viable option.

The use of modern imaging techniques has suggested that obturator hernia may be more common than previously suspected. In a series of 396 patients with suspected occult hernias, Nagahama found seven patients with symptomatic obturator hernia and another seven with asymptomatic obturator hernia, giving a frequency of 3.5% in this series.[834]

Operative management

Anderson (1900) described a groin approach to the sac in the space between the adductor longus and pectineus.[28] Milligan recommended an approach through an oblique incision, splitting the fibers of the external oblique with an extraperitoneal dissection to the hernia.[793] Both these routes are less traumatic to the patient but neither is adequate for bowel visualization and resection if needed. Either a midline incision with a supplementary thigh exploration or a Henry type extraperitoneal approach can be used.[494] Because the diagnosis is so rarely made with certainty before laparotomy, an abdominal incision has been employed in most reported series. Again, laparoscopy can be employed rather than a laparotomy. Either an extraperitoneal or an intraperitoneal approach can be used to identify and treat this hernia. The former method may be more easily done.

Repair by suturing or darning across the peritoneal opening has been employed in most cases.[4,1193] Prosthetic repair with tantalum gauze and the use of a tantalum gauze plug in a recurrent obturator hernia[901] have been described. Using adjacent peritoneum to suture across the defect or plug it is not recommended; such peritoneal repairs get reabsorbed and the hernia then recurs.[342]

In contemporary surgery an extraperitoneal patch with polypropylene mesh is recommended. The method of entry into the abdominal cavity can be either with a midline incision or with the use of laparoscopy (the extraperitoneal approach is preferred).[154,787]

Preoperatively

HEMODYNAMIC CONSIDERATION

If intestinal obstruction is present, appropriate intravenous fluid and electrolyte replacement is commenced and the patient resuscitated before anesthesia. If extensive bowel infarction is found, whole blood replacement may become necessary and a type and screen may be advisable preoperatively if this is a possibility. A nasogastric tube should be passed and the stomach contents aspirated prior to anesthesia if intestinal obstruction is present. A urinary catheter should be inserted also. This will allow the monitoring of the fluid status of the patient while providing that the bladder is not an impediment during the operative procedure.

SUTURE MATERIALS, PROSTHESES AND HEMOSTASIS

For details see Chapters 6 and 7.

The operation

POSITION OF PATIENT

The patient is laid on her back on the operating table and drapes are placed to allow a lower midline incision. This will also be appropriate for the laparoscopic approach. The drapes should be arranged so that access to the appropriate upper thigh can be gained if necessary.

OPEN INCISION AND EXPLORATION OF ABDOMEN

A lower midline abdominal incision is performed (Figure 20.5).

It is nearly always small intestine which is caught within the strangulated obturator hernia. Dilated bowel will be seen to pass into the pelvic cavity and thence into the obturator canal, from which the collapsed distal gut is found to emerge. At this point it is necessary to tilt the operating table into the head-down position.

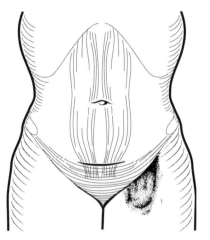

Figure 20.5 *Access is through a lower abdominal midline incision on the same side as the hernia.*

EXPOSURE

The intestinal contents within the pelvic cavity are packed off into the upper abdomen with warm wet packs. If the bowel above the obstruction is grossly dilated, it can be decompressed by retrograde milking of the contents to the stomach and aspiration through the nasogastric tube. The bowel above and below the loop caught within the hernia should be clamped with non-crushing clamps in case the obstructed loop has either perforated or is torn during delivery; in this way peritoneal contamination will be minimized (Figure 20.6).

THE SAC

This is formed by a narrow and usually small pouch of peritoneum lying within the tight confines of the obturator canal.

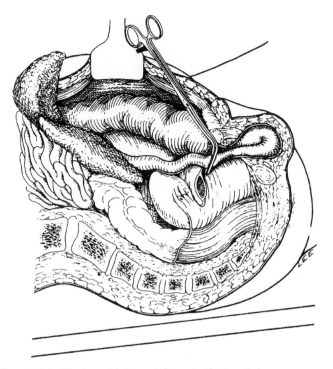

Figure 20.6 *The bowel is traced down to the hernial sac.*

Indeed, in some cases only part of the circumference of the bowel is caught within the hernia, forming a Richter type of strangulation (Figure 20.7).

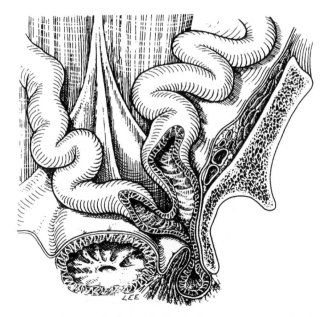

Figure 20.7 *The neck of the sac lies in the obturator canal, which is quite narrow.*

REDUCTION OF HERNIA

If the hernia cannot be reduced by gentle manipulation, the constricting ring should be stretched with the index finger; if this is not sufficient, then it must be divided taking particular care not to injure the obturator vessels and nerve which lie posterolaterally to the obturator foramen. These are avoided if any incision extending from the obturator foramen is made in an upward and medial direction.

EXPOSURE IN THIGH

These maneuvers will enable the occluded bowel to be released. If this is impossible, however, then the hernia must be exposed in the obturator region and its content carefully coaxed back by gentle pressure. A vertical incision is made medial to the femoral vein. The adductor longus is retracted medially and the pectineus pulled laterally or its fibers divided to enable the sac to be visualized (Figure 20.8).

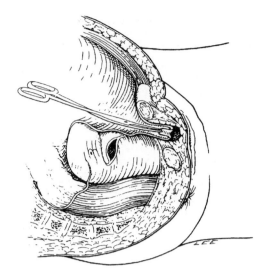

Figure 20.9 *The sac is invaginated, transfixed and excised.*

MESH REPAIR

The defect in the obturator membrane, which may be considerable, should be repaired using a patch of a prosthetic biomaterial placed deep to the peritoneum. The hernial sac is inverted and lifted. Then the adjacent peritoneum is freed from the pelvic parietes. The sac is opened and through this opening a mesh patch, sufficiently large to overlap the defect by 3.0 cm in each direction, is placed. The patch needs layering over the defect; suturing is usually unnecessary. The peritoneal sac is either excised and closed or left in situ so that the patch is left in the extraperitoneal plane (Figure 20.10).

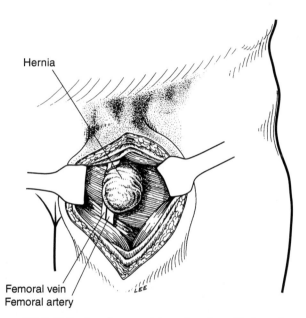

Figure 20.8 *If the hernia cannot be reduced readily into the abdomen, a thigh incision and dissection is needed. An incision is made below the inguinal ligament and the sac is exposed. The adductor longus is retracted medially and the pectineus laterally. The pectineus can be divided to make adequate exposure of the neck possible.*

When the strangulated gut has been delivered it must be carefully inspected. If gangrene of a small portion of the bowel has supervened, this area may be invaginated by a few seromuscular sutures. If the area is more extensive, resection must be performed.

INVERSION OF SAC

The sac is inverted by inserting a pair of artery forceps into it, grasping its fundus and applying steady traction (Figure 20.9). The fundus is opened and the peritoneum gently raised from the surrounding tissues by blunt dissection in the extraperitoneal plane. A plug of polypropylene mesh can be put into the hernia defect and the peritoneum closed over it; or preferably a full polypropylene or ePTFE mesh patch is applied in the manner of the Stoppa repair of inguinal hernias (see below). The use of a plug of Mersilene has been reported.[753]

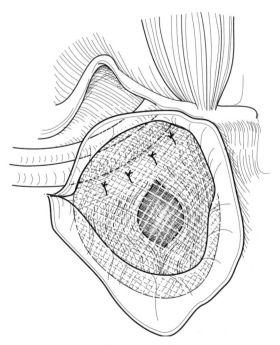

Figure 20.10 *Usually the defect is small and no formal repair is used. If the defect is large an extraperitoneal patch of mesh can be placed and the peritoneum closed over it. Another example of the 'ham sandwich' technique of hernia repair.*

OPEN EXTRAPERITONEAL APPROACH

The extraperitoneal approach (see Chapter 14) through a midline lower abdominal incision will give good access to the obturator area. Repair with mesh placed in the extraperitoneal plane can be used to make a repair if the defect is large.[1193]

LAPAROSCOPIC EXTRAPERITONEAL APPROACH

If the bowel is not excessively distended because of an obstruction, a laparoscopic approach is acceptable. In many cases, visualization of the area may be enhanced due to the magnification of the laparoscope. If a resection appears to be necessary, it may become necessary to convert to the open procedure. The initial attempt could be laparoscopic, however. This method would be identical to that of the TEP approach for the inguinofemoral hernias (see Chapter 16). The hernia should be reduced and the viability of the bowel determined. If viable, then a flat prosthetic mesh with a significant overlap of the area (>3 cm) should be placed. If polypropylene is used, no fixation is necessary.

The obturator foramen can be enlarged with this technique if this is needed. The same precautions as to the open method should be made.

Postoperative care

Early mobilization should be encouraged. If intestinal obstruction has been present, nasogastric aspiration and intravenous fluid replacement will be needed until the bowel regains its function.

SCIATIC HERNIA

A sciatic hernia is a protrusion of a pelvic peritoneum sac through either the greater sciatic foramen (above or below the piriformis) or the lesser sciatic foramen (Figure 20.11). The more

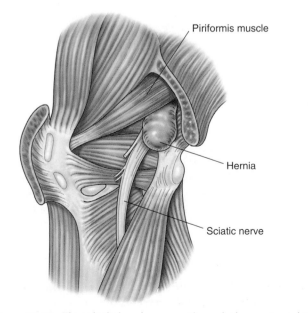

Piriformis muscle

Hernia

Sciatic nerve

Figure 20.11 *The sciatic hernia passes through the greater sciatic foramen either above or below the pyriformis muscle.*

common variety is through the greater sciatic foramen above the piriformis. The sac extends backwards and inferiorly deep to the gluteus maximus muscle. Sciatic hernias are very rare. In a series of 50 000 hernias from one hospital in Zaria, Nigeria, one sciatic hernia was reported.[61]

Watson in 1948 found 35 case reports[1194] and concurs that sciatic hernia is very rare. Sidney Black comprehensively reviewed the subject in 1995; he noted that although the Mayo Clinic from 1944 to 1974 repaired 30 000 hernias there was no sciatic hernia in the series.[128] Recently, Miklos reported 20 cases in a series of 1100 female patients that were operated upon because of chronic pelvic pain. This incidence of 1.8% in this group may indicate that this hernia may not be as rare as previously thought.[789]

Sciatic hernias may be either congenital or acquired. Congenital hernias present in children as reducible lumps in the buttock. Adult-acquired hernias are found equally in the sexes, herniation frequently being related to straining or heavy lifting. Without adequate repair these hernias may recur; indeed, a case in a 60-year-old woman which recurred three times was reported by Ivanov and colleagues in 1994.[541] Sciatic hernia related to wasting and weight loss in a young female was reported from the same unit in 1995.[541]

Clinical features

The symptoms of a sciatic hernia are very variable depending upon the structures involved in the hernia sac. If there are elements of intestinal obstruction, then abdominal distension, cramps and nausea are common. Many cases present first as undiagnosed intestinal obstruction and the true diagnosis is made only when the abdomen is opened.[1194] Non-specific pelvic pain of more than 6 months can be a presenting symptom of this hernia.[789] Some hernias present as bulges in the lower buttocks; bulges that characteristically are more pronounced when the patient stands, 'gurgle' and have bowel sounds in them, cause discomfort when the patient sits down and are reducible. Sciatic nerve compression can occur with pain and muscle weakness down the posterior of the lower limb. The hernia sac, and any contents, can be delineated by herniography but the investigation of choice is CT scanning.[400]

Operation

Although this hernia can be approached via a transgluteal approach, the operation is best performed through the main abdominal cavity. The patient is placed in the Trendelenburg position with the head tilted down. The abdomen is opened through a midline incision; the mouth of the hernia is situated just posterior to the broad ligament in the female and in a similar position anterolaterally to the rectum in the male. Often the hernial sac is readily identified by a loop of small intestine in the sac.

Firstly the contents are gently drawn out of the sac. If the neck is narrow it can be dilated under direct vision. If there is still difficulty with incarcerated intestine the neck can be carefully incised, taking care to avoid any underlying nerves, which must be visualized. External pressure on the buttock mass will expedite this process. Once the sac has been emptied of its contents forceps are inserted, the fundus grasped and the whole sac invaginated. The fundus is then incised, thus opening up the extraperitoneal space.

A large area of extraperitoneum is opened up by blunt dissection and a prosthetic mesh placed in to cover the defect widely. It is probably best to use a polypropylene sheet for this repair but an alternative is a polypropylene plug. The peritoneum is closed over the repair. This extraperitoneal repair is a further elaboration of the Stoppa operation for abdominal wall hernias.[212] The laparoscopic approach for this repair can also be utilized. The preperitoneal dissection will be similar to that of the open technique.[789] The mesh can be secured with endoscopic tacks (Figure 20.12).

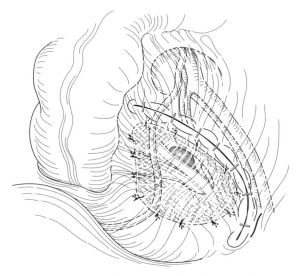

Figure 20.12 *The anatomic relationships of the sciatic hernia are shown as well as the proper positioning of the prosthesis used to repair this defect.*

PERINEAL HERNIA

Etiology

Perineal hernias are very rare. Acquired (incisional) perineal hernias occur in both males and females after abdominoperineal resection of the rectum and after pelvic operations for genital malignancy (radical prostatectomy and gynecological exenteration). These hernias can also be the source of chronic pelvic pain in females. These acquired forms of herniation can be extremely distressing.

Naturally occurring herniation through the pelvic floor is five times more common in older women (40–60 years) than in men. This sex difference is due to the broader female pelvis and antecedent obstetric damage to the pelvic floor. The hernia sac may protrude anterior or posterior to the superficial transverse perineal muscles. Anterior hernias proceed into the labium majus where they present as a 'gurgling' lump. In the male only posterior hernias have been described. Posterior hernias occur between the

levator ani and coccygeus muscles. If the internal fascia of the obturator internus muscle and the levator ani inferior fascia fail to fuse there is a potential space, the hiatus of Schwalbe, through which a hernia may protrude. Patients complain of a lower gluteal lump and discomfort. The hernia emerges below the inferior margin of the gluteus maximus, then extends anteriorly as a perineal lump. In the female the hernia extends into the labium majus – a pudendal hernia – where it causes discomfort. It passes through the pelvic triangle that is bounded by the bulbocavernosus, ischiocavernosus and transverses perinea muscles. The mass is readily palpable and usually easily reducible. Intestinal sounds in the lump may be noticed by the patient.

Diagnosis is simple. Herniography has been used to delineate the defect, the sac and contents. CT scanning will now be more commonly used to confirm the picture. Operative treatment is straightforward: with the patient in the Trendelenburg position the contents are coaxed from the hernia sac. The peritoneum of the sac and surrounding areas is raised and a prosthetic mesh patch inserted to cover the full extent of the levator floor. This operation is straightforward and similar to the Wells operation for rectal prolapse (Figure 20.13).

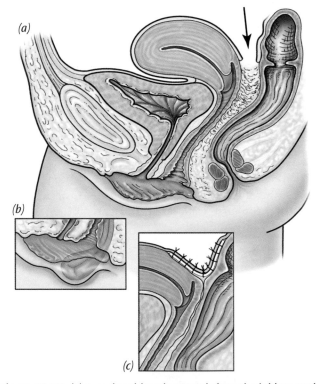

Figure 20.13 *(a) A perineal hernia extends into the labium majus through the potential space between the vagina and the rectum. It originates at the arrow. (b) Appearance of the bowel as a bulge at the labium majus. (c) Obliteration of the defect with prosthetic biomaterial prevents a recurrence. This can be placed with either an open or laparoscopic approach.*

The laparoscopic approach has been advocated for the diagnosis and treatment of these hernias also.[574] The hernia is reduced and the prosthetic mesh is placed as one would with the open technique. The peritoneum would be closed with absorbable sutures, tacks or staples.

SUPRAVESICAL HERNIA

Supravesical hernia was first described by Astley Cooper in 1804.[238] External supravesical hernias bulge through the transversus muscle aponeurosis and fascia transversalis in the most medial part of the myopectineal orifice of Fruchaud. They then present as very medial direct inguinal hernias or as interparietal hernias within the lower abdominal wall.[1061] The defects in the fascia transversalis are sometimes multiple, as in the original case with six hernial openings described by Astley Cooper in 1804; two of these hernias were in the supravesical fossae (Figure 20.14). Skandalakis and his colleagues have also described two separate patients with multiple hernias.[1059,1060]

Anterior (external) supravesical hernia presents with a groin lump and are usually routinely repaired as groin hernias without special difficulty.

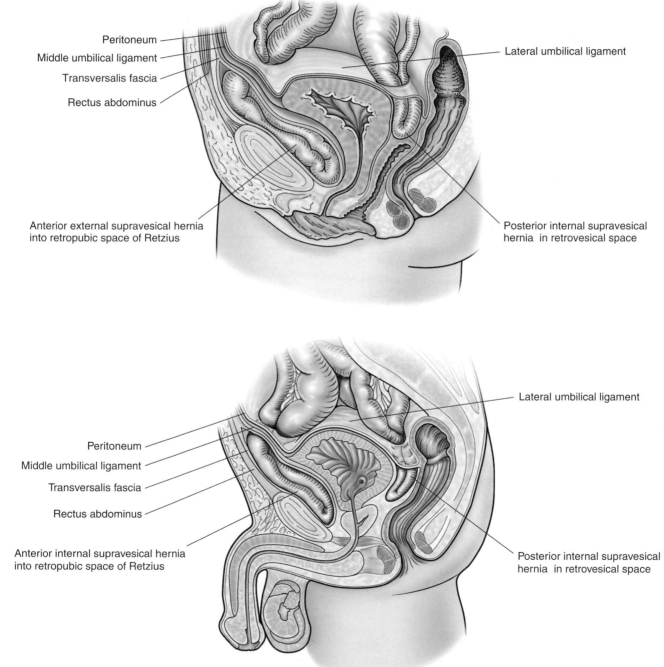

(a)

(b)

Figure 20.14 (a) Supravesical hernias occur through the parietal peritoneum either anterior to the bladder and extending into the retropubic space, or posterior to the bladder and uterus in the female and extending into the pararectal tissues. (b) Supravesical hernia in the male may present as a groin lump or plunge into the retropubic space. Repair using an extraperitoneal mesh technique can be employed.

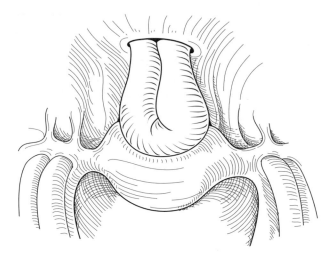

Figure 20.15 *Intestinal incarceration in anterior supravesical hernia.*

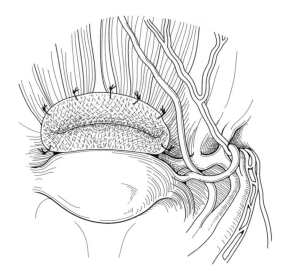

Figure 20.16 *Mesh repair of the hernia seen in Figure 20.15.*

Posterior (internal) supravesical hernias most commonly occur in the supravesical fossa whence a hernia sac extends anterior to the bladder and posterior to the pubis into the retropubic space of Retzius. A loop of small intestine can become incarcerated and obstructed in such a hernia (Figure 20.14b). Most reported cases have been in males and they usually present as urgent cases with obstruction, which sometimes is associated with bladder symptoms if the hernia reduces the bladder capacity.

Treatment is surgical because it is important to obliterate the sac to prevent recurrence. Internal (posterior) supravesical hernias traverse defects in the parietal peritoneum posterior to the bladder and into the pararectal tissue (Figure 20.15). The open inguinal approach is generally used for the repair of the external supravesical hernias. While the preperitoneal approach of Nyhus may be used for the internal supravesical hernias, the laparoscopic approach may be preferable as this allows complete visualization of the entire pelvic floor in great detail. Whichever approach is used, the hernia is reduced and is followed by the placement of a prosthetic biomaterial (Figure 20.16) as the tissues adjacent to the hernia are quite inadequate to effect an effective repair.

CONCLUSIONS

- Hernias that originate in the pelvis are quite rare and difficult to diagnose.
- Preoperative clinical examination can be unsatisfactory but the modern methods of radiologic evaluation will provide significant assistance for the accurate diagnosis of these entities.
- The repair of these hernias can be performed with open laparotomy, inguinal incisions or laparoscopy depending upon the level of suspicion and the viability of the involved intestine.
- Recurrence is uncommon.

21

Spigelian hernia

DEFINITION

Spigelian hernias occur through slit-like defects in the anterior abdominal wall adjacent to the semilunar line which extends from the tip of the ninth costal cartilage to the pubic spine at the lateral edge of the rectus muscle inferiorly. The semilunar line is formed by the division of the lamellae of the internal oblique to form the rectus sheath. Anteriorly throughout its length, the semilunar line is reinforced by the aponeurosis of the external oblique. Posteriorly in the cephalad two-thirds it is reinforced by the transversus abdominis muscle which is muscular almost to the midline in the upper abdomen. This musculo-aponeurotic support prevents herniation which is, therefore, very rare above the umbilicus. In the lower third or so the posterior rectus sheath is deficient where the internal oblique and transversus form the thin margin of the arcuate fold of Douglas, halfway between the umbilicus and the pubis. Most Spigelian hernias occur in the lower abdomen where the posterior rectus sheath is deficient, but hernias have been recorded all along the semilunar line (Figure 21.1).

Morphologically, some direct inguinal hernias (parainguinal hernias) are hernias through the semilunar line below and medial to the inferior epigastric vessels. There is no useful purpose in including this more frequent variety of hernia under the heading 'Spigelian hernia'.[281,1141] Because of the frequency of direct hernia, this 'low Spigelian hernia' may be more frequent than actually reported due to the inappropriate labelling of these type of hernias. This hernia will be easier to treat than the direct hernia due to the small orifice of the hernia.

The hernial ring is a well-defined defect in the transversus aponeurosis. The hernial sac, surrounded by extraperitoneal fatty tissue, is often interparietal (interstitial) passing through the transversus and the internal oblique aponeuroses and then spreading out beneath the intact aponeurosis of the external oblique, or lying in the rectus sheath alongside the rectus muscle[20,153,1076] (Figures 21.2 and 21.3).

The diagnosis of a Spigelian hernia is difficult; few doctors suspect it, it has no characteristic symptoms, and the hernia may be interparietal with no obvious mass on inspection or palpation. The introduction of both ultrasonography and computed tomography has greatly aided the diagnosis of this uncommon hernia. Because of these modalities the number of Spigelian hernias that have been proven has increased in the last two decades.

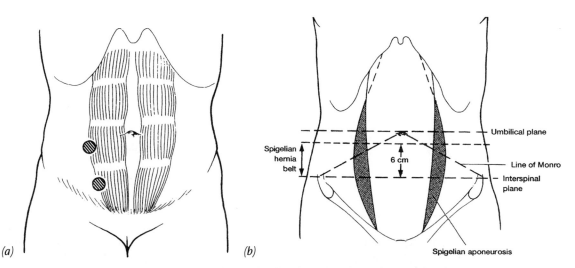

(a)   (b)

Figure 21.1 (a) Spigelian hernias occur through the semilunar line just lateral to the rectus muscle. They are more frequent in the lower abdomen at or below the fold of Douglas. (b) The sites of Spigelian hernias. (After Spangen, 1984.)

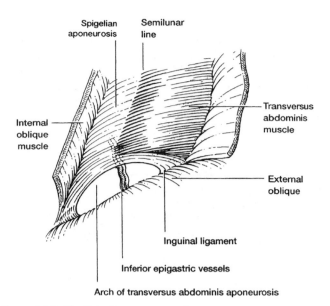

Figure 21.2 *The Spigelian aponeurosis.*

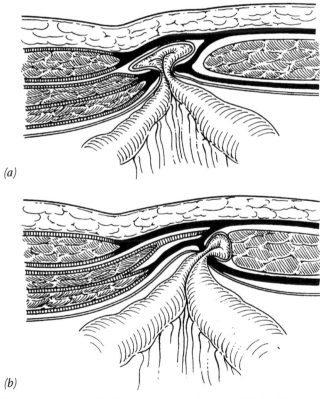

(a)

(b)

Figure 21.3 *(a) A Spigelian hernia may be interstitial with a palpable mass at the linea semiluna. (b) A Spigelian hernia may be occult, herniation occurring into the rectus sheath.*

HISTORICAL NOTE

The semilunar line was described by Adriaan van Spieghel (Spigelius, 1578–1625),[1081] who held the Chair of Anatomy and Surgery in Padua in the early 17th century; however, the hernia that is named for him was first described by Klinkosch in

1764.[604] Sir Astley Cooper recognized the hernia and described three cases in 1807. By 1827, Sir Astley Cooper had collected 23 cases of Spigelian hernia of which 19 occurred below the umbilicus. He wrote a precise description of his findings and launched the theory that the neurovascular openings in the Spigelian fascia may become enlarged permitting herniation: 'Vascular openings are situated in the semilunar line, viscera can find an easy exit through these openings.'[238,240] Today, however, this is considered of relative minor significance in the etiology of these hernias.

ANATOMIC BASIS

The detailed anatomic basis for Spigelian hernia was unravelled by Anson and his associates.[1238] They recognized the predisposition to herniation of the semilunar line and drew attention to the 'banding' of the abdominal wall muscles at this site. In a series of dissections of adult cadavers they demonstrated that in 22% the lateral abdominal wall muscles form bands or fascicles at the semilunar line and that there are slit-like deficiencies in the aponeurosis between these fascicles. Extraperitoneal fat and peritoneum can become extruded through these musculo-aponeurotic defects. Most of the hernias of the semilunar line are described as occurring at or below the level of the arcuate fold of Douglas, and this corresponds with the distribution of the defects in the muscles as described by Anson.

The Spigelian aponeurosis is widest between 0 and 6 cm cranial to the interspinous plane and 85–90% of the hernias occur within this 'Spigelian hernia' band.[1075] This aponeurosis is a congenital area of weakness in the abdominal wall. Aging and weight loss are recognized etiologic factors of these hernias. Paralysis of the muscles of the abdominal wall may also be a contributing factor in some cases.

INCIDENCE

Two cases of Spigelian hernia have been reported in girls under 1 year old; in one case the hernia reduced spontaneously after repair of a congenital diaphragmatic hernia and then spontaneously closed.[1181] Two cases of childhood Spigelian hernia related to the neuropathy caused by a mediastinal neuroblastoma were reported in Japan.[613] Other causes of Spigelian hernia in childhood are trauma and abdominal wall surgery. The ratio of males to females in children is 2.1:1 – quite different from the ratio in adults. One report suggests that there may be an association between the congenital Spigelian hernia and cryptorchidism.[18]

Spigelian herniation is most frequently found in adults in the age range 40–70 (mean 50.5) years. In adults the male to female ratio is 1:1.18.[1076] Spigelian hernias may be related to stretching in the abdominal wall caused by previous surgery or scarring. These hernias appear to peak in the 4th, 5th and 7th decades.[1199]

Richter's type strangulation is reported, the sharp fascial margins of the aperture predisposing to this complication.[1043,1076] Spigelian hernia has been described as a complication of chronic ambulatory peritoneal dialysis (CAPD).[333]

Spigelian hernias are uncommon; the incidence reported in the literature is less than 1% of all abdominal hernias treated surgically. Stuckej *et al.* (1973) reported 43 cases, the biggest series from one department, and estimated the incidence to be about 0.1% of all abdominal hernias.[1104] Spangen (1976), in a classic thesis, has reviewed the literature exhaustively.[1074] He reviews 744 patients operated on for Spigelian hernia; the mean age was 50 years (49.5 for women and 50.5 for men) and the ratio of women to men was 1.4:1. The hernia was bilateral in 24 patients and the ratio of right to left was 1.6:1. In 10 cases there was more than one hernia on one side. Most of the hernias were located below the umbilicus, only 28 being situated in the upper abdomen.[1074]

Since that report in 1976, there have been several reports, some with several patients that have confirmed the characteristics of the Spigelian hernia (Table 21.1). It appears from the world's literature that the age has not changed. The sex ratio is similar (4:3 female to male) with less than 5% of these hernias being bilateral and less than 5% occur under the age of 16 years. The reported incidence of incarceration is approximately 27%.

Table 21.1 *Reports on the Spigelian hernia*

Author (year)	Number of hernias
Artioukh (1996)	19
Guivarc'h (1998, 1999)	16
Gullmo (1980, 1984)	13
Kienzle (1978)	12
Ponka (1980)	19
Rodighiero (1996)	11
Spangen (1984)	45
Stirnemann (1982)	12

DIAGNOSIS

Spigelian hernias are of interest because of the diagnostic confusion they cause. The emerging hernial sac can be deflected by the overlying, intact, external oblique aponeurosis, so that it lies interstitially and tends to be pushed laterally where it may present as a swelling adjacent to the iliac crest and may easily be palpated at the anterosuperior iliac spine. Rarely the hernia can enter the rectus sheath to lie alongside the rectus muscle in an acute presentation it can be confused with a spontaneous rupture of the rectus muscle or with a hematoma in the rectus sheath (Figure 21.3b).

Patients may complain of a lump, which often disappears when they lie recumbent; they may have symptoms of acute or subacute intestinal obstruction; or they may have a variety of vague abdominal discomforts. Spigelian hernias may lie interparietally between the flank muscle layers or within the rectus sheath and not be easily palpable.[1076] Often the last is worse at

the end of a day's work and is relieved when the patient assumes the recumbent position. The local discomfort can be quite severe, but is sometimes only a feeling of 'something there that shouldn't be'.[1179] On occasion, the pain is vague or dyspeptic and can be confused with peptic ulceration. It has been suggested that neuralgic pain is a consequence of local pressure on peripheral nerves as they pass through aponeurosis (Figure 21.4). Incarceration of the bladder and a Meckel's diverticulum in a Spigelian hernia has been reported.[307,1031]

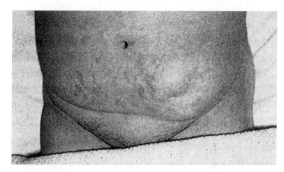

Figure 21.4 *The patient may have a classical lump when she stands up. The lump is painful if the patient stretches and disappears if she lies down.*

Classic features are localized pain made worse by stretching the arm on the affected side above the head to put the external oblique aponeurosis under tension, by abdominal straining, by defecation or by athletic exertion. Localized pain is associated with point tenderness and a reducible abdominal wall mass. If the hernia has incarcerated contents the pain is quite intense. If the contents are intestinal, signs and symptoms of intestinal obstruction may be present.

It is essential to examine the patient with the abdominal muscles relaxed; tense muscles compress an interparietal hernia and render it inconspicuous. The patient should also be examined standing because, although the external oblique muscle is tense, the general extent of the hernia may be felt on profile in this position. Despite the best efforts of the clinician, however, the diagnosis can be very difficult to make if the hernia is reduced at the time of examination. If the patient is tender at the site of the hernial orifice, a high index of suspicion must be made. This is not a pathognomonic finding, however.

Plain radiographs of the abdomen are generally not particularly helpful to confirm this diagnosis. Herniography has been used in the past but is not highly diagnostic and does carry some risk of the procedure.[450,452]

Ultrasonic scanning has been advocated by Spangen.[1076] With this aid he was able to obtain the correct diagnosis in 19 of 24 cases studied. Ultrasonic scanning of the semilunar line should be undertaken in all cases of obscure abdominal pain associated with bulging of the belly wall in the standing patient. Deitch and Engel have confirmed the usefulness of ultrasound in the diagnosis of abdominal wall defects.[281] Ultrasound provides the diagnosis easily and cheaply in our experience and is recommended as the first-line imaging investigation. The advantages of high-resolution real-time ultrasonography are the ability to perform the examination in both the supine and upright positions and while the patient performs a Valsalva maneuver. Other provocative techniques include a cough or sit-ups, which will increase the intra-abdominal pressure so that the hernia is more easily demonstrated. It is a sensible precaution to always ultrasonically scan the semilunar lines on both sides because herniation is frequently multiple.[178,825,1132] The use of ultrasonic guidance for the reduction of an incarcerated Spigelian hernia has been recorded as a case report.[1133]

Scanning by CT, performed with close thin sections, can visualize a Spigelian hernia. This is now the most reliable imaging technique to make the diagnosis (Figure 21.5).[179,510,1228] The use of oral contrast medium during the examination is recommended so that any bowel content can be identified.[1228] The increasing availability of the magnetic resonance imaging (MRI) may be of benefit in the preoperative evaluation of these difficult cases.[1130]

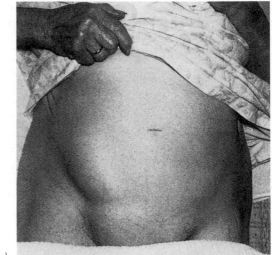

(a)

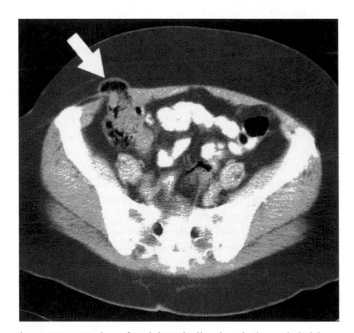

Figure 21.5 *CT view of a right Spigelian hernia (arrow). (With permission from the British Journal of Surgery.)*

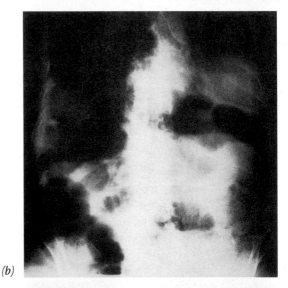

(b)

Many Spigelian hernias go unrecognized on clinical examination, even after both ultrasound investigation and CT scanning. If the diagnosis is still in question, the next procedure will be the laparoscopic examination.[191] The use of an exploratory laparotomy in these circumstances is not justified as the diagnosis (and treatment) can be done with the less invasive technique. If laparoscopy is not available, the use of intraoperative ultrasonography can be helpful, particularly in obese patients.[710]

The differential diagnosis includes appendicitis and appendiceal abscess, a tumor of the abdominal wall or a spontaneous hematoma of the rectus muscle or even acute diverticulitis.[967]

Spigelian hernias are treacherous and have a real risk of strangulation. For this reason, operation is advised for all cases (Figure 21.6).

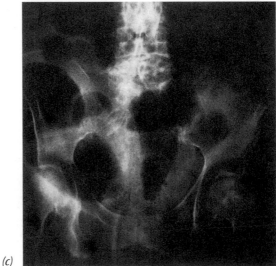

(c)

Figure 21.6 *(a) An elderly woman with a strangulated Spigelian hernia and bilateral femoral hernias; (b) an abdominal film shows the features of intestinal obstruction and a gas-filled loop in the Spigelian hernia; (c) gas is also seen in a loop of small gut in the left femoral hernia.*

PREOPERATIVELY

Suture materials

For details see Chapter 3.

Anesthesia

General anesthesia is preferred, but local infiltration anesthesia can be employed. If the latter is used, the operating surgeon must remember that the parietal peritoneum is very sensitive and manipulation of it can cause the patient much discomfort unless the anesthesia is adequate (see Chapter 8). Of course, the laparoscopic method requires a general anesthetic.

THE OPERATION

Position of patient

The patient is laid on his back on the operating table.

DRAPING

Drapes are placed so as to allow easy access to the hernia and to the abdominal cavity if bowel resection becomes necessary in patients with strangulated or obstructed intestine.

The open operation

If the traditional open approach is chosen, a transverse incision (gridiron) over the protrusion gives an excellent exposure. Only in the occasional very large hernia is it necessary to construct an elliptical incision and to remove the intervening redundant skin and subcutaneous tissue with the sac (Figure 21.7). If there is no obvious hernia protrusion, or if the diagnosis is in doubt, a midline or paramedian incision over the hernia itself is advisable. In that instance, a preperitoneal exploration could be

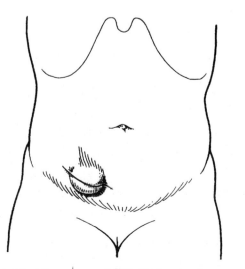

Figure 21.7 An oblique incision over the hernia gives access

performed quite adequately. To accomplish this the rectus muscle is retracted medially and the posterior sheath is incised longitudinally to reach the Spigelian aponeurosis.

The dissection is deepened to the external oblique aponeurosis. The hernial sac may lie deep to the aponeurosis, between it and the internal oblique, or it may be within the sheath of the rectus muscle. In either of these situations it is necessary to incise the aponeurosis and split it in the direction of its fibers to expose the peritoneal sac (Figure 21.8). If the gridiron incision is chosen it will be necessary to incise the anterior portion of the rectus sheath to provide exposure of the spigelian aponeurosis so as not to overlook an intravaginal herniation.

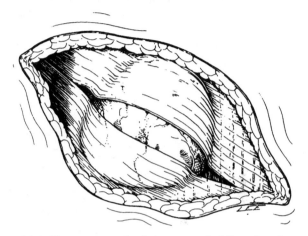

Figure 21.8 The aponeurosis of the external oblique is split to deliver the hernial sac.

Spigelian hernia defects may be multiple, therefore it is essential in every case to palpate the adjacent semilunar line fascia from the peritoneal surface to exclude other hernial orifices. To overlook a second Spigelian hernia would require that the patient undergo a second operation that should have been avoided.

The sac

This is always present, even if the hernia is small. It may be globular or mushroom shaped. The most common content of the sac is omentum, which may be adherent, but small or large intestine may be found. The appendix, stomach, gall bladder, endometrium, ovary and ectopic testicle have all been described in Spigelian hernia sacs.[1076]

Excision of sac

Once the sac has been adequately exposed, one option at that point would be to open it, so that its contents can be reduced. One could then excise the redundant part and close the neck of the sac with either pursestring suture or by a continuous suture according to size (Figure 21.9). Generally, however, the need to eliminate the sac is unnecessary. Most surgeons would simply invert the sac alone. This is particularly important if one

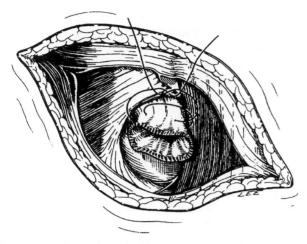

Figure 21.9 *The sac is opened and the contents reduced, then the neck of the sac is closed with a transfixion suture of absorbable polymer. Redundant sac is excised.*

chooses to proceed with a plug repair to decrease the risk of adhesions or fistulization.[1011]

Closure

To repair this hernia without the use of a prosthetic biomaterial the opening in the internal oblique and transversus muscles is closed with a continuous suture of polypropylene or another permanent suture material (Figure 21.10). The external oblique aponeurosis is sutured with the suture used for the deeper layers. The subcutaneous fat can be closed with an absorbable suture.

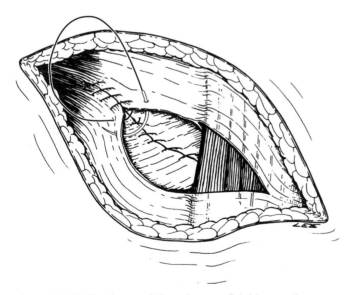

Figure 21.10 *The deep and then the superficial layers of aponeurosis are separately closed with continuous sutures of polypropylene. A suction drain may be used.*

The use of a prosthetic patch of this hernial orifice is frequently used as an integral part of the repair. The biomaterial can be placed in the preperitoneal space in the manner of the

Rives–Stoppa repair. This is probably the best location for the mesh but one may also repair the hernia with interrupted sutures and place the mesh above the fascia. Usually, however, the surgeon merely places the mesh and secures it to the fascial edges with a permanent suture. As with the other ventral hernias, this incurs a risk of re-herniation beneath the prosthesis itself.

The use of a plug to repair six Spigelian hernias has been reported with success. This repair mimics the plug repair of the groin and can be performed under local anesthesia.[1011]

The skin can be closed by whatever preference the surgeon dictates. Sutures, staples or subcuticular suturing all provide an excellent cosmetic result.

The laparoscopic operation

The laparoscopic technique has been used with success in several reports.[21,191,219,351,374,395,568,1134] The preoperative considerations would not differ from that of the open technique or that of the usual incisional hernia. The one exception may be the patient that is suspected of bowel infarction, in which case it may be preferable to proceed with the open approach.

The choice of trocar locations can differ but generally a midline port can be used for the initial location of the laparoscope. At least two additional trocars will be placed on the contralateral side of the abdomen to the hernia. Some surgeons may prefer to place one trocar on the contralateral side and the second operating trocar in the upper quadrant of the ipsilateral side of the hernia. The size of the trocars can be all 5 or 10 mm based upon the preference of the surgeon as well as the instrumentation and laparoscope sizes (Figure 21.11).

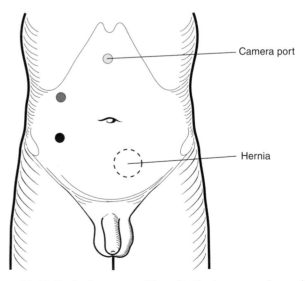

Figure 21.11 *Typical trocar positions for the laparoscopic repair of a left sided Spigelian hernia. Occasionally an additional trocar will be necessary on the left side of the abdomen.*

Once abdominal access is obtained, the site of the hernial orifice is readily identified. The presence of any incarcerated tissue must be reduced. This may require that the hernial ring be incised to provide a large enough orifice to reduce the contents safely. The tissue can be inspected to assure that there is viability. Once this is done, the operation will proceed in an identical manner as that of the traditional laparoscopic ventral herniorrhaphy (see Chapter 23). All of the reports referenced above employed the use of a prosthetic biomaterial with the single exception of Carter, who closed the hernial orifice with Vicryl® sutures. The use of a prosthetic is preferred as this will provide a tension-free repair. As this is placed in the intraperitoneal position, the use of ePTFE is recommended.

POSTOPERATIVE CARE

If there has been extensive handling and dissection of the small gut and omentum during the operation, postoperative management with nasogastric suction and parenteral fluids may be needed until normal peristalsis is established.

Early ambulation and breathing exercises are essential. The postoperative problem that most frequently arises is respiratory embarrassment due to the wound pain and the newly raised intra-abdominal pressure. With the use of prosthetic materials in the repair of the Spigelian hernia the amount of postoperative pain is diminished. These patients become ambulatory more rapidly because of this fact. In the majority of cases, these operations can be accomplished as an outpatient surgery.

CONCLUSIONS

* Spigelian hernias are clinically elusive often until strangulation occurs. Various radiologic imaging techniques allow the preoperative assessment of the semilunar line.
* Operation should always be advised. Apart from the discomfort these hernias cause, they strangulate frequently and for this reason particularly they should be repaired.
* The choice of repair can be tissue, open prosthetic or laparoscopic herniorraphy. Recurrences are rare.

22

Incisional hernia – the 'open' techniques (excluding parastomal hernia)

HISTORICAL NOTE

Incisional hernia is iatrogenic and its incidence has increased with each increment of abdominal surgical intervention. An incisional hernia is the most perfect example of a 'surgeon-dependent variable'. The recent introduction of continuous ambulatory peritoneal dialysis has been followed by its own unique harvest of incisional hernias.[202,333] Laparoscopic surgery has also added a new entity: 'Port Site' hernia[347] (Chapter 18, page 238). Although the latter is becoming infrequent with the advent of smaller ports and the instrumentation that is currently available.

The development of abdominal surgery in the 19th century – the excision of an ovarian cyst by McDowell in 1809,[768] partial gastrectomy by Billroth in 1881,[123] cholecystectomy by Langenbuch in 1882[632] – has been followed by operations to manage the incisional hernias which followed as complications. Gerdy repaired an incisional hernia in 1836 and Maydl another in 1886.[528] Judd in 1912[558] and Gibson in 1920[402] both described repair techniques based on extensive anatomic dissection of the scar and adjacent tissues. Prosthetic materials were introduced early on: autografts of fascia lata by Kirschner in 1910,[601] and fascial strips by Gallie and Le Mesurier in 1923.[382] Tendons, cutis and whole skin grafts, both homografts and heterografts, have been advocated and found to have problems. Non-biological prosthetics that have been used in the past include stainless steel and tantalum gauze. More recently polypropylene (Marlex, Prolene), polyester (Mersilene) and ePTFE (DualMesh Plus) have been introduced and are the materials of choice for many surgeons (these are reviewed in Chapter 7).

The ideal prosthetic material has yet to be discovered. The visionary Theodore Billroth stated more than a century ago, 'If we could artificially produce tissues of the density and toughness of fascia or tendon, the secret of radical cure of hernia would be discovered'.[1002] The currently available products, however, are generally excellent alternatives to the native tissues when the repair of these hernias is undertaken.

SYMPTOMS AND SIGNS

An incisional hernia is defined by Pollock and his colleagues as 'A bulge visible and palpable when the patient is standing and often requiring support or repair'.[650]

Sixty percent of patients with incisional hernias do not experience any symptoms; however, symptoms that predicate medical advice include difficulty in bending, cosmetic deformity, discomfort from the size of the hernia, persistent abdominal pain and episodic subacute intestinal obstruction. Incarceration persisting to acute intestinal obstruction and strangulation necessitate emergency surgery.

Spontaneous rupture of incisional hernia is an unusual but life-threatening complication. This complication is more likely in infra-umbilical hernia. It may be exacerbated by friction of clothes or corsetry.[481] Hernias after gynecological and obstetric interventions are most at risk.[1038]

The demonstration of small incisional hernias may be very difficult. Patients with tiny protrusions of extraperitoneal fat and a small peritoneal sac may complain of a tender lump which is not always there but which causes quite severe localized pain when it is present. Physical examination of the patient supine and relaxed usually reveals the cause. Ultrasound examination is a useful diagnostic test and will often reveal an impalpable defect, particularly in the obese patient. However, the sonographic examination of the abdominal wall is dependent upon a skilled interpreter. It is sometimes difficult to differentiate between a hernia and subcutaneous fat or small bowel in the hernia versus in close proximity to a weakened anterior fascia. In most situations and particularly for massive complex incisional hernias the CT scan may be much more efficient and accurate in defining the defect and planning the preoperative preparation of the patient and the operation chosen.

INCIDENCE

The overall incidence of incisional hernias is difficult to estimate. Homans, in 1887, reported that 10% of abdominal operations were followed by incisional hernias;[512] more recent studies give lower incidences – probably only 2% of all abdominal operations are followed by incisional hernia, although series which include only 'major laparotomy' wounds yield higher incidences. Certainly the reported incidence of this complication has fallen in the past 10 years, during which major sepsis has diminished, non-irritant, non-absorbable sutures have been introduced and the technique of wound closure has been emphasized. Incisional hernias are slightly more frequent in males than females (55:45) (see Table 3.2).

Until recently there were very few studies with adequate follow-up of laparotomy wounds to determine the real incidence of incisional hernia. Stanton, in 1916, reported 500 consecutive laparotomies followed up for 5–7 years. Over this period a total of 24 postoperative hernias were found (4.8%). In 260 clean cases only three incisional hernias developed, whereas in 186 contaminated cases 18 hernias developed.[1083]

Although the incidence of burst abdomen has been reduced by mass closure techniques, incisional hernia remains an important problem. The strength of the abdominal wall resides in the aponeurotic layers, the linea alba and the rectus sheath. These layers are slow to heal and only regain adequate strength after 120 days from wounding.[315] On a theoretical basis, most incisional hernias would be expected to be apparent before this healing is complete. The reports of onset of incisional hernia which occur in the standard textbooks are usually based on the information gleaned from patients having repair operations for symptomatic incisional hernias, hence they probably over-emphasize these large and early onset hernias. For instance, Akman (1962) estimated that 97% of incisional hernias were apparent at 5 years.[13]

Long-term prospective studies of laparotomy wounds were unknown until Hughes and Ellis separately raised the question of late wound failure in the early 1980s. Ellis and colleagues from the Westminster Hospital followed up 363 patients who had undergone laparotomy but who had sound wounds without herniation when examined at one year. When reviewed between 2½ and 5½ years later, 21 patients (5.8%) had developed incisional hernias.[156,332,474,822,824]

Mudge and Hughes from Cardiff have published an important continuation of their study of incisional hernia.[822] During the years 1972–1973, 831 patients aged over 40 years undergoing major abdominal surgery were entered into a long-term study. Of 564 patients surviving and being willing to enter the study at the end of one year, 337 patients were followed up for a further nine years. Of the remainder, 128 patients had died and 99 patients had an incomplete follow-up for various reasons. All the patients were questioned regarding symptoms and incapacity.

Of the 564 patients 62 (11%) had developed incisional hernias by the definition of Pollock. Of these 62 patients developing incisional hernias, details of the original operative closure technique were known for 52 and for 408 patients who did not develop hernias. The incidence of hernia in patients having nylon closure to both peritoneum and linea alba was 11 of 143 (7.7%); for catgut to peritoneum and nylon to linea alba, 24 out of 196 developed incisional hernia (12%); for catgut to both layers, 11 out of 100 developed incisional hernias (14%); of four patients having nylon through and through tension sutures,

two developed incisional hernias. When the 337 completing the 10-year follow-up are scrutinized 37 (11%) developed an incisional hernia and 13 of these (35%) first appeared at 5 years or later. One in three of these hernias caused symptoms.

More than half the incisional hernias first appeared more than one year after the initial operation. These 10-year results confirm that there is a continued attrition of the healed laparotomy wound, with incisional hernias developing up to and after 10 years. When the distress and disability of the hernias is considered, those that develop in the first 3 years after laparotomy cause the most symptoms; they are also the larger hernias and are more likely to require repairs.[474]

These findings from two independent groups in London and Cardiff confirm each other, the failure rate of abdominal wounds being about 6% at 5 years rising to 11% at 10 years.

Akman's earlier statement that 97% of incisional hernias are apparent at one year after the original surgery is not confirmed by these long-term studies. Moreover, without full-scale prospective follow-up the incidence of incisional hernia will be underestimated.

The number of incisional hernias coming to surgical operation is lower than their overall incidence. Over the 15 years mid-1970 to mid-1985, 277 incisional hernia repairs were undertaken in Stockton-on-Tees. During the same period approximately 19 000 abdominal operations were performed which, if recent British reports are broadly correct, should have been followed by a much greater (10%) harvest of incisional hernias. Fortunately not all incisional hernias warrant an operation. The incidence of incisional hernias resulting from various operative procedures is given in Table 22.1.

Currently it is believed that up to 13% of laparotomy incisions will eventually develop hernias. In the Systematic Review of Hodgson 2000 et al.[506] (see Chapter 6), it was concluded that abdominal fascial closure of midline laparotomy wounds with a continuous, non-absorbable suture results in a significantly lower rate of incisional hernia than using either non-absorbable or interrupted techniques. The recent adoption of the laparoscopic techniques for the treatment of intra-abdominal pathology will undoubtedly decrease the occurrence of the midline incisional hernias. However, this change will probably require a new generation of surgeons to emerge from the training programs.

ETIOLOGIC FACTORS

The important causative factors include sepsis (60% of patients developing an incisional hernia within the first year after surgery have had significant wound infection); the placement of drainage tubes through the original incision; a previous operation through the same incision within 6 months; initial closure with catgut alone ('inept methods of suture');[734,1113] steroid and other immunosuppressant therapy; and inflammatory bowel disease. Obesity is an important risk factor both for the occurrence of the original incisional hernia and for the likelihood of recurrence of the hernia after repair.[156,913] Early wound dehiscence is frequently followed by incisional herniation. Needle puncture

Table 22.1 *Incisional hernia: initial operative procedures*

Procedure	Akman (1962) Total no. 500 patients (%)	Ponka (1980) Total no. 794 patients (%)	Devlin (1982) Total no. 214 patients (%)
Hysterectomy and other gynecological interventions	18.6	34	19
Cholecystectomy and biliary tract operations	9.6	21	11
Appendicectomy	43.8	16	16
Colorectal operations*	7.6	9	9
Gastric operations	4.2	11	30
Cesarean section	4.2	2	12

*Colorectal operations are not defined separately by Akman: the figure quoted is the sum of 'laparotomy other than specified' and 'non-specified (i.e. non-urologic and non-gynecologic) pelvic operations'.

incisional hernias are described as 'satellites' of a main wound failure. These hernias may be related to the sawing effect of non-absorbable sutures on the aponeurosis.[526] Less significant factors include age and sex, anemia, malnutrition, hypoproteinemia, diabetes, type of incision, postoperative intestinal obstruction[740] and postoperative chest infection. Two recent retrospective reviews which included multifactorial regression analysis of putative risk factors, such as sex, age, smoking, chronic lung disease, obesity, sight, surgeon's experience, closure method and suture material have found that size of the hernia[503] and obesity[740] were the prime factors involved in recurrence after incisional hernia repair. Many of these hernias recurred early with re-medial time between the primary operation and the first symptoms of hernia being within a year. Fifty-five percent of incisional hernias occur in men. Incisional hernias are infrequent under the age of 40 years and their incidence increases with age. There is an association between the development of incisional hernias and the occurrence of the post-thrombotic syndrome.[823]

Of particular importance as an etiologic factor is the wound drain. Ponka records that of 126 patients with herniation through a subcostal incision for biliary surgery, all had drains delivered through the wound at the time of the initial operation.[913]

Midline incisions are at greater risk than paramedian incisions.[65] However, no matter which anatomic type of incision is made, the choice of suture material is crucial. Kirk compared paramedian incisions closed with two layers of catgut with midline incisions closed with nylon; the crucial difference was not the anatomy of the incision but the choice of suture – the nylon closed incisions were significantly better than those closed with catgut.[600]

Lower midline incisions seem to be at greater risk than upper midline incisions (but this may be a faulty finding; inadequate suture techniques as well as physiological factors need assessing). Many of the lower midline incisions are done for gynecological interventions and the subsequent hernias are often not included in purely 'surgical' follow-up data; hence, there may be under-recording of the true overall incidence of this problem. Table 22.2 shows the site of some incisional hernias. The incidence of these hernias has been changed with the findings of other laparoscopic authors, which is also shown in this table.[665] Additionally, the locations of these hernias has

Table 22.2 *Site of incisional hernias*

Site	Akman (1962) n = 500 (%)	Ponka (1980) n = 794 (%)	LeBlanc (2000) n = 100 (%)
Midline:			80
lower abdomen	33	26	
upper abdomen	5.4	16	
Subcostal: right and left	–	16	2
Paramedian: right and left	9.6	11	
Transverse and muscle-splitting right lower quadrant: McBurney, etc.	21	9	2
Peristomal	–	4	
Vertical:			
right upper quadrant	–	4	
right lower quadrant	–	3	
Vertical: midline xiphoid to pubis	–	11	
Left lower quadrant (prior colostomy)			3
Pfannenstiel			2
Renal transplant incision			1

become altered with the newer operations that have evolved with the current treatments of the medical problems of the patient.

The one clear conclusion is that catgut alone is an unreliable method of closing a laparotomy wound. Of 107 paramedian wounds closed with two layers of catgut in the Leeds trial, there was an early wound failure rate of 14%; of 107 wounds closed with two layers of catgut reinforced by all-layers nylon tension sutures, the wound failure rate was 4.8% ($P < 0.05$). Interrupted mass Smead–Jones closure with monofilament 28 s.w.g. wire gave a wound failure rate of 0.92% (method 1 vs. method 3, $P < 0.001$).[428]

Mass suture with wire is the most secure method, but wire is difficult to handle and is uncomfortable for the patient. Closure with catgut either alone or with tension sutures removed at 14 days was associated with a considerable incidence of late incisional herniation. No late incisional hernias developed in the cases closed with interrupted wire.[428] Additionally, there was a higher incidence of hematoma, wound infection and sinuses when catgut was used.

The newer absorbable polymer sutures polyglactin (Vicryl) and polyglycolic acid PGA (Dexon) have been subjected to trial and are reported as less good than non-absorbables. The longer life polymer polydioxanone (PDS) is under evaluation. A controlled trial of PDS versus polyamide (nylon) in the closure of 233 major laparotomy wounds failed to show any statistically significant difference. The patients were randomized to either suture, a mass-closure technique was used and patients were followed up to 6 months. There were two wound failures in the PDS group and more sepsis in the PDS group. There were no wound sinuses in either group.[407]

Late hernias occur just as frequently in patients whose wounds are sutured with catgut, absorbable polymer and non-absorbable filament. At present there is no explanation of why mature collagen should yield to form a hernia so long after healing has occurred. There is no etiological factor to account for these late hernias[474,822] although the concept of collagen failure, metastatic emphysema, may offer an explanation (see page 46).

Epigastric incisional hernias are recently reported as a complication of median sternotomy wounds for cardiac surgery. The risk factors identified include male sex, obesity, wound infection, aortic valve replacement and left ventricular failure.[267]

In children, either a layered or a mass closure with polyglycolic acid sutures gives acceptable results and a low failure rate. Non-absorbable sutures are unnecessary in children.[605] For some unknown reason the risk of failure in children is greatest in those undergoing pyloromyotomy (Ramstedt's) operation for hypertrophic pyloric stenosis.[147] Early incisional hernias in children are likely to resolve spontaneously. The late development of incisional hernias occurs rarely in children.[587]

PRINCIPLES OF OPEN REPAIR

The following principles should be followed:

1 Whenever possible the normal anatomy should be reconstituted. In midline hernias this means the linea alba must be firmly reconstructed; in more lateral hernias there should be layer-by-layer closure as far as possible. However, the use of sutures with the repair of these hernias is associated with a rate of recurrence that is at least as high as 43%.[715] For this reason, it may not be feasible or desirable to reconstitute the linea alba . This is not always possible with the larger hernias and certainly not done with the laparoscopic repair.

2 Only tendinous/aponeurotic/fascial structures should be brought together. In situ darning over the defect without adequate mobilization and apposition of the aponeurotic defect gives a 100% recurrence rate.[474]

3 The suture material must retain its strength for long enough to maintain tissue apposition and allow sound union of tissues to occur. A non-absorbable material must therefore be used.

4 The length of suture material is related to the geometry of the wound and to its healing. Using deep bites at not more than 0.5 cm intervals, the ratio of suture length to wound length must be 4:1 or more.[540,549]

5 Repair of an incisional hernia inevitably involves returning viscera to the confines of the abdominal cavity with a resultant rise in intra-abdominal pressure. It is important to minimize this. Preoperative weight reduction is the first precaution. This, unfortunately, is generally not possible. Therefore the surgeon will usually be forced to repair these hernias with little consideration for the increase in the intra-abdominal pressure. In the majority of situations, this is not a clinical issue as few patients will experience an increase in intra-abdominal pressure that is clinically significant.

6 Every care must be taken to prevent abdominal distension due to adynamic ileus which will lead to additional stress on repair suture lines. For this reason, handling of the viscera should be minimized.

7 Postoperative coughing can put an additional unwarranted strain on the suture lines. Hence, pulmonary collapse, pulmonary infection and pulmonary edema must be avoided. Restriction of preoperative smoking, chest exercises, weight reduction and avoidance of excessive blood or fluid replacement (and their hemodynamic effects on the heart) are important components in the successful repair of an incisional hernia.

8 The repair must be performed aseptically; inoculated bacteria, traumatized tissue and hematoma should not be features of these wounds.

Drawing these eight points together, appropriate preparation for operation includes measures to reduce the risk of subsequent infection: all skin lesions and erosions should be resolved before surgery: pulmonary function should be optimized. A carefully planned procedure using a tension-free repair with prosthetic reinforcement is recommended in appropriate patients.[1013]

In epigastric incisional hernia repair it should be remembered that the linea alba is broad in the epigastrium – at least as broad as the xiphoid cartilage is wide – therefore efforts to draw the rectus muscles close together are unanatomic and doomed to disruption. Most of the side-to-side tension in the linea alba in the epigastrium is generated in the anterior rectus sheath which consists of two laminae, the anterior lamina being the external oblique arising from the lower ribs. The short span of this muscle makes this layer relatively inelastic and unstretchable to the midline for repair.[56] Division of one anterior rectus sheath longitudinally over the rectus muscle will allow a medial flap to be turned into suture to the contralateral fellow flap (Figure 22.1).[152] Alternatively, longitudinal incision of the medial scarred margins of both the rectus sheaths, the longitudinal 'releasing operation' of Gibson (1916),[402] allows the rectus muscles to spring into a straight line to cover the defect.[733,1233] The defect in the anterior sheath can be repaired with an onlay fascia lata graft or nowadays preferably with an onlay polypropylene (Marlex) mesh.[152,466,1158] A nylon darn is an alternative

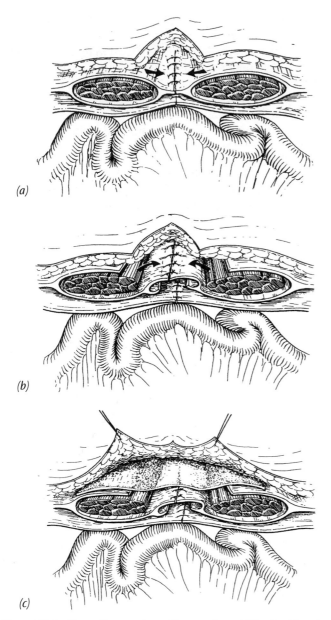

Figure 22.1 *Chevrel's procedure. Closure of a midline incisional hernia may be under considerable tension (a). This tension can be relieved by a longitudinal rectus relieving incision. The medial rectus margin can then be turned in as aponeurotic flaps to repair the defect (b). The anterior rectus sheath is replaced by mesh in the extraparietal (extra-aponeurotic) plane (c).*

technique to reinforce the anterior rectus sheath. The darn should only be used if one layer of aponeurotic repair can be accomplished, by turning in the rectus sheath for instance.[525]

INCISIONAL HERNIA FOLLOWING APPENDECTOMY

Incisional hernias related to appendectomy are reported in all series. Etiological factors include severe postoperative wound sepsis and the placement of a drain through a grid-iron appendectomy wound. These hernias occurring through the red

muscle in the flank are difficult to repair adequately. If there is a well-developed fibrous margin to the defect this can be used as the basis of a Mayo-type overlap repair. Direct suture of these hernias, suturing red muscle, often fails and if an adequate overlap cannot be constructed, extraperitoneal mesh or mesh reinforcement of the external oblique aponeurosis is advised.

PNEUMOPERITONEUM AS AN AID IN SURGICAL TREATMENT OF GIANT HERNIAS

Management of giant incisional hernia is often compromised by obesity, intrahernial adhesions and contraction in the volume of the abdominal cavity – the hernial contents have lost their 'right of domain'. Long operations to free the adhesions and brutal reduction of the contents can lead to ileus, pulmonary restriction and cardiac embarrassment. After these operations, if the patient does not succumb to the cardiorespiratory complications the persistent ileus will lead to disruption of the repair.

The use of pneumoperitoneum before attempting definitive repair of giant hernias was originally suggested by Moreno in 1940.[805] The advantages of the technique are:

- Stretching of the abdominal wall, creating a larger cavity into which the hernial contents can be replaced.
- Reduction of edema in the mesentery, omentum and viscera in the hernial sac, creating less mass to be reduced.
- Stretching of the hernial sac leading to elongation of adhesions, making dissection and reduction easier.[465]
- Increased tone of the diaphragm, allowing preoperative respiratory and circulatory adaptation to the elevation of the diaphragm.[371]

The technique of pneumoperitoneum is simple: under local anesthetic an epidural catheter, an intracath or a ureteric pigtail catheter, is introduced into the peritoneal cavity. The site of puncture should be kept well away from the hernia or its margins to avoid damaging viscera fixed by adhesions. The optimum site is probably through the linea alba. Successful abdominal puncture is marked by a lessening of the pressure required to advance the needle. The catheter can then be easily threaded into the peritoneal cavity and its position checked radiologically after injection of a small quantity of contrast medium.[941] The catheter is fixed into position and about 500 ml of gas or air is injected via a micropore filter.[60] Graduated amounts of gas or air are injected on successive days, 500 ml at a time once, twice or thrice a day, until a daily volume of about 2.5 liters is obtained. Caldironi and colleagues used nitrous oxide in 41 patients with giant incisional hernias. A laparoscopic insufflator was used to top up the pneumoperitoneum every other day for a mean of 5.5 days, a total volume of 23.2 liters of nitrous oxide being injected. The volume introduced at each session was 1000/1500 ml greater than the previous session and the procedure was well tolerated in all but one patient. The good results of the subsequent repairs (only two recurrences in 40 repairs at a mean 25 months follow-up) attests to the success of this technique.[167] The abdomen will inevitably be blown up like a balloon and much patient reassurance may be needed. If the patient develops discomfort, shoulder tip pain, tachycardia or dyspnea, the rate of insufflation can be reduced; indeed, if severe symptoms occur gas or air can be withdrawn. No attempt is made to prevent the hernial sac distending; distension of the hernial sac is helpful, stretching adhesions and allowing contents to reduce spontaneously prior to operation. Unfettered distension of the peritoneal sac may reveal subsidiary hernial protrusions, enabling a more adequate surgical repair to be planned and undertaken. There is a profound need for this technique in the surgical armentarium but while this has been found to be of significant benefit in South America and some parts of Europe, the experience with this technique in the United States is limited.

In practice, the patient is ready for operation at about 2 weeks after induction of the pneumoperitoneum, the end point being judged by the tension of the abdominal wall, which should feel as tight as a drum, especially in the flanks.[83] The patient should be operated on at this stage – if possible most of the dissection should be performed with the hernial sac unpunctured and distended. Puncture of the sac at operation will allow easy reduction of contents and the slack parietes will facilitate repair. Air is only slowly absorbed from the peritoneal cavity and often after the first two or three days absorption is so reduced as to become inconsequential.

Contraindications to pneumoperitoneum include abdominal wall sepsis, prior cardiorespiratory decompensation and strangulation of hernial contents. Complications, which are very rare, include visceral puncture, hematoma and the risk of an embolism into a solid organ if the liver or spleen is needled prior to insufflation. Mediastinal and retroperitoneal surgical emphysema are rare complications.

INDICATIONS FOR OPERATION

Incisional hernias produce symptoms of discomfort and pain, and often recurrent colic if subacute obstructive episodes occur. Such symptoms are reason enough for operative intervention. Irreducibility and a narrow neck are further indications for surgery. Obstruction and strangulation are absolute indications.

CONTRAINDICATIONS TO ELECTIVE OPERATION

Extreme obesity can be a contraindication to surgery. Obese patients frequently have cardiorespiratory decompensation and diabetes, making weight reduction essential prior to surgery.[1047] Subcutaneous and intra-abdominal obesity make the open repair more difficult and postoperative complications more likely. The laparoscopic repair seems to be the more effective and less morbid operation for the obese patients. In the particularly high-risk patients, the use of invasive monitoring such as a Swan–Ganz catheter and the monitoring that the intensive care units provide will allow such patients to undergo these operation without undue risks in these modern times.

Continuing deep sepsis in the wound is also a contraindication to repair surgery. Such cases frequently have a history of more than one repair attempt, and the wound may be indurated with many sinuses in it. If the sepsis is longstanding, calcification may be present. Usually wounds with continuing infection contain buried and heavily infected non-absorbable material; it is best to open these wounds, remove all the foreign material, drain all the pockets of pus. The wound is then left to granulate over. Only when the wound has been without deep sepsis for 6–9 months should repair surgery be undertaken.

Skin infections and intertrigo beneath a vast incisional hernia are common, and require vigorous preoperative treatment. Operation should be delayed until the skin is sound.

CHOICE OF OPERATIVE TECHNIQUE

It is usually preferable to make an accurate assessment of the anatomy of the hernia prior to surgery. How big is the defect? Does the size of the defect increase or decrease on movement? Are the contents easily reducible? If the hernia contents are incarcerated, this may not be possible.

The sac and fibrous margins of the sac are examined with the patient supine and at ease, and then standing erect.

Finally the patient is laid flat again, and as much of the sac as possible is reduced and held reduced by the examining surgeon. The patient is then asked to sit up while the surgeon continues to hold the hernia reduced. In some hernias, particularly upper midline ones, the margins of the defect close together on movement and the contraction of the abdominal wall will then hold the sac reduced (Figure 22.2). These maneuvers may provide the surgeon with the information necessary to decide upon the operation that should be used, whether a prosthesis is mandatory and if there is a possibility that the laparoscopic method should be performed rather than the open repair.

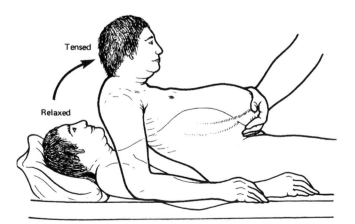

Figure 22.2 *Examination of an incisional hernia. The anatomy of the sac must be known. The patient is examined laid and relaxed, and with the muscles tensed. Do the margins of the sac close or open during activity? Is there a tissue defect?*

Layer-by-layer closure

If the sac is small, does not protrude and become pendulous in the erect patient, and if the margins can be approximated easily when the patient is relaxed and draw themselves together when the patient tenses the muscles, there is relatively normal anatomy and a layer-by-layer anatomic repair should be done. Akman and Obney, from the Shouldice clinic, recommended a layer-by-layer closure with an overlap. If the operation is performed under local anesthetic the patient can be encouraged to breathe in synchronously with the suturing, enabling a tight first layer of repair. Subsequent layers overlap the aponeurosis and reinforce this. This repair is generally considered in patients that have a defect size that measures 4 cm or less. Even this consideration may need to be tempered in patients with very weak fascia or incisional hernias with multiple defects.

Prosthetic mesh operation

If the aponeurotic margins of the defect cannot be approximated in the conscious patient and do not spontaneously draw together when the patient moves, it is probable that there is a tissue defect (or loss) and that a prosthetic operation will be required. At operation, if the fascial defect(s) is greater than 4 cm, a prosthesis is recommended. The prosthetic biomaterials that are available at the time of this publication are described in Chapter 7.

An important note of caution: unless the margins of the defect can be approximated in the conscious patient do not attempt a layer-by-layer repair. The sutures will cut out and the result will be failure. Some form of prosthetic repair is mandatory if there is a persisting tissue deficit in the relaxed conscious patient.[397]

Anesthesia

Small incisional hernias without a tissue defect can be repaired using a local anesthetic; however, for larger hernias and for the laparoscopic repair full general anesthesia is necessary. Muscle relaxants will assist in reducing the contents of the sac and drawing together the margins of the defect during the repair. In some circumstances, the use of spinal or epidural anesthesia may be considered but this would depend upon the location of the hernia site and the surgeon's familiarity with the choice of that anesthesia method.

THE OPEN OPERATION

Position of patient

If the hernia is located in the midline or lateral aspects of the anterior abdominal wall, the patient is placed in the supine position on the operating table.

The incision

An elliptical incision is made to enclose the cutaneous scar. The incision must generally be extended at either end to give adequate access to all the margins of the defect. The direction of this initial incision will depend on the shape of the original scar through which the hernia has come.

Care should be taken not to excise too much skin: at this stage the minimum excision of cutaneous scar tissue is done (Figure 22.3).

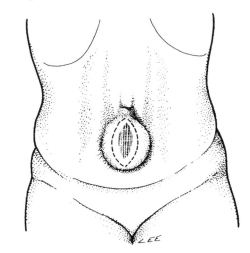

Figure 22.3 *Elliptical incisions are made on either side of the hernial cicatrix.*

Removal of overlying redundant tissue

The redundant skin and scar are separated from the underlying hernial sac, which is often just subcutaneous especially near the fundus of the hernia. Redundant skin and scar tissue are removed (Figure 22.4). This is a significant difference between the open

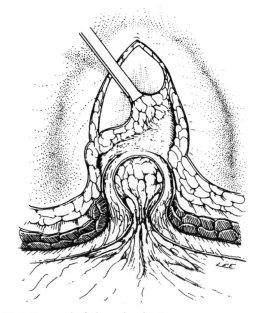

Figure 22.4 *Removal of the redundant scar.*

and the laparoscopic method. Some surgeons prefer this open approach so that the redundant skin can be removed. Generally, however, the cosmetic result of the laparoscopic repair is acceptable without the resection of the redundant tissue.

If the hernia is very large the skin and underlying peritoneal sac may be virtually fused into one layer near the fundus of the hernial protrusion. When removing the redundant skin, care is necessary to avoid damage to the hernia contents which may be adherent over wide areas of the inside of the sac (Figure 22.5).

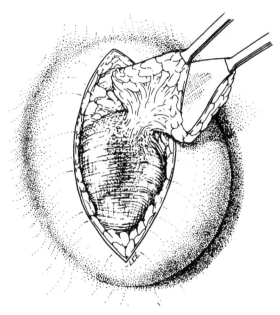

Figure 22.5 *Care must be taken not to remove too much skin and not to damage the hernial sac. The cutaneous cicatrix is often closely adherent to the sac.*

Exposure

The hernia is dissected from the surrounding subcutaneous fat. The surgeon may choose to use the scalpel blade, scissors, and/or the electrocautery pencil for this dissection. The coverings of the hernia are stretched scar tissue merging into the stretched abdominal wall aponeurosis at the circumference of the protrusion and a variable amount of extraperitoneal fatty tissue (Figure 22.6).

The scar tissue is incised in an elliptical fashion around the hernial neck, where it merges with the stretched aponeurosis. The peritoneal hernial sac is thus defined all around at its attachment to the muscle/aponeurotic layer (Figure 22.7).

Managing the peritoneal sac

If intestinal obstruction or strangulation is present the sac must be opened and its contents explored. The advent of laparoscopic techniques for incisional hernia repair has revealed that at least one-third of hernia sacs contain visceral contents which are adherent to the sac itself. For this reason it is recommended

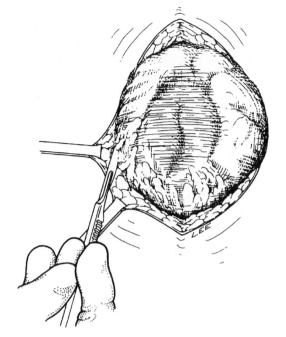

Figure 22.6 *The sides of the hernial sac are dissected to the aponeurotic margins of the defect.*

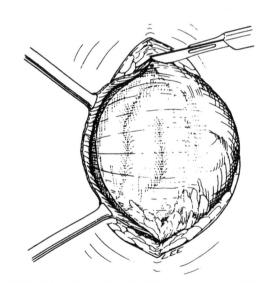

Figure 22.7 *The peritoneal sac is defined at its neck; this clearly identifies the aponeurotic defect.*

that all sacs are opened, adhesions of the contents divided, the viscera returned to the peritoneal cavity and then the sac is completely excised except for a marginal cuff which is used to supplement the fascial closure.

Opening the peritoneal sac

The sac should be opened near its neck as shown. The presence of a great deal of extraperitoneal fat may make this difficult because the peritoneal sac is deeply buried in layers of fat which are often surprisingly vascular.

The peritoneum is often very thin over the fundus of the sac and the cavity is frequently loculated here by adhesions between the sac and its contents. Such adhesions are less marked at the neck of the sac. The peritoneum is usually less adherent and is thin at this point (Figure 22.8).

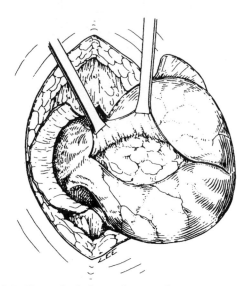

Figure 22.8 *The neck of the sac is opened.*

Contents of the sac

The sac may contain almost any intraperitoneal viscus, but usually omentum, small bowel and transverse colon are found.

Unless the hernia is strangulated and the small bowel non-viable, any adhesions are divided and the small bowel is returned to the abdominal cavity. Strangulated small bowel or omentum can be resected at this stage. The diagnostic decision is now made as to what should be done about very adherent and frequently partially ischemic omentum. If there is any doubt about omentum it is best excised; to return omentum of doubtful viability to the peritoneal cavity invites the formation of adhesions (Figure 22.9).

Particular care must be taken in manipulating and dissecting any colon in the sac. If the colon is strangulated it should be resected. Depending upon the experience of the surgeon and the local practice, the colon could be re-anastomosed primarily or an end colostomy with either a mucus fistula or a closed distal stump could be performed. If it is not strangulated it should be mobilized and returned to the peritoneal cavity. Any densely adherent hernial sac should be trimmed and left adherent to the bowel and returned to the peritoneal sac rather than risk perforating the bowel in a tedious dissection. The greatest care must be taken to avoid puncturing the colon. If the colon is punctured, a minor injury could generally be closed with sutures. A substantial injury must be treated by one of the methods outlined above. If a colostomy is created, the re-anastomosis of the colon and repair of the hernia can be performed at a later operation after full patient evaluation and colon antibacterial preparation (Figure 22.10).

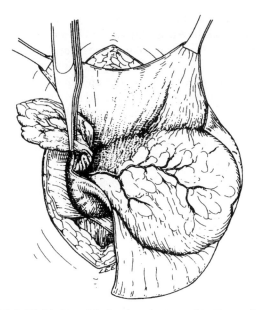

Figure 22.9 *Viable bowel is freed and returned to the peritoneal cavity. If the peritoneal sac is closely attached to the bowel, most particularly the large bowel, no attempt should be made to dissect it free. Damaging the bowel is a hazard to be avoided; such fragments of adherent sac should be left alone and replaced in the peritoneal cavity. On the other hand, adherent omentum of doubtful viability is best excised.*

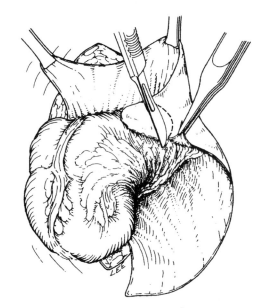

Figure 22.10 *Completion of clearing the contents from the sac.*

Excision of sac and suture of peritoneum

The redundant peritoneum of the sac is now excised and the peritoneal edges are united with a continuous suture. In the upper part of the wound it will be seen that the peritoneal layer is strengthened by the incorporation of the posterior layer of the rectus sheath, which is, of course, deficient below the semilunar fold of Douglas, halfway between the umbilicus and the pubes. In many patients, such as those with very large fascial defects, the closure of the peritoneum will not be possible. A suction drain can be placed down to this suture line (Figure 22.11). Wide drainage is used to eliminate dead space and fluid accumulation.[1013]

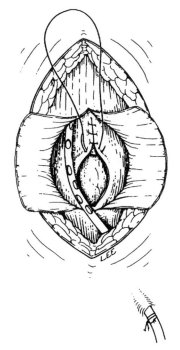

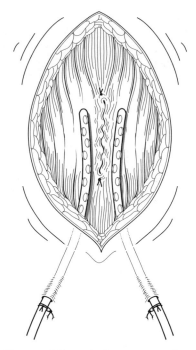

Figure 22.12 *Closure of the anterior aponeurosis, rectus sheath. Only normal aponeurosis can be used in this type of repair. Some surgeons elect to avoid the use of suction drains.*

Figure 22.11 *Now that the peritoneum is identified, it can be closed. Redundant peritoneum is first excised. A suction drain is placed down to this suture line. Some surgeons elect to avoid the use of suction drains.*

Closure of aponeurotic layer

The aponeurosis must be dissected until normal aponeurosis and not scar tissue is identified. Then the full thickness of the margins of all the aponeurotic layers (i.e. the abdominal wall in midline and paramedian areas) are approximated and held together by sutures until healing is complete (Figure 22.12). Occasionally this is not possible due to the size of the fascial defect. The closure of massive defects of the abdominal wall with sutures alone can result in a significant amount of tension on the midline of the repair. This has a recurrence rate of 43% or higher.[715] In the situation in which the use of a prosthesis is not an option, one may desire to use the techniques that provide relaxing incisions to the abdominal wall tissues laterally. Multiple small incisions to the anterior fascia of Clotteau–Prémont (Figure 22.13) or the bilateral large incisions that include the fascia, subcutaneous tissue, and skin of Welti–Eudel (Figure 22.14) will generally permit the re-approximation of the midline with significantly less tension than a direct sutured closure (Figures 22.15 and 22.16). It is apparent that these techniques merely incise the lateral tissue(s) so that there is a release of the tension caused by the re-approximation of the midline in the patient with retracted musculofascial tissues.

A permanent suture is started at each end of the defect. Suturing is continued towards the center of the defect, one suture alternating with the other and slowly being used to draw

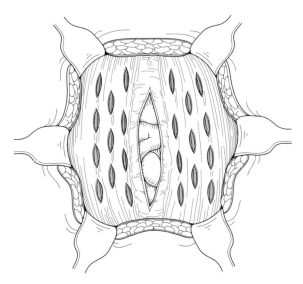

Figure 22.13 *Multiple small incisions in the anterior fascia to allow closure of the midline of the abdomen.*

together the margins of the defect. Stitch intervals of no more than 0.5 cm are used and bites must be taken more than 2.5 cm from the edges to be sutured (Figure 22.17). Alternatively, because of the availability of sutures of sufficient length, the suture could be started at one end and completed at the other end of the incision. Additional closure of further layers can be performed so that the completed closure resembles a darn.

Depending upon local custom, the subcutaneous fat is either left unclosed or is closed in layers with absorbable sutures. The skin margins are now approximated. Skin closure must be effected without any tension, but undue redundant

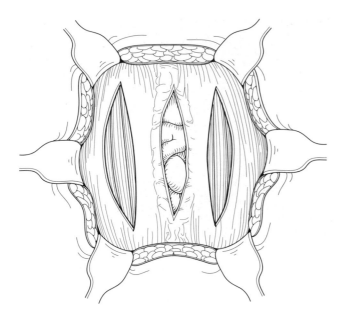

Figure 22.14 *Single long incisions in the anterior fascia to allow closure of the midline of the abdomen.*

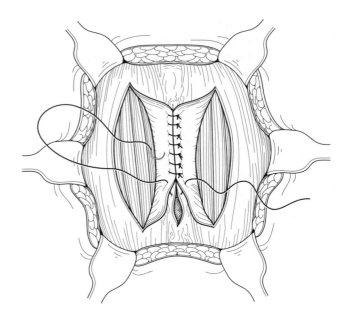

Figure 22.16 *Completed closure of the hernia and the midline of the abdominal wall using the Welti-Eudel method.*

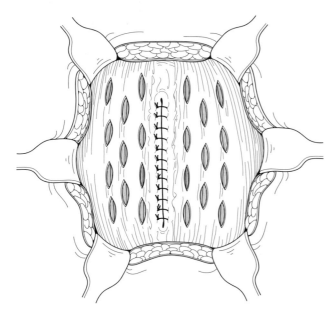

Figure 22.15 *Completed closure of the hernia and the midline of the abdominal wall using the Clotteau-Prémont method.*

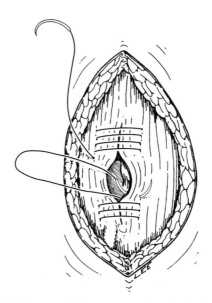

Figure 22.17 *Closure of the aponeurosis, suturing from each end simultaneously to distribute the load. Notice the drains.*

skin can be excised at this stage. This may be accomplished with sutures or skin staples.

POSTOPERATIVE CARE

Immediate active mobilization is the key to rapid convalescence.

In the absence of extensive handling of the intestines there is no postoperative adynamic ileus and no need for encumbrances such as nasogastric suction or intravenous drips. The patient is made to take deep breaths; breathing exercises and, where necessary, chest percussion are given. As soon as possible the patient gets up and walks. Fluids are given for the first day, then a light

diet started. These patients can experience a significant amount of pain, which will require parenteral analgesia. If this can be controlled with oral sedatives and the patient does not experience a significant ileus, a minimal hospital stay can be expected. Generally, the length of stay will be 3–5 days depending upon the size of the hernia, the amount of dissection required, and the number of co-morbid conditions of the patient.

OPEN PROSTHETIC REPAIR

This technique is applicable to the large diffuse incisional hernia when there is a tissue defect demonstrated preoperatively.

To a large extent, especially in the USA, the repair of approximately 90% of incisional hernias is repaired with a biomaterial of some type. Alternatively, on-table pneumoperitoneum can be used, which assists in defining the real margins of the defect and may also reveal the presence of occult hernias.[1217] This same effect is accomplished with the laparoscopic method of repair discussed in Chapter 15.

Incision and dissection

The elliptical incision, removing the skin cicatrix, is used as previously described. The dissection is carried down to the neck of the sac. If the sac needs to be opened – because it is irreducible or its contents are compromised – this is done and the peritoneal opening is then closed. If the sac does not need to be opened, and opening the sac should be avoided if possible, it is imbricated with running absorbable sutures. The steps taken from this point forward vary greatly depending upon the surgeon's preferred method for location of the mesh, the strength of the repair, and the need to re-approximate the midline of the abdomen.

If the hernia is in or near the midline, the anterior rectus sheath on either side should be mobilized by a lateral releasing incision.[707] The anterior rectus sheath is then reflected inward, sutured together and reinforced with a nylon darn to form the posterior layer. The lateral edges are then brought to within 3 cm of each other and sutured together to form the anterior layer (Figure 22.18).

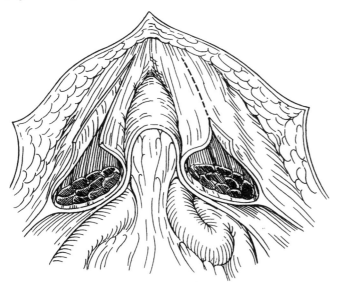

Figure 22.18 *Bilateral longitudinal releasing incisions on the anterior layer of the rectus sheath.*

If the peritoneum is deficient, for instance in a flank hernia, and cannot be closed over the viscera, the greater omentum should be mobilized to lie over the intestines. The plain polypropylene and polyester meshes should never be in direct contact with the intestine, because of the risk of adhesion formation and fistulation.[652] There is also a risk of mesh erosion into the bowel with these types of meshes (Figure 22.19). On

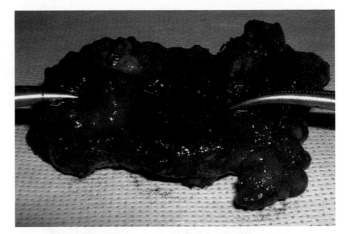

Figure 22.19 *Erosion of a piece of PPM that had been used in an incisional hernia repair into the ileum which presented as a fistula. The hemostat in the right points to the mesh while the one on the left to the end of the bowel.*

the other hand, there has never been a reported case of this complication as a result of the use of ePTFE patches. The newer meshes with the incorporated 'anti-adhesive' agents may diminish this complication with the PPM and POL meshes but there are no long-term studies to verify this fact as these complications are seen many years after the insertion of them (see Chapter 7).

The mesh should be fixed to aponeurosis around the margins of the defect. The greatest difficulty is usually to make the tension of the mesh equal all around the defect it is to repair. There are several different approaches:

1 The mesh is placed over the defect (onlay) and sutured in position (Figure 22.20) (see video clip 'Onlay incisional hernia repair').

2 The mesh is carefully cut to size and finally 'railroaded' into position at the correct tension. Wagman (1985) recommends a 'through all layers' suturing of the mesh. In this technique, first sutures are placed through all layers and the peritoneum

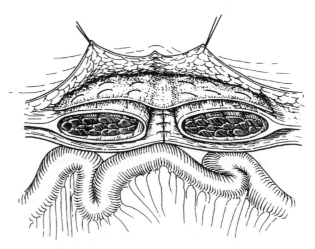

Figure 22.20 *Repair using a mesh onlay. Alternatively, a continuous suture may be used along the edge of the prosthesis but this may increase seroma formation.*

and aponeurosis are closed. Then the sutures placed through all layers of the parietal muscle wall are pushed through the mesh which is 'railroaded' into position and fixed in the extraparietal plane[1176] (Figure 22.21).

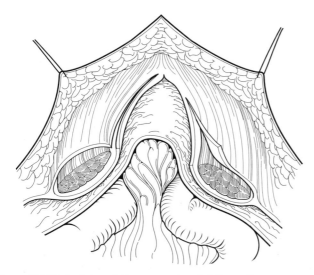

Figure 22.21 *Repair by onlay mesh with all-layers fixation. The mesh is 'railroaded' down previously inserted sutures and fixed extraparietally.*

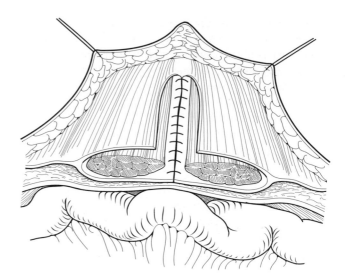

Figure 22.23 *Initial closure of the posterior sheath which serves to protect the bowel from contact with the prosthetic biomaterial.*

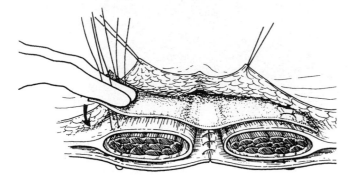

Figure 22.22 *Incision of the rectus sheath bilaterally to expose the posterior rectus sheath.*

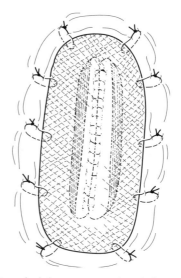

Figure 22.24 *Transfacial sutures are placed circumferentially to secure the prosthesis to the abdominal wall.*

3 Rives–Stoppa repair – This repair is the forefather of the laparoscopic repair. In this technique (sublay) the prosthesis is placed in the preperitoneal (and retromuscular) space so that it does not contact the bowel. Each rectus sheath is incised along its medial border and opened in the midline to expose the anterior and posterior aspects of the rectus muscle (Figure 22.22), which by blunt dissection is mobilized to its entire width along the length of the defect. The mesh is then placed posterior (retro-) to the rectus muscles, after first closing the posterior leaf of the sheath/peritoneum with monofilament nylon (Figure 22.23). The mesh is then sutured to the abdominal wall with the placement of transfascial sutures (Figure 22.24). Alternatively the mesh is secured with interrupted absorbable sutures between the edges of the mesh and the underlying posterior rectus sheath/peritoneum. The

layered closure is completed by approximation of the anterior rectus sheath over the prosthesis (see video clip 'Sublay incisional hernia repair').

4 Chevrel's procedure – The technique that has been developed by Jean-Paul Chevrel combines some of the concepts above.[215] He incises the anterior rectus sheath and closes this to itself in a three-layer fashion to reconstitute the midline of the abdomen. He then places an onlay of a polyester mesh to reinforce the repair (Figure 22.21). This is feasible with even the very large incisional hernias. The use of fibrin glue for this repair was associated with improved results.[214]

5 Percutaneously placed sutures – A similar approach that is nearly identical to the laparoscopic placement of the transfascial sutures through small skin incisions was described by Devlin in 1994.[297] The mesh is placed in the preperitoneal space without the dissection of the prefascial tissues. This avoids the potential complications of tissue

slough and infection that can be seen with these larger dissection planes of tissue. The mesh can be placed quite accurately and flat with equalized tension around the entire periphery of the prosthetic. This is shown in Figures 22.25–22.27.

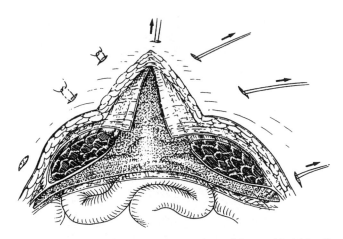

Figure 22.27 *When all the sutures are in position and held in clips the mesh is slid into position in the extraperitoneal plane deep to the musculo-aponeurotic layer of the abdominal wall. The sutures are then tied securely using robust non-slip knots. The stab wounds are then closed with subcuticular strands. (Reproduced with permission from Devlin and Nicholson, 1994.)*

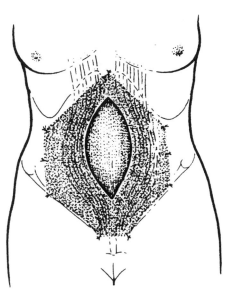

Figure 22.25 *A large piece of mesh is cut so that it overlaps the margins of the defect by at least 2 cm, or over 3 cm if possible – the larger the overlap the better. The mesh should be cut with a chevron shape to go down into the pelvis behind the pubis and inguinal ligaments, and above with an inverted chevron so that it fits up to the costal margin. (Reproduced with permission from Devlin and Nicholson, 1994.)*

Whichever technique is employed, the mesh must overlap each margin of the aponeurotic defect by some 3–4 cm and must be well fixed to the aponeurosis. Multiple methods have been used to secure the prosthetics to the fascia. This can be achieved by using continuous 'quilting' sutures, at least three lines, all around the defect, although some have used as few as one continuous suture. The direct fascia-to-prosthetic one-layered closure with only one suture is discouraged. This technique uses only one running suture that secures the edge of the fascia to the edge of the prosthetic biomaterial. This is fraught with multiple recurrences between the sites of the sutures and therefore cannot be recommended. The most effective method of suture fixation appears to be the transfascial sutured technique similar to that of the Rives–Stoppa repair and the stab wound incisions. However, the use of some of the newer prosthetic biomaterials such as the Kugel patch® may allow the placement of that product with minimal or no sutures at all. Long-term follow-up studies have yet to be reported, however.

Preparation and insertion of mesh

The preparation of the mesh is critically dependent upon the method chosen to suture the prosthetic into place. One method will require that the mesh is cut so that it is 4 cm longer and some 8 cm wider than the defect (Figure 22.28).

The mesh is applied as an onlay to the external surface of the aponeurosis, or the external surface of the anterior rectus sheath if method 1 is being used, and fixed with polypropylene sutures. Generally several lines of sutures are placed.

The farthest one is placed first, at the margin of the mesh, which should be at least 4.0 cm from the edge of the aponeurotic defect and preferably covering the whole width of the posterior rectus sheath. The sutures should take good bites of the aponeurosis and mesh at intervals of not more than 0.5 cm (Figure 22.29).

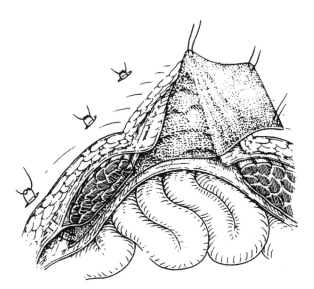

Figure 22.26 *A series of tiny stab wounds is made 2 cm or more from the margins of the defect. Sutures are passed through each stab wound, through the full thickness of the abdominal wall and through the mesh. The lowermost sutures should pick up the pectineal ligament and the mesh. The sutures are held in clips and not tied until all the sutures are in position. (Reproduced with permission from Devlin and Nicholson, 1994.)*

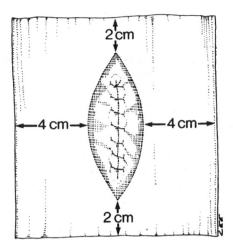

Figure 22.28 *The dimensions of the mesh for repair of a midline defect.*

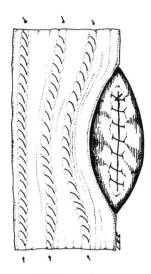

Figure 22.30 *Three parallel lines of quilting are used on either side of the defect.*

With the mesh spread taut by traction by an assistant, a second line of interrupted sutures 1 cm closer to the margins of the defect is placed, and finally a third line of sutures at the margin of the defect may be required (Figure 22.30).

The mesh is now put into the contralateral side using the same technique. In lower midline hernias it is extremely important to fix the mesh inferiorly. This can only be achieved effectively by using non-absorbable sutures to Cooper's ligament, which implies that repair for hernias with a suprapubic component must be effected by method 3, i.e. the extraperitoneal, retromuscular route. Without such fixation there is a high incidence of suprapubic 'bulge' or recurrence. The obvious reason is the fascia is above and not behind the prosthesis thereby negating the intra-abdominal pressure forces on the fascia directly (Figure 22.31). The laparoscopic technique will also place and fixate the prosthesis in this position in this situation.

A fine suction drain catheter is now placed to lie superficial to the mesh and behind the rectus muscle (Figures 22.32 and 22.33).

A technique of stapling the mesh in position has been described.[1176] After placing the mesh in the preperitoneal space deep to the abdominal wall muscles, it is fixed in place with an articulating stapler at multiple points. The disadvantage of this technique is possible injury to bowel underlying the posterior rectus sheath/peritoneum. The medial edges of the anterior sheaths are then approximated and closed; this can be facilitated by multiple buttonholes in the anterior rectus sheath. The mesh will be used as a one-piece appliance to cover the entire fascial defect and provide at least a 3 cm overlap of the defect.

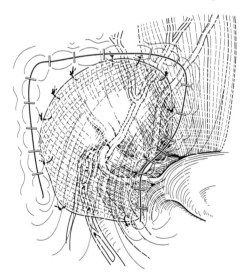

Figure 22.31 *The prosthesis must be secured to Cooper's ligament in the hernias that are very close to the public bone. There is too little fascia to assure firm fixation of the biomaterial.*

Closing the defect

The closure of the defect will have been affected prior to, or after the biomaterial is in place, depending on the technique

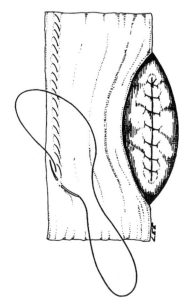

Figure 22.29 *Quilting the mesh into position.*

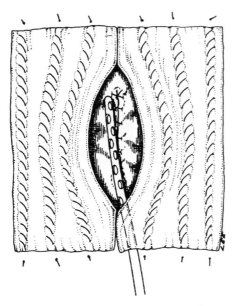

Figure 22.32 *Fine suction drainage is always used.*

employed. In those patients in which it has not been possible to re-approximate the midline, there is a potential for respiratory function to be compromised. This is seldom a clinical problem but must be anticipated with the very large defects in very obese patients.

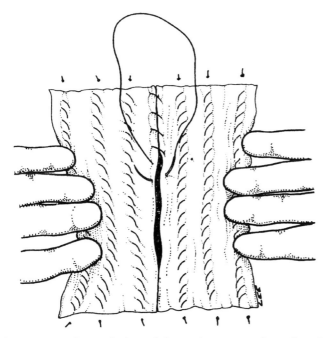

Figure 22.33 *The two halves of the mesh are sutured together at the correct tension.*

The subcutaneous fat can be tacked down to the underlying aponeurosis to obliterate the 'dead space'. Skin closure may be done with sutures (continuous or interrupted) placed through the skin or in the subcuticular manner. The use of skin staples is probably the most common method to re-approximate the skin, however.

INFECTED INCISIONAL HERNIA

The infected incisional hernia is a very difficult problem to treat effectively. The options that are available will depend greatly if a fistula exists, a prosthetic biomaterial has been used to repair the hernia, the size of the fascial defect and the amount of skin that can be used to cover the repair. Several methods have been proposed in the past including that of Ton's device.

In 1967, Ton reported the use of a novel extractable prosthesis to manage the multiple recurrent and the fistulizing incisional hernia.[1131] Doeven has reported the use of this device in the non-infected incisional hernia.[308]

The device is a U-shaped loop of metal, one leg of the loop is perforated throughout its length, the other solid. The device is manufactured in a variety of sizes (Figure 22.34).

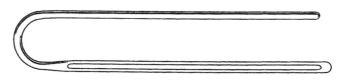

Figure 22.34 *The Ton device.*

The concept is three-fold: (a) to use strong non-absorbable sutures for the repair; (b) to distribute the load to the aponeurosis through the rods and thus prevent the sutures cutting out; (c) to allow all the non-absorbable material to be removed and thereby eliminate sepsis and ongoing sinuses.

Sutures are placed around the solid limb and tied through the perforated limb. When healing is complete the U-loop is removed through a small incision; removal of the loop means removal of the sutures too – they slip off the solid limb and are pulled from the wound in the perforated limb (Figures 22.35–22.37).

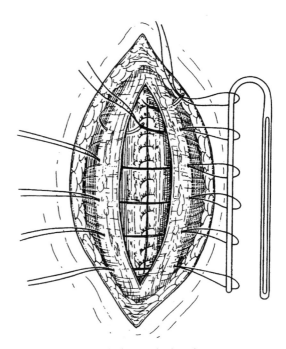

Figure 22.35 *The Ton technique; placing the sutures.*

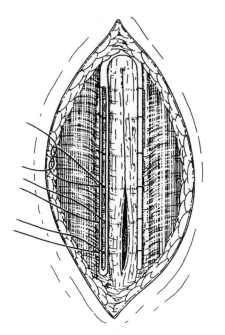

Figure 22.36 *The Ton technique; fixing the device in place.*

This device is not used extensively today. Because of the frequency of the use of prosthetic biomaterial in the repair of these hernias, one must deal with these in the treatment of any infection. Generally, the polypropylene products can be opened and drained. The mesh will become granulated to allow the placement of a split thickness skin graft once this has covered the mesh. It is seldom necessary to remove the prosthetic in this

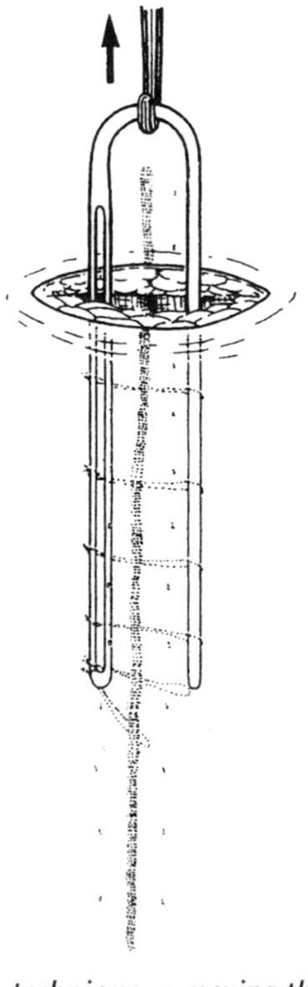

Figure 22.37 *The Ton technique; removing the device under local anesthetic.*

situation. Similarly, the polyester materials can be treated by this conservative approach.

If the prosthetic that has repaired the fascial defect is based on ePTFE, it is seldom possible to preserve the prosthetic in the patient. If the infection occurs early, it is best to remove the patch and repair the hernia with some other technique. If the infection occurs after the in-growth has secured the ePTFE to the tissues, it may be possible to sequentially excise the portion of the patch that is infected and close the patch to itself. Occasionally only one excision will allow the infection to be eradicated and the hernia repair and prosthesis left intact. In other cases, the surgeon could return the patient to the operating room to continue to remove the inner portions of the patch and close the patch again. If the patient is not septic, this could occur every 7–10 days to allow the native tissues to adapt to the increased tension caused by the resection of the inner portions of the prosthesis. The sequential nature of this method will also decrease the likelihood of intra-abdominal hypertension caused by a tight closure of the midline. Ideally, the midline can be re-approximated at the time that the entire patch is excised.

Another approach could be to replace an ePTFE prosthesis with a polypropylene mesh and allow this to granulate in the manner described above. The major disadvantage of this approach is the fact that the intestine will be in direct contact with the very adhesiogenic biomaterial. However, in a severely septic patient, this may be a prudent option.

With the introduction the biological prosthesis, Surgisis ES® and Surgisis Gold®, one of these products may be used in this situation. These are described in Chapter 7. The prior synthetic biomaterial can be removed and replaced with one of these prosthetics. These can be sewn in place by one of the techniques described earlier in this chapter. This will allow the closure of the fascial defect with another prosthetic that is resistant to infection. This is a new device and the experience with it in this situation is anecdotal.[658]

RESULTS

The past results of the sutured repairs have not changed significantly in the past four decades. There are wide discrepancies in the recurrence rates. The reported results of incisional hernia repair vary; recurrence rates from 1.6% (layered steel wire) in the Shouldice clinic and 0% (Marlex mesh) from Usher in Houston compete with 19% from Warrington (releasing incision and suture) and 46% from the Westminster Hospital (keel and mass nylon technique)[5,13,37,397,1158] (Table 22.3).

There are reports of excellent results with tissue repairs but they are not as successful as repairs that include the use of a prosthesis. Table 22.3 details a few of the past and several of the more recent published series. These studies have shown a rate of recurrence that is consistently improved with the use of a synthetic biomaterial as an element to the open repair of incisional and ventral hernias.

Table 22.3 *Results of incisional hernia repair*

Reference	No. of patients	Recurrence rate (%)
Suture or layer techniques		
Obney (1957)	192	12.5
Young (1961)	15	6.6
Akman (1962)	500	1.6
Maguire and Young (1976)	32	18.8
Jenkins (1980)	50	8.0
George and Ellis (1986)	81	46.0
Graft techniques		
Usher (1962)	156	10.2
Hamilton (1968)	43	7.0
Usher (1970)	48	0.0
Larson and Harrower (1978)	53	11.3
Lewis (1984)	50	6.0
Pless (1993)	32	28
van der Lei (1989)	11	18
Molloy (1991)	50	8
Matapurkar (1991)	60	0
Liakakos (1994)	102	8
Tissue repairs		
Obney (1957)	192	12.5
Maguire and Young (1976)	32	18.8
George and Ellis (1986)	81	46.0
Chevrel and Flament (1990)	417	24.0
Hesselink (1993)	298	36.0
Chevrel (1997)	153	18.3
Flament (1999)	181	24.9
Luijendijk (2000)	97	43.0
Open prosthetic repairs		
Usher (1962)	156	10.2
Chevrel and Flament (1990)	326	16.3
Liakakos (1994)	102	8.0
Chevrel (1997)	326	4.0
Flament (1999)	474	5.7
Luijendijk (2000)	84	24

CONCLUSIONS

- The striking conclusion is that specialists who have developed an interest and experience in these operations have significantly better results than non-specialists.
- Important predictors of recurrence are hematoma and wound infection, and obesity.
- The choice of operative technique is critical. If there is no tissue loss and the defect is less than 4 cm, layer-by-layer closure or the overlap operation used at the Shouldice clinic gives good results.
- If there is any tissue loss, a defect greater than 4 cm or any risk factors prosthetic mesh reinforcement is always needed.

23

Laparoscopic incisional and ventral hernioplasty

INTRODUCTION

Laparoscopic incisional and ventral herniorrhaphy (LIVH) was first described in the published literature in 1993.[669] The concepts of this technique are equivalent to the prosthetic repair of inguinal hernias and emulates the features of the Rives–Stoppa repair of incisional hernia. The open repair of hernias that develop on the anterior abdominal wall is not an effective method of repair and has recurrence rates of 25–56%[503,715] if no prosthetic biomaterial is utilized. The use of a prosthetic biomaterial of some type lowers this re-herniation rate to 11–24%.[652,503,715] The rate of recurrence with the laparoscopic approach has been reported from 0–11% in the experiences of the reported series.[374,492,630,665] Currently the published results of this procedure have demonstrated a success rate that appears to warrant its continued growth. The current average recurrence rate as reported in the literature by experts for the LIVH is 3.3%. At the time of writing approximately 20–25% of these hernias are repaired by this technique in the USA.

The repair of incisional and ventral hernias by this approach should be considered a technique that should be performed by high-volume laparoscopic surgeons. The surgeon should be adept at performing the more common laparoscopic operations and also be comfortable to perform the more complex laparoscopic procedures. The assistance of another surgeon during this operation is felt to be of great benefit, if not mandatory, on most occasions. This chapter will present the concepts, technical aspects and results of the LIVH as it is currently performed. There are variations of the technique that are presented within this chapter, as is common to every surgical procedure. This methodology is continuing to evolve and undoubtedly will be modified as newer prosthetic biomaterials and instrumentation are developed in the future. A laparoscopic modification of the 'component separation technique' using the laparoscope for the initial dissection has been described.[721] While this method does not use a prosthesis nor is it a true solely laparoscopic repair, there are likely to be further operative changes in this hernioplasty.

PREOPERATIVE EVALUATION

In general, if a patient is a medically appropriate candidate for open herniorrhaphy, then he or she could be considered a candidate for the laparoscopic approach. Patients that have significant cardiac decompensation may experience physiological abnormalities during the procedure because of the insufflation, and resulting decrease in the venous return, of the abdominal cavity.

The size of the fascial defect can be a consideration in the indication of this operation. Generally almost all hernias are candidates for the LIVH. Even the smaller hernias in obese individuals could be repaired with this technique. The incidence of recurrence of these hernias is so great that the use of a prosthetic biomaterial is preferred. The laparoscopic approach will afford the best visualization of the abdominal wall to identify the often overlooked additional defects that are not seen by the open technique. One may opt to use the open approach in a thin patient if it is apparent that the defect is 3 cm or less. The rate of recurrence is quite low for the open repair in these patients. In the obese patient, however, many laparoscopic surgeons prefer to repair all of the incisional and ventral hernias laparoscopically.

A very large fascial defect that nearly encompasses the entire anterior abdominal wall may pose a difficult problem. A laparoscopic approach, however, may be feasible. The decision to attempt the laparoscopic method should be based upon the experience of the surgeon, the number of prior operative procedures, mesh repairs, the type of prosthetic utilized in any previous repair(s) and the location of the potential sites. However, there are currently no 'hard and fast' rules about this issue. In those patients with very large defects, a reasonable option would be to commence the operation laparoscopically and convert to an open repair if that appears to be the best alternative. More often than not, this proves to be unnecessary. A probable exception to this sequence is those individuals that exhibit a 'loss of domain' of the abdominal contents. In these patients it is usually impossible to actually enter the abdomen behind the abdominal wall musculature because this musculature has been displaced laterally. In these cases, conversion to the open method would occur earlier rather than later. More commonly, however, prudence dictates that the entire procedure should be of the open type rather than even attempting the laparoscopic approach.

Morbid obesity can occasionally become a limiting factor. In such patients, the trocars may not be of sufficient length to maintain an adequate access to the abdomen cavity. It could become necessary to convert to the open repair because a working channel through the abdominal wall cannot be maintained.

The open end of the trocars will be continually withdrawn into the excessive fatty tissue. This eliminates the working channel and/or results in insufflation of the subcutaneous tissue, which further obscures the view of the abdominal cavity. This can be overcome with the use of longer trocars that are available.

Absolute contraindications to the use of the laparoscopic method would be the presence of an acute surgical abdomen and/or an intra-abdominal infection from any source. The use of a prosthetic biomaterial in the site of an overt infection precludes the use of such a product. Because the laparoscopic repair requires its use in all but the smallest of defects, one should perform an open repair of the hernia in that circumstance. Similarly, while the presence of incarcerated bowel does not prevent the performance of the procedure, strangulation of the bowel may necessitate an open hernioplasty.

Because the most common incision of the abdomen is placed in the midline, most incisional hernias occur in the midline. When a surgeon begins to perform laparoscopic incisional herniorrhaphy, it is recommended that he or she should repair midline defects initially to gain confidence in use of the laparoscopic technique. Once this is accomplished, the presence of a non-midline defect or multiple defects that are not adjacent to each other should not preclude the use of laparoscopy. Appropriate positioning of the patient and accurate placement of the trocars will permit an approach to the entire abdominal cavity in most cases.

Previous intra-abdominal surgery is a major consideration in the evaluation of a patient for the laparoscopic procedure. The number and type of earlier operations will influence the choice of patient position, the method of abdominal entry, trocar placement, and the position of the monitors. This preoperative assessment will allow the surgeon to plan the operative procedure and the operative suite based upon these findings. Any previous open laparotomies will, of course, be associated with more potential for adhesion formation than procedures that were performed laparoscopically. Additionally, in those patients in whom a previous incisional hernia repair included the implantation of any 'unprotected' polypropylene prosthesis (see Chapter 7) can be expected to have dense scarring in all areas in which the material was exposed to the intra-abdominal contents. This should not deter experienced surgeons from attempting a laparoscopic approach because as many as one-third of these patients will not have any adhesions at all. It is important to note, however, that the difficulty of the procedure can be greatly magnified because of the dissection of the tenacious scarring that is encountered involving the prosthesis and the bowel and/or omentum. The risk of enterotomy is significantly increased in such instances.

Patients in whom there is an additional need for a surgical procedure such as a cholecystectomy, fundoplication of the stomach, inguinal herniorrhaphy or biopsy of an intra-abdominal or retroperitoneal structures are special subsets that deserve careful consideration. Hernia repairs in such cases are discussed later in this chapter.

Laparoscopic incisional herniorrhaphy should be individualized in patients with known ascites because it is impossible to close the trocar sites in a consistently watertight manner that averts ascitic leaks. Moreover, these patients usually have a metabolic problem (e.g. chronic renal failure or hepatic disease) that can cause poor healing and predispose them to development of a hernia at the trocar sites. The use of the 5 mm trocars, however, has made this less problematic and these patients may also be considered on occasion. Special trocars that do not cut into the abdominal muscle but dilate the tissues to enter through the wall of the abdomen should be used in these patients. The site of entry will be smaller than the actual trocar itself after it is removed thereby further minimizing the risk of leakage of ascitic fluid or subsequent herniation.

LIVH patients are admitted to the day-surgery unit of the hospital because they can usually be considered for discharge on the day of surgery. The number and type of comorbid conditions of the patient, the type and location of the hernia(s), the presence of incarceration and the amount of adhesiolysis required will influence the decision of timing of discharge from the hospital. Many patients now undergo laparoscopic incisional hernia repair in an ambulatory surgery center. Appropriate laboratory testing should be obtained prior to entry on the day of surgery. Patients are routinely given a preoperative dose of either a first generation cephalosporin or a fluoroquinolone unless the biomaterial that will be implanted contains antimicrobial agents (e.g. DualMesh® Plus).

INTRAOPERATIVE CONSIDERATIONS

Patient preparation and positioning

LIVH repair requires the use of general anesthesia to achieve the necessary degree of relaxation and sedation. In most cases, it is not necessary to use an orogastric or nasogastric tube unless the site of entry is in the vicinity of the stomach. A urinary drainage catheter is not used if the procedure is felt to be short in length. If the operative site is close to the bladder (e.g. very low midline hernias or concomitant inguinal hernia repairs) or if the procedure will be prolonged it is then advisable to insert a urinary drainage catheter. Insertion of a nasogastric tube for procedures in which extensive dissection of the bowel is necessary may help to reduce the postoperative ileus that is likely to develop. It is seldom necessary to leave this tube beyond the intraoperative phase of the procedure, however.

Most patients will be placed in the supine position. Operations upon lateral defects of the abdominal wall, such as those in a subcostal or flank incision, will be facilitated by use of a semidecubitus or full decubitus position. The use of a 'bean-bag' in these instances will greatly aid in the positioning of the patient. The additional use of the tilt capabilities of the operating table will assist in the manipulation of the bowel during dissection. Steep Trendelenberg or reverse Trendelenberg positions will cause the abdominal contents to move into positions that will make visualization of the contents of both the hernia and the abdomen easier. The patient's arms should be tucked in close to the body to allow sufficient room to move around the patient; this is especially important if the defect is in the lower abdomen. Occasionally this may not be feasible due to the size of the individual but, in general, it is preferred when possible. Use of a protective transparent adhesive drape is optional.

Abdominal entry

It is understood that the method of access into the abdomen should always be the safest approach possible. Many surgeons use the open type of Hassan entry because it is familiar to them. An open entry such as this could result in a poor seal around the trocar, which makes maintenance of insufflation pressures difficult resulting in inadequate visualization throughout the procedure. This method also requires the use of a larger trocar thereby posing a risk of herniation at that site in the future despite the best attempts at fascial closure. On the other hand, these problems are infrequent and the use of this larger trocar will facilitate the introduction of the prosthetic biomaterial into the abdominal cavity.

In the patient with a primary ventral hernia or a single small defect, a Veress needle could be considered for insufflation before introduction of the first trocar. A 'safe' area for needle insertion is usually in the right upper quadrant because it is generally free of adhesions of bowel and omentum. A site in the upper mid-line could also be used if it can be placed far enough away from the hernia so as not to interfere with the repair of the hernia.

Another method to gain access into the abdominal cavity uses an 'optical' trocar for abdominal entry. Two such devices are the Non-bladed trocar (Ethicon Endosurgery, Inc., Cincinnati, Ohio) and the Visiport® trocar (US Surgical Corporation/Tyco International, Norwalk, CN). These trocars are designed to provide visualization of each layer of the abdominal wall as the trocar passes through them. This is accomplished because the laparoscope is inserted into the trocar and these structures are seen as the trocar is passed. The former is available in 5, 10, and 12 mm sizes (Figure 23.1) while the latter is only available in the 10 mm size (Figure 23.2).

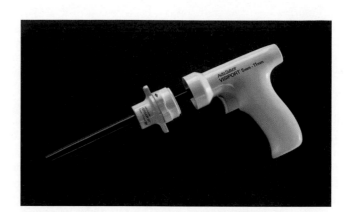

Figure 23.2 *United States Surgical Corporation/Tyco International, Inc. Visiport* trocar. This is to be used with a 10 mm laparoscope. *Trademark of United States Surgical. Copyright © 2002 United States Surgical. All rights reserved. Reprinted with the permission of United States Surgical, a division of Tyco Healthcare Group LP.*

necessary trocars. After the insertion of each additional trocar, the laparoscope should be placed through it to inspect the abdomen. The new view that is afforded from that vantage point will identify the optimal location of the sites of the other trocars. Additionally, the collections of these different views are important to identify any bowel that may be at risk during adhesiolysis. This is extremely important because, in some cases, neither the surgeon nor the assistant will appreciate the proximity of the bowel from only the view that is available from an individual trocar position.

When determining the best locations for the trocar positions, the selection should avoid the problem of 'mirror imaging' during the manipulation of the instruments from the side in direct opposition to the viewing laparoscope (Figures 23.3 and 23.4). This produces an image of any manipulation that is

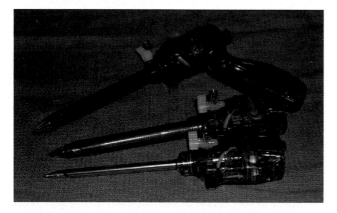

Figure 23.1 *Ethicon Endosurgery® Non-Bladed Trocars, 5, 10, and 12 mm. As noted in the photo, these are available with and without a pistol-grip and with or without threads.*

In the majority of patients with an incisional hernia the view of the abdomen is, at least partially, obscured by adhesions. To enhance visualization and to free up enough space for placement of additional trocars, blunt dissection of these adhesions is often done with the laparoscope itself placed through the initial trocar. The primary goal after the insertion of each of the additional trocars will be placement of the final number of

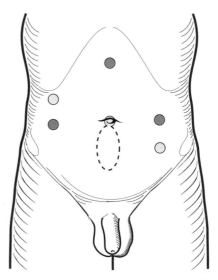

Figure 23.3 *Typical trocar positions for a lower midline hernia. The dark circles represent the location of the initial trocars. The upper midline trocar will accommodate the laparoscope. The other circles represent the location of additional trocars if these are needed to complete the procedure.*

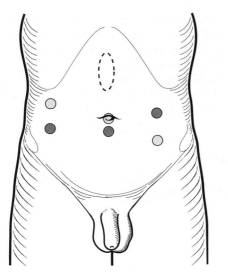

Figure 23.4 *Typical trocar positions for an upper midline hernia. The representations of the trocar sites mimic that of Figure 23.3.*

viewed from that port that is opposite the action taken. That is, a move of the laparoscopic instrument to the left will be seen as a move to the right and vice versa. Placement of the camera in the midline of the abdomen will avoid this problem. An alternative is the insertion of an additional trocar on the ipsilateral side of the location of the camera. With practice many surgeons can overcome this technical problem without the use of additional trocars. Most of this difficulty can be eliminated if the assistant surgeon can use the instruments from his or her side of the patient. One should not hesitate to insert additional trocars when this problem cannot be corrected easily to ensure the safety of the operation.

Instruments

The choice of laparoscope (0, 30, or 45 degree) used for incisional hernia repair depends upon the familiarity of the operating team with the instruments, the planned position of the trocars, and the habitus of the patient. While the 0° laparoscope is the primary choice of one of the authors (K.A.L.), the majority of surgeons utilize the 30° laparoscope because it will allow good visualization of the undersurface of the abdominal wall. Additionally, one may view to the left and right of the operative field without changing the location of the optics. This is particularly beneficial in thin patients with good muscle tone. The 45° laparoscope is seldom necessary for this operation. If the optics of the camera and system are optimal, the 5 mm laparoscopes will perform as well as do the 10 mm ones. A benefit of the smaller scopes is that they utilize smaller trocars, which diminishes postoperative pain and minimizes the risk of herniation at the site of the trocar.

The most significant and potentially fatal complication of laparoscopic incisional herniorrhaphy is an injury to the bowel. This will occur during the dissection of the adhesions that are frequently encountered. The method of dissection is critically important in order to minimize the risk of injury to the intestine. If the adhesions encountered are few and rather filmy, one may use the scissors with the additional application of electrocautery.

This should only be done if there is absolute certainty that there is no bowel adjacent to the area that will be affected by the lateral extension of the electrocautery burn. The transection of the falciform ligament is an example of this situation. In most patients dissection of omentum and/or bowel from abdominal wall will be required. This is most safely accomplished with the use of an ultrasonic dissection device. The Harmonic® scalpel (Ethicon Endosurgery®, Inc, Cincinnati, Ohio) or the Ultrashears® (US Surgical Corporation/Tyco International) are available for this task. Both devices have scissor-like jaws that disperse an ultrasonic level of heat with very minimal lateral spread of that heat. This factor significantly increases the safety in the dissection of the intestine. This should not allow the surgeon to become complacent in the use of an energy source within the abdominal cavity. The use of any type of an energy source can result in an injury to the intestine if used improperly. It is recommended that if the intestine is densely adherent to the abdominal wall or to polypropylene biomaterial from a prior failed repair, the use of scissors without cautery should be preferred.

Not uncommonly, the hernia contents are known to be incarcerated preoperatively and cannot be reduced with dissection and traction. In such cases, the fascial defect must be enlarged to allow reduction of the involved organs. Electrocautery scissors are used if the fascia is thick. Sometimes the ultrasonic dissector will be sufficient to cut the tissue but this is infrequent. Generally, a 2 or 3 cm incision into the fascia will suffice. The size of this incision is not that important because the resulting defect size will be covered by the prosthesis.

Prosthetic biomaterials

There are currently many different products that are available for the repair of incisional hernias. The polypropylene biomaterials are prone to adhesion formation and pose a significant risk of fistulization. Most surgeons will choose a biomaterial that has been manufactured with some method to shield the intestine from coming into direct contact with the polypropylene or polyester material. There are expanded polytetrafluoroethylene products or composites of these materials available as well. These products are described in detail in Chapter 7.

Adhesiolysis and identification of the fascial defect(s)

Before insertion of the prosthesis, the entire fascial defect(s) must be uncovered (Figure 23.5). This usually requires removal of all the adhesions (Figure 23.6) within the abdomen especially those attached to the anterior wall (see video clip). It is best to dissect all of the adhesions that may potentially interfere with the appropriate positioning of the prosthetic material. It is also important to ensure that the parietal surface of any prosthetic material is in direct contact with the fascia and not with adipose tissue or omentum. Any fatty tissue that is interposed between the abdominal fascia and the prosthesis will inhibit the appropriate ingrowth of tis-sue and subsequent incorporation of the biomaterial. A technical problem can develop if all of the adhesions are not adequately removed in the area of the final location of the prosthesis. If it becomes apparent that the adhesions are inhibiting the final attachment of the patch then the procedure must be temporarily delayed to allow for the additional adhesiolysis. This process can be particularly difficult once the patch is partly attached to the abdominal wall, hampering visualization and further dissection.

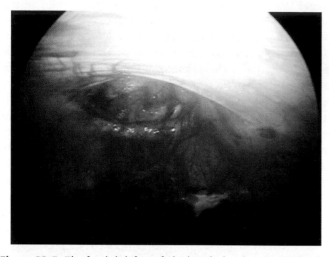

Figure 23.5 *The fascial defect of the hernia has been completely freed from the contents of the hernia and the adjacent adhesions.*

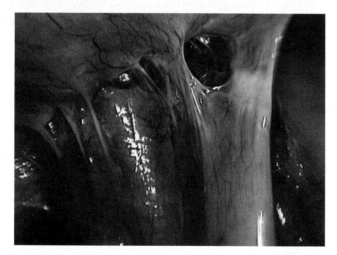

Figure 23.6 *Typical appearance of the adhesions of the small intestine and the omentum (to the right of the bowel) to the anterior abdominal wall.*

Dissection of the hernia sac is difficult and can result in bleeding while not producing any appreciable benefits for the patient. Therefore, it is not necessary to remove it. Some surgeons apply electrocautery or argon beam to the site of the peritoneal lining of the hernia sac in an effort to obliterate it and thereby reduce seroma formation. It is not known whether this has the desired effect. Closure of the fascial defect is also unnecessary because the security of the herniorrhaphy depends upon an adequate overlap of the fascial defect by the prosthesis and adequate patch fixation. In most patients closure of the linea alba is not possible because of the significant loss of tissue from the effects of longstanding herniation. There have not been any

reports of clinical respiratory difficulties due to the lack of the re-approximation of the midline of the abdomen nor has the postoperative cosmetic result been unacceptable to either the patient or the surgeon.

It is essential that the measurement of the hernia defect is accurate. This size of the defect will determine the size of the prosthetic. If this measurement is performed with the abdomen fully insufflated the resulting size determination will be artifactually larger than the proper measurement. The size of the defect must be measured with the insufflation pressure reduced from the working amount of 14–16 mmHg to near zero. Reducing the pressure prevents the inflation artifact that occurs because this measurement is done on the external surface of the abdominal wall rather than on the interior surface. After desufflation, the defect is outlined on the skin over the abdomen with a skin-marking pencil (Figure 23.7). If the choice of prosthetic size is made based on the measurement in the insufflated position, it is likely that the prosthesis will be much larger than is required. Use of that material can be exceedingly difficult because the lateral trocar sites can be covered with the biomaterial. One must then trim the patch as it lies within the abdomen, which is cumbersome. The entire circumference of the defect should be identified to ascertain its maximum dimensions. To ensure adequate coverage with the prosthesis, 6 cm is added to the maximum measurements in all directions. In other words, if the defect were 7 cm × 12 cm, the minimum patch size would be 13 cm × 18 cm. The choice of the prosthesis will be made based on the available sizes that are manufactured. In many cases, this will provide coverage in excess of the 3 cm requirements. This is felt to be advantageous. If the patient is morbidly obese, it is preferred that a larger overlap, even as much as 5 cm be used to disperse the intra-abdominal pressure over a larger surface area to diminish the risk of recurrence. We also believe that it is preferable to cover the entire length of the original incision even though only a portion may have an actual hernia defect. This will avoid the future recurrence of the hernia either above or below the actual repair of the original hernia. Several different techniques may be used before patch insertion to ensure that the prosthesis will be oriented properly and cover the defect adequately.

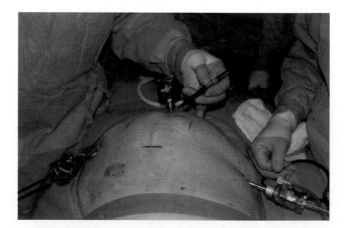

Figure 23.7 *The surgeon is placing superficial marks on the skin to delineate the edges of the fascial defect of the hernia. This is most easily done with the abdomen fully insufflated.*

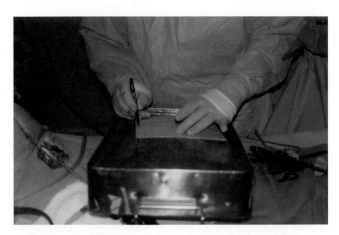

Figure 23.8 *Placement of the marks that will identify the midpoints of the axes of the patch. It is best if this is done on a flat surface as illustrated.*

A common approach is to tie ePTFE sutures (CV-0) at either side of the midpoint of the long axis of the patch and mark both sides of the midpoint of its short axis with a marking pencil prior to its insertion into the abdominal cavity.[655] It is important to mark both sides of the midpoints of the prosthesis (Figures 23.8 and 23.9). This can be done with a marking pencil if this is possible to do so; if the biomaterial does not allow this, then one may mark these points with sutures. Once the prosthetic is inserted, the surgeon will need to visualize both surfaces of the biomaterial to assure the correct axial orientation along the abdominal wall. Some surgeons mark the short axis by placement of a contrastingly colored non-absorbable suture, such as Prolene® or Ethibond®. Others place four or more sutures at the corners or periphery of the patches prior to insertion. The more sutures that are placed into the prosthesis prior to insertion the more likely that there will be a tangle of suture material that can be cumbersome to separate and pull through the abdominal wall. The use of sutures in this repair continues to be discussed. Some surgeons do not believe that transfascial sutures are necessary[185] but others feel that this is absolutely indicated.[655,886,939] Currently available data and prostheses will continue to evolve and the final decision on the use of sutures will be made in the future.

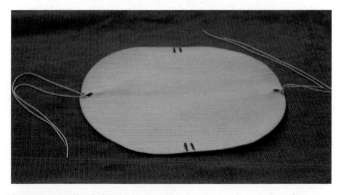

Figure 23.9 *The initial two sutures have now been placed at the midpoints along the long axis of the biomaterial. The two marks along the other axis are apparent.*

The patch with any attached sutures is rolled or folded for introduction into the abdomen. The method of folding the patch is simplest if the material is folded into sequential halves after the prior fold.[660] As shown in Figures 23.10–23.13, the sutures are placed into the first fold and the subsequent folds result in a smaller size of the biomaterial. Early in the learning curve, it is suggested that 10 mm or 12 mm ports be utilized to insert the patches. As experience is acquired, one will find that the use of only 5 mm trocars will suffice. Some of the prostheses that are available today, such as the polypropylene or polyester based biomaterials, require the use of the larger trocars for their insertion into the abdominal cavity. With those products that can be compressed adequately, such as DualMesh® Plus (which is 50% air by volume), one can pull them into the abdomen with the use of the 5 mm ports. In these instances, the skin incision at the site of patch introduction should be made larger than that which is necessary for placement of the trocar itself (typically 7–8 mm). Generally, particularly for the larger patches, a grasping instrument is passed through a trocar on the opposite side of the abdomen, which is then passed outward through a trocar on the other side. The trocar through which the

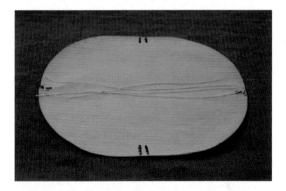

Figure 23.10 *Placement of the initial two sutures inside of the patch. Note the marks at the midpoints of the prosthesis.*

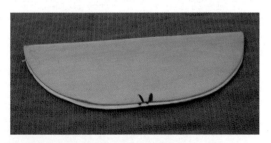

Figure 23.11 *The prosthesis is then folded in half to include the initial two sutures in the fold.*

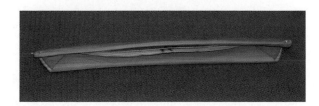

Figure 23.12 *The prosthesis is then folded in half again.*

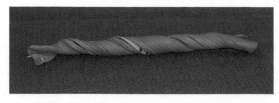

Figure 23.13 *The final fold makes the prosthesis small enough to wring it into the tight roll that is needed for insertion.*

instrument is exited is then removed (Figure 23.14). The tightly rolled and/or twisted biomaterial will be grasped by the instrument and pulled into the abdominal cavity (Figures 23.15 and 23.16). The assistant surgeon can assist this maneuver by maintaining the 'twist' of the patch as it is introduced. The pliability of the abdominal wall musculature will accommodate the insertion of even the largest of the ePTFE patches available (24 cm × 36 cm). This maneuver can, of course, be duplicated with the larger trocars. If the larger trocars are used, however, the smaller patches can frequently be inserted directly through the trocar rather than by the above method.

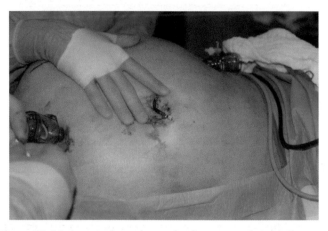

Figure 23.14 *A contralateral grasping instrument is passed across the abdomen through a trocar which has been removed.*

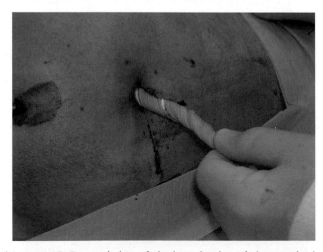

Figure 23.15 *External view of the introduction of the prosthesis by pulling it into the abdominal cavity.*

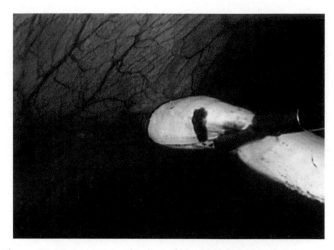

Figure 23.16 *Laparoscopic view of the introduction of the prosthesis. It is best to use a self-retaining instrument with large teeth to accomplish this task.*

Placement of the prosthesis

Once the insertion of the prosthetic is done, the patch must be returned to its original flattened shape. The biomaterial is placed onto the viscera whereupon the surgeon and the assistant will then assist each other in the manipulation of the biomaterial to completely flatten it as much as is feasible. This will facilitate the fixation of the material to the abdominal wall. If this is not possible it may be easier to unroll the prosthesis after one or both of the initial sutures have been passed through the abdominal wall. It is preferable, however, to do this only if the above method fails because the maneuverability of the prosthesis will be impaired once the fixation is initiated.

If one has chosen to use only two initially placed sutures, these are now pulled through the entire abdominal wall with use of a sharp suture-passing instrument inserted through a small skin incision (Figure 23.17). There are several different devices that are available for this purpose. These two sutures are placed along the long axis of the defect taking care to center the

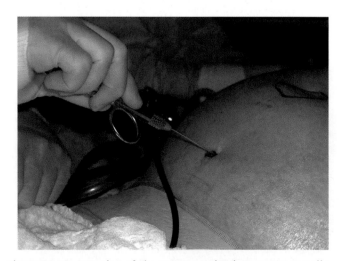

Figure 23.17 *Insertion of the suture-passing instrument to pull the initial sutures out of the abdomen.*

prosthesis over the defect. If necessary, the laparoscope can be placed into another port to confirm that it is centered with the necessary 3 cm minimum overlap and drawn tautly. If these two facts cannot be confirmed then one or both of these sutures must be repositioned. Once the optimal position is achieved, the sutures are tied. Even in large patients, the knots can usually be pulled down to the level of the fascia. It is important to make sure that these and all the subsequent sutures are tied sufficiently tight to pull them to the fascia without any laxity. It is sometimes necessary to enlarge the skin incision slightly to allow the surgeon enough room to properly tie the suture down to the fascial level. If this is difficult, the use of a laparoscopic knot-pusher can facilitate the tying of the knots. An additional method of confirmation will be simply to examine each suture laparoscopically once tied or at the completion of the entire procedure. If the suture is loose then it must be cut and replaced.

The next step will be to confirm that the correct orientation along the short axis of the patch is correct. The surgeon and the assistant will grasp the previously marked midpoints on either side of the biomaterial. The material is then positioned over the desired final location. Either the assistant or the surgeon then uses a spiral tacker or other fixation device to attach the midpoint of one side placing only one or two tacks at that time. The tacking instrument is then given to the other surgeon and the unattached midpoint is likewise secured with one or two tacks. Inspection of the position of the biomaterial is again performed usually by moving the laparoscope to one of the other trocars to visualize the position of the biomaterial from different angles before the insertion of the additional tacks and sutures that will permanently secure the patch. After this inspection, the tacks are deployed along the periphery of the prosthesis by inserting them 5–6 mm from the edge of the patch, 1–1.5 cm apart (Figure 23.18).[655] Newer alternatives to these tacks are either the Salute® (Onux Medical, Inc., Hampton, NJ) or the Endoanchor® (Ethicon® Endosurgery, Inc., Cincinnati, OH).

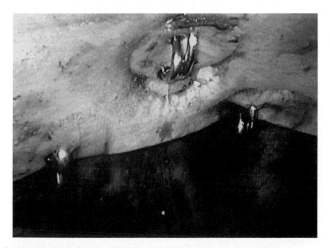

Figure 23.18 *Proper distance of the Onux Salute constructs along the periphery of the patch. These are to be placed 1 cm apart with an inner alternating row.*

Several authors have identified the need to place transfascial sutures to ensure adequate fixation of the biomaterial.[282,655,665,939]

It is generally believed that the insertion of the tacks are merely an initial step and serve mainly to approximate the prosthesis to the abdominal wall to ensure adequate tissue ingrowth. In one study the rate of hernia recurrence without the use of these transfascial sutures resulted in a recurrence of 13% while there were no recurrences seen in those patients that had the use of sutures.[665] Tacking is followed by placement of non-absorbable sutures (e.g. ePTFE) of size 0. These sutures will be placed through all musculofascial layers of the abdominal wall and tied above the fascia in a manner similar to the tying of the initial two sutures. During the insertion of the sutures, one should avoid clamping of any portion of the suture material that will remain within the patient. If this occurs, the suture will be permanently weakened and may fracture at that site which can lead to failure of the suture and a recurrence of the hernia.

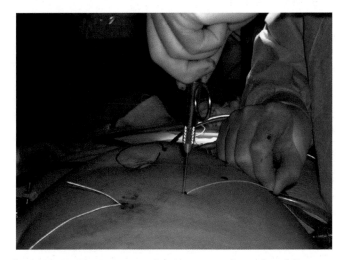

Figure 23.19 *The suture-passing instrument is used to deliver the additional transfascial sutures.*

Using the view of the laparoscope, the planned sites of suture placement are marked at intervals of 5 cm apart. A mark is made with the skin-marking pen at these points whereupon a no.11 scalpel blade is used to make a 1–2 mm skin incision at each of these points. Then at each site a suture is passed through the skin incision with one of the many fascial closure or suture-passing devices that are available (Figure 23.19). The suture passer pierces the patch at the appropriate place. The assistant (from the opposite side of the abdomen) retrieves the suture with a grasping instrument and the suture is released (Figure 23.20). The device is now withdrawn into the subcutaneous tissue and reinserted through the patch approximately 1 cm from the previous puncture site. The previously inserted suture is retrieved from the assistant and withdrawn from the abdomen onto the skin (Figure 23.21). The two tails of the suture are grasped with a hemostat and the suture is cut with sufficient length to allow for the tying of the suture. These maneuvers are repeated then along the entire edge of the patch (Figure 23.22). Once the sutures are tied the patch should lay flat and obliterate the fascial defect. A final examination of the prosthetic is performed to insure that all sutures are tight and

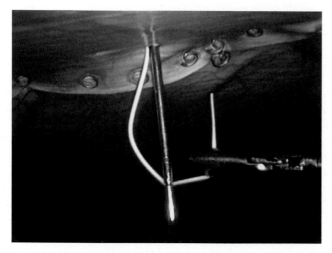

Figure 23.20 *Retrieval of the newly introduced transfascial by the suture-passing instrument.*

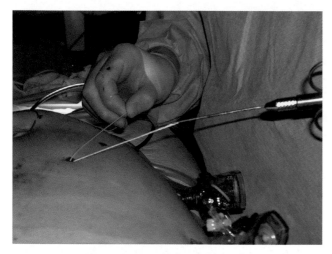

Figure 23.21 *Removal of the transfascial suture from the abdomen. This will be subsequently tied by the surgeon.*

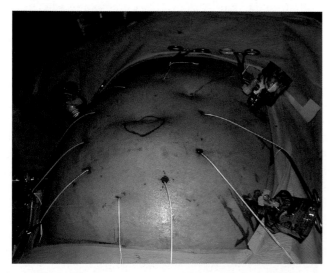

Figure 23.22 *The final appearance of the abdomen after the placement of all of the transfascial sutures.*

that all edges of the patch are secured (Figure 23.23). Any laxity of the sutures will require that these be replaced with others that provide sufficient fixation without looseness.

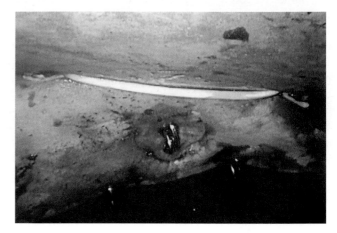

Figure 23.23 *The completed fixation of the prosthesis. The transfascial suture puncture sites should be 1.5–2 cm apart.*

Alternatively, if more than two sutures are placed initially then these are then pulled out sequentially with the same manner that has been described above. It is important to assure the position of these additional sutures so that the prosthetic biomaterial will cover the defect(s) adequately and lay as flat as possible.

When the sutures are tied down, a dimple of the skin may develop at the site of the incision where the suture has been passed. This is caused by the fixation of the subcutaneous tissue that may have been grasped by the knots of the suture. This dimple can be removed by placing a fine pointed hemostat or sturdy skin hook into the incision to lift the skin away from the suture (Figure 23.24). It is important to inspect the abdominal wall with the abdomen fully insufflated after the completion of the suture fixation so that any dimples are removed. If this is not done, the cosmetic result will be unacceptable to the patient.

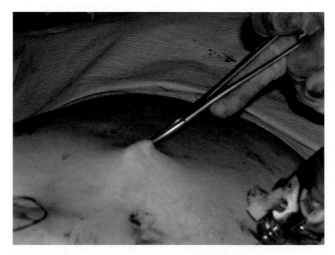

Figure 23.24 *Insertion of a hemostat to separate the subcutaneous tissue from the transfascial suture. This will eliminate the puckering of the skin that can occur with these sutures.*

Rather than placing the additional sutures as described above, in some centers, an additional row of staples are placed near the fascial edges. The result is two concentric rows of tacks that secure the prosthesis. This 'double-crown' technique is popular in some centers.[185] Current follow-up data appears to be favorable but longer term data will be necessary to verify its effectiveness.

After the removal of the trocars and closure of the skin incisions, an abdominal binder is frequently used and left in place for at least 72 h. It is believed that the use of this binder aids in the prevention of a postoperative seroma at the site of the hernia. It assists in the management of postoperative pain and does not appear to affect the respiratory effort of the patient.

IMMEDIATE POSTOPERATIVE CONSIDERATIONS

Approximately 50% of these patients can be discharged on the same day of surgery. Generally this will be the patient that has a single defect, a hernia dimension of less than 25 cm^2, few adhesions and no incarcerated contents of the hernia. The average length of stay is 1–2 days[282,665,886,939] (see Table 23.3). Patients can consume liquids the day of surgery and resume taking any regular medications immediately. Oral and parenteral sedatives are given as needed. Postoperatively, many patients will experience some degree of abdominal distension, which is usually proportional to the extent of adhesiolysis and the extent of bowel involvement. However, most patients can resume a regular diet the day after the operation. Occasionally, some patients will experience prolongation of the ileus. This should be managed by the usual methods; which would include a nasogastric tube when necessary.

Pain may be used as the guide to determine when patients can resume their normal activities. They are allowed to shower the next day. Patients may return to their daily activities, including work, as soon as they can do so without marked pain. The majority of patients are able to drive within a week and resume job-related activities in 7–14 days. Most surgeons do not restrict the activities of these patients but allow the level of pain to dictate the increase in the level of activity.

After removal of the binder, many patients will note a firm bulge at the hernia site. The bulge may represent a seroma in the first few weeks, but subsequently this area represents the cicatrical event that occurs in the majority of these patients. Seroma formation occurs in up to 43% of these cases.[282,492,665] However, it is rarely, if ever, necessary to aspirate these fluid collections, as they will generally resolve without intervention. Aspiration will also expose the patient to a risk of the introduction of infection into the seroma. One method to reduce the incidence of postoperative seromas involves the use of electrocautery to the hernia sac itself at the time of the original surgery.[1144] In a randomized study, the incidence of postoperative seromas was reduced from 25% to 4% when this was applied ($P < 0.025$). More research would be needed to confirm these findings as there is a risk of a full thickness burn to the skin with the use of this energy source.

LATE POSTOPERATIVE CONSIDERATIONS

In most patients with the cicatrical 'bulge' and/or seroma at the hernia site, resolution will be noted within 2 months, depending on the size of the hernia and its contents. Occasionally the skin of the abdominal wall that overlaid the hernia will become erythematous within 4–6 days postoperatively, usually in association with a distinct surface firmness but with little tenderness and without the presence of fever, chills, or leukocytosis (Figure 23.25). This situation, which is seen in approximately 5–7% of patients, can persist for a few weeks and can be most unsettling. This is believed to be the result of resorption of fatty tissue or the hernia sac that was left in place during the initial operation. This appears to be particularly common after the repair of hernias that had minimal soft tissue between the skin and peritoneal sac and/or a significant amount of incarcerated tissue. No treatment is necessary unless there is a strong suspicion of infection.

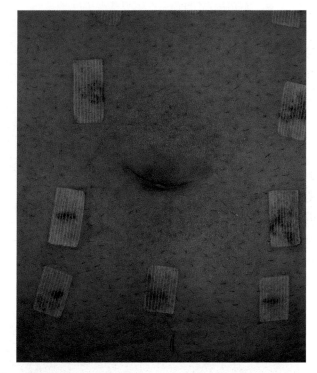

Figure 23.25 *Non-infected postoperative erythema that can be seen in some patients after LIVH.*

Usually within 2–3 months, the abdominal wall will have completed its postoperative changes (Figures 23.26 and 23.27). Infrequently, an apparent seroma can still be felt. Ultrasonography or CT scan could evaluate this finding if there is a concern regarding the possibility of a recurrence of the hernia.

In less than 2% of the patients prolonged pain (>3 months) at the site of the transfascial sutures will occur. Usually this can be treated effectively with non-steroidal anti-inflammatory drugs or direct injections of xylocaine or other local anesthetic. If this problem persists despite these maneuvers, the surgeon might consider performing a laparoscopic examination to inspect the patch, tacks and sutures. This is rarely necessary but occasionally transection of the offending suture will be necessary to effect a permanent relief of these symptoms.

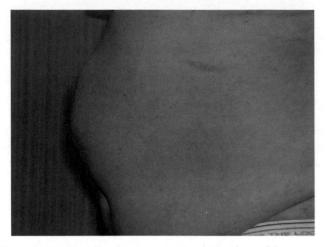

Figure 23.26 *Preoperative appearance of a patient with a large incisional hernia following a laparotomy for trauma.*

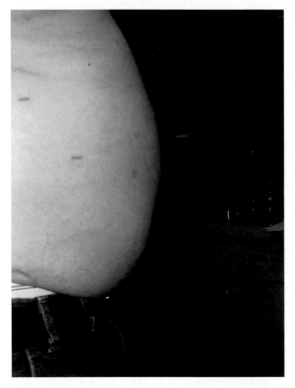

Figure 23.27 *Postoperative appearance of the same patient in Figure 23.26 after 3 months.*

HERNIORRHAPHY OF INFREQUENT DEFECTS

The majority of incisional and ventral hernias will occur in the midline of the abdomen. One will encounter other hernias that offer a particular challenge whether repaired by the open or the laparoscopic technique. One such hernia is that which lies very

high in the midline, perhaps at the exit site of a mediastinal drainage tube used for open-heart surgery. Repair of this defect may require that the prosthetic patch be placed near or onto the diaphragm. For a defect in the pericardial area, it is advisable to use only sutures to secure the patch in order to avoid penetration of tacks into the myocardium or development of pericarditis requiring removal of the tacks. It may be difficult to achieve an adequate amount of counter pressure necessary for the tacking device to provide adequate penetration of the tacks. Should this occur, non-absorbable sutures should be placed. Additionally an oversized patch is recommended to provide a greater overlap than usually required due to this fixation problem.

Hernias that extend to the symphysis pubis or are associated with an inguinal hernia can also present a challenge. To repair these defects, it will be necessary to attach the lower part of the patch to Cooper's ligament. To accomplish this it will be necessary to dissect the preperitoneal space similar to the laparoscopic transabdominal preperitoneal inguinal hernia repair. This must be done to provide for strong fixation of the patch to the muscle wall of the lower abdomen and the periosteum of the pubis because transfascial sutures cannot be placed in this location. Additionally, interposing preperitoneal fat and peritoneum that remains between the patch and muscle will compromise subsequent tissue attachment. After the patch is secured, the preperitoneal flap can be secured it in its usual position to the maximum extent possible.

Incisional 'hernias' that occur after nephrectomy or an anterior approach to the spine are usually not true hernias as they generally do not exhibit a well-defined fascial defect. The repair of these deformities is not currently established in the literature. Surgeons that do attempt to repair these deformities must pay particular attention to the positioning of the patient. Patients with such defects should be placed in a lateral decubitus position on a 'bean bag'. Defects along the upper flanks that involve denervated musculature rather than a true fascial lesion require a very large patch that is secured tightly with more than the usual number of sutures to achieve an acceptable cosmetic result. The laxity of the muscles will frequently require that sutures be placed above the rib margin to secure the prosthetic biomaterial. Additionally, one may need to place sutures onto the diaphragm to ensure fixation. It is frequently beneficial to place additional trocars through the biomaterial itself (Figure 23.28) to allow for the accurate placement of all of the methods of fixation. In the few patients that have undergone this repair by one of the authors (K.A.L.), the results are encouraging but longer term follow-up is necessary (see Chapter 19).

Many patients who present for laparoscopic incisional hernia repair may also require surgical treatment of a concomitant illness. This most commonly will include cholelithiasis, inguinal hernia, gastroesophageal reflux disease, or a need for biopsy of an intra-abdominal or retroperitoneal structure. This has been reported.[492,665] Most commonly the primary procedure is not the incisional hernia repair and, as such, will be performed initially. If the primary operation can be completed without contamination, the hernia repair could then be performed. If contamination does occur, a prosthetic hernia repair should not be done. An open repair without the insertion of a prosthetic material

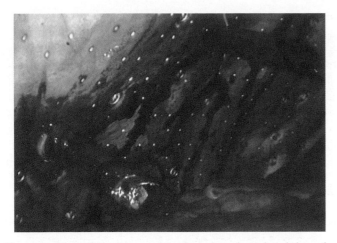

Figure 23.28 *Additional trocars that have been introduced through a prosthesis. This will provide better precision for the operation.*

could be considered but should be individualized to the patient's risk factors, prior operations and/or prior hernia repairs. Preoperative discussions with the patient should have examined this possibility. In those individuals in whom the hernia repair can be attempted subsequent to the primary procedure, placement of additional trocars may be necessary. The surgeon could plan on the future trocars at the initiation of the primary procedure but should not compromise the first procedure by the inappropriate positioning at that point. Any additional necessary trocars should be placed in the locations most appropriate for the herniorrhaphy once the decision is made to proceed with the second procedure. One should not avoid using more trocars when deemed necessary to carry out the second operation in a safe and effective manner.

RESULTS

There have been five reports that have compared the open method of repair with the laparoscopic method. These have compared many aspects of these two options for the repair of incisional and ventral hernia repair. The operative times are not significantly different between the two procedures. As shown in Figure 23.29 the cumulative average for either operation is approximately 92 min.[184,282,886]

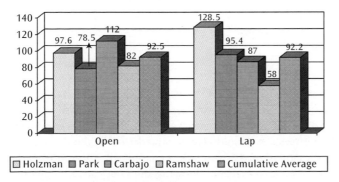

Figure 23.29 *Comparison of operative times of open and laparoscopic incisional and ventral herniorrhaphy.*

There were a myriad of postoperative complications seen in both arms of these studies and also in the one reported by DeMaria. As shown in Table 23.1 the most common complications following the open repair groups were bowel obstruction, ileus, seroma and infections. Comparatively, the most common complications in the laparoscopic groups were ileus and seroma. In all of these comparative analyses, the incidence and severity of the complications were less in the laparoscopic group. A notable exception to this statement is the development of seromas. This complication is felt by many notable surgeons to be an occurrence that is so common in the laparoscopic repair that it should be considered an expected finding rather than a complication. The true incidence is probably much higher than that which is shown in the literature.

The most dreaded complication in the laparoscopic herniorrhaphy is the enterotomy. This is the obvious exception to the above comment as this complication was more frequent in the laparoscopic group. Ramshaw's series had an incidence of 2.6% compared to that of 0.6% in the open group. While not statistically significant, it should reinforce the need for vigilance in the avoidance of this complication. Should this occur and is recognized, the injury should be repaired, of course. The next decision is whether or not to proceed with the repair of the hernia itself. The use of a prosthesis is to be avoided. A primary repair will be associated with a high risk of recurrence. Therefore, many experts recommend that the primary repair be avoided and the patient be returned to the operating room in several days. There are few reports that describe this treatment.[657]

There was a statistically significant difference in the length of hospitalization in three of the five papers. As shown in Table 23.2, the patients are sent home more rapidly with the minimally invasive procedure. This has proven to account for the decrease in the costs associated with this repair compared to the open method. The shortened hospitalization decreases the expenses for the repair of incisional hernia by approximately US$3000–4000.[282,511] This is noted despite the fact that these repairs used the ePTFE as a prosthesis.

There have been many other publications that have described this operation. Several are listed in Table 23.3 and include only those studies that have included 50 or more patients. Most of these series include the early experience of the authors in the compilation. The complication rates in these papers ranged from 5–24%, which is similar or better to that of the open repair. Length of hospitalization was consistent with the above studies and averaged a mean of 2 days. Recurrences ranged from 0–11%. The recurrence rates from the five comparative studies are also detailed in Table 23.1. It is apparent that the results with the laparoscopic technique are better than the open method. The notable exception is that of DeMaria in which there was a single recurrence in the laparoscopic group. Nevertheless, a rate of recurrence for the incisional hernia repair compares very favorably with the open prosthetic repair (see Chapter 22, Table 22.3).

Careful review of patients during the development phase of the operation enabled the identification of factors that influenced the 9% recurrence rate in LeBlanc's series.[665] In all of the

Table 23.1 *Percentage comparison of complications associated with open prosthetic incisional and ventral herniorrhaphy*

	Carbajo		Holzman		Park		Ramshaw		DeMaria	
	Open	Lap	Open	Lap	Open	Lap	Open	Lap	Open	Lap
Bowel obstruction	–	3	12.5	0.5	–	–	–	–	11	–
Cardiac	–	–	4.1	–	–	–	–	–	–	–
Cellulitis	6.7	–	–	–	–	–	3.4	2.5	–	–
Cerebrovascular accident	–	–	–	–	–	–	0.6	–	–	–
Deep venous thrombosis	–	–	–	–	–	–	–	–	5.6	–
Enterotomy – recognized	–	–	–	–	–	–	–	1.3	–	–
Enterotomy – unrecognized	–	–	–	–	–	–	0.6	1.3	–	–
Fistula	–	–	–	–	–	–	–	–	–	4.8
Genitourinary	–	–	6.1	–	–	–	2.3	2.5	–	–
Hematoma	20	3	–	–	10.2	–	–	–	–	–
Hypoxia	–	–	6.3	0.5	–	–	–	–	–	–
Ileus	–	–	12.5	–	–	5.4	8.1	6.3	–	4.8
Infection of mesh	–	–	–	–	–	–	3.6	2.9	–	–
Infection (other)	–	–	4	0.5	–	–	–	–	33	9.6
Intestinal injury	–	–	4	–	–	–	–	–	–	–
Phlebitis	10	–	–	–	–	–	–	–	–	–
Protracted pain	–	–	–	–	4.1	3.6	–	–	–	–
Pulmonary embolus	–	–	–	–	–	–	0.6	–	–	–
Recurrence rate	6.7	0.0	12.5	10.0	34.7	11.0	20.7	2.5	0.0	4.8
Re-operation	–	–	–	–	–	–	–	–	–	9.6
Respiratory distress	–	–	–	–	–	1.8	0.6	1.3	–	–
Seroma	67	13	–	–	3.6	3.6	6.9	2.5	22	43
Serosal injury	–	–	–	–	–	–	0.6	2.3	–	–
Skin necrosis	3.3	–	–	–	–	–	–	–	–	–
Wound infection	–	–	6.3	–	2	–	–	–	–	–

Table 23.2 *Comparison of hospitalization length of stay (days) between open and laparoscopic incisional and ventral herniorrhaphy*

	Carbajo*		Holzman		Park*		Ramshaw		DeMaria*	
	Open	Lap	Open	Lap	Open	Lap	Open	Lap	Open	Lap
Average	9.06	2.23	4.9	1.6	6.5	3.4	2.8	1.7	4.4	0.8
Range	3–21	1–15	–	–	2–26	1–17	–	–	0.5–14	0.5–3

*Indicates statistical significance.

patients that developed a recurrence, the method of fixation of the prosthesis was either staples or tacks alone. In this subset of patients, the rate of recurrence was 13% while there were no recurrences in the patients in which we used additional transfascial sutures. This is currently the only data in the literature that documents the need for these transfascial sutures. An additional finding is that in five of these nine patients with the recurrent hernia, it appeared that the amount of overlap of the prosthetic was not at least 3 cm. The combination of these findings has caused the recommendation of the use of at least a 3 cm overlap and the use of the transfascial sutures in addition to the tacks. It should also be noted that in the comparative studies mentioned earlier in this chapter, all of the patients that developed a recurrence following the laparoscopic repair did not have the additional transfascial sutures placed as part of the method of fixation.

Table 23.3 *Reported large series (more than 50 patients) of laparoscopic incisional and ventral hernia repairs (n = 1047)*

Series	No. of patients	Complication rate (%)*	Hospital stay (days) Mean except where noted	Follow-up (months) Mean except where noted	Recurrence rate (%)†
Kyzer	53	11	3 (Median)	17 (Median)	0
Park	56	18	3	24	11
Ramshaw	79	19	2	21	3
LeBlanc	100	14	1	51	9
Heniford	100	14	2	23	3
Franklin	112	5	1–12 (range)	30	1
Toy	144	24	2	7	4
Heniford	407	13	2	23	2

*Does not include hernia recurrence.

†Does not include patients with recurrence after removal of the prosthesis used in the repair (because of infection or other problem).

Adapted from LeBlanc *et al.* American Journal of Surgery 2000;180:193–197, with permission from Excerpta Medica, Inc.

CONCLUSIONS

- Laparoscopic repair of incisional hernias of the abdominal wall is gaining in popularity. There are a few significant technical mandates of this operation, which will result in favorable outcomes.

- The rates of both complications and recurrence following this method of incisional and ventral herniorraphy appear to be fewer than that associated with the open prosthetic repair.
- Long-term follow-up to date suggests that this may be the procedure of choice in the future but it continues to evolve.

24

Parastomal hernia

Parastomal hernias may present as problems of stoma care, difficulty with appliances or irrigation, a significant cosmetic deformity; or as straightforward complications of a hernia, intestinal obstruction or strangulation. The presence of a large protrusion itself may make repair a necessity irrespective of its other side effects. Herniation is less frequent with ileostomy than colostomy but the overall incidence of parastomal herniation is difficult to quantify.

PARACOLOSTOMY HERNIA – INCIDENCE AND ETIOLOGY

Burns, in 1970, found 16 paracolic hernias among 307 colostomates, an incidence of 5%.[164] Other authors quote figures of 5–50% (Table 24.1). Burgess and colleagues in the north of England reviewed their experience of permanent colostomy with abdominoperineal resection for rectal cancer in the decade 1970–1980. A total of 124 operations were performed and six patients (5%) developed paracolostomy hernias, but only one of these hernias required surgical correction.[161]

In 1981, Wara et al. reviewed their experience of herniation about temporary transverse colostomy and reported 3.9% incidence of parastomal herniation.[1191]

Contrary to previous surgical dogma[429,1129] the risk of stomal herniation is not reduced if the stoma is brought through the rectus muscle.[708,871] The extraperitoneal technique of stoma formation described by Goligher does not slightly lessen the risk of parastomal hernia either.[708]

The worst parastomal hernias occur if the stoma is brought out through a laparotomy wound. Indeed, it should be a principle of colon surgery never to place a stoma in a laparotomy wound because of the risks of infection, dehiscence, herniation and difficulties with appliance fitting.[429,521,894,1129,1131]

Table 24.1 *Percentage of patients developing paracolostomy hernia*

Study	Date	Number of end colostomies performed	Percentage of patients developing paracolostomy hernias*
Birnbaum	1952	569	4.71
Green	1966	318	2.5
Burns	1970	307	5.2
Saha et al.	1973	200	1.0
Kronberg et al.	1974	362	11.6
Harshaw et al.	1974	99	9.1
Marks and Ritchie	1975	227	10.1
Kodner	1978	–	50
Abrams	1979	248	1.6
Burgess et al.	1984	124	4.8
Cevese et al.	1984	183	16
Pearl et al.	1985	88	2.5 (Only early complications reviewed. This report is difficult to decipher because it does not include the actual figures involved)
Phillips et al.	1985	243	5
		52	12
Sjodahl et al.	1988	79	10
Londono-Schimmer et al.	1994	203	36.7
Ortiz et al.	1994	4	48.0

*The duration of follow-up varies in different series.
289 operations were performed but only 203 patients available for review at 10 years.[708]

PARA-ILEOSTOMY HERNIA – INCIDENCE AND ETIOLOGY

The incidence of para-ileostomy hernia is between 5% and 10% and of para-ileal conduit stomas in urological practice 5–10%.[750]

Lubbers and Devlin reviewed their experience of permanent ileostomy in the years 1970–1980; the incidence of para-ileostomy hernia was five out of 102 (5%).[712]

Williams *et al.*, in a study of 28 ileostomies using clinical and radiological CT evaluation, found the rate of herniation to be 35% and the same whether the ileum exited through or lateral to the rectus muscle.[1213] Parastomal hernias occur most usually alongside the mesentery of the emergent gut. Thus in the conventional right lower quadrant ileostomy the hernia initially presents along the mesenteric attachment at the superomedial aspect of the stoma. Nevertheless, the most optimum site for ileostomy management is to site the stoma on the top of the infra-umbilical mound of the rectus muscle with the stoma constructed so that the bowel exits through the rectus muscle.[292,871,894]

TYPES OF HERNIA

The anatomy of the herniation is variable. For convenience, four principal types may be identified:

1   *Interstitial.* In this instance there is a hernial sac lying within the muscle/aponeurotic layers of the abdominal wall. This may contain omentum, small or large intestine. In these cases the stoma is asymmetrical, and is edematous and cyanotic if its vascular supply is compromised (Figure 24.1).

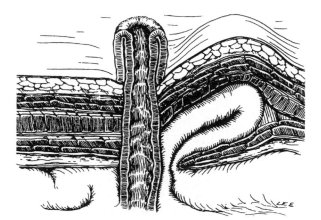

Figure 24.1 *An interstitial parastomal hernia.*

2   *Subcutaneous.* In this instance there is herniation alongside the stoma with a subcutaneous sac containing omentum, small or large intestine. This is the commonest form of paracolostomy hernia and not infrequently colon situated just proximal to the stoma is found in the sac.

Such a tangled-up stoma is very difficult to irrigate (Figure 24.2). The interstitial and subcutaneous hernias are considered to be variants of a sliding hernia. Because the ring of tissue that surrounds the contents of the hernia can be quite narrow, these hernias are particularly at risk for incarceration and strangulation.

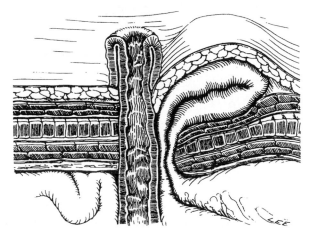

Figure 24.2 *A subcutaneous parastomal hernia.*

3   *Intrastomal.* This is a problem of spout ileostomies only. A loop of intestine may herniate alongside the stoma and lie between the emergent and the everted layer of the stoma. Intestinal obstruction has been described in such hernias by Cuthbertson and Collins[260] (Figure 24.3).

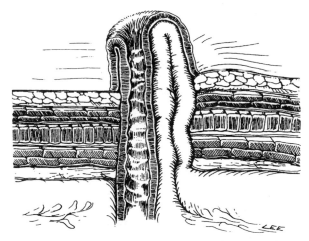

Figure 24.3 *An intrastomal hernia.*

4   *Perstomal or prolapse.* All stomas can prolapse, but transverse colostomies prolapse three times more frequently than any other stoma. A prolapsed stoma contains a hernial sac within itself; other viscera, especially small gut, can enter this sac and even become strangulated. Large perstomal hernial sacs are often seen in neonates who have a transverse colostomy for anorectal agenesis (Figure 24.4).

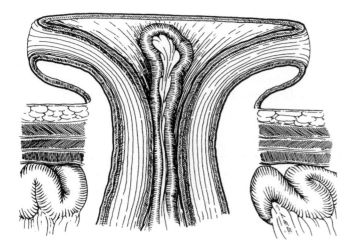

Figure 24.4 *Prolapse or perstomal herniation.*

Strangulated small bowel requiring resection has been found in the hernial sac of a prolapsed terminal colostomy.[263] A similar strangulated small bowel hernia can be found in large prolapsed transverse colostomy. The treatment should be to expedite the closure of a transverse colostomy or to excise and refashion the bowel into an end stoma.

PREDISPOSING FACTORS

A variety of factors are responsible for the development of parastomal herniation. These may be:

- *'Operator-dependent'* – a disproportionately large aperture in the abdominal wall, placement of the stoma in the laparotomy incision or postoperative parastomal infections. The placement of the ostomy site lateral to the rectus abdominis muscle is associated with nearly an eight-fold increase in the incidence of herniation.[1058]
- *'Patient-dependent'* – cachexia due to advanced malnutrition or malignancy, senility or excessive obesity. Obesity and the presence of other abdominal wall hernias are important risk factors for the development of paracolostomy herniation. The latter observation suggests that paracolostomy hernia in the older patient could be a further example of failure of the transversalis fascia.[708] Other risk factors that have been noted are diabetes mellitus, chronic steroid usage, and advanced age.

PRINCIPLES OF MANAGEMENT

An accurate diagnosis and assessment of the anatomy of the hernia is essential. Therefore, the patient must be examined (a) recumbent and relaxed; (b) with the muscles tense; and (c) in the erect position. Investigation of the detailed anatomy with CT scanning is useful to delineate large parastomal defects in the abdominal wall. CT scanning can also detect small

impalpable defects around ileostomies that present with dysfunction.[1130]

An accurate assessment of the anatomy of the hernia should be made. Alternative stoma sites should be considered if relocation of the stoma is needed. Care must be taken if a decision to re-site a stoma is made; the help of a stoma care nurse (enterostomal therapist) is invaluable.[292]

The patient who has had cancer surgery must be screened for recurrence before surgery is advised. Similarly, it is prudent to exclude recrudescent inflammatory bowel disease before undertaking operation in patients with ileostomies although it should be noted that the risk of para-ileostomy herniation is similar in patients with ulcerative colitis and Crohn's disease. An additional consideration that has become more commonplace is the life expectancy of the patient. An increasing number of patients of an advanced age are being seen with multiple medical problems that add to the risk of a general anesthetic. If these illnesses will significantly shorten the life of the patient (e.g. less than 2–3 years) or if these prohibit anesthesia, then one may not wish to proceed if there is no immediate need for surgical intervention.

There are four operative options to treat a parastomal hernia:

A local repair operation

The stoma is mobilized locally, the peritoneal sac identified and its contents reduced, and the peritoneum is closed. The musculoaponeurotic defect is stretched laterally with a retractor and closed with far and near non-absorbable sutures[513] (Figure 24.5). If the skin aperture is too large it can be reduced using the 'Mercedes' technique described by Todd[1129] (Figure 24.6).

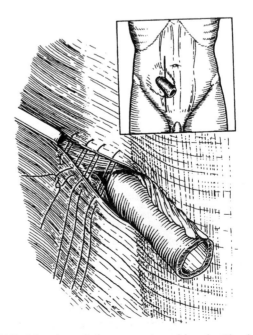

Figure 24.5 *A local repair for a parastomal hernia. The defect frequently extends into the muscle fibers, which does not hold sutures or repair adequately.*

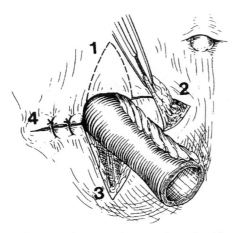

Figure 24.6 *The Mercedes operation to reduce the skin aperture around a stoma (Todd, 1978).*

Local repair operations for parastomal hernias cannot be recommended. Horgan and Hughes report two patients and in both of these the operation failed.[513] This experience was shared by H. Brandon Devlin who employed the technique twice; on both occasions the hernia recurred within 18 months. One of these patients had a further local repair – again followed by failure. This patient then had his stoma relocated with long-term success. In this patient the aponeurotic defect extended laterally into the banding of the internal oblique, a sort of Spigelian hernia, so that the lateral margin of the stoma incision extended into the fleshy internal oblique. Sutures into these red muscle bands are unlikely to hold and lead to lasting healing, particularly if the medial defect is splinted open by the emergent stoma.

Horgan and Hughes, 1986, conclude: 'We cannot recommend [in situ herniorrhaphy] as both patients treated in this manner had recurrence of their hernia within 2 years.[513] Prian *et al.*,[925] Cuthbertson and Collins[260] and the authors agree with this observation. In Rubin's series of 29 patients with a primary fascial repair for a primary hernia, the recurrence rate was 76%.[983] We do not recommend local repair of subcutaneous parastomal hernias.

Prosthetic repair by either an extraperitoneal or extraparietal route

Extraperitoneal placement of polypropylene mesh at open operation is a similar technique to the GPRVS operation for groin hernias. The mesh is laid around the stoma in the plane between the peritoneum and the parietal muscles. This is the recommended technique if mesh repair of a defect is needed.[389,972,983]

Intraperitoneal placement of polypropylene mesh around an emergent colostomy has been reported. This is a successful operative technique in the short term but long-term reservations about the intraperitoneal usage of polypropylene mesh must be noted.[165] Others have reported the use of the intraperitoneal polypropylene without complications.[983,1107]

Placement of the mesh in the subcutaneous plane involves mobilization of the stoma and fixation of the prosthesis to the external oblique, after threading the stoma through a window in the prosthesis. The advantage of subcutaneous placement is that no laparotomy is required. Rosin has used an incision directly over the hernia whereas Phillips has pioneered the use of this technique using a local circumstomal incision and he reports excellent results.[972,1088] A similar technique using a specially devised polypropylene ring set in a polypropylene mesh is used by de Ruiter and Bijen.[280]

The disadvantage of local techniques is the risk of contamination from the stoma. No matter how the stoma is sealed, there is a risk of contamination and of subsequent sepsis. If sepsis occurs troublesome sinuses follow; such sinuses may warrant removal of the mesh. However, modern polypropylene mesh is tolerant of sepsis and simple local infection will usually settle with the prosthesis remaining in place.[1088]

The extraperitoneal operation offers significant advantages avoiding sepsis.

Laparoscopy

Laparoscopy offers several advantages that encompass many of the attributes noted above. The laparoscopic approach offers the surgeon the ability to visualize the entire abdominal wall so that any incisional hernias may also be repaired at the same time. This technique requires that the prosthetic biomaterial be placed in the intraperitoneal position. The use of polypropylene has been described but we believe that the preferred biomaterial is ePTFE.[122,662,920,1171] The experience with this technique is in its infancy, therefore longer follow-up will be necessary to evaluate its effectiveness.

Stoma relocation

Stoma relocation may be carried out either with formal laparotomy or with limited transperitoneal transfer of the stoma. This is the most consistently satisfactory operation.[983] The disadvantage, of course, is that the patient may prefer the location of the original ostomy or wish to defer this more traumatic operation until one of the above has failed. A laparoscopic approach has not been described but will undoubtedly be used in the future. Pneumoperitoneum is a useful preoperative technique to secure increased intra-abdominal space and to stretch adhesions prior to operation on large peristomal hernia.

INDICATIONS AND CONTRAINDICATIONS TO SURGERY

Surgery is imperative in all cases of intestinal obstruction or strangulation related to parastomal hernia. Urgent emergency surgery is also absolutely indicated in all cases of paracolostomy hernia where perforation has occurred during irrigation.

Surgery is the treatment of choice when a parastomal hernia causes abdominal wall distortion and difficulties with fitting an appliance or irrigating a stoma. Surgery should also be considered if the stoma has become out of the patient's range of vision or if its site on a hernia bulge makes it unmanageable to elderly patients, especially those with arthritis. The disfigurement caused by a bulging parastomal hernia may warrant surgery for cosmetic reasons. In special circumstances, the repair may need to be accompanied by an abdominoplasty to permit a good fit of the appliance.

Contraindications to surgery include such general problems as cardiorespiratory failure, recurrent Crohn's disease, extreme obesity, disseminated malignancy or a short life expectancy from any disease process.

PNEUMOPERITONEUM

Preoperative pneumoperitoneum is a useful adjunct in the management of large parastomal hernias; this is described in detail on page 266.

TECHNIQUE OF EXTRAPERITONEAL PROSTHETIC REPAIR OF PARASTOMAL HERNIA

We prefer the use of preoperative cleansing of the colon with any of the available methods in use today. The use of antibiotics is arguable if a tissue repair alone or stoma relocation is performed but when a prosthesis is to be inserted this is particularly preferred (whether extraperitoneal or intraperitoneal). The patient is prepared with the stoma sealed with an adherent plastic film. The original laparotomy scar is excised and reopened (Figure 24.7).

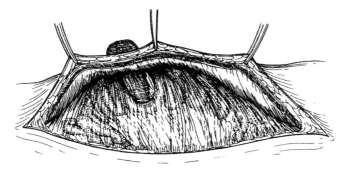

Figure 24.7 *Reopening the laparotomy incision.*

A plane of dissection is opened between the peritoneum and the parietal muscles lateral to the stoma. During this dissection the hernial contents are reduced if possible without opening the hernial (peritoneal) sac. This may not be possible. If the peritoneum is opened it is closed carefully around the stoma so that the mesh can be introduced into the extraperitoneal plane (Figure 24.8).

A sheet of polypropylene mesh is prepared, to repair the defect, with a hole in it to allow the egress of the stoma. A cut is made in the mesh so that it can be positioned. The polypropylene should fit snugly around the efferent bowel and should

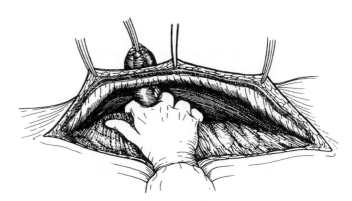

Figure 24.8 *Developing the extraperitoneal plane to the stoma.*

overlap the margins of the defect by at least 3 cm (Figure 24.9). The polypropylene is quilted into place (Figure 24.10). Suction drains are positioned. If there is any defect in the main wound, the margin of the mesh is extended medially to overlap and repair this defect, as described earlier. The wound is closed carefully as before.

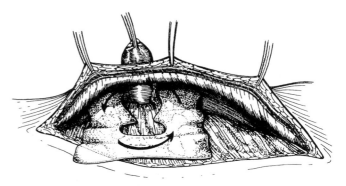

Figure 24.9 *Preparing the mesh to make the repair.*

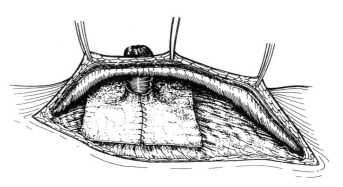

Figure 24.10 *Placing the polypropylene in place deep to the muscle layer and superficial to the peritoneum – in the extraperitoneal plane again like 'ham in a sandwich'.*

The use of a prosthetic material in this manner has been noted to allow recurrent herniation because of enlargement of the opening in the mesh in four out of five patients within 3 years.[280] This led these authors to utilize a prosthesis that contained a polypropylene ring that had a fixed opening of 20, 25 or 30 mm. This was used successfully in 13 out of 14 patients with no complications or recurrence of the hernia after a median follow-up of 18 months (range 5–35 months). One patient did develop a staphylococcus aureus infection that necessitated removal of the prosthesis. While this device represents an intriguing option in the repair of these difficult hernias, there have not been further studies to document its efficacy.

SUBCUTANEOUS PARASTOMAL HERNIA REPAIR

An adherent wound drape is used to occlude the stoma and restrict contamination.

Incision

An incision is made through the old incision and then laterally above and around the stoma, permitting the stoma to be raised on an 'L'-shaped flap (Figure 24.11). The incision is deepened to the aponeurosis (Figure 24.12). Alternatively a circumstomal incision may be used just around the stoma. The stoma is oversewn and temporarily closed[1088] (Figure 24.13).

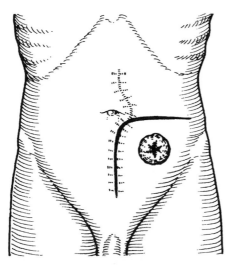

Figure 24.11 *An 'L' shaped incision is made; this allows the stoma to be raised on a flap.*

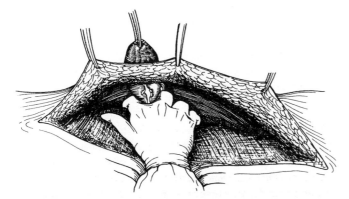

Figure 24.12 *Extraparietal repair; the incision is made and the stoma then approached in the subcutaneous layer.*

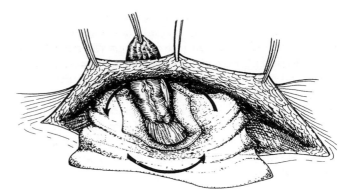

Figure 24.13 *The sac is reduced and the mesh introduced.*

Hernial sac

The sac is found, opened and its contents reduced. The peritoneum is closed. A defect in the aponeurosis is closed.

Mesh repair

The mesh is introduced around the stoma and quilted down to the aponeurosis (Figure 24.13). The mesh should extend 3 cm outside the margins of the aponeurotic defect. If possible, a cuff of mesh should surround the emergent stoma (Figure 24.14); this prevents later stoma prolapse. A prosthetic mesh with a polypropylene ring used around the stoma is useful here.[280] Suction drains may be inserted. Closure is as described previously.

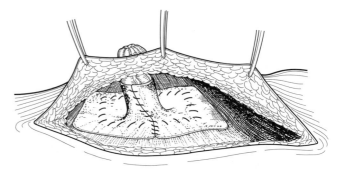

Figure 24.14 *The mesh surrounds the stoma and is fixed by quilting sutures to the underlying external oblique aponeurosis.*

INTRAPERITONEAL PROSTHETIC REPAIR

Open repair

The repair in this fashion has been described by Sugarbaker.[1106,1107] This method utilizes the old laparotomy incision for access to the abdominal cavity. Identification of the colon within the mass of herniated contents, mesentery and the accompanying adhesions is facilitated by the intraoperative insertion of either an endoscope or a large catheter. Either if these are placed into the stoma using sterilized endoscopes or catheters just after the skin preparation of the patient prior to draping. This is then moved into a position directly lateral to the ostomy and then covered by a plastic adhesive drape to seal this site and minimize the potential for contamination.

The abdomen is entered and the contents of the hernia are dissected free from the edges of the fascial defect. One must be careful to preserve the vascular supply to the colon during this dissection. It is not necessary to dissect or remove the peritoneal sac of the hernia itself. An accurate measurement of the defect will allow the appropriate sizing of the biomaterial. As stated earlier, a minimum of a 3 cm overlap is considered mandatory but if the hernia is very large or if the abdominal wall is quite lax, a larger mesh should be used.

The prosthesis can be fixed to the abdominal wall in a variety of methods. It is usually helpful if the colon is sutured to the lateral abdominal wall by either permanent or absorbable sutures (Figure 24.15). The mesh should be positioned to provide the necessary amount of overlap so that the intestine is 'lateralized' in relation to the exit of the stoma. The biomaterial will be more easily fixed at this point by the use of tacks or a Salute construct (see Chapter 7). The use of additional sutures provides the most assurance that the biomaterial will achieve permanent fixation. These can be placed intraperitoneally to avoid the possibility of contamination of the operative field by the contents of the ostomy. However, these can be placed transfascially quite safely by one of the suture passing instruments. Care must be exercised to place these sutures at a point that the ostomy appliance will not allow contact with the skin incisions by the output of the intestine (Figure 24.16).

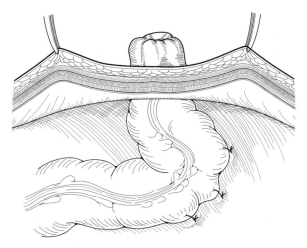

Figure 24.15 *Position of the lateralized colon onto the sidewall of the abdomen prior to the placement of the biomaterial. This must usually be sutured into place to maintain this position.*

The original description of this procedure varies slightly from the above and did not give an exact description of the prosthetic mesh that was used (although it appears that this was a polypropylene product). The 4-year follow-up of these seven patients did not reveal any problems related to the mesh. However, we share the concern of many that the use of an 'unprotected' biomaterial within direct contact may lead to long-term complications that are not necessarily apparent in a

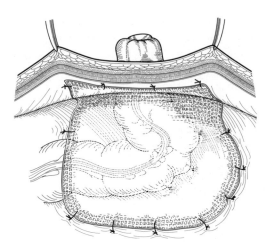

Figure 24.16 *Completed repair of the parastomal hernia. Note that the biomaterial covers the hernia defect as well as the lateralized intestine.*

4-year time frame. Because of this fact, the preferred biomaterial is that of a dual-surfaced ePTFE product (see Chapter 7).

As mentioned above, the results reported by the above technique in the seven patients in which the intraperitoneal placement of the patch was used were quite favorable. The series included two patients with urostomies and six of these repairs were in recurrent patients. There were no recurrences or complications after a minimum of 4 years of follow-up (the range was 4–7 years).[1107]

Laparoscopic repair

The laparoscopic repair of parastomal hernias has only recently been utilized as a method to repair these defects. The growth of laparoscopic incisional hernia repair has been extended into this area by a few authors. At the time of this writing there have been only four reports in the literature of this methodology.[122,662,920,1171] Each of these articles detailed a different technique involving few patients (Table 24.2).

Pocheron closed the hernial orifice and used the patch only as a reinforcing layer with no slit used to allow egress of the colon. Bickel created two strips of mesh, securing one to the abdominal wall and the other to the intraperitoneal colon. Voitk used a technique that mimicked that of open intraperitoneal repair described above. All of these authors used tacks alone to provide fixation to the abdominal wall. Although Bickel used polypropylene mesh (PPM) for the repair of that patient, they commented that the use of intraperitoneal PPM may lead to adhesion formation and that the use of a 'dual mesh non-adherent surface on one side' may be preferable.

LeBlanc used a technique identical to that which he uses for the usual incisional hernia repair[655,657,667] (see Chapter 22). The method was modified to create a slit within the DualMesh Plus® that led to a central ring that was cut into the patch (Figure 24.17). The biomaterial was then placed around the intraperitoneal intestine. This was secured to the abdominal wall with tacks and transfascial sutures (see video clip). A second prosthetic biomaterial with a central ring was then placed over this first one with the slit in an opposing direction and was also fixed

Table 24.2 *Laparoscopic parastomal reports*

Author and year	Number of patients	Prosthesis	Location of prosthesis	Length of hospital stay (days)	Length of follow-up (months)
Porcheron (1998)	1	ePTFE	Preperitoneal	4	12
Bickel (1999)	1	Polypropylene	Intraperitoneal	6	12
Voitk (2000)	4	Polypropylene	Intraperitoneal	2 (3 patients) 9 (1 patient)	
LeBlanc (2002)	3	ePTFE	Intraperitoneal	1 (all patients)	6–14

with tacks and sutures (Figure 24.18). The intent is to cover the first slit with the second patch so that the ring cannot enlarge and result in re-herniation as noted by de Ruiter.[280] Additionally, the increased thickness of the biomaterial seems to provide greater support to the abdominal wall at the unsightly site of the prior herniation. At the time of this writing the follow-up of 6, 8, and 14 months have resulted in excellent cosmetic results without complication or recurrence (Figures 24.19 and 24.20).[662]

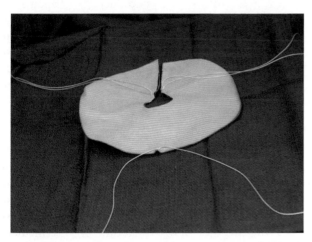

Figure 24.17 *Prosthesis with a slit and 3 cm hole to allow placement of the patch around the colon.*

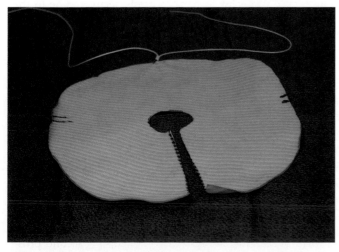

Figure 24.18 *The second prosthesis with a slit placed in the contralateral location to the one on the initial patch.*

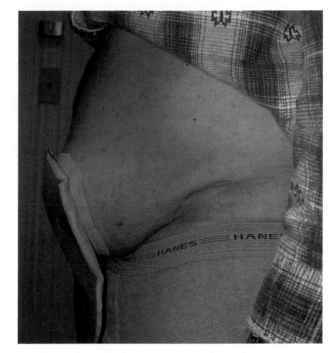

Figure 24.19 *Preoperative appearance of a patient that developed three months after an abdominoperineal resection.*

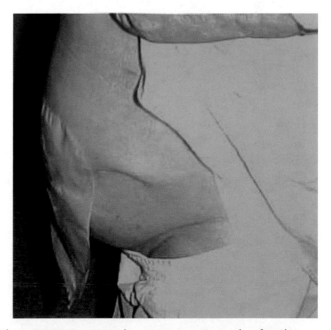

Figure 24.20 *Postoperative appearance 6 months after the laparoscopic repair of a paracolostomy hernia.*

TECHNIQUE OF STOMA RELOCATION

New stoma site

The new stoma site must be precise and careful. One in the upper abdomen overlying the contralateral rectus muscle and away from any old incisions and delves in the skin is preferred. Commonly, however, the location selected by the patient will be at the contralateral abdominal location. Preoperative consultation with the enterostomal nurse is considered essential to the identification of the ideal location. The site will be marked at that time.

A problem, which should be foreseen, is distortion of the abdominal wall by surgery after the operation has begun. The laxity of the musculature caused by anesthetic paralysis and the positioning of the patient on the operating table can result in a significant change in the habitus of the patient. Additionally the operative manipulation of the skin and muscle can result in lateral undermining of the tissues, which can eventuate in a poorly constructed stoma. Therefore, the stoma incision site is marked into each layer of the abdominal wall with the patient conscious.

The technique described by Turnbull and Weakley is recommended: the center of the disc of skin to be removed is injected with a speck of dye – methylene blue or patent blue violet – which similarly marks each layer of the abdominal wall at right angles to the skin[1147] (Figure 24.21).

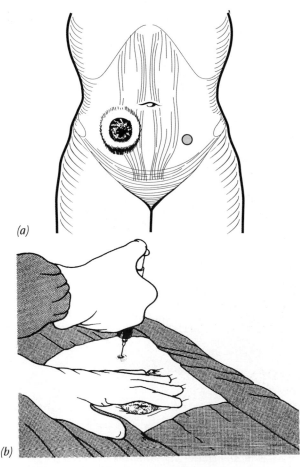

(a)

(b)

Figure 24.21 *Stoma relocation: marking the site.*

Mobilization of existing stoma

Preoperative colonic cleansing and antibiotic prophylaxis is necessary. In some patients it may be necessary to approach the operation via a midline laparotomy incision if they are obese or if the hernia has become obstructed and or incarcerated. This approach will greatly facilitate the operation. In many instances, however, a simple circumstomal skin incision can be used. A 'trick of the trade' is to carry this incision through normal skin about 1 mm from the point of mucocutaneous fusion. Preservation of the scar tissue at the point of mucocutaneous fusion facilitates subsequent closure of the stoma (Figure 24.22). The incision is deepened until the stoma is completely freed from the skin and subcutaneous tissue (Figure 24.23).

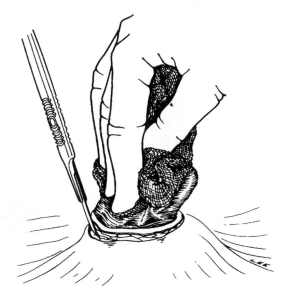

Figure 24.22 *Mobilizing the original stoma (1).*

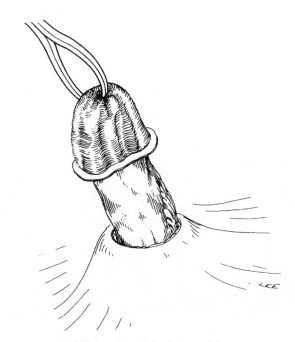

Figure 24.23 *Mobilizing the original stoma (2).*

Closure of stoma

The stoma is straightened out, an everted ileostomy being uneverted, and then closed.

A continuous circular suture of polypropylene is used, with small bites taken of the previously preserved scar tissue at the stoma margins. This suture is tied, closing the stoma off (Figure 24.24).

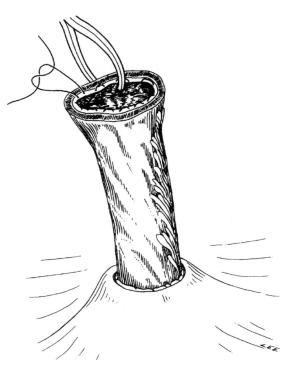

Figure 24.24 *Closing the stoma.*

If there is doubt as to the competence of this closure a second, inverting suture can be put in. It must be stressed that the stoma closure must be adequate if contamination is to be avoided (Figure 24.25).

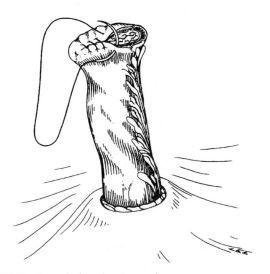

Figure 24.25 *Completing the stoma closure.*

One can also close the bowel using one of the linear stapling devices. This will avoid any contamination and generally results in a closed ostomy that is easier to manipulate than one that is sutured and then closed with a second inverting suture. Theoretically, the exposed end of the staple row can be a source of infectivity but this is uncommon after a good preoperative preparation and the use of antibiotics. One can cover the end of the staple line with a gauze soaked in an antibiotic solution if desired (see below).

Local antimicrobial chemoprophylaxis

At this stage, before any deep dissection is undertaken, the wound and the abdominal wall should be reviewed for inadvertent fecal contamination. Cleansing of the closed stoma, the wound and the abdominal wall with povidone–iodine solution and a change of gloves, drapes and instruments, at this stage converts the operation into a clean abdominal case (Figure 24.26). In the modern era of cost containment, the necessity of the extensive changes in gloves, gowns and instruments is undergoing a conscious revision. In many centers, if the preparation is good, only the instruments are discarded from the operative field without significant adverse sequalae.

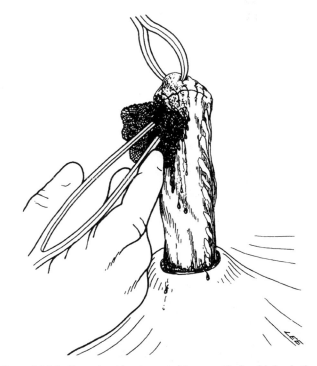

Figure 24.26 *Cleansing the stoma with an antimicrobial solution.*

Dissection of contents of hernia

The incision around the stoma is deepened and the subcutaneous herniated bowel mobilized and freed from the adjacent tissue.

After the bowel has been traced down to the external oblique/anterior rectus aponeurosis, the opening in the fascia is identified and the bowel is mobilized. If necessary, this opening can be enlarged by splitting the muscle laterally in the line of its fibers (Figure 24.27).

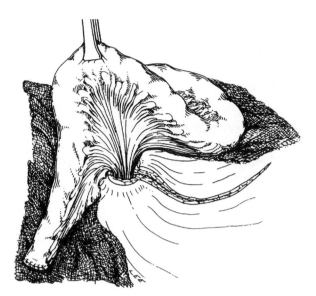

Figure 24.27 *Dissecting and freeing the hernial sac contents.*

Interstitial/intermuscular component

The deeper parts of the hernia are mobilized and freed, which involves the complete mobilization of the hernial contents and sac down to its junction with the parietal peritoneum. Once the contents have been mobilized, they are returned to the main peritoneal cavity (Figure 24.28).

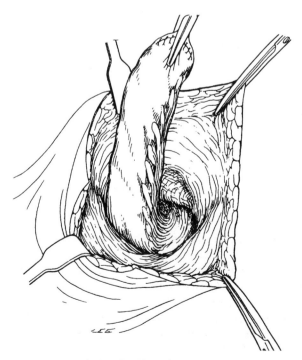

Figure 24.28 *Completing the dissection to the aponeurotic defect.*

The defect and the new stoma

At this stage a decision must be reached about the construction of the new stoma. If the hernial defect is large – it is in effect a major laparotomy wound – the abdomen can now be explored and the construction of the new stoma accomplished through it. If it is small or it does not afford access to the new stoma site, a midline laparotomy incision should have been chosen from the outset of the operation. To construct the new stoma it is necessary to be sure of the following:

* A very adequate length of intestine – ileum for ileostomy, colon for colostomy – must be mobilized so that the new stoma can easily be constructed with no degree of tension.
* There is no need to close 'lateral spaces' around a stoma in the upper abdomen. The stoma should be placed close to the middle of the rectus sheath; the 'spaces' on either side of it are then vast and are left entirely open. Postoperative strangulation of intestine in such a large defect is unlikely (Figure 24.29).

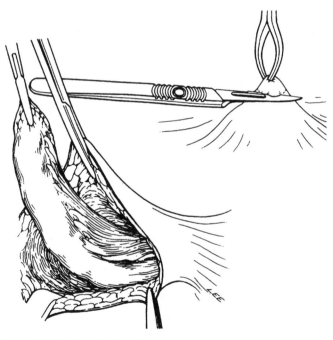

Figure 24.29 *Transferring the stoma to the new site.*

Closure of defect

The peritoneum can be closed with continuous suture but this is not mandatory. Each layer of fascia/aponeurosis is closed with interrupted or short runs of continuous absorbable suture such as Vicryl or PDS (Figure 24.30). One should also fix the intestine to the fascial edges during the placement of, at least, some of these sutures. Closure of the abdominal wall is crucial; you do not want to create a further parastomal hernia or leave a new hernia at the old stoma hernia site. It is sensible to reinforce the aponeurosis at both sites with polypropylene mesh.[972]

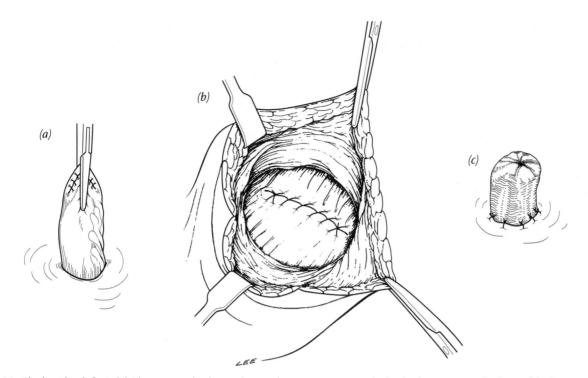

Figure 24.30 *Closing the defect. (a) The ostomy is elevated enough to create a stomal nipple that prevents leakage. (b) The stoma is matured with interrupted absorbable sutures. (c) The defect is closed.*

Closure of wound

The subcutaneous tissue is carefully closed with interrupted absorbable sutures. Suction drainage is seldom necessary but can be used; being placed down to the external oblique aponeurosis (Figure 24.31). The skin is closed with a subcuticular suture of PDS.

POSTOPERATIVE CARE

Appropriate stoma care should be instituted. Some degree of postoperative adynamic ileus may follow the surgery dependent upon the operative trauma incurred. This can be followed by hyperactivity of the stoma, which may necessitate intravenous fluid replacement for 24–72 h after operation. The resumption of meals and activity should be done in the manner exercised for operations of this magnitude.

RESULTS

Rubin *et al.* reviewed the results of the various methods of repair of the ostomy hernias.[983] There were a total of 68 hernia repairs in 55 patients. In this series, 53% underwent a fascial repair, 10% had a fascial repair with the reinforcement by a prosthetic mesh (57% intraperitoneally and 43% extraperitoneally), and 37% had relocation of the stoma. The overall rate of recurrence of the hernia was 63%. The primary repair of these hernias developed

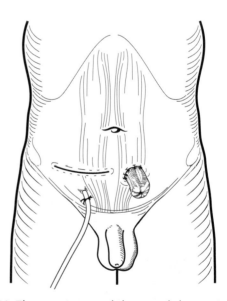

Figure 24.31 *The new stoma and the wound closure. A drain can be placed if deemed necessary.*

a recurrence in 76% of those repaired with fascia only but stoma relocation had a recurrence rate of 33%. There was a 50% recurrence rate with the use of a prosthesis. The recurrence rate for repair of recurrent parastomal hernias was 100% for fascial repair, 33% for a repair combined with a prosthetic mesh and 71% for stomal relocation. Complications were more frequent with stoma relocation (88% vs. 50%).

The use of a prosthetic in the repair of these hernias has become more popular. The reports of Sugarbaker and Rosin demonstrated the effectiveness of this repair (using an open laparotomy) as neither series noted a recurrence in their patients. The reports mentioned above using the laparoscopic method have also not been associated with a recurrence. Admittedly, the length of follow-up is short with the newer technique. More time and studies are needed to demonstrate the efficacy of the laparoscope but it would be assumed that the results should be similar to that of the open method.

CONCLUSIONS

- The best option for the patient with an ostomy is to achieve an appropriate location and prevention of the hernia at the outset. When faced with this type of hernia the most successful operation may be relocation of the stoma, but this is also the most traumatic and extensive.

- There are relatively few reports in the literature that clearly lead the surgeon to the appropriate operation when these hernias are encountered.
- The success of repair with a prosthetic biomaterial should allow us to consider this repair as the treatment of first choice even for primary hernia.
- An exception may be the young ileostomate. Stoma relocation may be advisable if a parastomal hernia develops. However, even in this situation, an initial attempt at primary prosthetic, whether open or laparoscopic, is preferred.
- If the patient is an inordinate anesthetic risk and should not undergo surgery, one can resort to a corset-type colostomy appliance.
- Further studies are needed to delineate the most appropriate method of repair for these difficult hernias as all repairs have a significant risk of recurrence.

25

Complications of hernia repair

INGUINAL HERNIA REPAIR

The complications of open elective hernia repair are remote when performed by a skilled surgical team and the risk it carries is so negligible that operation can be safely offered to nearly all patients. Improvements in treatment appear to depend on standardization of technique and the adherence to protocols. Nevertheless hernia surgery is generally taught and performed by surgeons with minimal attempts at standardization. In contrast, in the hernia clinics which standardize preoperative, operative, and postoperative management, results are consistently good. Such an environment facilitates teaching, performance, and reproducibility and can permit the performance of randomized studies.

Several large series of patients with groin hernias that have been studied using the laparoscopic technique have shown that the incidence of postoperative complications is usually low, minor and some unique to that procedure. Table 25.1 lists a few series that have itemized these complications. There are many other papers in the literature that have found that, in skilled hands, the untoward events following the laparoscopic approach are no more frequent than that of the open repairs (see Chapter 22). There are relatively few studies that evaluated the differences in the complications between the trans-abdominal preperitoneal repair (TAPP) and trans-abdominal peritoneal repair (TAP) repairs. Generally there is little difference between these two techniques; however, there appear to be fewer with the totally extraperitoneal repair (TEP) (Table 25.2). The majority of the complications that are noted with the laparoscopic method is influenced by the level of training that the surgeon has received and how far beyond the 'learning curve' that this experience extends.

OPERATION FAILURE

Recurrence

The chance of recurrence is related to the experience of the operator. This phenomenon is most clearly demonstrated by the results of the Shouldice clinic. In their early years the recurrence rate was similar to that in general hospitals, but with increasing experience and refinement of the technique they have had, for

Table 25.1 *Complications of laparoscopic inguinal herniorrhaphy*

Complication	Phillips[a]	Schmedt[b]	Feliu-Palà[c]	Van der Hem[d]
Recurrence	19 (1%)	55 (1%)	23 (2.3%)	2 (2%)
Total complications	141 (7%)	202 (3.7%)	79 (6.4%)	12 (12%)
Hematoma	45	–	34	2
Bleeding	–	34	2	–
Seroma	–	4	22	2
Neuralgia	35	–	1	1
Epididymitis/ orchitis	–	11	–	–
Urinary retention	20	26	4	–
Testicular pain	11	–	15	–
Chronic pain	6	1	–	–
Small bowel obstruction	4	7	–	–
Bladder injury	0	6	–	–
Bowel injury	0	9	–	–
Vascular injury	1	–	–	–
Nerve injury	–	25	–	–
Vas deferens injury	–	2	–	–
Trocar site infection	3	3	–	–
Transfusion	2	–	–	–
Trocar site hernia	2	47	–	–
Mesh infection	–	7	–	–
Other	10	18	1	4
Death*	2	–	–	–

* Liver failure (1), Myocardial infarction (1).
[a] Trans-abdominal preperitoneal repair (TAPP) in 1944 patients.
[b] TAPP in 5524 patients.
[c] Totally extraperitoneal repair (TEP) in 1227 patients.
[d] TEP in 104 patients.

Table 25.2 *TAPP versus TEPP*

Complication	Ramshaw[a]		Cohen[b]		Felix[c]	
	TAPP	**TEP**	**TAPP**	**TEP**	**TAPP**	**TEP**
Recurrence	5 (1.7%)	0	2 (1.8%)	0	–	–
Total	27 (11%)	3 (3.2%)	16 (20.5%)	9 (13.4%)	22 (5.6%)	7 (1%)
Seroma			4	6	4	2
Epigastric vessel injury	4	0	–	–	–	–
Enterotomy	1	0	–	–	–	–
Cystotomy	1	1	1	–	–	–
Paresthesia	6	0	–	–	–	–
Port site hernia	1	0	4	0	6	0
Urinary retention	14	2	–	–	–	–
Other	–	–	5	3	–	–

[a] Trans-abdominal preperitoneal repair (TAPP) in 290 patients and totally extraperitoneal repair (TEP) in 118 patients.
[b] TAPP in 78 patients and TEP in 67 patients.
[c] TAPP in 395 patients and TEP in 692 patients (not all complications were differentiated between these two repairs).

Table 25.3 *Etiology of hernia recurrence*

Technical failure (early)	Tissue failure (late)
Missed concomitant hernia, e.g. a femoral in an inguinal hernioplasty	Inadequate collagen replacement as the repair heals
Inadequate dissection and reduction of the peritoneal sac, e.g. leaving the stump of an indirect sac within the cord to develop, e.g. a femoral hernia years after an inguinal hernia repair	Inadequate tissue stretches to allow another adjacent defect
Inadequate restoration of the disordered anatomy, e.g. failure to reconstruct the deep ring snugly around the cord	Sepsis
Inadequate suture technique, e.g. sutures too close to the tissue margin or too far apart or pulled too tight	
Inadequate size of mesh to cover and overlap fascial margins of the posterior inguinal wall	
Wrong suture material. Aponeurosis must be closed with a non-absorbable suture	

some 30 years, consistently low recurrence rates for all types of hernia. To have general applicability a hernia operation must have a short learning curve and be capable of reproduction in the hands of general surgeons working in district hospitals. A highly technical operation, which can achieve good results only in the hands of experts, cannot be popularized for the large volume of hernia surgery that has to be carried out on a day-to-day basis.

The causes of recurrence can be broadly divided into two groups – technical failure at the time of operation or tissue failure over the years after successful surgery (Table 25.3).

Recurrence from a laparoscopic repair varies from 0% to 16% (see Chapter 15). The difficulty in the scientific evaluation with many of these series that have been reported in the past is that these have included those cases that were early in the experience of the surgeons. Better analysis of recurrence is to be found in the more recent articles listed in Tables 25.1 and 25.2. These have shown that this problem is reduced to approximately 2% or, more commonly, even less. The majority of the cases of recurrence are those that have resulted in misidentification of another hernia, the selection of too small a prosthetic mesh or inadequate fixation. Current practices will identify all areas of potential herniation, use a patch that covers the entire myopectineal orifice and assure proper fixation and/or positioning of the mesh. All of these considerations are not mutually exclusive but rather complement each other. In fact, with proper technique, fixation may be less of a factor in recurrence rates than previously thought.[585] However, more studies are needed to confirm this observation (see Figure 25.1).

Missed hernia

This is a most serious and most unforgivable technical failure. It casts serious doubts on the surgeon's competence. Furthermore, to the patient, a missed hernia which appears after the operation is an operative failure no matter what casuistry is advanced to disguise the truth. Even in the literature, casuistry is used to camouflage fact! The reporting technique for the Shouldice

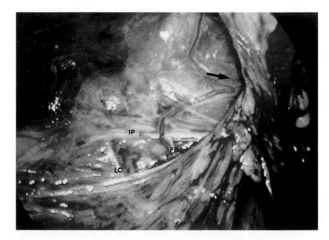

Figure 25.1 *After an accurate surgical dissection during a laparoscopic hernia repair, the femoral branch of the genitofemoral nerve and the lateral femoral cutaneous nerve have been identified as they approach and pass below the iliopubic tract: IP = iliopubic tract; LC = lateral femoral cutaneous nerve; FB = femoral branch of the genitofemoral nerve. The arrow indicates the enlarged deep inguinal ring, through which an indirect inguinal hernia found its outlet.*

clinic is the 'gold standard' again; they report any anatomic type of hernia appearing in the related part, e.g. the groin, after operation as a recurrence. Contrast this with another report which does not classify all operation failures as recurrences.[699]

The message is to thoroughly examine all the points of potential weakness at operation and repair all deficient areas. This is most important in incisional and groin hernias. In incisional hernias, small peritoneal protrusions alongside the main hernia defect, adjacent to the sites where sutures penetrated the aponeurosis at the time of laparotomy closure, are easily overlooked. These protrusions can extend and lead to recurrence subsequently. In the groin the small crescent of an indirect sac, if overlooked, can push its way down the cord and years later present as a 'recurrent indirect hernia'. This type of recurrence is easily recognized at re-operation – the sac is within the cord, it is virgin and unscarred by previous surgery – above all, no suture material is found in its wall. The femoral hernia occurring soon after an 'inguinal repair' is most often a 'missed hernia'. It is an excellent policy to open the peritoneal cavity and through the opening to palpate all the potential hernial sites bimanually from within the abdomen.

Glassow, in his review of 1500 femoral hernia repairs, notes that 359 of these cases had undergone a previous inguinal hernioplasty on the same side. While he acknowledges that some of these may be hernias missed at the earlier operation, he postulates that some could be due to an opening up of the femoral cone by the pull of the inguinal repair on the anterior margin of the femoral canal fascia transversalis. This possibility should be considered at primary surgery.[422] The inclusion of Cooper's ligament in the medial fascia transversalis repair will prevent this type of postoperative femoral hernia.

One of the very real benefits of the use of the laparoscope to repair hernias is the ability to closely inspect the inguinal floor. Occult hernias can be found in approximately 13–25% of patients that undergo this operation.[252,610] This may have been a problem in the past or in the 'learning curve' of the surgeon but currently this is a definite advantage of the laparoscopic technique.

Suture and mesh failure

For the Shouldice operation close deep bites distribute tissue tension more adequately than infrequent bites and should always be employed. In groin hernia repair the tension is greatest in the medial part of the direct area and, if the sutures show a tendency to cut out, a relaxing incision should be employed.[166] Localized defects (recurrences), particularly in the medial area of Hesselbach's triangle are most likely caused by too tight suturing under tension.

A careful examination of the small number of recurrences occurring at the Lichtenstein Clinic revealed that the majority had occurred at the pubic tubercle due to inadequate overlap by the mesh allowing a direct recurrence to creep between the edge of the mesh and the pubic tubercle.[25] Great emphasis is placed by the Lichtenstein surgeons on accurate sizing, meticulous suturing and secure placement of the mesh. Shifting, shrinkage and curling up of the edges of the mesh are critical factors for recurrence, which can be avoided by correct size, adequate overlap of the posterior wall and pubic tubercle and suture fixation.

Similarly, in the Shouldice operation recurrent direct hernias should not occur if the fascia transversalis repair and overlap are adequate, particularly as with the Lichtenstein operation at the medial pubic tubercle end. To ensure adequacy, all the posterior wall of the canal must be exposed and reviewed. With the Shouldice repair this cannot be accomplished unless the cremaster is removed to give an adequate anatomic dissection. With the tension-free hernioplasty using the Lichtenstein technique, fenestration of the cremaster to search the spermatic cord for the indirect sac is adequate and excision of the cremaster is not required. Additionally, the posterior wall must be fully assessed both visually and by digital testing, using a finger deep to the fascia transversalis or intraperitoneally to discover any small defects.

Femoral hernia may occur after inguinal repair; these hernias must be regarded (at least from the patient's perspective) as recurrences, although some perhaps are hernias overlooked at the initial intervention. The overall incidence of femoral hernia after Shouldice inguinal hernia repair is less than 0.5% in the series from the Shouldice clinic. Indifferent surgery leading to too great a tension on the anterior femoral sheath and inguinal ligament could also be responsible. Over the years the Shouldice clinic have significantly reported a decrease in this complication, pointing to the value of experience and specialization in hernia surgery.

Late repair failure

The reason why late musculo-aponeurotic failure occurs after hernioplasty (and after primary laparotomy closure) is unknown. However, all series demonstrate this phenomenon, which must be related to a continuing disease process rather than incompetent surgery. Reference has been made elsewhere to the work of Peacock and Madden and of Read and his associates demonstrating collagen malsynthesis in some patients.[892,943] Berliner has studied the structure of fascia transversalis. He has demonstrated a paucity of and fragmentation of elastic tissue fibers at the deep ring in cases of indirect inguinal herniation and around the fascial defect in direct hernia cases.[117] These changes are similar to those reported in patients with Marfan's and Ehlers–Danlos syndromes. The attrition rate and long-term failure rate in hernia repairs suggest that collagen metabolic dysfunction may be responsible. The absence of a late failure rate (up to 10 years of follow-up) in the mesh types of repair for primary inguinal hernia leads to the inescapable conclusion that replacement of the transversalis fascia by a prosthetic material overcomes any potential metabolic synthetic dysfunction.[1050]

First-time recurrent hernia can usually be readily repaired using the Lichtenstein technique, laparoscopic repair or Shouldice operation as described.

When there is much scarring and multiple hernias, particularly if femoral and inguinal hernias are simultaneously present, the extraperitoneal prosthetic technique or laparoscopic repair is advised.

WOUND COMPLICATIONS

The complications of open hernioplasty wounds are (a) bruising; (b) hematoma; (c) sepsis; and (d) sinus formation. Prompt and uncomplicated wound healing is most important in elective hernia repair. If wound healing is compromised, sepsis may involve the fascial repair with persistent sinuses or more extremely with failure of the repair.

Bruising

Bruising is very common after abdominal wall and groin hernia repair. Hemostasis must be meticulous, particularly after repair using local anesthetic infiltration if adrenaline is included in the anesthetic infiltration. Skin discoloration following inguinal hernia repair is common.[928] Pye and colleagues studied 351 patients over a 3-year period. They observed a flair consisting of a reddened area around the wound, which blanched on digital pressure and subsequently turned yellow before fading, in one-third of patients. However, only 7.4% of these patients developed wound sepsis.

Generally bruising is of no consequence. In the groin it may track down into the scrotum, becoming most pronounced some 3 or 4 days after operation. Edema of the scrotum may compound the patient's anxiety and discomfort. An expectant policy is correct: reassurance, a scrotal support and time always lead to a successful resolution and in the longer term bruising leaves no sequelae.

Hematoma

Hematoma formation in a hernioplasty wound can spell disaster for the enterprise. Hematoma is the precursor of infection and this must be avoided at all costs. Meticulous hemostasis using fine neat exact ligatures of 3-0 polyglycolic acid (Dexon) or 3-0 polyglactin (Vicryl) is employed. For minor vessels diathermy is used.

Bassini, in 1887, advised that after closing the aponeurosis of the external oblique a tube drain should be placed in the wound and brought out through the outer end of the wound. He later particularly advised a drain in cases where dissection had been difficult or when the isolation of a large sac caused much trauma and predisposed to bleeding. Modern suction drains are very efficient and in complex inguinal hernia, inguinoscrotal, recurrent repairs, or when heparin prophylaxis is mandated by intercurrent medical conditions, fine-bore suction drains confer a significant benefit. The suction drain is only required for 24 h postoperatively. In a controlled trial of fine suction drains in groin hernia repairs, the complication rate was reduced from 48.7% to 17.6% when a fine-bore drain was used.[98]

In incisional or umbilical hernias in adults, especially in the obese, multiple fine-bore suction drains are an obligatory precaution against hematoma formation, with the ever present risk of consequent infection. Hemostasis and subcutaneous fat closure are essential to successful hernioplasty. Hematoma and its bedfellow seroma can be eliminated by careful hemostasis, the elimination of 'dead space' and the judicious use of closed suction drains.

Sepsis

Skin closure should respect the integrity of the skin as an antibacterial barrier. Sutures should never penetrate the skin. Skin is closed with microporous adhesive tape or a subcuticular absorbable suture. Our preference for all hernioplasty wounds is a clear polymer subcuticular suture. This is easy to insert, does not require removal and does not cause sinuses. Colored PDS should not be used as a subcuticular suture; there have been reports of the color leaching out of the suture with tattooing of the wound.

Sepsis after simple clean hernia repair is a most important short-term complication and cause of prolonged hospital stay. More importantly, it is a determinant of recurrence. In the Shouldice experience, where the wound infection rate is 1.8%, recurrence is four times as likely in an infected as in an uninfected case.[418] Fear of infection in prosthetic and mesh materials used for the Lichtenstein technique and other mesh repairs is not justified.[408] Gilbert and Felton, in a co-operative multicenter prospective study of 2493 inguinal hernia repairs carried out by 65 surgeons using mesh repair, observed a wound infection rate of less than 1%. More than 70% of the wound infections occurred in patients over the age of 60 and prophylactic antibiotics had no effect on the infection rate. Removal of biomaterials from infected wounds was not necessary in any case and generally is not recommended, nor did recurrence occur in any infected wound.

Sinus formation

Sinus formation is rare. Using polypropylene sutures or polypropylene mesh to repair hernias simplifies the therapeutic response to sepsis. These prosthetics are biologically inert and, being monofilament, bacteria are not trapped in the interstices, if pore size is adequate (see page 76). They need never be removed on account of acute sepsis. Despite their presence in the wound, the wound will granulate and heal if it is kept cleansed. Braided polyester sutures or meshes, on the other hand, are prone to sinus formation.

LAPAROSCOPIC TECHNIQUE

The most common of the complications that occur in laparoscopic hernia repair can be attributed to:

- Inadequate knowledge of the anatomy of the preperitoneal space.
- Inappropriate use of tacks or staples to secure mesh (when used tacks and staples should only be placed into the pectineal ligament, above the iliopubic tract and the anterior abdominal areas).

- Use of the transabdominal rather than the totally extraperitoneal or vice versa when the other procedure is the more appropriate route for hernia repair.
- Use of balloon dissection to expand the preperitoneal space in patients with previous lower abdominal surgery.

This suggests that with training and a better understanding of the laparoscopic approach to hernia repair, serious complications are likely to be no more frequent than with open hernia repair.

The most common and significant complications are listed in Tables 25.1 and 25.4–25.7. These can be subdivided into those complications that are specific to laparoscopy, those related to the mesh products, those related to the methods of fixation or closure of the peritoneum and those typical of inguinal hernia repair.

Table 25.4 *Complications related to laparoscopy*

Intraperitoneal penetration of the dissection balloon
Insufflation of the intra-abdominal cavity
Inadequate dissection of the preperitoneal space
Laceration of the inferior epigastric vessels

The method of entry into the preperitoneal space is accomplished with an open technique in most centers in the extraperitoneal but not the transperitoneal method. A Veress needle is frequently used in the latter method. If the balloon is used to dissect the preperitoneal space, one can occasionally pass the device into the abdominal cavity in those patients with little thickness to the posterior rectus sheath. If this occurs it is preferable to convert to the TAPP technique as the violation of the peritoneum will make the continuous insufflation of the preperitoneal space quite difficult. If the peritoneum is inadvertently torn in the dissection of the preperitoneal space either with the balloon or one of the dissection instruments, then the carbon dioxide will have free access to the intra-abdominal cavity. While this is generally of little consequence if the tear is minute, the insufflation of the abdomen will markedly diminish the working space in the preperitoneal area. Usually, this can be overcome in experienced hands. Again, if it is a considerable problem the procedure could be converted to a TAPP repair.

Inadequate dissection of the preperitoneal space can occur with either the TEP or TAPP and whether or not a dissection balloon is used in the former. While this, in and of itself, is not a true complication it can lead to the development of one. One may not appreciate a femoral hernia should the Cooper's ligament be adequately visualized. If the dissection is not placed laterally sufficiently, then the prosthetic mesh will not lie flat in the space. This can result in a wrinkle, which will predispose the patient to the development of intra-abdominal adhesions even if the peritoneum was never violated. Additionally, a wrinkled mesh may not cover the entire myopectineal orifice such that the patient may experience a recurrence of the hernia.

Laceration of the epigastric artery or vein is an avoidable complication. Careful dissection initially so that these vessels are maintained in the normal anatomic position will avert this problem in most circumstances. If during the dissection (particularly during a TAPP repair) these are injured control will require ligation of them. This can sometimes be done with a surgical clip commonly used in laparoscopic cholecystectomy. Transfascial sutures placed with a suture-passing device will provide the surest method of ligation, however. The use of the electrocautery for control of this hemorrhage is discouraged. These patients will typically develop a significant ecchymosis over the lower abdomen and should be warned of such an occurrence. Conversion to an open laparotomy should rarely be necessary to control this type of bleeding.

The potential complications related to the mesh prosthesis are limited (Table 25.5). These are uncommon and are not generally related to technique. Migration of the mesh has been seen in the early experiences of the attempts at plugging the hernia defect. This resulted in movement of the prosthetic mesh or pieces of the meshes into the scrotum although there were anecdotal reports of migration into the peritoneal or extraperitoneal cavities. In the modern era of laparoscopy, this is not seen.

Table 25.5 *Complications related to the mesh prosthesis*

Migration of the mesh
Shrinkage of the mesh
Adhesions
Infection

Shrinkage of all of the prostheses that are used in the repair of hernias is a physiological phenomenon and, as such, is virtually unavoidable. Prosthetic biomaterials are known to experience a reduction in the size of the original implant by as much as 25–60%. This is seen in all meshes regardless of the type of product. It is actually incorrect to state that there is shrinkage as the phenomenon is a result of the normal healing process and cicatrization with scar contraction. Generally, this is not a clinically significant problem, particularly for the repair of inguinal hernias. However, it must be remembered that this event will occur with all prosthetic biomaterials despite the manner of insertion or fixation into the patient.

Adhesions are also a natural consequence of the healing process. The inflammatory response that the prosthetic devices generate will result in proliferation of the fibroblastic and/or foreign body response at the cellular level that will encourage the development of adhesions. The polypropylene biomaterials are well known for this occurrence both experimentally and clinically.[664,666] This is particularly evident in the situation that the mesh is wrinkled rather than flat. Therefore, it is important that the surgeon tries to assure that any flat prosthetic biomaterial lies as flat as possible wherever it is placed to avoid the potentiation of any adhesions. This phenomenon is seen both with the open and laparoscopic repairs of hernias.

Infection is rarely seen with the laparoscopic repair of inguinal hernias. Nevertheless, it is imperative that there is attention given to this risk. This can occasionally be treated with antibiotics alone, however, a fistula can develop at the site of the mesh which will make this treatment ineffective. In that situation, one must remove the biomaterial. An open approach is favored. The laparoscopic method would be very difficult and fraught with potential injury to the preperitoneal structures.

Table 25.6 *Complications related to the methods of fixation*

Injury to nerves
Injury to arteries or veins
Inadequate fixation of the prosthetic biomaterial
Skin puckering
Osteitis pubis

The complications listed in Table 25.6 are infrequent but are very troubling when they occur. Management of these problems can be quite difficult. The avoidance of misplacement of the fixation devices will be the best assurance against these complications. Thorough familiarity of the anatomic structures in the preperitoneal space will be the best prevention of the problems.

The most common reported injuries to nerves are the genitofemoral and lateral femoral cutaneous nerves. These sensory nerves pass underneath the iliopubic tract (Figure 25.1). Any method of fixation that is placed beneath that structure will potentially penetrate these nerves. If that occurs, the patient will have immediate pain in the ipsilateral hemiscrotum and proximal thigh or the lateral thigh respectively. If the patient complains of this in the immediate postoperative period, it is best to return to the operating room with haste. The offending tack, staple or suture can be removed laparoscopically. This will result in complete elimination of the symptoms. There is no benefit in a trial of conservative management and the institution of this therapy may result in permanent injury to these nerves.

There have been anecdotal reports of injury to the obturator and femoral nerves. These injuries are avoidable. The fixation devices should not be placed near the vicinity of these structures. These patients will experience severe pain and motor problems in these motor nerves. Immediate removal is indicated. In all of these cases, the re-exploration can be performed with the laparoscopic technique. In fact, this is preferred, as this will magnify the field, which will enhance one's ability to visualize the location of the offending fixator.

The inferior epigastric artery and vein are vulnerable to injury during the dissection of the preperitoneal space. Usually this is only a minor problem of the tributaries of these vessels. The hemorrhage that occurs with this is typically controlled without intervention. Should one of these vessels be cut during dissection or if these are punctured with the fixation device, significant bleeding will result. Control of this hemorrhage will be complicated by the fact that the blood in the field of vision may obscure the ability to control this site. Usually, however, this can be temporarily stopped with direct manual compression with a dissection instrument. This will allow time to suction the blood if necessary and bring the necessary instruments into the operative field. One may elect to place a metal clip onto the vessel for control. This is frequently easily done. However, this may require additional dissection in the hematoma that may be present. This will be difficult. A better option is usually the placement of a transfascial suture with a suture-passing device around the injured vessel. This is nearly always effective and can be done in the presence of a hematoma.

Inadequate fixation of the prosthetic biomaterial is a very uncommon occurrence. This was seen in the early days of laparoscopic inguinal hernia repair because of the attempt at plugging the defect with multiple pieces of mesh. It is important to assure that the mesh is placed flat against the myopectineal orifice so that there are no wrinkles. Any wrinkling of the mesh will predispose the patient to the risk of the development of adhesions at the site of every wrinkle. This is usually avoidable. At the present time, there is a move away from the use of any fixation of the meshes, which would make the inadequacy of fixation by the instrumentation irrelevant. Future concern may become evident if meshes placed in this manner should migrate away from the site of initial placement.

A less common problem is that of skin puckering which can occur in the thin patient. The fixation device can penetrate past the muscular layer of the anterior abdominal wall and grasp the subcutaneous tissue of the patient. This can be a subtle event at the time of surgery. One must be aware of this possibility, as this will result in a very real cosmetic deformity postoperatively. The abdominal surface should be inspected at the completion of the placement of the fixation devices to identify any evidence of skin puckering. If this is found, manually pulling on the skin adjacent to that site and elevating the skin and subcutaneous tissue away from that device can easily correct it. That is all that is required but one must remember that these patients may complain of a vague pain or 'sticking' at the site of this occurrence for several weeks after the operation. This generally resolves without intervention, however, the patient must be reassured.

Osteitis pubis can be a more gradual and persistent problem. This will result by the inflammatory reaction of the bone and periosteum of the pubis where the fixation is placed. This is an unpredictable problem and may present at various times in the postoperative period. Remedies include non-steroidal anti-inflammatory medications, direct injection with a local anesthetic or short-term steroid use. These are effective and removal of the device is rarely necessary.

Table 25.7 *Miscellaneous complications*

Perforation of the peritoneum
Inadequate closure of the peritoneum
Trocar herniation
Bladder injury
Seroma

Table 25.7 lists extremely infrequent complications. Perforation and inadequate closure of the peritoneum can result in similar complications. A perforation can be unrecognized at the time of the operative procedure. This is unusual, however, but the abdomen will usually fill with the carbon dioxide making the procedure technically more difficult. Minute perforations may be difficult to identify and impossible to close. The larger obvious tears in the peritoneum should be closed. If one experiences a very large defect, it may be preferable to convert to the TAPP so that the peritoneum may be closed with assurance this is properly done. If this is inadequate, the patient will be exposed to the risk of postoperative herniation through any opening with a resultant bowel obstruction.

Trocar herniation should now be a rare event. This is very unusual with the use of the 5 mm trocars but they are known to occur. The TEP operation minimizes this risk, as there is intact peritoneum over the site of penetration of the trocar. Trocars larger than the 5 mm should have fascial closure as the incidence of herniation is as high as 6% with these trocars.

Injury to the urinary bladder can occur in a variety of methods. The bladder can be inadvertently cut during the dissection especially if the patient has a history of prostatic hypertrophy and a thin bladder wall or diverticulum. The bladder can also be involved as part of a sliding hernia and be incorporated in the repair of the hernia with the fixation device. A very rare injury can occur with the use of the dissection balloon. In this instance, the bladder neck can become separated from the urethra. In this case, the patient may experience symptoms of retention immediately. The emergence of hematuria in the postoperative period should lead one to suspect a bladder injury. In either case, this should either be repaired or bladder drainage may suffice depending upon the injury that is found. A non-acute injury to the bladder has been reported when a polypropylene mesh migrated into the bladder after a TAPP femoral hernia repair.[498]

Seroma of the inguinal canal is not uncommon and can be confused with a recurrent hernia by both patient and doctor. Two to twenty-two percent of patients will present with this problem some 1–2 weeks after totally extraperitoneal or transperitoneal hernia repair. A well-defined mass, which lacks a cough impulse, is palpable in the inguinal region of these patients. Its presence can be confirmed with ultrasonography if the pathology is unclear. In the presence of a seroma, the best treatment is observation alone. These will generally resolve in 2–6 weeks depending on the size of the original hernia. Infrequently this can be treated by needle aspiration of the serous fluid but this will incur the risk of infecting the seromatous collection and conversion into an abscess with probable involvement of the prosthetic biomaterial. Infrequently a lipoma of the cord, either missed or newly developed will present as a mass in the groin after this operation. This too can be confused with a recurrence or a seroma. The sonographic exam will help delineate the difference. Unless symptomatic no treatment is necessary.

SCROTAL COMPLICATIONS

Ischemic orchitis and testicular atrophy

The major blood supply of the testis is the testicular artery, a branch of the abdominal aorta. The testicular artery joins the spermatic cord at the deep ring. Additional blood supply to the cord is via the cremasteric artery, a branch of the inferior epigastric. This artery is variable in its course, sometimes entering the cord structures through the deep ring but more frequently emerging through the fascia transversalis in the posterior wall of the inguinal canal to enter the inferior portion of the cremaster muscle and then ramify through the cord coverings. A third arterial supply, the artery to the vas deferens, enters the cord at the deep ring; the artery to the vas is a branch of the superior vesical artery which is, in turn, a branch of the anterior

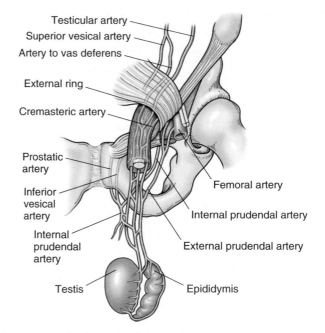

Figure 25.2 *Blood supply of the testicle. The main supply is from the inguinal canal vessels, testicular and cremasteric, but the pudendal and vesical systems contribute importantly. Every effort should be made to preserve these superficial anastomoses.*

division of the internal iliac. These three arteries form an anastomosis in the cord proximal to the testicle. At the superficial inguinal ring the cord receives additional arterial blood supply from the internal and external pudendal arteries (Figure 25.2).

During operations, all these arteries are exposed to risk. The testicular artery can be damaged in the abdomen if an extraperitoneal approach to the groin is employed, at the deep ring or in the cord during anterior mobilization. The cremasteric artery, when it pierces the posterior wall of the canal away from the deep ring, must be dissected and divided to effect an adequate repair of the fascia transversalis in the posterior wall of the inguinal canal. If the cord has to be dissected to remove a lipoma or if the vas is closely adherent to a thickened hernial sac, the artery to the vas and the testicular artery are put at risk. All these arteries communicate freely with one another. This extensive anastomosis is a boon to the inguinal surgeon, for if only one of the supplies to cord and testicle are divided the testicle will survive and function on the remaining vessels. As a general rule, if the cord is being extensively mobilized, for instance in the Shouldice operation, provided the testicle is left undisturbed in the scrotum the pudendal and scrotal anastomosis will ensure its viability. However, the combination of mobilization from the scrotum and ligation of the vessels in the canal will jeopardize testicular life. If transection of the cord is contemplated, for instance to close a multiple recurrent inguinal defect, care must be taken to preserve the distal anastomotic supply to the scrotal contents. As a general rule, the testicular blood supply will be adequate if the cord medial to the pubic tubercle is left undisturbed. *Never* deliver the testicle from the scrotum during hernioplasty in either child or adult.[160] Other identifiable risk factors include previous groin or scrotal surgery, in particular a clumsy vasectomy operation which may result in disruption of the distal collateral blood supply to the testes, dissection of distal sacs with similar effects on scrotal blood supply, and concomitant scrotal surgery.[952]

The testicular veins emerge from the back of the testis and receive tributaries from the epididymis. They then unite with one another and form a convoluted plexus, the pampiniform plexus, which forms the bulk of the cord and ascends anterior to the vas. About the superficial ring these veins coalesce to form three or four veins in the cord as it traverses the inguinal canal. These veins enter the abdomen at the deep ring, where they further coalesce to generally form two veins which ascend retroperitoneally. On the right the testicular veins drain to the inferior vena cava and on the left to the renal vein. The testicular veins are valved.

The testicular veins are vulnerable during groin surgery. In the inguinal canal they are thin walled and easily torn as structures are dissected out of the cord. The same caveats apply to the testicular venous drainage as do to the arterial supply. If the testicle is undisturbed in the scrotum, adequate venous drainage is maintained even if the testicular veins themselves are ligated proximally, as may be done in a varicocele operation.

Thrombosis of the testicular veins may complicate hernioplasty. This leads to transient scrotal and testicular edema, but provided the scrotal venous anastomoses are intact this edema generally settles spontaneously.

Lymphatics from the scrotal contents pass within the cord generally as four to eight trunks accompanying the veins into the abdomen to the lateral and preaortic nodes. Lymphatic interference at surgery can precipitate postoperative hydrocele.

A syndrome of avascular inflammation may complicate inguinal hernioplasty in infants, children and adults. In infants and children, the condition most frequently follows episodes of incarceration or strangulation of the hernia. In these patients, raised pressure in the sac leads to obstruction of the testicular vessels with venous engorgement and inflammation of the testicle. In infants and children, sac strangulation is usually at the external ring which is aponeurotic and relatively rigid. After reduction of the hernia, or herniotomy, the testicle remains firm and tender, there may be scrotal edema and slight fever. The situation resolves spontaneously, but often with some inevitable testicular atrophy, although the epididymis is spared the mass loss that occurs is in the testis. This syndrome complicates up to 10% of strangulated infantile inguinal hernias. The risk of this and the subsequent testicular atrophy is an additional reason for advising prompt operation for inguinal hernias in infants and children.[927]

Testicular atrophy as a complication of elective herniotomy in male children should occur in less than 1% of cases, although this incidence may rise if the surgeon is inexperienced or a low-volume operator.

In adults, the complication of ischemic orchitis and testicular atrophy occurring after operation can raise more sinister problems than the spontaneous, non-iatrogenic complication in the child. Men of all ages who suffer this complication are very unhappy, even though their life-threatening hernia has been cured and even though the atrophy of one testicle does not diminish testosterone levels, or reduce sexuality or fertility.[1183]

In adults, the ischemic orchitis syndrome classically commences some three or four days after surgery but may become manifest soon after hernioplasty. Then the cord becomes swollen and tender as it emerges subcutaneously from the external ring. A tender painful testicle develops, often with minimal if any scrotal edema. A low fever and occasional leukocytosis occurs. The severity of the signs vary greatly; sometimes there is gross swelling and discoloration of the scrotum. The signs are not related to the ultimate outcome.

The condition sometimes completely resolves, but in up to half the cases a progressive testicular atrophy develops. The atrophy can take up to 12 months to become fully established. This is important to remember, for when a patient with bilateral hernias develops this complication during his reproductive years the second side should not be operated until the final outcome of the ischemia is settled. The atrophic testicle is ultimately painless and non-tender. The cord becomes foreshortened as the swelling resolves and the testicle is then drawn up into a high subinguinal position. Such malposition inevitably becomes permanent.

The sequence is the development of a swollen, painful and tender cord as it emerges from the superficial inguinal ring and is palpable and very tender over the pubis. The testicle then swells in the scrotum. Fruchaud operated on such cases and described the venous infarction of the cord and testicle.[376] The cord is infarcted and then becomes foreshortened and the swollen testicle is drawn up in the scrotum. The thickening and shortening of the cord distinguishes the testicular infarction syndrome from a simple hematoma in the scrotum, i.e. that following trauma or a reactionary hemorrhage after a vasectomy. The process of testicular infarction is sterile and suppuration does not occur. Very rarely the testicle may become necrotic and necessitate orchidectomy. It is important not to introduce infection by an ill-judged operation.

Histologically, in the established case there is atrophy of the seminiferous tubules. The supporting Sertoli cells and Leydig cells which produce testosterone remain normal. Atrophy of the testicle after ischemic orchitis is not associated with an increased incidence of malignancy.

Similar atrophy, demonstrated on serial biopsy, follows elective division of the cord in the closure/repair of inguinal hernias provided the cord and testicle distal to the pubic tubercle are left undisturbed (preserving the pudendal anastomosis).[134]

In primary Shouldice repairs the incidence is small; the Shouldice clinic reports a 1% incidence in 28 760 repairs,[424] while Wantz reports a 0.36% incidence in 2240 Shouldice operations.[1184] In operations for recurrent hernias, the incidence is as high as 5%.[531] Extensive dissection of the fundus of large scrotal indirect hernias predisposes to this complication, suggesting that dissection which disturbs the pudendal/scrotal anastomosis at the external ring is important in pathogenesis.[1183] This problem is quite uncommon with the laparoscopic method but is known to occur.[1023]

The extensive dissection required to repair a recurrent hernia using an anterior approach hazards the testicular vessels with a much higher incidence of testicular ischemia – up to 5% in some series. This is a very powerful argument for employing the extraperitoneal (preperitoneal) approach, which does not entail risk to the scrotal/pudendal anastomosis when operating on recurrent groin hernias.

In all complete or scrotal indirect hernias care should be exercised in dissecting the distal sac. Indeed, it is not necessary to remove all the sac; it is adequate to identify the neck of the sac, divide it and close the proximal peritoneum leaving the distal sac unclosed in situ. No complications of the sac are consequent on this maneuver. This is the procedure of choice in the circumstances.

Ischemic orchitis is generally held to be surgeon-dependent (i.e. a failure of technique), the surgeon being blamed for damaging the cord, closing the external ring too tightly or snugging the deep ring too narrowly around the vas, the veins and the testicular artery.[367,1189] You cannot make the deep ring too tight because the superolateral boundary of the deep ring is soft and pliant; the ring is in reality a 'U' shaped sling, not a rigid band as a wedding ring. The superficial ring cannot be incriminated because in anterior hernioplasty it is not tightened; the external oblique is merely re-assembled.[1189] The rich collateral circulation of the testes indicates that too tight a closure of the internal ring is not the correct hypothesis and histological examination of the testis reveals that anemic infarction is not the pathology, i.e. necrosis does not take place. Constriction of the deep veins at the level of the deep ring does not produce testicular venous congestion unless the collateral venous circulation has been interrupted, either at the time of surgery or by previous scrotal operation. Nevertheless, reconstruction of the internal ring by adequate closure is essential to reduce the incidence of indirect recurrences. The cause of ischemic orchitis is now generally attributed to surgical trauma to the testicular veins, which may amount to little more than merely stretching during operation. The pathogenesis can be explained entirely on the basis of testicular vein thrombosis. Thus, extensive dissection of the cord is not recommended. Koontz reports: 'Atrophy of the testicle sometimes follows a simple primary operation for inguinal hernia repair in which neither the collateral nor the primary circulation has been molested as far as the surgeon is aware. The same surgeon may operate on two entirely similar hernias in exactly the same way, in different patients, and atrophy of the testicle will occur in one and not the other.'[616] The almost chance incidence and unpredictability of this condition is a further argument against simultaneous bilateral primary inguinal hernia repair in a young man and the argument for a laparoscopic repair.

Wantz hypothesizes that the most important etiologic factor is trauma to the pampiniform veins, leading to progressive thrombosis of the venous drainage and hence true infarction (L. infarcire, to stuff) of the testicle and its appendages. This thesis fits the clinical course of the syndrome, with the slow onset of pain and swelling at first in the cord and then in the testicle, followed by gradual resolution and atrophy. Non-traumatic and meticulous dissection of the inguinal canal and cord, nondisturbance of the cord or removal of extensive lipomas within the cord, avoidance of dissection of the cord or scrotal contents distal to the pubic tubercle and leaving the distal sac in indirect hernias in situ are technical details that minimize the risk of this complication. Anomalies of testicular blood supply are bound to occur and these may lead to sporadic cases following

the most perfect and experienced surgery. In repairing the deep ring during sutured repairs due care must be given to placing the peritoneal stump deep to the suture line and then carefully reconstructing the deep ring around the medial side of the cord so that the venous drainage is not impeded.

If the complication occurs an expectant policy is advised; analgesics and a scrotal support enable the condition to settle. Antibiotics have no role in this abacterial inflammation. Anticoagulants have a theoretical but untested place on the therapeutic menu. Re-exploration is very unlikely to achieve any benefit. Chronic pain is not a feature of the condition.

The effect of testicular atrophy on fertility was studied by Yavetz and colleagues.[1226] Among 8500 patients attending a fertility clinic during the period 1979–1990, 565 men (6.65%) reported an incident of inguinal hernioplasty, with or without subsequent atrophy of the testes. Additional pathology was present in 41 men and these were excluded from the study, as were 96 who had undergone bilateral hernia repair. Of the remaining 428 patients, 49 (11.4%) were found to have atrophy of one testis. Semen quality (sperm concentration, motility and morphology) of these patients was markedly reduced in comparison to that of fertile men. Thus, in cases where hernioplasty was followed by atrophy of the testes, the sperm characteristics and Sertoli cell function were damaged, although there were no changes in luteinizing hormone or testosterone levels. These results indicate the serious consequences for fertility in young men previously having hernia repair, which resulted in testicular atrophy.

Injury to the vas deferens

The vas deferens should only rarely be damaged during primary hernia repair in adults. It should never be injured in children (see pages 139–140). This is a rare event with the TAPP or TEP repair.[1023] In recurrent hernias the vas, like the vessels, may be traumatized, particularly if an anterior approach is used to repair a multiply recurrent hernia. Vas transection should immediately be repaired using a magnifying loop or microscope to achieve adequate end-to-end apposition with a row of interrupted circumferential suture of very fine Prolene. Matsuda and colleagues studied 724 patients attending a male infertility clinic.[756] Unilateral obstruction of the vas deferens occurred in 12 of 45 patients (27%) who were subfertile and gave a history of inguinal hernia repair during childhood. The diagnosis was made by palpation of the scrotal contents as a suitable noninvasive method. Moreover, half of the 12 patients had dysfunction of the contralateral testes and successful vasovasotomy was possible only in five, with pregnancy later occurring in only two cases. This series points to the disastrous long-term consequences of damage to the vas occurring after childhood hernia repair. This problem is quite uncommon with the laparoscope but is known to occur.[1023]

Hydrocele

Postoperative hydrocele complicates Shouldice repair of an inguinal hernia in approximately 1% of cases. It is rare with the laparoscopic technique. The hydrocele is lax and resolves spontaneously. Obney, from the Shouldice clinic, analyses their experience of postoperative hydrocele and observes that the greatest incidence of hydrocele at the clinic occurred in 1948, a year in which a now abandoned policy of extensive stripping of the fat out of the spermatic cord was used.[862] History repeating itself! Halsted made this observation 50 years earlier.

Provided the cord is not maltreated, hydrocele is very infrequent. Postoperative hydrocele usually requires no treatment. If it is troublesome, sterile aspiration allows it to resolve.

Hydrocele as a complication of a distal retained hernial sac, left deliberately to avoid distal dissection (see page 174), also occurs. Again, these hydroceles resolve as the cord lymphatics regain their function postoperatively. Surgical interferencewith these hydroceles can hazard the blood supply of the testicle – a hazard that leaving the distal sac in situ is intended to avoid. Slitting the anterior wall of the distally retained sac for a short distance without traumatizing any cord structures may alleviate this problem.

Genital edema

Edema of the penis and scrotum is a common sequel to groin hernia repair in men. It generally settles spontaneously within 72 h of operation. After preperitoneal mesh placement for bilateral recurrent or giant hernias, more extensive edema of the pubic area, penis and scrotum is common. Although sometimes this appears horrific to the patient, it always settles spontaneously. Reassurance and a scrotal support is all that is required.

Impotence

Men frequently complain of impotence in the immediate aftermath of a hernia repair. No organic cause for this can be identified, and firm counseling usually resolves the problem. Patients can be assured that hernia repair does not compromise sexual efficiency.

SPECIAL COMPLICATIONS

Nerve injury

The iliohypogastric (L1), ilio-inguinal (L1) and genitofemoral (L1 and L2) nerves are liable to trauma during open inguinal hernioplasty (Figure 25.3). Virtually all patients have some numbness in an area inferior and medial to the incision after operation. The ilio-inguinal and iliohypogastric nerves penetrate the internal oblique laterally and then run deep to the external oblique aponeurosis 2 or 3 cm cephalad to the superficial inguinal ring. The iliohypogastric nerve supplies the skin of the lower abdomen. The ilio-inguinal nerve penetrates the internal oblique near the anterior part of the iliac crest, then it enters the inguinal canal to run deep to the cord and emerge from the superficial inguinal ring. It provides cutaneous

sensation to the root of the penis, the side of the scrotum and a variable area of the upper medial thigh. The size of the ilio-inguinal nerve is in inverse proportion to that of the iliohypogastric nerve. The iliohypogastric and ilio-inguinal nerves are purely sensory.

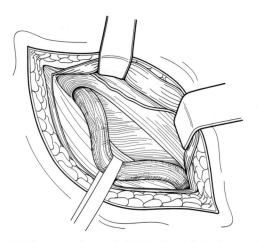

Figure 25.3 *The normal neural distribution of the inguinal canal.*

The genitofemoral nerve is a mixed nerve, the genital branch giving a motor supply to the cremaster and the femoral branch a sensory supply to the upper more medial part of the skin of the femoral triangle. The genital branch enters the inguinal canal through the deep ring. In addition to the motor supply to the cremaster, the nerve carries sensation from a variable area of the scrotum and base of the penis. The femoral branch passes behind the inguinal ligament and enters the femoral sheath lateral to the femoral artery. It then pierces the anterior femoral sheath and fascia lata to supply the skin of the upper medial thigh.[1100] There is considerable overlap between the sensory areas supplied by each of these nerves.

The ilio-inguinal nerve is most at risk when the external oblique is first opened to isolate the spermatic cord. The iliohypogastric nerve lying above the canal is vulnerable during dissection and particularly vulnerable if a relaxing incision is needed in the anterior rectus sheath.

Attitudes to these nerves during hernioplasty vary. Division of any one causes little if any permanent disturbance because of the degree of overlap of their sensory functions. The motor function of the genitofemoral nerve is effectively abolished by dissection and division of the cremaster, with loss of its suspensory function and the cremaster reflex in the inguinal canal during the Shouldice operation. Because fenestration, and not excision, of the cremaster muscle is all that is required for the mesh tension-free hernioplasty, it is to be expected that complications arising from damage or division of the genitofemoral nerve will not occur with such frequency after this operation. If damage has occurred, an area of numbness is almost always complained of; this invariably settles in months. An attempt should be made to protect the function of the ilio-inguinal and iliohypogastric nerves, but if these nerves are damaged or stretched they should be cleanly divided and ligated to prevent regenerative penetration of adjacent mesodermal scar tissue and neuroma formation. Neuroma formation can cause persistent postoperative pain and require ablation by phenol injection or operation.

When the extraperitoneal approach with extensive mesh reinforcement is being employed for recurrent herniation, it is important to identify and avoid the femoral nerve. Injury to this nerve or a suture snagging it will result in paresis of the extensors of the thigh. The femoral nerve should not be at risk during primary anterior hernioplasty when the fascia transversalis is reconstructed medial to the deep ring. However, sutures through the fascia transversalis lateral to the deep ring and emergent cord are very dangerous; they are prone to catch the nerve and should never be used. They are unnecessary anyway, the object of anterior repair being to restore the normal shutter mechanism of the deep ring medial to the cord. Sutures on the lateral side only destroy this shutter mechanism. The deep ring should always be reconstructed from the medial side under direct vision.

In the extraperitoneal repair of recurrent hernia with polypropylene mesh, there is often much scar tissue to be transversed and dissected. The femoral nerve lies on the psoas muscle lateral to the femoral sheath. It is covered by dense fascia and can scarcely be at risk of injury by dissection. However, laterally placed sutures to fix the prosthesis may catch it if care is not taken.

Chronic residual neuralgia can be the end result of nerve damage.[1189] The consequences of such damage are accompanied by a range of vegetative, and potentially medicolegal, manifestations. Two types of pain can be attributed to nerve damage:

1 Nociceptive pain due to proliferation of nerve fibers outside the neurolemma can result in a burning pain. In specialist centers with appropriate expertise this condition can be treated by genitofemoral or ilio-inguinal neurectomy.[581] Kennedy and colleagues treated 23 patients over a 9-year period, who had been symptomatic for an average of 3.3 years and had previously undergone 3.1 operations before referral. Of the patients, 15 underwent L1 to L2 paraspinus nerve block and 13 had pain relief; three patients had persistent neuralgia associated with significant orchialgia. This series supports the concept of early referral for neurectomy in selected cases.
2 Deafferentiation resulting in delayed-type hyperesthesia. Selective nerve-block is often successful in alleviating this problem.

Wantz, in giving advice as to the avoidance of chronic residual neuralgia, advises the intentional division of the sensory nerves which may be necessary in up to 25% of inguinal hernioplasties.[1189] The nerve that is most at risk during laparoscopic herniorrhaphy is that of the lateral femoral cutaneous nerve. It lies posterior to the iliopubic tract and can be skewered by the placement of a fixation device such as a tack or staple. Modern surgeons have long recognized this possibility and do not place such devices below that structure. Consequently, this is very uncommon but there are a few patients that can have an abnormal neural anatomy in which these nerves are above rather than below the iliopubic tract (see above).

Persistent postoperative pain

Persistent pain at or adjacent to the pubic tubercle and nearby bone is sometimes a complaint after successful hernioplasty. Periostitis of the pubis, adductor strain, nerve entrapment, strain of the origin of abdominal muscles, the rectus, pectineus or conjoint tendon are all mentioned. The differential diagnosis between each of these entities is almost impossible. Deep sutures through the periosteum of the pubic tubercle can lead to periostitis; it was a complication frequently reported when biological derived sutures, silk, catgut and tendon, were employed in hernioplasty. There are no reports of this periostitis with modern polymer suture materials. Periosteal suture should be avoided and is unnecessary anyway.

If pain at the pubic tubercle persists and if there is local bone tenderness, a radiograph of the bone should be advised to exclude osteitis. If no bone pathology is identified, injection with local anesthetic and corticosteroids invariably alleviates the symptoms. This, too, is very rare with the laparoscopic repair but should be treated initially with medications such as non-steroidal anti-inflammatory drugs, steroids or sometimes Gabapentin help.

Femoral vein compression

Compression of the femoral vein can occur if sutures or a prosthesis are placed too far laterally in repair of a femoral hernia or in a Cooper's ligament type repair of an inguinal hernia. Edema of the lower limb and pulmonary embolus could be in the presenting signs of femoral vein compression.[150] The diagnosis can be confirmed by phlebography or venous Duplex scanning.[851] Systemic anticoagulation and re-operation should be undertaken immediately.[358] There is a real risk of major pulmonary embolism occurring in these circumstances.

The femoral vein is also at risk of being snagged by a suture during repair of the fascia transversalis to the iliopubic tract/ anterior femoral sheath during both inguinal and femoral hernia repair. If sutures are placed too deeply or carelessly the vein will be injured and blood will well up and fill the space deep to the repair. Removal of the suture and firm pressure usually stems the venous leak.

Urinary retention

Urinary retention is reported by up to 30% of male patients in the immediate aftermath of a groin hernia repair operation. Usually, simple methods such as mobilization and the upright posture or standing by a running-water tap resolve the problem. However, if retention persists a once-only catheterization is advised before the bladder becomes too distended.

Caution is advised in older men with bladder neck obstruction. If there is a history to suggest prostatism, this should be evaluated and treated before hernioplasty. Cramer and colleagues reported on the outcome in 44 patients who had symptomatic prostatic obstruction that required either transuretheral or open prostatic resection within 12 months of hernia repair.[251] Twenty-seven of these patients had prostatectomy prior to hernia repair, 16 had hernia repair prior to prostatectomy, and one had simultaneous prostatectomy and hernia repair. No urinary tract infections occurred after hernia surgery when prostatectomy was performed first. However, in five of 16 patients urinary tract infection occurred after hernia surgery when prostatectomy was delayed. This incidence of urinary tract infection (31%) correlated with the need for, and duration of, bladder catheterization as a result of prostatic obstruction. Cramer thus recommended that, in cases of inguinal hernia and symptomatic prostatic obstruction, prostatectomy should be performed first to reduce the incidence of urinary tract infection consequent upon catheterization with no additional risk related to the hernia. This is an important recommendation because inguinal hernia is found in 25% of prostatectomy patients and 11–30% of inguinal hernia patients develop prostatic symptoms. Both inguinal hernia and prostatic enlargement are common conditions, occurring in 3% and 50% of men over the age of 65 respectively.

Early mobilization prevents urinary retention. General anesthesia, increasing age, and moderate volumes of perioperative fluid administration increase the incidence of postoperative urinary retention.[905] In a retrospective study of 295 patients, Petros and colleagues found the incidence to be 19% in patients having general anesthesia versus 8% in those undergoing spinal anesthesia, 14% in patients under the age of 53 versus 27% in those over the age of 53, and 16% in those having less than 1200 ml of perioperative fluid administration versus 25% in those receiving more than this amount. By avoiding general anesthesia altogether, Finlay and colleagues virtually eliminated urinary retention in a series of 880 patients after adopting spinal anesthesia.[357] The Shouldice clinic reports that catheterization is required less than once in 1000 postoperative patients.[530] Many have used the argument against general anesthesia because the incidence of this problem may be increased during the repair of inguinal hernias. The laparoscopic approach invariably is accomplished under a general anesthetic and the incidence of this complication is approximately 0.6% (Table 25.1). Regardless of the operative procedure that resulted in this event, the current appropriate initial treatment usually consists of several daily doses of tamsulosin, which is very effective in eliminating this problem once it occurs.

Osteitis pubis

Osteitis pubis is a rare complication of hernioplasty. The condition is well known as a complication of a urological and gynecological procedures and is a condition recognized in athletes.[559,682] The pathogenesis is unclear but is probably related to periosteal trauma which seems to be the initiating event. The inflammatory process generated then leads to pelvic pain, which can radiate from the pubic area to the adductor region and over the ischial tuberosities. This is disabling and results in a waddling gate, intermittent fever and sometimes anorexia or weight loss.

Radiological appearances include widening of the symphysis pubis, loss of definition of the adjacent cortical surfaces followed by periosteal new bone formation and finally sclerosis of bone and bony fusion of the symphysis. Rarely the condition is associated with osteomyelitis in which case the remedy is antibiotic treatment rather than anti-inflammatory medication. However, the distinction is difficult and relies on bone biopsy. Unless there are good grounds for suspecting infection the condition should be treated as inflammatory.

Osteitis pubis as a complication of open herniorrhaphy is extremely rare, with only a few cases reported in the literature.[480] Although the condition is self-limiting, conservative measures with physical rest and anti-inflammatory drugs may take several months to resolve the condition.

Laparoscopic herniorrhaphy has also been reported to result in the complication of osteitis pubis both secondary to mesh infection and as a prima facie inflammatory pathology.[725]

In the initial trials of the laparoscopic approach to inguinal hernia repair the relative frequency of this complication was unknown.[725] Subsequent studies do not report this problem (Tables 25.1 and 25.2). It is believed that this is a very rare event.

INCISIONAL AND VENTRAL HERNIA REPAIR

The repair of these hernias by the laparoscopic technique continues to increase in popularity. Because of this, it is important that the potential complications are familiar to the surgeon. Some of these are quoted in Chapter 23, Table 23.1, which lists the comparison of the complications of the open versus laparoscopic procedure. Table 25.1 lists complication and recurrence rates from other authors. There are several complications that are common to both the open and laparoscopic operations. These are also addressed above and in this section. Table 25.8 delineates the more common complications that have been reported in the literature. While there are many other articles about this operation, these represent the larger and most current evaluations of this procedure.

The incidence of complications that are noted with the laparoscopic procedure compares favorably with the open technique. In the large series noted in Table 25.8, the total complication rates (excluding recurrence) vary from 13–38%. One series has reported this rate as low as 5%.[374] A compilation of these statistics reveals an average complication rate of approximately 18%. The most common of these will be a clinically significant postoperative seroma in 2–43%. However, one study that very closely studied patients for this problem after this operation found that 100% of the patients developed a seroma that was found on sonographic testing even though not all were apparent clinically.[1109] The marked variation in the incidence of this finding is related to the variances in the definition of the seroma. Some authors define this as significant if one is found while others note its presence only if it is quite large and/or symptomatic (see below).

A postoperative ileus is another common finding that will vary in the definition if the patient develops a 'prolonged' ileus. This incidence will vary from 2–8% and is one of the more commonly reported complications. Its main significance is the differential diagnostic dilemma of a possible unrecognized intestinal injury. The incidence of this dreaded complication should ideally be zero but can be as high as 2%.[113,219,492,671,939] This entity must also be differentiated from a postoperative bowel obstruction. This is a relatively infrequent problem, however. There have been reports that have noted this to be due to postoperative adhesions.[113,671] An interesting finding that is unique to this technique is the obstruction that is caused by the migration of the small bowel between the patch and the abdominal wall. This has been reported in two series and is probably related to the inadequate penetration of the staples or tacks.[113,185] Proper technique of placement of these fixation devices as well as the use of transfascial sutures should prevent this complication. It has not been reported in any series in which transfascial sutures were also placed to fix the prosthesis to the abdominal wall.

Infection of the prosthetic product is another dreaded problem. In the experience of one of the authors (K.A.L.), the infection followed the aspiration of postoperative seromas.[282,665] Subsequent to that initial series, we do not aspirate seromas unless they have been present for many months. This, however, is exceedingly rare. Nevertheless, infection that involves the prosthesis occurs in 0–3.6% of the patients.[886] Its avoidance is preferred. The use of preoperative antibiotics such as cephalexin or a prosthetic with an impregnated antimicrobial such as DualMesh® Plus is recommended (see Chapter 7). The very low rate of trocar infections is typical of all laparoscopic procedures. Here, again, however, one must be alert to the possibility of a more ominous problem. The initial presentation of an infection that involves the prosthetic material can be the finding of a trocar site infection or localized cellulitis.

Because of the use of fixation devices and/or transfascial sutures there is a risk of injury to the inferior epigastric vessels. This is generally apparent during the operation but, if not, it can be responsible for postoperative hematomas that are seen in up to 3% of the patients.[184] Patients that have chronic renal failure are predisposed to the development of hematomas unrelated to injury to these vessels.[671]

There are a variety of uncommon complications of this operative technique. Many are related to general anesthesia and the other complications that can be seen after any intra-abdominal operation and are, therefore, not unique. However, another complication that is peculiar to any laparoscopic operation is the development of a postoperative trocar site hernia. This is infrequently reported but as noted in Table 25.8, it can occur in 0.25–0.5% of the patients. This can occur in the acute setting, in the experience of one of the authors (K.A.L.) in the one patient that we have seen such a complication. Although the exact type of hernia is not significant, a few are known to be Richter's type of hernias. The frequency of this will decline with the increased use of trocars that are smaller than 10 mm.

Recurrence

The laparoscopic repair appears to have a low rate of recurrence particularly when compared to that of the open technique. It varies from 0–11% in the literature (Table 25.8 and Chapter 22, Table 22.3). The cumulative average of the reports in

Table 25.8 *Complications of laparoscopic incisional and ventral hernia repair*

Complication	Ben-Haim[a]	Chowbey[b]	Heniford[c]	LeBlanc[d]
Total	24 (24)	77 (38)	53 (13)	47 (18)
Recurrence	2 (2)	2 (1)	14 (3.4)	13 (6.5)
Prolonged ileus	4 (4)	–	9 (2.2)	16 (8)
Seroma > 6 weeks	11 (11)	65 (32)	8 (1.97)	15 (7.5)
Suture site pain > 8 weeks	–	–	8 (1.97)	2 (1)
Significant intestinal injury	7 (7)	–	5 (1.23)	2 (1)
Bowel obstruction	3 (3)	–	–	1 (1)
Cellulitis of trocar site	–	5 (2.5)	5 (1.23)	–
Mesh infection	–	–	4 (0.98)	4 (2)
Hematoma or bleeding	1 (1)	3 (1.5)	3 (0.74)	1 (0.5)
Urinary retention	–	2 (1)	3 (0.74)	–
Fever of undetermined origin	–	–	3 (0.74)	–
Respiratory distress	–	–	2 (0.49)	–
Intra-abdominal abscess	–	–	1 (0.25)	–
Trocar site herniation	–	–	1 (0.25)	1 (0.5)
Conversion to open operation	7 (7)	–	8 (2)	2 (1)
Other	–	–	–	3 (1.5)

[a] Average follow-up of 14 months in 100 patients.
[b] Average follow-up of 34 months in 202 patients.
[c] Average follow-up of 23 months in 407 patients.
[d] Average follow-up of 36 months in 200 patients.
The numbers in parentheses are percentages. These may not total accurately because some of the patients had more than one complication.

the literature is approximately 3.3%. In our own series of 200 patients, the recurrence rate was 6.5%.[671] However, an analysis of our initial 100 patients and our second 100 patients revealed that this rate had dropped to four percent. In fact, the etiology of these two groups of patients differed. In the first group, either inadequate fixation or an inadequately large prosthetic biomaterial was felt to be responsible for all of the recurrences. One patient did require removal of the patch because it became infected after the recurrence. This has also been reported in other series.[113,185,492] In Heniford's series, 43% of the recurrences were seen in patients that did not have the use of transfascial sutures.

In our second group of patients, however, these etiologies did not play a role in the recurrence. Two of the four recurrences were due to the development of a prosthetic infection that resulted in explantation of the patch. These hernia defects were then repaired primarily with permanent sutures but later recurred. Another 'recurrence' was seen in a patient that had a repair of an upper midline incisional hernia. This patient returned with a new hernia that had developed beneath the prior repair. At re-operation, the original repair was intact. Because of this experience, it is recommended to cover as much of the original incision that has developed the hernia. This may require that the patch extend to the level of Cooper's ligament in the pelvis to protect the very low midline near the pubis. This will prevent the future development of a parapubic hernia at that site.

The fourth recurrence was seen in our second 100 cases developed at the point of a transfascial suture. A laparoscopic instrument clamped this suture during the operative procedure. It was found to have fractured at that site, which allowed the patch to separate from the abdominal wall quickly (prior to tissue penetration). It is, therefore, critical to avoid grasping any portion of any suture that will remain within the patient to minimize this risk of recurrence.

While not a true recurrence, a new entity has been described that may be more recognized in the future. Two cases of a 'tack' hernia have been found.[671] Figure 25.4 shows a hernia that has developed between two transfascial sutures. Figure 25.5 shows two small fascial defects that correspond to the site of the

adjacent tacks. It is difficult to prevent the development of these new hernias. It is hoped that a modification in the placement of these fixation devices and sutures will prevent this new hernia from occurring. One should place the transfascial sutures no more than 4–5 cm apart with at least a 1.5–2 cm bridge between the punctures used to introduce them. Additionally, the additional tacks should be staggered along the edge of the patch with no more than a one cm distance apart (Figure 25.6). These two modifications are hoped to disperse the intra-abdominal forces and hopefully prevent these hernias.

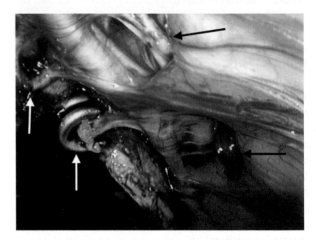

Figure 25.5 *The fascial defects (black arrows) that are caused by the extrusion of two tacks (white arrows) are shown.*

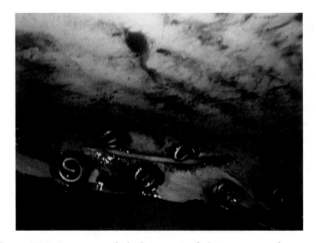

Figure 25.6 *Recommended placement of the two rows of staggered tacks with a transfascial suture.*

To the laparoscopic surgeon, the approach to any recurrent laparoscopically repaired hernia will be to attempt another laparoscopic repair. Usually only a small portion of the prior mesh will have become dislodged. One will merely re-expose the entire hernia defect as before. Another patch should be applied that has wide margins over the fascial defect (<5 cm). It is important to apply more fixation devices and sutures to this new repair because there will be no tissue penetration between any surface of the patch that contacts the original patch. This, of course, only applies to the ePTFE products. If a polypropylene mesh was used before, the placement of another PPM will

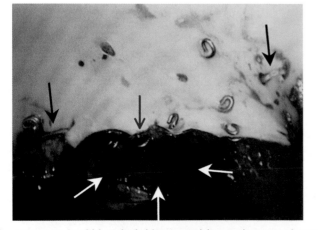

Figure 25.4 *A 'tack' hernia (white arrows) is seen between the two transfascial sutures (black arrows). The offending tack is shown by the blue arrow.*

allow in-growth across both meshes due to the macroporous nature of these products. An attempt to re-secure the loose patch or mesh will not succeed in repairing the recurrence.

Intraoperative hemorrhage

This uncommon complication is usually due to an injury to the inferior epigastric vessels. Other sources of intraoperative bleeding can originate from omental or mesenteric vessels. These latter structures can usually be controlled with electrocautery, ultrasonic shears, metal clips or sutures. There is usually no difficulty in identifying this bleeding. The epigastric blood vessels are usually injured during the placement of the fixation devices or the transfascial sutures. The exact site of penetration cannot be visualized at that time because the patch is in place against the abdominal wall. The easiest method to stop the hemorrhage from these is to place one or two transfascial 'figure-8' sutures using one of the many suture-passing instruments. Infrequently, the procedure must be converted to the open operation to stop hemorrhage.[113]

A disastrous vascular complication is that which can occur by penetration of a major vessel such as the iliac artery or vein by an operative trocar. This potential exists with all laparoscopic procedures but has not been reported with the laparoscopic incisional hernia repair. It is, nevertheless, known to occur even with the use of the 'optical' trocars.

Conversion to the open operation

In and of itself, a conversion to the open operation should not be considered a complication. It is generally the result of a complication such as a recognized bowel injury. Various reports have listed this as necessary in up to 7% of the cases.[113] Other reasons for a laparotomy are extensive adhesions or bleeding. The typical incision will be placed in the midline. One should attend to the problem that forced the conversion and then repair the hernia in an appropriate manner.

Recognized intestinal injury

This has always been a risk of intestinal injury during the adhesiolysis that is required to repair incisional hernias. With the laparoscopic repair, this is especially dangerous because 90% of these operations follow from incisional hernias.[671] The adhesions that are often encountered in this repair can obscure the view of the bowel that can be part of the adhesions and/or incarcerated in the hernia itself. The incidence of a recognized injury is generally one percent but has been reported to occur in four percent of the patients.[113,492,671,939] Avoidance of this problem is preferred. One should use enough trocars so that access and visualization is optimized at all times (see Chapter 15).

The method of repair of the intestine will be influenced by the severity of the injury. If the lumen has not been violated, one may choose either to close the serosa with sutures or with an intestinal stapling device and proceed with the planned hernia repair with placement of the prosthetic. An equally acceptable technique may be merely not repairing this injury at all. There does not appear to be any benefit or risk of any of these three choices.[671] The utmost concern should be the absolute assurance that the injury is only serosal and not intraluminal.

The full thickness injury will require repair. The method chosen will be made based upon the organ involved, the skill level of the surgeon and the location and size of the perforation. These injuries can be closed either with sutures in a one or two layer repair or with the stapling devices. One will perform this in the manner most appropriate to one's level of laparoscopic sophistication. The critical issue is the determination that the closure is secure and that there are no other injuries. The decision that must then be made is whether or not to proceed with the original hernia repair in an open or laparoscopic manner. Because of this latter concern, many surgeons prefer to convert to the open operation to fully visualize the entire intestinal tract. Generally, however, this is not necessary if there exists an isolated injury. It may be safe to repair this perforation and still repair the hernia with a prosthetic biomaterial because the bacterial flora of the gut does not contain skin contaminants. It has been suspected that these organisms are not capable of infecting the patch with such a small inoculum but this has not been substantiated in the laboratory.

It is recommended to prepare the patient for the potential of this complication. I (K.A.L.) prefer to repair the injury and not repair the hernia at that time because of medico-legal concerns and of the high rate of recurrence with the primary repair that would be required without a prosthetic biomaterial. The patient will be returned to the operating room less than a week later for this hernioplasty with a biomaterial. This might have been necessary anyway because the size of the hernia defect may preclude a primary repair. If the choice is made to convert to the open operation, a possible prosthesis that could be used may be the porcine small intestinal submucosa product, Surgisis Gold® (see Chapter 7).

Ileus

The incidence of this problem varies in the different series from 0–8%.[1134] It seems, however, that this may occur less than that of the open procedure.[886,939] The definition of this entity may be a source of this difference. Most do not list this as a complication if the patient does not require any type of intervention, such as a nasogastric tube. The frequency with which this is seen has led several authors, including us, to conclude that this should not be considered a complication. Rather, this postoperative occurrence is expected to occur in most patients due to the intra-abdominal procedure that has taken place.

Generally, the treatment of this condition is mere limitation of oral intake. Should the patient develop emesis that is uncontrolled with anti-emetics, one should insert a nasogastric tube. This usually results in the rapid resolution of the problem. The significant concern, however, is that this may represent an early sign of an unrecognized bowel injury that is becoming manifest by the appearance of an ileus. If this is a concern, an appropriate workup should be initiated (see below).

Unrecognized intestinal injury

This is the most feared complication of the laparoscopic repair of these hernias. It has been reported in 1–3% of the patients.[113,612,630,939] It may be no more common than that of the open repair, however.[886,939] There is a very high mortality rate if this occurs. Death can be unsettlingly rapid in many cases. There does not seem to be an increase in the risk of bowel injury in the presence of extensive adhesions or incarceration.[671] However, logic dictates that this possibility is probably more frequent in these situations.

The clinical signs of this complication can sometimes be lacking at the early stages of the presentation. One of the early indications will be the occurrence of an ileus. Herein lies the difficulty in diagnosis. The normal postoperative course of these patients will be the occurrence of a mild temperature elevation that is so often associated with atelectasis. If the patient experiences a significant temperature increase, such as to 101°F, that is associated with an ileus, further testing will be needed. Physical examination should provide information as to which direction to proceed with the patient. If there is no evidence of a minor infection such as bronchitis, pneumonia, or urinary tract infection, the surgeon must proceed with further work-up rapidly. The usual laboratory tests such as a complete blood count (CBC) and liver function studies will help indicate if there is underlying sepsis as the white count will usually become elevated and the early sign of sepsis that can be seen with an elevation of the total bilirubin. If the patient appears to have signs of an acute abdomen, operative intervention should be undertaken without any further diagnostic evaluation.

Radiologic examination should be performed immediately if the concern shifts to the unrecognized bowl injury. The free carbon dioxide that can be found following any laparoscopic operation should be absorbed within 3 days. One of the authors (K.A.L.) has personally seen 'free air' as late as 7 days without any bowel injury, but this is very unusual. A large amount of free air on the upright view of the abdomen should be viewed with much trepidation. If there is only a minimal amount of free air but the suspicion remains high, the next test must be CT scan of the entire abdomen and pelvis. This will more accurately depict the amount of air in the abdomen. The presence of ascites should be assumed to indicate free fluid that has come from the lumen of some portion of the intestine with subsequent peritoneal reaction.

At this point, the surgeon *must* explore the abdomen urgently, if not, emergently. The level of suspicion will determine the method of choice. At a minimum, a laparoscopic examination should be done. This can provide an accurate assessment of the abdomen. Others will start with the laparotomy. The finding of discolored or bile stained fluid will confirm an injury. One could examine the bowel and repair any enterotomy laparoscopically if the skill level will allow this technique. Most often, even in skilled hands, conversion to laparotomy will be the best

option. This will permit an extensive evaluation of all of the intra-abdominal contents. Any and all potential and real sites of injury can be identified and repaired. The choice of repair is not critical as long as the repair is sound. If there is an injury to the colon, primary repair or temporary colostomy can be decided based upon the amount of contamination and the clinical condition of the patient.

Hematoma

Most published series have shown that this is an infrequent problem. Others have noted this complication in as many as 9% of patients.[1145] However, this report only included eleven patients. It may be less common than the incidence in the open operation.[184,886] The treatment of this should be similar to that of the open procedure. The dilemma, however, is the fact that the closed procedure does not usually provide for egress of the hematoma through a skin incision. To properly drain this collection, the surgeon will violate the intact skin that covers not only the hematoma but also the prosthetic biomaterial (in most cases). This can predispose the patient to the risk of the development of an infection that will involve the prosthetic biomaterial.

If the collection is not too large and the patient is relatively asymptomatic, one can elect to simply follow this expectedly. The patient will undoubtedly develop a fair amount of ecchymosis beneath the skin in the immediate area and/or the areas dependent to that site. While this may take several weeks to completely resolve, it will usually do so without intervention.

If this becomes significantly symptomatic, one should return the patient to the operative suite and drain this under sterile conditions with the use of prophylactic antibiotics. Generally the collection of blood is not liquified enough to allow percutaneous drainage and an incision must be made over the hematoma. This should be closed at the completion of the drainage if there is any contact between the hematoma and the prosthetic material. The placement of a drain is not recommended because of the risk of introducing bacteria via the drain site subsequent to the procedure.

Seroma

The development of a seroma is very commonplace following all incisional hernia repairs (Table 25.7). The published reports vary greatly in the incidence of this complication. The larger series note an incidence from 2% to 32%.[219,492,671] It is interesting that in Chowbey's report in which he used PPM as the prosthetic mesh for the repair, the incidence of seroma was 32% but in Franklin's series, the incidence was one percent using the same biomaterial. Similarly, using ePTFE, the variation of this problem ranges from 2% to 43%.[282,492] The wide differences in these reports are more likely due to the definition of a 'clinically significant' seroma by the different authors. Susmallian and colleagues closely followed patients with ultrasonography after this operation in which ePTFE was used.

In this study, *all* of the patients were noted to develop at least a small seroma.[1109]

There should be little surprise that this entity occurs. This operation leaves intact the peritoneal surface of the hernia sac. It continues to secrete fluid that will accumulate within this dead-space. The best treatment may be an attempt to prevent the development of the fluid collection following the operation. The use of an abdominal binder will compress the sac and minimize or even eliminate the fluid accumulation. Some surgeons are reluctant to use this 'belt' for fear of compromising respiration of the patient but this is unfounded. There has not been a single report of this complication with the use of this apparatus. I (K.A.L.) have used this for over five years in these patients without a single complication related to its use. Additionally, this binder helps relieve some of the postoperative pain by stabilizing the abdominal wall.

The treatment of this problem is controversial. The majority of surgeons experienced in this procedure do not recommend treating this seroma unless forced to do so. These seromas will invariably resorb. A few have aspirated these seromas and have experienced the development of postoperative infections involving the patch.[282,939,1134,1135] It is not always clear, however, if these infections were preceded by seroma aspiration. However, in our early series, we did have infections following aspiration of seromas. Since then, we do not aspirate them for fear of introducing infection. Our experience parallels others that most will resolve without intervention within 10–12 weeks.[185,493]

If one is compelled to aspirate these seromas, such as those that are present for many months or are quite large, one should precede this with an ultrasonic or CT examination to validate that this collection is not, in fact, a recurrence of the hernia. This will prevent perforation of the bowel if the mass is not fluid. Once this is assured, then under strict aseptic technique one may aspirate the seroma fluid. Cultures of that fluid should be performed to assure that there are no bacteria within the seroma at the time of aspiration. If the culture is positive,

appropriate antibiotics should be given and the patient watched closely for worsening infection. There are some surgeons that do not hesitate to aspirate these seromas when necessary.[1109]

Infections

INFLAMMATORY RESPONSE

Approximately 15% of patients will develop a significant erythematous reaction at the site of the hernia sac approximately 5–7 days postoperatively (Figure 25.7). This is due to the inflammatory reaction that develops as a consequence of the operative dissection. This may be due to the energy sources (e.g. electrocautery or the ultrasonic scalpel) that are utilized during that phase of the operation. Usually when this problem occurs, the patient will have required a large amount of dissection due to a large hernia defect that contains bowel and/or omentum. There will undoubtedly be remnants of fatty tissue within the hernia that necrose and undergo resorption, which causes this reaction. No treatment is necessary. This is a self-limiting process that is unassociated with pain, fever or leukocytosis. It can last over 30 days, however.

TROCAR SITE INFECTIONS

This type of infection is more commonly referred to as trocar cellulitis and occurs in up to 2.5% of patients.[493] There has been no demonstrable predilection for one site or another. A localized erythematous area will be seen early at that site, which will probably be more painful than expected. This can drain pus if not treated early in its development. Drainage should be regarded with concern because this may signify that the infection involves the prosthesis rather than a simple superficial infection at the trocar site. One should be quick to obtain either an ultrasound or preferably a CT scan to evaluate the hernia sac for air or air/fluid levels indicative of an abscess.

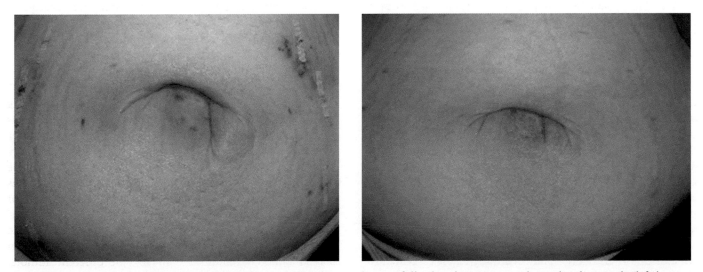

Figure 25.7 *This patient exhibits the postoperative erythema that can be seen following the LIVH procedure. The view on the left is at 7 days while the view on the right is at 30 days.*

One may need to open the skin incision if it appears that there may be a collection of fluid beneath the skin that may be involved with the infection. Needle aspiration prior to that may obviate the need to open the incision if there is no production of pus. Any fluid that is obtained should be sent to the laboratory for Gram stain and preferably culture. This usually responds simply to the use of antibiotics that are appropriate to treat the skin flora, such as a first generation cephalosporin. This should be given for 7–14 days depending upon the severity of the condition.

SUTURE SITE INFECTIONS

This is even a less frequent finding than trocar site infections. The majority of surgical literature recommends the use of non-absorbable transfascial sutures to secure fixation of the prosthesis.[492,665,671] These are placed at the periphery of the patch via incisions that are generally 2–3 mm in length. One will typically note a firm area at the site of the suture incision within 7 days, which can be followed by erythema and/or drainage. Because of this, it is difficult to diagnose at this stage, one should initiate treatment as soon as this is suspected. Here, again, an attempt at aspiration at the site may be beneficial. A first generation cephalosporin is recommended in this situation.

DEEP INFECTION INVOLVING THE BIOMATERIAL

This is, of course, the most feared complication of this procedure (other than unrecognized enterotomy). This will occur in up to 5% of the patients. Generally, however, the incidence of this complication is 1% or less.[282,492,665,671,886,975] Rather than a rapid onset of infection, these patients usually undergo a slow progression of the infection. Because of this, it is particularly difficult to make the diagnosis in some of these patients as these infections can be indolent and not become manifest for several months. Frequently, this diagnosis is suspected when the patient's pain is more at the site of the hernia defect rather than at the periphery of the patch sites of fixation. Another presentation will be the patient that has increasing levels of pain rather than declining levels of pain. Erythema may not become evident in the early development of the infection. A persistent elevation of the patient's temperature could also be an early indication of an infection. Leukocytosis will frequently be significant in these patients. Rarely, the first indication of this problem will be the development of drainage of pus at a trocar site.[671]

At any time in the postoperative period that one becomes suspicious of this infection, a white cell count and a CT scan should be obtained. The CT scan, the most sensitive test, may demonstrate fluid either above or below the biomaterial. It must be remembered that a seroma is a very frequent finding after this operation.[1109] Therefore, the mere presence of a fluid collection does not prove that an infection is present. The presence of air within the hernia sac can be seen as late as 10 days in some cases. However, one should assume that the carbon dioxide has been absorbed within 7 days. In that instance, should there still be a question regarding an infection in the hernia sac,

needle aspiration with Gram stain and culture will be helpful. If there is an air/fluid within the hernia sac, the surgeon must also rule out the existence of a missed enterotomy as the source of the infection (see above).

If the patient is not in extremis, an attempt at non-removal of the prosthesis may be made. This is usually only an option if the biomaterial used in the repair was made of polypropylene. One should initiate treatment similar to that of an infection following an open repair of the hernia. The presence of any pus indicates the need for open drainage, which is best done in the operating room. A midline incision will provide adequate exposure of the repair and access to the abdominal cavity if there is a need to explore the patient for an intra-abdominal infection. The wound should be left open and treated with frequent dressing changes. The antibiotic choice will be based upon culture results. Empiric Gram-positive, Gram-negative, and anaerobic coverage should be used until this is available.

The wound will granulate successfully (with PPM) in approximately 90% or more of these cases. The use of vacuum assisted suction apparatus upon the wound may speed up the process considerably. Once there is complete coverage of the prosthesis by granulation tissue a skin graft may be applied. In a few patients, however, contraction of the wound will allow primary closure of the skin. It is generally preferable to leave this prosthetic biomaterial in place rather than attempting to excise it. The PPM prostheses, as well as the polyester products, are all associated with an intense adhesive reaction to the intestinal organs. Therefore, an attempt at removal of these can be associated with a significant risk of injury and resultant fistulization.

The laparoscopic repair of incisional and ventral hernias most often is performed using a product that is either a solid sheet of expanded polytetrafluoroethylene (ePTFE) or a composite product that contains ePTFE. These products will be considered identical in the presence of infection because of the need to treat the ePTFE biomaterial. The ePTFE biomaterial limits the effectiveness of the antibiotic and drainage therapy that can be tried above when PPM is used. When an infection is seen following the use of ePTFE, an aggressive attempt at open drainage may occasionally be successful when combined with appropriate antibiotics. This is rarely successful, however.[665]

Occasionally only the central portion of the ePTFE prosthesis will be infected. This is usually apparent when only that portion exhibits a lack of tissue penetration. The lateral portions of the patch will be firmly adherent to the fascia. In this instance, an attempt may be made to excise the infected prosthesis and close the uninvolved portion primarily. This should only be done in the operating room and using pressure lavage during the operative procedure. The subcutaneous tissues and skin would then be loosely approximated. It is important that the biomaterial will not remain exposed after the closure of these tissues. Continued antibiotic coverage for four weeks will be necessary if it appears that this regimen is effective. If this site exhibits continued drainage of infected material and has positive cultures (or if the patient worsens clinically), one should proceed rapidly with excision of all of the prosthetic biomaterial. However, if this does not occur, the surgeon may continue to attempt treatment in this manner.

More commonly, however, the entire prosthetic is infected. The quickest remedy is to proceed with removal of the entire patch. This situation is problematic as there is generally a large fascial defect that remains following the removal of the biomaterial that served as the repair of the hernia. In the smaller hernias (e.g. those <4 cm), one may be able to affect a primary closure of the defect with a monofilament non-absorbable suture. Closure with very wide margins of an interrupted suture in a 'figure-8' pattern is preferred. These sutures will act as internal 'retention' sutures. If possible, one should then close the midline again over these sutures or incorporating these into a running closure of the fascia with another non-absorbable monofilament suture. Because of the resultant tension on this repair there will be high rate of recurrence of the hernia. Additionally, there is a risk of the development of an abdominal compartment syndrome if there is a significant pressure increase within the abdomen.

If a compartment syndrome appears to be a significant risk then the method of closure is dictated by the clinical status of the patient. If the patient is maintaining a good hemodynamic status, a sequential excision of the patch may allow for the eventual reconstitution of the midline primarily. In this case, the patient will be returned to the operating room at scheduled intervals to debride and lavage the wound. The surgeon could then excise approximately 25% of the central portion of the prosthesis and close the patch at the end of the procedure by sewing the edges together. If the patient continues to improve clinically then he or she can be returned to the operating room within 5–7 days for a repeat of the above surgical procedure. Lesser amounts of the central portion should be excised if any concern exists of the development of a compartment syndrome. After a few such interventions and removal of all of the remaining prosthesis, the midline will be closed with a non-absorbable monofilament suture as described above. The use of retention sutures may sometimes be advisable at the full closure of the abdomen. It can be anticipated that as many as 50%, if not greater, of these patients will develop a recurrence in the future.

The above option can certainly be modified depending on the condition of the patient. The advantage of the ePTFE product is that the re-operations will usually not be complicated with the intense adhesions that are seen with the macroporous meshes. At any time that the patient exhibits signs of severe sepsis because of the presence of the biomaterial, it must be removed completely at that time. The situation is now more difficult but there are still a few remaining options.

One may choose to leave the entire abdominal cavity open and institute treatment with the vacuum suction apparatus. These patients will generally have enough intestinal adhesions that the risk of evisceration is minimal. These devices are changed two to three times per week. The results with the use of such a therapeutic device can be quite dramatic. If PPM is in place, as mentioned earlier, it will granulate and the patient could be closed primarily when appropriate or a skin graft may be applied. Typically, however, ePTFE will have been used and the hope of granulation tissue is absent.

Use of one of the absorbable prosthetics to bridge the fascial defect may be successful with the smaller hernias but the larger defects will generally exert too much tension upon the product so that these biomaterials will disintegrate rather rapidly. These could be used early in the treatment phase of the ill patient with close monitoring of the fascial edges and a plan to provide other methods of closure.

A new option that seems to hold promise is the use of a collagen based product (see Chapter 7). These are natural biomaterials that can be used to bridge the fascial margins and effectively repair the original defect. This material is designed to allow the migration of the patient's fibroblasts over the collagen fibers that make up this product. The patient's own fibroblasts will then produce their own native collagen to create a 'neofascia' which will then provide a permanent closure of the defect. These products are relatively new and have not had a published report related to its use in this manner. It should be noted that these products cannot be used in the presence of an intestinal fistula as this will result in resorption of the product.

Alternatively, the surgeon could employ the services of a plastic surgeon to provide coverage of the abdominal contents will a large 'free flap' of tissue that contains skin, subcutaneous tissue and muscle. This is generally not a practical option because it is a tremendous undertaking in patients that are usually very aged and very sick.

Finally, the surgeon could simply close the skin that is available over the hernia thereby leaving the hernia intact. This is recommended if the patient is so significantly ill that a quick solution is required. However, this can be quite difficult if the skin has contracted so much that there will not be ample tissue to re-approximate it. Once the infection has been successfully treated another attempt at hernia repair could be done. If another prosthesis is used, one should wait 6–9 months before this is attempted because of the risk of re-infection. Longer-term antibiotic prophylaxis is recommended both preoperatively and postoperatively.

MORTALITY FROM ELECTIVE HERNIA REPAIR

The mortality rate for elective hernia repair must be carefully separated from the mortality rate for emergency hernia repair. Emergency hernia repair for incarceration and strangulation carries a substantial mortality, especially in the older age groups. Iles, in 1969, compared the mortality rate for elective inguinal hernioplasty in public hospitals in North America with the results from the Shouldice clinic: in public hospitals the death rate was 4.1 per 1000 compared with the Shouldice clinic rate of 0.5 per 1000.[531] Many factors may account for this great difference in the perioperative death rate between the American public hospitals and the Shouldice clinic: early ambulation and local anesthesia, different patient selection, and the fact that all the Shouldice patients are motivated to seek the best medical care for their hernioplasty. In 1974, Ponka reported a perioperative death rate of 0.5% in a series of 200 patients over 70 years old undergoing elective hernia repair.[916] Rutledge (1980) reports one operative death in 758 Cooper's ligament repairs – a 65-year-old man suffering a fatal myocardial infarction.[1000] In a 2-year period, 1986–1987, Gilbert repaired 175 hernias in patients over the age of 65 years;[404] 58% of the patients were ASA grade 3, having severe systemic disease which limited activity but was not incapacitating, and most of this comprised vascular disease. The majority of patients (124) underwent local anesthesia or epidural anesthesia (34). Strict protocols were adhered to with preoperative control of systemic medical conditions, careful choice of anesthesia, and the avoidance of perioperative complications. There were no deaths, even though 19 patients presented as an emergency with an incarcerated hernia. In a study of hospital costs and morbidity in octogenarians undergoing surgery, Gardner and Palaski confirmed that death was a result of complications of the primary disease rather than the general surgical condition such as hernia.[386]

In contrast, there is a considerable mortality related to strangulated inguinal hernias. The Confidential Enquiry into Perioperative Deaths in the UK estimate the death rate for adults with strangulated groin hernias to be 7.0%.[155] More recently, the report of the National Confidential Enquiry into Perioperative Deaths 1991–1992 studied the year 1990 for the management of strangulated hernia.[177] During that year 210 English residents died as a result of complications of inguinal hernias, and a further 120 died following complications of femoral hernia. Several recommendations were made as a result of this report:

- First, the experience of the anesthetist and surgeon attending the patient should be matched to the ASA grade of the patient, i.e. elderly frail patients should be attended by consultants.
- Second, patients must be prepared adequately for surgery by adequate and timely resuscitation.
- Third, prompt access to emergency operating theaters must be available, and high-dependency units should be available for intensive care and postoperative management of these frequently unstable patients.
- Finally, some patients may be too ill for surgery and a more humane approach to their care should be considered. This should be a consultant's decision.

Laparoscopic repair hernias have a very low mortality rate. There are only a few reports of mortality following laparoscopic incisional hernia repair due to unrecognized intestinal injury.[612] In fact, this is a very real occurrence that is not found in most reports, as those who report their findings are experienced surgeons. Despite the rarity of reported deaths with this operation, it is known to occur. Extreme vigilance for the possibility of an unrecognized injury to the intestine must be shown to avoid this outcome.

References and Further Reading

1. Abrams BL, Alisikafi FH, Waterman NG. Colostomy: a new look at morbidity and mortality. Annals of Surgery 1979; 45: 462.
2. Abramson JH, Gofin J, Hoppe C, Makler A. The epidemiology of inguinal hernia. A survey in western Jerusalem. Journal of Epidemiology and Community Health 1978; 32: 59–67.
3. Ackerman LV. Tumours of the retroperitoneum mesentery and peritoneum. In: Atlas of Tumour Pathology. Washington DC: Armed Forces Institute of Pathology, 1954: 134–135.
4. Adams HD, Smith DC. Obturator hernia. Journal of the American Medical Association 1948; 948–950.
5. Adamson RJW. A case of bilateral hernia through Petit's triangle with two associated abnormalities. British Journal of Surgery 1958; 46: 88–89.
6. Adler MW. Randomized controlled trial of early discharge for inguinal hernia and varicose veins. Annals of the Royal College of Surgeons of England 1977; 59: 251–254.
7. Adye B, Luna G. Incidence of abdominal wall hernia in aortic surgery. American Journal of Surgery 1998; 175: 400–402.
8. Agbakwuru E, Arigbabu AO, Akinola OD. Local anaesthesia in inguinal herniorrhaphy: our experience in Ile-Ife, Nigeria. Central African Journal of Medicine 1995; 41: 405–409.
9. Ahmed A, Ahmed M, Nmadu PT. Spontaneous rupture of infantile umbilical hernia: report of three cases. Annals of Tropical Paediatrics 1998; 18: 239–241.
10. Aird I. The association of inguinal hernia with traumatic perforation of the intestine. British Journal of Surgery 1935; 24: 529–533.
11. Aird I. Companion in Surgical Studies, 2nd edn. Edinburgh: Churchill Livingstone, 1957.
12. Akita K, Niga S, Yamato Y, Munata T, Sato T. Anatomic basis of chronic groin pain with special reference to sports hernia. Surgical and Radiological Anatomy 1999; 21: 1–5.
13. Akman PC. A study of 500 incisional hernias. Journal of the International College of Surgeons 1962; 37: 125–142.
14. Alexander MAJ. How to select suitable procedures for out-patient surgery: the Shouldice Hospital experience. American College of Surgeons Bulletin 1986; 71: 9–11.
15. Allegra SR, Broderick PA. Desmoid fibroblastoma. Intracytoplasmic collagen synthesis in a peculiar fibroblastic tumour: light and ultrastructural study of a case. Human Pathology 1973; 4: 419–429.
16. Allen PIM, Zager M, Goldman M. Elective repair of groin hernias in the elderly. British Journal of Surgery 1987; 74: 987.
17. Allen RP, Condon VR. Transitory extraperitoneal hernia of the bladder in infants (bladder ears). Radiology 1961; 77: 979–983.
18. Al-Salem AH. Congenital Spigelian hernia and cryptorchidism: cause or coincidence? Pediatric Surgery International 2000; 16: 433–436.
19. Alsarrage SAM, Godbole CSM. A randomized trial to compare local with general anaesthesia for inguinal hernia repair. Journal of the Kuwait Medical Association 1990; 24: 31–34.
20. Altman B. Interstitial presenting as Spigelian hernia. British Journal of Surgery 1960; 48: 60–62.
21. Amendolara M. Videolaparoscopic treatment of Spigelian hernias. Surgical Laparoscopy and Endoscopy 1998; 8: 136.
22. American Society of Anaesthesiologists. Classification of Physical Status, 1985.
23. Amid PK. Driving after repair of groin hernia. British Medical Journal 2000; 321: 1033–1034.
24. Amid PK, Shulman AG, Lichtenstein IL. Selecting synthetic mesh for the repair of groin hernia. Postgraduate Medical Journal 1992; 4: 150–155.
25. Amid PK, Shulman AG, Lichtenstein IL. Critical suturing of the tension free hernioplasty. American Journal of Surgery 1993; 165: 369–372.
26. Amid PK, Shulman AG, Lichtenstein IL. Local anaesthesia for inguinal hernia repair: step-by-step procedure. Annals of Surgery 1994; 220: 735–737.
27. Amid PK, Shulman AG, Lichtenstein IL. Simultaneous repair of bilateral inguinal hernias under local anaesthesia. Annals of Surgery 1996; 223: 249–252.
28. Anderson GR. Obturator hernia. Liverpool Medico-Chirurgical Journal 1900; 20: 271–275.
29. Ando H, Kaneko K, Ito F, Seo T, Ito T. Anatomy of the round ligament in female infants and children with an inguinal hernia. British Journal of Surgery 1997; 84: 404–405.
30. Andren-Sandberg A, Ihse I. False hernias through parametric defects. Acta Chirurgica Scandinavica 1981; 147: 381–384.
31. Andrew DR, Williamson KM. Meckel's diverticulum – rare complications and review of the literature. Journal of the Royal Army Medical Corps 1994; 140: 143–145.
32. Andrews BT, Burnand KG, Ferrar D. Putting a finger on the deep inguinal ring. Journal of the Royal College of Surgeons of Edinburgh 1996; 41: 90–92.
33. Andrews NJ. Presentation and outcome of strangulated external hernia in a district general hospital. British Journal of Surgery 1981; 68: 329–332.
34. Andrews WE, Topuzlu C, Mackay AG. Special indications for preperitoneal hernioplasty. Archives of Surgery 1968; 96: 25–26.
35. Andrews WE. Imbrication of lap joint method: a plastic operation for hernia. Chicago Medical Recorder 1895; 9: 67–77.
36. Angelini GD, Butchart EG, Armistead SH, Breckenridge IM. Comparative study of leg wound skin closure in coronary artery bypass graft operations. Thorax 1984; 39: 942–945.
37. Annandale T. Reducible oblique and direct inguinal and femoral hernia. Edinburgh Medical Journal 1876; 21: 1087–1091.
38. Anon. Advice about driving after herniorrhaphy. British Medical Journal 1980; 280: 1134–1135.
39. Anson BJ, Morgan EH, McVay CB. Surgical anatomy of the inguinal region based upon a study of 500 body halves. Surgery, Gynecology and Obstetrics 1960; III: 707–725.
40. Archampong EQ. Preoperative diagnosis of strangulated obturator hernia. Postgraduate Medical Journal 1968; 44: 140–143.

41. Archampong EQ. Strangulated obturator hernia with acute gangrenous appendicitis. British Medical Journal 1969; 1: 230.

42. Archampong EQ, Naaeder SB, Darko R. Changing pattern of intestinal obstruction in Accra, Ghana. Hepatogastroenterology 2000; 47: 185–193.

43. Armitage EN, Howat JM, Long FW. A day surgery programme for children incorporating anaesthetic outpatient clinic. Lancet 1975; ii: 21–23.

44. Armstrong DN, Kingsnorth AN. Local anaesthesia in inguinal herniorrhaphy: influence of dextran and saline solutions on duration of action of bupivacaine. Annals of the Royal College of Surgeons of England 1986; 68: 207–208.

45. Arnaud JP, Eloy R, Weill-Bousson M, Grenier JF, Adloff M. Resistance et tolerance biologique de 6 prostheses 'inertes' utilisees dans la reparation de la paroi abdominale. Journal de Chirurgie, Paris 1977; 113: 85–100.

46. Arnbjornsson E. A neuromuscular basis for the development of right inguinal hernia after appendectomy. American Journal of Surgery 1982; 143: 367–369.

47. Arnbjornsson E. Development of right inguinal hernia after appendectomy. American Journal of Surgery 1982; 143: 174–175.

48. Arregui ME. Preperitoneal repair of direct inguinal hernia with mesh. Presented at Advanced Laparoscopic Surgery: The International Experience. Indianapolis, Ind., May 20–22, 1991.

49. Arregui ME. A laparoscopic perspective of the anatomy of the peritoneum, preperitoneal fascia, transversalis fascia and structures in the space of Bogros. Postgraduate General Surgery 1995; 6: 30–36.

50. Arregui ME, Navarrette J, Davis CJ et al. Laparoscopic inguinal herniorrhaphy: techniques and controversies. Surgical Clinics of North America 1993; 73(3): 513–527.

51. Arroyo A, Garcia P, Perez F, Andreu J, Candela F, Calpena R. Randomized clinical trail comparing suture and mesh repair of umbilical hernia in adults. British Journal of Surgery 2001; 88: 1321–1323.

52. Artandi C. A revolution in sutures. Surgery, Gynecology and Obstetrics 1980; 150: 235–236.

53. Artioukh DY, Walker SJ. Spigelian herniae: presentation, diagnosis and treatment. Journal of the Royal College of Surgeons of Edinburgh 1996; 41: 241–243.

54. Ashby EC. Chronic obscure groin pain is commonly caused by enthesopathy: 'tennis elbow' of the groin. British Journal of Surgery 1994; 81: 1632–1634.

55. Ashley GT. Hernia in East Africa – an anatomical analysis of 700 cases. East African Medical Journal 1954; 31: 315–319.

56. Askar O. Surgical anatomy of the aponeurotic expansions of the anterior abdominal wall. Annals of the Royal College of Surgeons of England 1977; 59: 313–321.

57. Askar O. A new concept of the aetiology and surgical repair of para-umbilical and epigastric hernias. Annals of the Royal College of Surgeons of England 1978; 60: 42–48.

58. Askar OM. Aponeurotic hernias. Recent observations upon para-umbilical and epigastric hernias. Surgical Clinics of North America 1984; 64: 315–354.

59. Association of Anaesthetists of Great Britain and Ireland. Recommendations for Standards of Monitoring during Anaesthesia and Recovery, revised edn. London: AAGBI, 1994.

60. Astudillo R, Merrell R, Sanchez J, Olmedo S. Ventral herniorrhaphy aided by pneumoperitoneum. Archives of Surgery 1986; 121: 935–936.

61. Attah M, Jibril JA, Kalayi GD, Nmadu PT. Congenital sciatic hernia. Journal of Pediatric Surgery 1992; 27: 1603–1604.

62. Atwell JD. Inguinal hernia and the testicular feminization syndrome in infancy and childhood. British Journal of Surgery 1962; 49: 367–371.

63. Atwell JD. Inguinal hernia in female infants and children. British Journal of Surgery 1962; 50: 294–297.

64. Atwell JD, Burn JMS, Dewar AK, Freeman NV. Paediatric day case surgery. Lancet 1973; ii: 895–897.

65. Ausobsky JR, Evans M, Pollock AV. Does mass closure of midline laparotomies stand the test of time? A random controlled clinical trial. Annals of the Royal College of Surgeons of England 1985; 67: 159–161.

66. Badoe EA. Acute intestinal obstruction in Korie Bu Teaching Hospital, Accra: 1965–1969. Ghana Medical Journal 1970; 9: 283–287.

67. Badoe EA. External hernia in Accra – some epidemiological aspects. African Journal of Medical Science 1973; 4: 51–58.

68. Badruddoja M, Bush IM, Angres G, Ansari SA, Schwartz MP, Sullivan KP. The role of herniography in undiagnosed groin pain. In: Arregui ME, Nagan RF, eds. Inguinal Hernia: Advances or Controversies? Oxford: Radcliffe Medical Press, 1994: 323–331.

69. Badylak S, Kokini K, Tullius B, Whitson B. Strength over time of a resorbable bioscaffold for body wall repair in a dog model. Journal of Surgical Research 2001; 99: 282–287.

70. Bailey J. The economics of day surgery. In: Guidelines for Day Case Surgery. London: Royal College of Surgeons of England, 1992.

71. Baillie RC. Incarceration of a Meckel's inguinal hernia in an infant. British Journal of Surgery 1959; 46: 459–461.

72. Bain IM, Bishop HM. Spontaneous rupture of an infantile umbilical hernia. British Journal of Surgery 1995; 82: 35.

73. Bakwin H. Indirect inguinal hernia in twins. Journal of Pediatric Surgery 1971; 6: 165–168.

74. Balique JG, Alexandre JH, Arnaud JP et al. Intraperitoneal treatment of incisional and umbilical hernias: intermediate results of a multicenter prospective clinical trial using an innovative composite mesh. Hernia 2000; 4 (Suppl): S10–S16.

75. Ballantyne A, Jawaheer G, Munro FD. Contralateral groin exploration is not justified in infants with a unilateral inguinal hernia. British Journal of Surgery 2001; 88: 720–723.

76. Bamberger PK. Revisiting Amyand's hernia in the laparoscopic era. Surgical Endoscopy 2001; 15: 1051.

77. Barie PS, Mack CA, Thompson WA. A technique for laparoscopic repair for herniation of the anterior abdominal wall using a composite mesh prosthesis. American Journal of Surgery 1995; 170: 62–63.

78. Barile A, Erriquez D, Cacchio A, DePaulis F, Di Cesare E, Masciocchi C. Groin pain in athletes: role of magnetic resonance. Radiological Medicine 2000; 100: 216–222.

79. Barker AK, Smiddy FG. Mass reduction of inguinal hernia. British Journal of Surgery 1970; 57: 264–266.

80. Barkun JS, Wexler MJ, Hinchley EJ, Thibeault D, Meakins JL. Laparoscopic versus open inguinal herniorrhaphy: preliminary results of a randomized controlled trial. Surgery 1995; 118: 703–710.

81. Baron HC. Umbilical hernia secondary to cirrhosis of the liver. Complications of surgical correction. New England Journal of Medicine 1960; 263: 824.

82. Barron J. Pectineus fascia for femoral hernia repair. Quoted by Ponka JL, Brush BE, Problems of femoral hernia. Archives of Surgery 1971; 102: 417–423.

83. Barst HH. Pneumoperitoneum as an aid in the surgical treatment of giant hernia. British Journal of Surgery 1972; 59: 360–364.

84. Barwell NJ. Recurrence and early activity after groin hernia repair. Lancet 1981; 2: 985.

85. Barwell NJ. Personal letter, 1984.

86. Barwell NJ. Results of conventional inguinal hernia surgery in England. In: Buchler MW, Farthmann EH, eds. Progress in Surgery. Karger, Basel and London, 1996; 21: 100–104.

87. Barwell NJ, Schumpelick V, Wantz GE, eds. Inguinal Hernia Repair. Basel: Karger, 1995.

88. Baskerville PA, Jarrett PE. Day case inguinal hernia repair under local anaesthesia. Annals of the Royal College of Surgeons of England 1983; 65: 224–225.

89. Bassini E. Neue operations–Methode zur Radicalbehandlung der Schenkelhernia. Archiv für Klinische Chirurgie 1894; 47: 1–25.

90. Bassini E. Nuova technica per la cura dell'ernia inguinali. Societa Italiana di Chirurgica 1887; 4: 379–382.

91. Bassini E. Nuova technica per la cura radicale dell'ernia. Atti del Associazione Medica Italiano Congresso 1887; 2: 179–182.

92. Bassini E. Ueber die Behandlung des Leistenbruches. Archiv für Klinische Chirurgie 1890; 40: 429–476.

93. Battle WH. Abstract of a clinical lecture on femoral hernia. Lancet 1901; i: 302–305.

94. Baumer CD. Groin hernia. British Journal of Surgery 1971; 58: 667–669.

95. Bayley AC. The clinical and operative diagnosis of Maydl's hernia: a report of five cases. British Journal of Surgery 1970; 5: 687–690.

96. Bay-Nielsen M, Kehlet H. Establishment of a national Danish Hernia data base: preliminary report. Hernia 1999; 3: 81–83.

97. Bay-Nielsen M, Kehlet H, Strand L et al. Prospective nationwide quality assessment of 26,304 herniorrhaphies in Denmark. Lancet 2001; 358: 1124–1128.

98. Beacon J, Hoile RW, Ellis H. A trial of suction drainage in inguinal hernia repair. British Journal of Surgery 1980; 67: 554–555.

99. Beattie WM. Distinguishing direct and indirect inguinal hernias. British Medical Journal 1980; 1: 1321.

100. Beets GL, Dirksen CD, Go P, Geisler FEA, Baeten CGMI, Kotstra G. Open or laparoscopic preperitoneal mesh repair for recurrent inguinal hernia? Surgical Endoscopy 1999; 13: 323–327.

101. Beets GL, Van Geldere D, Baeten CGMI, Go PMNYH. Long-term results of giant prosthetic reinforcement of the visceral sac for complex recurrent inguinal hernia. British Journal of Surgery 1996; 83: 203–206.

102. Behnia R, Hashemi F, Stryker SJ, Ujicki GT, Policka SM. A comparison of general versus local anaesthesia during inguinal herniorrhaphy. Surgery, Gynecology and Obstetrics 1992; 174: 277–280.

103. Belcher DW, Nyame DK, Wurapa FJ. The prevalence of inguinal hernia in adult Ghanaian males. Tropical and Geographical Medicine 1978; 30: 39–43.

104. Belham GJ, Emery RJ, Cheslyn-Curtis S, Ralphs DNL. Early discharge despite post-operative pyrexia after inguinal herniorrhaphy in unselected patients. British Journal of Surgery 1985; 72: 973–975.

105. Bellis CJ. Immediate return to unrestricted work after inguinal herniorrhaphy. Personal experiences with 27,267 cases, local anaesthesia, and mesh. International Surgery 1992; 77: 167–169.

106. Bellón JM, García-Carranza A, Jurado F, García-Honduvilla N, Carrera-San Martin A, Buján J. Peritoneal regeneration after implant of a composite prosthesis in the abdominal wall. World Journal of Surgery 2001; 25: 147–152.

107. Bendavid R. A femoral 'umbrella' for femoral hernia repair. Surgery, Gynecology and Obstetrics 1987; 165: 153–156.

108. Bendavid R. Femoral hernias: primary versus recurrence. International Surgery 1989; 74: 99–100.

109. Bendavid R. New techniques in hernia repair. World Journal of Surgery 1989; 13: 522–531.

110. Bendavid R. The space of Bogros and the deep inguinal circulation. Surgery, Gynecology and Obstetrics 1992; 174: 355–358.

111. Bendavid R. Femoral hernias: why do they recur? Problems in General Surgery 1995; 12(2): 147–149.

112. Bender E, Sell H. Small bowel obstruction after laparoscopic cholecystectomy as a result of a Maydl's herniation of the small bowel through a trocar site. Surgery 1996; 119: 480.

113. Ben-Haim M, Kuriansky J, Tal R et al. Pitfalls and complications with laparoscopic intraperitoneal expanded polytetrafluoroethylene patch repair of postoperative ventral hernia. Surgical Endoscopy 2002; 16: 785–788.

114. Bennett C. Appendiceal pus in a hernia sac simulating strangulated inguinal hernia. British Medical Journal 1919; 2: 75.

115. Berger P. La hernie inguino-interstitielle et son traitment par la cure radicale. Revue de Chirurgie, Paris 1902; 25: 1.

116. Bergstein JM, Condon RE. Obturator hernia: current diagnosis and treatment. Surgery 1996; 119: 133–136.

117. Berliner S, Burson L, Kate P, Wise L. An anterior transversalis fascia repair for adult inguinal hernia. American Journal of Surgery 1978; 135: 633–636.

118. Berliner SD. Inguinal hernia: a handicapping condition? Journal of the American Medical Association 1983; 249: 727.

119. Berliner SD. An approach to groin hernia. Surgical Clinics of North America 1984; 64: 197–213.

120. Berliner SD. When is surgery necessary for a groin hernia? Postgraduate Medicine 1990; 87: 149–152.

121. Bhatti IH. A case of strangulated inguinal hernia in a 37 day old infant. British Journal of Surgery 1963; 5: 452–453.

122. Bickel A, Shinkarevsky E, Eitan A. Laparoscopic repair of paracolostomy hernia. J Laparoendoscopy and Advanced Surgical Technique 1999; 9(4): 353–355.

123. Billroth T. Clinical Surgery. Extracts from reports of surgical practice between the years 1860–1876. Translated from the original by C.T. Dent. London: New Sydenham Society, 1891.

124. Binns JH, Cross RM. Hernia uteri inguinalis in a male. British Journal of Surgery 1967; 54: 571–575.

125. Birnbaum W, Ferrier P. Complications of abdominal colostomy. American Journal of Surgery 1952; 83: 64–67.

126. Birth M, Friedman RL, Melullis M, Weiser HF. Laparoscopic transabdominal preperitoneal hernioplasty: results of 1000 consecutive cases. Journal of Laparoendoscopic Surgery 1996; 6: 293–300.

127. Bjork KJ, Mucha P, Cahill DR. Obturator hernia. Surgical Gynecology and Obstetrics 1988; 167(3): 217–222.

128. Black S. Sciatic hernia. In: Nyhus LM, Condon RE, eds. Hernia, 4th edn. Philadelphia: Lippincott, 1995.

129. Blanchard, St-Vil D, Carceller A, Bensoussan AL, DiLorenzo M. Repair of the huge umbilical hernia in black children. Journal of Pediatric Surgery 2000; 35: 696–698.

130. Blodgett JB, Beattie EJ. The effect of early post-operative rising on the recurrence rate of hernia. Surgery, Gynecology and Obstetrics 1947; 84: 716–718.

131. Bloodgood JC. The transplantation of the rectus muscle in certain cases of inguinal hernia in which the conjoined tendon is obliterated. Bulletin of the Johns Hopkins Hospital 1898; 9: 96–100.

132. Blumberg NA. Infantile umbilical hernia. Surgery, Gynecology and Obstetrics 1980; 150: 187–192.

133. Bogojavalensky S. Laparoscopic treatment of inguinal and femoral hernia (videopresentation). 18th Annual Meeting of the American Association of Gynecological Laparoscopists, Washington DC, 1989.

134. Bohde YG. Condition of the testicle after division of cord in treatment of hernia. British Medical Journal 1959; 1: 1507–1510.

135. Boley SJ, Kleinhams S. A place for the Cheatle/Henry approach in pediatric surgery? Journal of Pediatric Surgery 1966; 1: 394–397.

136. Bourke JB. Strangulated femoral hernia in a female child of three years and nine months. British Journal of Surgery 1968; 55: 880–881.

137. Bourke JB, Lear PA, Taylor M. Effect of early return to work after elective repair of inguinal hernia: clinical and financial consequences at one and three years. Lancet 1981; 2: 623–625.

138. Bower H. A safety net cast over new surgery. Hospital Doctor 1996; 16 May.

139. Bowley DMG, Butler M, Shaw S, Kingsnorth AN. Dispositional pessimism predicts delayed return to normal activities after inguinal hernia surgery. Surgery 2003; 133: 141–146.

140. Bowley DMG, Kingsnorth AN. Umbilical hernia, Mayo or mesh? Hernia 2000; 4: 195–196.

141. Brandt WE. Unusual complications of hernia repairs: large symptomatic granulomas. American Journal of Surgery 1956; 92: 640–643.

142. Brenner A. Zur radical operation der Leisten-hernien. Zentralblatt fur Chirurgie 1898; 25: 1017–1023.

143. Brenner J. Mesh materials in hernia repair. In: Schumpelick V, Wantz GE, eds. Inguinal Hernia Repair. Basel: Karger, 1995.

144. Brereton RJ. Hernia repair in children. Lancet 1980; i: 156.

145. Bridger P, Rees M. What a difference a day makes. Health Service Journal 1995; 20 April: 22–23.

146. Bringman S, Ek Å, Haglind E, Heikkinen T-J, Kald A, Kylberg F, Ramel S, Wallon C, Anderberg B. Is a dissection balloon beneficial in bilateral, totally extraperitoneal, endoscopic hernioplasty? A randomized, prospective, multicenter study. Surgical Laparoscopy, Endoscopy and Percutaneous Techniques 2001; 11(5): 322–326.

147. Bristol JB, Bolton RA. The results of Ramstedt's operation in a district general hospital. British Journal of Surgery 1981; 68: 590–592.

148. Britton BJ, Morris PJ. Local anaesthetic hernia repair. An analysis of recurrence. Surgical Clinics of North America 1984; 64: 245–256.

149. Bronsther B, Abrams MW, Elboim C. Inguinal hernias in childhood – a study of 1,000 cases and a review of the literature. Journal of the American Medical Women's Association 1972; 27: 522–535.

150. Brown RE, Kinateder RJ, Rosenburg N. Ipsilateral thrombophlebitis and pulmonary embolism after Cooper's ligament herniorrhaphy. Surgery 1980; 87: 230–232.

151. Browse NL. Distinguishing direct and indirect inguinal hernias. British Medical Journal 1980; 1: 1270.

152. Browse NL, Hurst P. Repair of long, large midline incisional hernias using reflected flaps of anterior rectus sheath reinforced with Marlex mesh. American Journal of Surgery 1979; 138: 738–739.

153. Bryant AL. Spigelian hernias. American Journal of Surgery 1947; 73: 396–397.

154. Bryant TL, Umstot RK Jr. Laparoscopic repair of an incarcerated obturator hernia. Surgical Endoscopy 1996; 10: 437–438.

155. Buck N, Devlin HB, Lunn JN. The Report of a Confidential Enquiry into Perioperative Deaths. London: Nuffield Provincial Hospital Trust and the King Edward's Hospital Fund for London, 1987.

156. Bucknall TE, Cox PJ, Ellis H. Burst abdomen and incisional hernia: a prospective study of 1129 major laparotomies. British Medical Journal 1982; 284: 931–933.

157. Bucknall TE, Ellis H. Abdominal wound closure. A comparison of monofilament nylon and polyglycolic acid. Surgery 1981; 89: 672–677.

158. Bull WT. Notes on cases of hernia which have relapsed after various operations for radical cure. New York Medical Journal 1891; 53: 615–617.

159. Burd RSA, Heffington SH, Teague JL. The optimal approach for management of metachronous hernias in children: decision analysis. Journal of Pediatric Surgery 2001; 36: 1190–1195.

160. Burdick CG, Gillespie DHM, Higinbotham NL. Fascial suture operations for hernia. Annals of Surgery 1937; 106: 333–345.

161. Burgess P, Matthew VV, Devlin HB. A review of terminal colostomy complications following abdominoperineal resection for carcinoma. British Journal of Surgery 1984; 71: 1004.

162. Burn JMB. Responsible use of resources: day surgery. British Medical Journal 1983; 286: 492–493.

163. Burney RE, Jones KR, Coon JW, Blewitt DK, Herm A, Peterson M. Core outcomes measures for inguinal hernia repair. J Am Coll Surg 1997; 185: 509–515.

164. Burns FJ. Complications of colostomy. Diseases of the Colon and Rectum 1970; 13: 448–450.

165. Byers JM, Steinberg JB, Postier RG. Repair of parastomal hernias using polypropylene mesh. Archives of Surgery 1992; 127: 1246–1247.

166. Calcagno D, Wantz GE. Suture tension and the Shouldice repair. Lancet 1985; ii: 1446.

167. Caldironi MW, Romano M, Bozza F, Pluchinotta AM, Pelizzo MR, Toniato A, Ranzato R. Progressive pneumoperitoneum in the management of giant incisional hernias: a study of 41 patients. British Journal of Surgery 1990; 77: 306–308.

168. Callesen T, Bech K, Kehlet H and the Hvidovre Hernia Group. The feasibility, safety and cost of infiltration anaesthesia for hernia repair. Anaesthesia 1998; 53: 31–35.

169. Callesen T, Bech K, Kehlet H. One thousand consecutive inguinal hernia repairs under unmonitored local anesthesia. Anesthesia and Analgesia 2001; 1373–1376.

170. Callesen T, Kehlet H. Post-herniorrhaphy pain. Anesthesiology 1997; 87: 1219–1230.

171. Callesen T, Klarskov B, Bech K, Kehlet H. Short convalescence after inguinal herniorrhaphy with standardized recommendations: duration and reasons for delayed return to work. European Journal of Surgery 1999; 165: 236–241.

172. Callisen H. Herniorum rariorum bigna acta societas medicae hafniae. Haanniae 1777; 2: 321.

173. Calne RY. Repair of bilateral hernia: a technique using Merselene mesh behind the rectus abdominis. British Journal of Surgery 1967; 54: 917–920.

174. Cameron AEP. Accuracy of clinical diagnosis of direct and indirect inguinal hernia. British Journal of Surgery 1994; 81: 250.

175. Campbell HE. The incidence of malignant growth in the undescended testicle: a reply and re-evaluation. Journal of Urology 1959; 81: 663–668.

176. Campbell RC, Dudley HAF. Hospital stay of patients undergoing minor surgical procedures. Lancet 1964; 2: 403–405.

177. Campling EA, Devlin HB, Hoyle RW, Lunn JN. The Report of a National Confidential Enquiry into Perioperative Deaths 1991/1992. London, 1993.

178. Campos L, Sipes E. Laparoscopic hernia repair: use of a fenestrated PTFE graft with endo-clips. Surgical Laparoscopy and Endoscopy 1993; 3(1): 35–38.

179. Campos SM, Walden T. Images in clinical medicine: Spigelian hernia. New England Journal of Medicine 1997; 336: 1149.

180. Cannon DJ, Casteel L, Read RC. Abdominal aortic aneurysm, Leriche's syndrome, inguinal herniation and smoking. Archives of Surgery 1984; 119: 387–389.

181. Cannon DJ, Read RC. Metastatic emphysema. A mechanism for acquiring inguinal herniation. Annals of Surgery 1981; 194: 270–276.

182. Cannon SR, Ralphs DNL, Bolton JP, Wood JJ, Allan A. Early discharge following hernia repair in unselected patients. British Journal of Surgery 1982; 69: 112–113.

183. Caplan G, Board N, Paten A, Tazclaar-Molinia J, Crowe P, Yap SJ, Brown A. Decreasing length of stay: the cost to the community. Australia and New Zealand Journal of Surgery 1998; 68: 433–437.

184. Carbajo MA, Martin del Olmo JC, Blanco JI et al. Laparoscopic treatment vs open surgery in the solution of major incisional and abdominal wall hernias with mesh. Surgical Endoscopy 1999; 13: 250–252.

185. Carbajo MA, Martin del Olmo JC, Blanco JI et al. Laparoscopic treatment of ventral abdominal wall hernias: preliminary results in 100 patients. Journal of the Society of Laparoscopic Surgeons 2000; 4: 141–145.

186. Carbonell JF, Sanchez JLA, Peris RT, Ivorra JC, Delbano MJP, Sanchez C, Araez JIG, Greus PC. Risk factors associated with inguinal hernias: a case control study. European Journal of Surgery 1993; 159: 481–486.

187. Carey LC. Acute appendicitis occurring in hernias: a report of 10 cases. Surgery 1967; 61: 236–238.

188. Carnett JB. Inguinal hernia of the caecum. Annals of Surgery 1909; 49: 491–515.

189. Carrieri P, Nardi S, Basuku GC, Vitali A, Nistri R. The involvement of the urinary tract in inguinal hernias. Annals Italia Chirugia 1998; 69: 795–797.

190. Carriquiry LA, Pineyro A. Pre-operative diagnosis of non strangulated obturator hernia, the contribution of herniography. British Journal of Surgery 1988; 75: 785.

191. Carter JE, Mizes C. Laparoscopic diagnosis and repair of Spigelian hernia: report of case and technique. American Journal of Obstetrics and Gynecology 1992; 167. 77–78.

192. Carter JE. Surgical treatment of chronic pelvic pain. Journal of the Society of Laparoendoscopic Surgeons 1998; 2(2): 129–139.

193. Castelein RM, Saunter AJM. Lumbar hernia in an iliac bone graft defect. Acta Orthopaedica Scandinavica 1985; 56: 273–274.

194. Castleden WM. Meckel's diverticulum in an umbilical hernia. British Journal of Surgery 1970; 57: 932–934.

195. Catterina A. L'operatione di Bassini der la cura radicale dell'ernia inguinale. Bolognia, Italia: L. Capelli, 1932.

196. Catterina A. Bassini's Operation. London: Lewis, 1934.

197. Celsus AC. Of Medicine. Translated by James Grieve, London 1756.

198. Cevese P, D'Amico D, Biasiato R et al. Peristomal hernia following end colostomy: a conservative approach. Italian Journal of Surgical Science 1984; 14: 207–209.

199. Chamary VL. Femoral hernia: intestinal obstruction is an unrecognized source of morbidity and mortality. British Journal of Surgery 1993; 80: 230–232.

200. Champault GG, Rizk N, Catheline JM, Turner R, Boutelier P. Inguinal hernia repair – totally preperitoneal laparoscopic approach versus Stoppa operation: randomized trial of 100 cases. Surgical Laparoscopy and Endoscopy 1997; 7(6): 445–450.

201. Chan CK. Femoral hernia repairs: the Shouldice experience in the 1990s. Presented at the meeting 'Hernia in the 21st Century', sponsored by the American and European Hernia Societies, June 2000, Toronto, Canada.

202. Chan MK, Baillod RA, Tanner RA et al. Abdominal hernias in patients receiving continuous ambulatory peritoneal dialysis. British Medical Journal 1981; 283: 826.

203. Chang FC, Farha GJ. Inguinal herniorrhaphy under local anaesthesia. Archives of Surgery 1977; 112: 1069–1071.

204. Charlton JE. Monitoring and supplemental oxygen during endoscopy. British Medical Journal 1995; 310: 886–887.

205. Chatterjee SK. Spontaneous rupture of umbilical hernia with evisceration of small intestine. Journal of the Indian Medical Association 1972; 59: 287.

206. Cheatle GL. An operation for radical cure of inguinal and femoral hernia. British Medical Journal 1920; 2: 68–69.

207. Cheatle GL. An operation for inguinal hernia. British Medical Journal 1921; 2: 1025–1026.

208. Cheek CM, Black NA, Devlin HB, Kingsnorth AN, Taylor RS, Watkins DFL. Groin hernia surgery: a systematic review. Annals of the Royal College of Surgeons of England 1998; 80 (Suppl 1): S1–S80.

209. Cheek CM, Williams MH, Farndon JR. Trusses in the management of hernia today. British Journal of Surgery 1995; 82: 1611–1613.

210. Chen KC, Chu CC, Chou TY, Wu CJ. Ultrasonography for inguinal hernias in boys. Journal of Pediatric Surgery 1999; 34: 1890–1891.

211. Cheselden W. The Anatomy of the Human Body, 12th edn. London: Livingston, Dodsley, Cadell, Baldwin and Lowndes, 1784.

212. Chevrel JP, ed. Chirurgie des Parois de l'Abdomen. Berlin: Springer-Verlag, 1985.

213. Chevrel JP, Flament JB, eds. Les éventrations de la paroi abdominale. In: Association Française de Chirurgie. 92nd French Congress on Surgery. Paris, France: Masson, 1990.

214. Chevrel JP, Rath AM. The use of fibrin glues in the surgical treatment of incisional hernias. Hernia 1997; 1: 9–14.

215. Chevrel JP. Traitement des grandes éventrations médianes par plastie en paletot et prothèse. Nouvelle Presse Medicale 1979; 8: 695–696.

216. Chilvers C, Pike MC, Foreman D, Fogelman K, Wadsworth MEJ. Apparent doubling of frequency of undescended testis in England and Wales 1962–1981. Lancet 1984; ii: 330–332.

217. Chin T, Liu C, Wei C. The morphology of the contralateral internal inguinal ring is age-dependent in children with unilateral inguinal hernia. Journal of Pediatric Surgery 1995; 30: 1663–1665.

218. Chou TY, Chu CC, Diau GY, Wu CJ, Gueng MK. Inguinal hernia in children: US versus exploratory surgery and intraoperative contralateral laparoscopy. Radiology 1996; 201: 385–388.

219. Chowbey PK, Sharma A, Khullar R, Baijal, Vashistha A. Laparoscopic ventral hernia repair. Journal of Laparoendoscopy and Advanced Surgical Technique 2000; 10(2): 79–84.

220. Chung-Kuao Chou, Liu GC, Chen LT, Jaw TS. The use of MRI in bowel obstruction. Abdominal Imaging 1993; 18: 131–135.

221. Ciampolini J, Shandall AA, Boyce DE. Adult hernia surgery in Wales revisited: impact of the guidelines of the Royal College of Surgeons of England. Annals of the Royal College of Surgeons of England 1998; 80: 335–338.

222. Cilley RE, Krummel TM. Disorders of the umbilicus. In: O'Neill JA, Rowe MI, Grosfeld JL, eds. Pediatric Surgery, 5th edn. St Louis: Mosby, 1998: 1037–1041.

223. Clain A. Traumatic hernia. British Journal of Surgery 1964; 51: 549–550.

224. Cleland J, Mackay JY, Young RB. The relations of the aponeurosis of the transversalis and internal oblique muscles to the deep epigastric artery and the inguinal canal. Memoirs and Memoranda in Anatomy 1889; 1: 142.

225. Cloquet J. Recherches anatomiques sur les hernies de l'abdomen. These, Paris, 1817, 133: 129.

226. Cloud DT, Reed WA, Ford JL, Linkner LN, Trump DS, Dorman GW. The 'Surgicenter': a fresh concept in outpatient pediatric surgery. Journal of Paediatric Surgery 1972; 7: 206.

227. Coe RC. Changing methods best way to cut costs. American Medical News 1981; 24: 5.

228. Coetzee T, Phillips WR. Torsion of a myomatous uterus incarcerated in an umbilical hernia. British Journal of Surgery 1960; 48: 342–344.

229. Cohen RV, Alvarez G, Roll S, Garcia ME et al. Transabdominal or extraperitoneal laparoscopic hernia repair? Surgical Laparoscopy and Endoscopy 1998; 8: 264–268.

230. Cole GJ. Strangulated hernia in Ibadan. Transactions of the Royal Society of Tropical Medicine and Hygiene 1964; 58: 441–447.

231. Cole P. The filigree operation for inguinal hernia. British Journal of Surgery 1942; 29: 168–181.

232. Coley WB. The operative treatment of hernia with a report of 200 cases. Annals of Surgery 1895; 21: 309–437.

233. Colles AA. Treatise on Surgical Anatomy. Dublin: Gilbert and Hodges, 1811.

234. Colville JAC, Power RE, Hickey DP, Lane BE, O'Malley KJ. Intermittent anuria secondary to a stone in a ureterofemoral hernia. Journal of Urology 2000; 164: 440–441.

235. Condon RE, Nyhus LM. Complications of groin hernia and of hernia repair. Surgical Clinics of North America 1971; 51: 1325–1336.

236. Condon RE. In: Nyhus LM, Condon RE, eds. Hernia, 4th edn. Philadelphia: Lippincott, 1989.

237. Condon RE. Reassessment of groin anatomy during the evolution of preperitoneal hernia repair. American Journal of Surgery 1996; 172: 5–8.

238. Cooper A. The Anatomy and Surgical Treatment of Inguinal and Congenital Hernia I. London: T. Cox, 1804.

239. Cooper A. The Anatomy and Surgical Treatment of Hernia II. London: Longman, Hurst, Rees and Orme, 1807.

240. Cooper A. Lectures on the Principles and Practice of Surgery III. London: Simpkin and Marshall, 1827.

241. Cooper JL, Nicholls AJ, Simms IM. Genital oedema in patients treated by continuous ambulatory peritoneal dialysis: an unusual presentation of inguinal hernia. British Medical Journal 1983; 286: 1923–1924.

242. Cope Z. The Early Diagnosis of the Acute Abdomen, 4th edn. London: Oxford University Press, 1972.

243. Copeman WSC, Ackerman WL. Fibrositis of the back. Quarterly Journal of Medicine 1944; 13: 37–40.

244. Corbitt J. Laparoscopic herniorrhaphy: A preperitoneal tension-free approach. Surgical Endoscopy 1993; 7: 550–55.

245. Corbitt JD. Laparoscopic herniorraphy. Surgical Laparoscopy and Endoscopy 1991; 1: 23–25.

246. Corcione F, Cristinzio G, Maresca M, Cascone U, Titolo G, Califano G. Primary inguinal hernia: the held-in mesh repair. Hernia 1997; 1: 37–40.

247. Costanza MJ, Heniford BT, Area MJ, Mayes JT, Gagner M. Laparoscopic repair of recurrent ventral hernias. American Surgeon 1998; 64: 1121–1127.

248. Coulter A, McPherson K. Socioeconomic variations in the use of common surgical operations. British Medical Journal 1985; 291: 183–187.

249. Cox KR. Bilateral pre-vascular femoral hernia. Australian and New Zealand Journal of Surgery 1962; 31: 318–321.

250. Craig RDP. Strangulated obturator hernia. British Journal of Surgery 1962; 49: 426–428.

251. Cramer SO, Malangoni MA, Schulte WJ, Condon RE. Inguinal hernia repair before and after prostatic resection. Surgery 1983; 94: 627–630.

252. Crawford DL, Hiatt JB, Phillips EH. Laparoscopy identifies unexpected groin hernias. American Surgeon 1998; 64(10): 976–978.

253. Criado FJ. A simplified method of umbilical herniorrhaphy. Surgery, Gynecology and Obstetrics 1981; 153: 904–905.

254. Cronin K, Ellis H. Pus collections in hernial sacs. British Journal of Surgery 1959; 46: 364–367.

255. Crump ED. Umbilical hernia. 1. Occurrence of the infantile type in Negro infants and children. Journal of Pediatrics 1952; 40: 214–223.

256. Cubillo E. Obturator hernia diagnosed by computed tomography. American Journal of Roentgenology 1983; 140: 735–736.

257. Cumberland O. Ueber die Verschliessung von Bauchwunden und Brustpforten durch versenkte Silberdrahtnetze. Zentralblatt fur Chirurgie 1900; 27: 257.

258. Cuschieri A. Minimal Access Surgery: Implications for the NHS. Edinburgh: HMSO, 1994.

259. Cushing H. The employment of local anaesthetics in the radical cure of certain cases of hernia with a note on the nervous anatomy of the inguinal region. Annals of Surgery 1900; 31: 1.

260. Cuthbertson AM, Collins JP. Strangulated paraileostomy hernia. Australian and New Zealand Journal of Surgery 1977; 47: 86–87.

261. Czeizel A, Gardonyi J. A family study of congenital inguinal hernia. American Journal of Medical Genetics 1979; 4: 247–254.

262. Czerny V. Studien zur Radikalbehandlung der Hernien. Wiener Medizinische Wochenschrift 1877; 27: 497–500.

263. Daniell SJ. Strangulated small bowel hernia within a prolapsed colostomy stoma. Journal of the Royal Society of Medicine 1981; 74: 687–688.

264. Daum R, Meinel A. Die operative Behandlung der kindlichen Leistenhernie: Analyse von 3 Fällen. Chirurgica 1972; 43: 49–54.

265. Davey WW. Companion to Surgery in the Tropics. Edinburgh and London: Livingstone, 1968.

266. Davey WW, Strange SL. The stomach as a content of inguinal and femoral hernias. British Journal of Surgery 1954; 41: 651–658.

267. Davidson BR, Bailey JS. Incisional herniae following median sternotomy incisions – their incidence and aetiology. British Journal of Surgery 1986; 73: 995–997.

268. Davies JOF, Barr A. Survey of hospital treatment of uncomplicated herniorrhaphy. British Journal of Surgery 1965; 52: 569–573.

269. Davies M, Najmaldin A, Burge DM. Irreducible inguinal hernia in children below two years of age. British Journal of Surgery 1990; 77: 1291–1292.

270. Davies N, Thomas MG, McIlroy B, Kingsnorth AN. Early results with the Lichtenstein tension-free hernia repair. British Journal of Surgery 1994; 81: 1478–1479.

271. Davis PR. The causation of herniae by weight lifting. Lancet 1969; ii: 155–157.

272. De Boar A. Inguinal hernia in infants and children. Surgery 1957; 75: 920–927.

273. DeBord JR, Bauer JJ, Grischkan DM, LeBlanc KA, Smoot Jr. RT, Voeller GR. Laboratory and clinical findings after implantation of standard and antimicrobial agent impregnated. Expanded polytetrafluoroethylene patches for hernia repair. Hernia 1999; 4(3): 189–193.

274. De Chauliac G. La Grande Chirurgie composée en 1363. Revue avec des notes, une introduction sur le moyenage. Sur la vie et les oeuvres de Guy de Chauliac par E. Nicaise. Paris: Felix Alcan, 1890.

275. DeCou JM, Gauderer MW. Inguinal hernia in infants with very low birth weight. Seminars in Pediatric Surgery 2000; 9: 84–87.

276. De Garengeot RJC. Traite des Operations de Chirurgie, 2nd edn. Paris: Huart, 1731: 369–371.

277. De Gimbernat A. Nuevo metodo de operar en la hernia crural. Madrid: Ibarra, 1793.

278. De Giuli M, Festa V, Denoye GC, Morino M. Large post-operative umbilical hernia following laparoscopic cholecystectomy: a case report. Surgical Endoscopy 1994; 8: 904–905.

279. De Grood PMRM, Harbers JBM, Van Egmond J, Crul JF. Anaesthesia for laparoscopy – a comparison of five techniques including propofol, etomidate, thiopentone and isoflurane. Anaesthesia 1987; 42: 815–823.

280. De Ruiter P, Bijnen AB. Successful local repair of paracolostomy hernia with a newly developed prosthetic device. International Journal of Colorectal Disease 1992; 7: 132–134.

281. Deitch EA, Engel JM. Spigelian hernia. Archives of Surgery 1980; 115: 93.

282. DeMaria EJ, Moss JM, Sugerman HJ. Laparoscopic intraperitoneal polytetrafluoroethylene (PTFE) prosthetic patch repair of ventral hernia. Surgical Endoscopy 2000; 14: 326–329.

283. Department of Health and Social Security. Hospital Plan. London: HMSO, 1964.

284. Department of Health. Press release 94/251, 1994.

285. Department of Health. Press release 95/82, 1995.

286. Deshpande PV. Testicular gangrene in infancy due to incarcerated inguinal hernia. British Journal of Surgery 1964; 51: 237–238.

287. Detmar DE, Buchannan-Davidson DJ. Ambulatory surgery. Surgical Clinics of North America 1982; 62: 685–704.

288. DeTurris SV, Cacchione RN, Mungara A, Pecoraro A, Ferzli GS. Laparoscopic herniorrhaphy: beyond the learning curve. Journal of the American College of Surgeons 2002; 194(1S): 65–73.

289. Deva AK, Quinn MJ, Nettle WJS. The difficult problem of a groin lump in a morbidly obese patient. Australian and New Zealand Journal of Surgery 1993; 63: 664–665.

290. Devlin HB. Time for the economist and the surgeon to rub shoulders. Health and Social Services Journal 1980; Jan. 11.

291. Devlin HB. Hernia. In: Russell RCG, ed. Recent Advances in Surgery II. Edinburgh: Churchill Livingstone, 1982.

292. Devlin HB. Stoma Care Today. Medicine (Oxford), 1985.

293. Devlin HB. The economics of day case surgery. In: Guidelines for Day Case Surgery. London: Royal College of Surgeons of England, 1985.

294. Devlin HB. Management of Abdominal Hernias. London: Butterworth, 1988.

295. Devlin HB. History of Surgical Procedures. Sonderdruck aus Hygeine in Chirurgischen Alltag. Berlin: De Gruyter, 1993.

296. Devlin HB, Gillen PHA, Waxman BP, Macnay RA. Short stay surgery for inguinal hernia: experience of the Shouldice operation 1970–1982. British Journal of Surgery 1986; 73: 123–124.

297. Devlin HB, Nicholson S. Hernias of the abdominal wall and pelvis: incisional hernias and parastomal herniation. In: Keen G, Farndon J, eds. Operative Surgery and Management, 3rd edn. Oxford: Butterworth Heinemann, 1994.

298. Devlin HB, Russell IT, Muller D, Sahay AK, Tiwari PN. Short stay surgery for inguinal hernia. Lancet 1977; i: 847–849.

299. Deysine M. Hernia repair with expanded polytetrafluoroethylene. American Journal of Surgery 1992; 163: 422–424.

300. Deysine M. Umbilical hernias. In: Bendavid R, Abrahamson J, Arregui M, Flament JB, Phillips E, eds. Abdominal Wall Hernias: Principals and Management. New York: Springer–Verlag, 2001.

301. Deysine M, Grimson RC, Soroff HS. Inguinal herniorrhaphy: reduced morbidity by service standardization. Archives of Surgery 1991; 126: 628–630.

302. Deysine M, Soroff HS. Must we specialize herniorrhaphy for better results? American Journal of Surgery 1990; 160: 239–241.

303. Dierking GW, Dahl JB, Kanstrup J, Dahl A, Kehlet H. Effect of pre- vs postoperative inguinal field block on postoperative pain

after hernoirrhaphy. British Journal of Anaesthesia 1992; 68: 344–348.

304. Dieudonné G. Plug repair of groin hernias: a 10-year experience. Hernia 2002; 5: 189–191.

305. Dillon E, Renwick M. The antenatal diagnosis and management of abdominal wall defects: the Northern Regional experience. Clinical Radiology 1995; 50: 855–859.

306. Dion YM, Morin J. Laparoscopic inguinal herniorraphy. Canadian Journal of Surgery 1992; 35: 209–212.

307. Dixon E, Heine JA. Incarcerated Meckel's diverticulum in a Spigelian hernia. American Journal of Surgery 2000; 180: 126.

308. Doeven JJ. Results of treatment of incisional hernias with extractable prostheses. Archivum Chirurgicum Neerlandicum 1975; 27: 245–255.

309. Doherty VC, O'Donovan TR, Hill GJ. Current Status of Ambulatory Surgery in the United States in Out-Patient Surgery, 3rd edn. Philadelphia: Hill George J Saunders, 1988.

310. Doig CM. Appendicitis in umbilical hernial sac. British Medical Journal 1970; 2: 113–114.

311. Doolin W. Inflamed appendix in a hernial sac. British Medical Journal 1919; 2: 239.

312. Doran FSA, Lonsdale WN. A simple experimental method of evaluation for the Bassini and allied types of herniorrhaphy. British Journal of Surgery 1949; 36: 339–345.

313. Doran FSA, White M, Drury M. The scope and safety of short stay surgery in the treatment of groin herniae and varicose veins. British Journal of Surgery 1972; 59: 333–339.

314. Douglas DM. The healing of aponeurotic incisions. British Journal of Surgery 1952; 40: 79–82.

315. Douglas DM, Forrester JC, Ogilvie RR. Physical characteristics of collagen in the later stages of wound healing. British Journal of Surgery 1969; 56: 219–222.

316. Downs SH, Black NA, Devlin HB, Royston CMS, Russell RCG. Systematic review of the effectiveness and safety of laparoscopic cholecystectomy. Annals of the Royal College of Surgeons of England 1996; 78: part II.

317. Ducharmé JC, Bertrand R, Chacar R. Is it possible to diagnose inguinal hernia by X-ray? Journal of the Canadian Association of Radiologists 1967; 18: 448.

318. Dulucq JL. Treatment of inguinal hernia by insertion of a subperitoneal patch under pre-peritoneoscopy. Chirurgie 1992; 118(1–2): 83–85.

319. Dulucq JL. Treatment of inguinal hernias by insertion of mesh through retroperitoneoscopy. Postgraduate Surgery 1992; 4(2): 173–174.

320. Dutta CR, Katzarski M. The anatomical basis for the inguinal hernia in Ghana. Ghana Medical Journal 1969; 8: 185–186.

321. Duvie SO. Femoral hernia in Ilesa, Nigeria. West African Journal of Medicine 1988; 8: 246–250.

322. Eames NWA, Deans GT, Lawson JT, Irwin ST. Herniography for occult hernia and groin pain. British Journal of Surgery 1994; 81: 1529–1530.

323. Eaton AC. A controlled trial to evaluate and compare sutureless skin closure technique (op-site skin closure) with conventional skin suturing and clipping in surgery. British Journal of Surgery 1980; 67: 857–860.

324. Edelman DS, Misiakos EP, Moses K. Extraperitoneal laparoscopic hernia repair with local anaesthesia. Surgical Endoscopy 2001; 15: 976–980.

325. Editorial. Development of practice guidelines. Lancet 2000; 355: 82–83.

326. Edwards H. Discussion on hernia. Proceedings of the Royal Society of Medicine 1943; 36: 186–189.

327. Edwards H. Inguinal hernia. British Journal of Surgery 1943; 31: 172–185.

328. Ekberg O, Lasson A, Kesek P, Van Westen D. Ipsilateral multiple groin hernias. Surgery 1995; 115: 557–562.

329. Ekwueme O. Strangulated external hernia associated with generalised peritonitis. British Journal of Surgery 1973; 60: 929–933.

330. Elechi EN. External abdominal wall hernias: experiences with elective and emergency repairs in Nigeria. British Journal of Surgery 1987; 74: 834–835.

331. Ellis H. Famous Operations. Pennsylvania: Harwell Publishing Media, 1984.

332. Ellis H, Gajraj H, George CD. Incisional hernias, when do they occur? British Journal of Surgery 1983; 70: 290–321.

333. Engeset J, Youngson GG. Ambulatory peritoneal dialysis and hernial complications. Surgical Clinics of North America 1984; 64: 385–392.

334. Erichsen CJ, Vibits H, Dahl JB, Kehlet H. Wound infiltration with ropivacaine and bupivacaine for pain after inguinal herniotomy. Acta Anesthesiologia Scandinavica 1995; 39: 67–70.

335. Esposito C, Montupet P. Laparoscopic treatment of recurrent inguinal hernia in children. Pediatric Surgery International 1998; 14: 182–184.

336. Esposito TJ, Fedorak I. Traumatic lumbar hernia. Case report and review of the literature. Journal of Trauma 1994; 37: 123–126.

337. Estrada A, Yun Choel-Heui, Van Kessel A, Li B, Hauta S, Laarveld B. Immunomodulatory activities of oat β-glucan in vitro and in vivo. Microbiology and Immunology 1997; 41(12): 991–998.

338. EU Hernia Trialists Collaboration. Laparoscopic compared with open methods of groin hernia repair: systematic review of randomized controlled trials. British Journal of Surgery 2000; 87: 860–867.

339. Evans AG. The comparative incidence of umbilical hernias in colored and white infants. Journal of the National Medical Association 1941; 33: 158.

340. Evans RG, Robinson GC. Surgical day care: measurements of the economic pay off. Canadian Medical Association Journal 1980; 123: 873–881.

341. Faille RJ. Low back pain and lumbar fat herniation. The American Surgeon 1978; 44: 359–361.

342. Fakim A, Walker MA, Byrne DJ, Forrester JC. Recurrent strangulated obturator hernia. Annales Chirurgiae et Gynaecologiae 1991; 80: 317–320.

343. Fallis LS. Direct inguinal herniation. Annals of Surgery 1938; 107: 572.

344. Farquharson EL. Early ambulation with special reference to herniorrhaphy as an out patient procedure. Lancet 1955; ii: 517–519.

345. Farrakha M. Laparoscopic treatment of ventral hernia. Surgical Endoscopy 2000; 14: 1156–1158.

346. Fawcett AN, Rooney PS. Inguinal canal lipoma. British Journal of Surgery 1997; 84: 1169–1170.

347. Fear RE. Laparoscopic: a valuable aid in gynecologic diagnosis. Obstetrics and Gynecology 1968; 31: 297–304.

348. Feliu-Palà X, Martin-Gomez M, Morales-Conde S, Fernández-Sallent. The impact of the surgeon's experience on the results of laparoscopic hernia repair. Surgical Endoscopy 2001; 15: 1467–1470.

349. Felix EL. A unified approach to recurrent laparoscopic hernia repairs. Surgical Endoscopy 2001; 15: 969–971.

350. Felix E, Scotts S, Crafton B et al. Causes of recurrence after laparoscopic hernioplasty. Surgical Endoscopy 1998; 12: 226–231.

351. Felix EL, Michas C. Laparoscopic repair of Spigelian hernias. Surgical Laparoscopy and Endoscopy 1994; 4: 308–310.

352. Ferguson AH. Oblique inguinal hernia. Typic operation for its radical cure. Journal of the American Medical Association 1899; 33: 6–14.

353. Ferzli GS, Massad A, Albed P. Extraperitoneal endoscopic inguinal hernia repair. Journal of Laparoendoscopic Surgery 1992; 2: 281–285.

354. Ficarra BJ. Hernia: masquerader of surgical disorders. Surgical Clinics of North America 1971; 51: 1401–1414.

355. Fingerhut A, Hay JM. Seventh annual meeting of the French Association for Surgical Research (ARC), and first French–German joint meeting with the permanent working party on clinical studies (CAS) of the German Surgical Society, 27th March, 1993 in Paris, France: Shouldice or not Shouldice? Late results in a controlled trial in 1,593 patients. Theoretical Surgery 1993; 8: 163–167.

356. Fingerhut A, Millat B, Bataille N, Yachouchi E, Dziri C, Boudet M-J, Paul A. Laparoscopic hernia repair in 2000. Update of the European Association for Endoscopic Surgery (EAES) consensus conference in Madrid, June 1994. Surgical Endoscopy 2001; 15: 1061–1065.

357. Finley RK, Miller SF, Jones LM. Elimination of urinary retention following inguinal herniorrhaphy. American Surgeon 1991; 57: 486–489.

358. Fitzgerald P, Mehigan IE. A complication resulting from the use of a rigid inlay in repair of an inguinal hernia. British Journal of Surgery 1959; 46: 422.

359. Fitzgibbons RJ, Camps J, Cornet DA et al. Laparoscopic inguinal herniorrhaphy. Results of a multicenter trial. Annals of Surgery 1995; 221: 3–13.

360. Fitzgibbons RP. Laparoscopic inguinal hernia repair. In: Zucker KA, ed. Surgical Laparoscopy Update. St Louis: Quality Medical Publishing, 1993: 373–934.

361. Flament JB, Avisse C, Palot JP, Delattre JF. Biomaterials. Principles of implantation. In: Schumpelick V, Kingsnorth A, eds. Berlin: Springer-Verlag, 1999.

362. Flanagan LJR, Bascom JV. Herniorrhaphies performed upon out-patients under local anaesthesia. Surgery, Gynecology and Obstetrics 1981; 153: 557–560.

363. Flanagan LJR, Bascom JV. Repair of groin hernia: out-patient approach with local anaesthesia. Surgical Clinics of North America 1984; 64: 257–268.

364. Flich J, Alfonso JL, Delgrado F, Prado MJ, Cortina P. Inguinal hernias and certain risk factors. European Journal of Epidemiology 1992; 8: 277–282.

365. Fölscher DJ, Jamali FR, Leroy J, Marescaux J. Utility of a new sort, non-woven polypropylene mesh for the transabdominal extraperitoneal laparoscopic hernia repair: preliminary results. Hernia 2000; 4: 228–233.

366. Fon LJ, Spence RAJ. Sportsman's hernia. British Journal of Surgery 2000; 87: 545–552.

367. Fong Y, Wantz GE. Prevention of ischaemic orchitis during inguinal hernioplasty. Surgery, Gynecology and Obstetrics 1992; 174: 399–402.

368. Fonkalsrud EW, De Lorimier AA, Clatworthy HW. Femoral and direct inguinal hernias in infants and children. Journal of the American Medical Association 1965; 192: 597.

369. Ford JL, Reed WA. The Surgicentre: An innovation in the delivery and cost of medical care. Arizona Medicine 1969; 26: 801–804.

370. Forrest I. Current concepts in soft connective tissue wound healing. British Journal of Surgery 1983; 70: 133–140.

371. Forrest J. Repair of massive inguinal hernia with pneumoperitoneum and without mesh replacement. Archives of Surgery 1979; 114: 1087–1088.

372. Franco P. Traite des hernies contenant une ample declaration de toutes leurs especes et autres excellentes parites de la chirurgie, assauoir de la pierre, des cataractes des yeux, et autres maladies, desquelles comme la cure est perilluese, aussi est elle de' peu d'hommes bien exercee. Lyon: Thibauld Payan, 1561.

373. Frankau C. Strangulated hernia: a review of 1487 cases. British Journal of Surgery 1931; 19: 176–191.

374. Franklin ME, Dorman JP, Glass JL, Balli JE, Gonzales JJ. Laparoscopic ventral and incisional hernia repair. Surgical Laparoscopy and Endoscopy 1998; 8(4): 294–299.

375. Friedman DW, Boyd CD, Norton P, Greco RS, Boyarsky AH, Mackenzie JW, Deak SB. Increases in Type III collagen gene expression and protein expression in patients with inguinal hernias. Annals of Surgery 1993; 218: 754–760.

376. Fruchaud H. Anatomie Chirurgicale des Hernies de l'Aine. Paris: G. Doin, 1956.

377. Fruchaud H. Le Traitement Chirurgicale des Hernies de l'Aine chez l'Adulte. Paris: G. Doin, 1956.

378. Fry ENS. Hypoglycaemia in children undergoing operations. British Medical Journal 1976; 2: 639.

379. Fung A. Inguinal herniotomy in young infants. British Journal of Surgery 1992; 79: 1071.

380. Gallegos NC, Dawson J, Jarvis M, Hobsley M. Risk of strangulation in groin hernias. British Journal of Surgery 1991; 78: 1171–1173.

381. Gallie WE, Le Mesurier AB. Living sutures in the treatment of hernia. Canadian Medical Association Journal 1923; 13: 468–480.

382. Gallie WE, Le Mesurier AB. The transplantation of the fibrous tissues in the repair of anatomical defects. British Journal of Surgery 1924; 12: 289–320.

383. Ganesaratnam M. Maydl's hernia: report of a series of seven cases and review of the literature. British Journal of Surgery 1985; 72: 737–738.

384. Gans SL. Sliding inguinal hernia in female infants. Archives of Surgery 1959; 79: 109.

385. Garcia AA, Perales NJ, Schiefenbusch ME, Marquez JL, Polo HE, Cacha LG. Inguinal bladder hernias: a report of two cases. Actas Urologia Espana 1999; 23: 625–628.

386. Gardner B, Palasti S. A comparison of hospital costs and morbidity between octogenarians and other patients undergoing general surgical operations. Surgery, Gynecology and Obstetrics 1990; 171: 299–304.

387. Gardner B, Palasti S. A comparison of hospital costs and morbidity between octogenarians and other patients undergoing general surgical operations. Surgery, Gynecology and Obstetrics 1993; 177: 126–130.

388. Garland EA. Femoral appendicitis. Journal of the Indiana State Medical Association 1955; 48: 1292–1296.

389. Garnjobst W, Sullivan ES. Repair of paraileostomy hernia with polypropylene mesh reinforcement. Diseases of the Colon and Rectum 1984; 27: 268–269.

390. Gaster, J. Hernia: One day repair. Darien, Connecticut: Hafner, 1970.

391. Gaunt ME, Tan SG, Dias J. Strangulated obturator hernia masquerading as pain from a total hip replacement. Journal of Bone and Joint Surgery 1992; 74b: 782–783.

392. Gaur DD. Venous distension in strangulated femoral hernia. Lancet 1967; i: 816.

393. Gazayerli MM. Anatomic laparoscopic repair of direct or indirect hernias using the transversalis fascia and iliopubic tract. Surgical Laparoscopy and Endoscopy 1992; 2: 49–52.

394. Gazayerli MM, Arregui ME, Helmy HS. Alternative technique: laparoscopic iliopubic tract (IPTR) inguinal hernia repair with inlay buttress of polypropylene mesh. In: Ballantyne GH, Leahy PF, Modlin IR, eds. Laparoscopic Surgery. Philadelphia: WB Saunders, 1993.

395. Gedebou TM, Neubauer W. Laparoscopic repair of bilateral spigelian and inguinal hernias. Surgical Endoscopy 1998; 12: 1424.

396. Geis WP, Saletta JD. Lumbar hernia. In: Nyhus LM, Condon RE, eds. Hernia, 3rd edn. Philadelphia: Lippincott, 1989.

397. George CD, Ellis H. The results of incisional hernia repair: a twelve year review. Annals of the Royal College of Surgeons of England 1986; 68: 185–187.

398. Ger R. The management of certain abdominal herniae by intra-abdominal closure of the neck of the sac. Annals of the Royal College of Surgeons of England 1982; 64: 342–344.

399. Ger R, Monroe K, Duvivier R, Mishrick A. Management of indirect hernias by laparoscopic closure of the neck of the sac. American Journal of Surgery 1990; 159: 371–373.

400. Ghahremani GG, Michael AS. Sciatic hernia with incarcerated ileum – C.T. and radiographic diagnosis. Gastrointestinal Radiology 1991; 16: 120–122.

401. Gianetta E, DeCian F, Cuneo S *et al.* Hernia repair in elderly patients. British Journal of Surgery 1997; 84: 983–985.

402. Gibson CL. Operation for cure of large ventral hernia. Annals of Surgery 1920; 72: 214–217.

403. Giglio M, Medica M, Germinale F, Raggio M, Campodonice F, Stubinski R, Carmignan G. Scrotal extraperitoneal hernia of the ureter: case report and literature review. Urology International 2001; 66: 166–168.

404. Gilbert AI. Hernia repair in the aged and infirmed. Journal of the Florida Medical Association 1988; 75: 742–744.

405. Gilbert AI. An anatomic and functional classification for the diagnosis and treatment of inguinal hernia. American Journal of Surgery 1989; 157: 331–333.

406. Gilbert AI. Inguinal hernia repair: biomaterials and sutureless repair. Perspectives in General Surgery 1991; 2: 113–119.

407. Gilbert AI. Sutureless repair of inguinal hernia. American Journal of Surgery 1992; 163: 331–335.

408. Gilbert AI, Felton LL. Infection in inguinal hernia repair considering biomaterials and antibiotics. Surgery, Gynecology and Obstetrics 1993; 177: 126–130.

409. Gilbert AI, Graham MF. Symposium on the management of inguinal hernias. 5. Sutureless technique: second version. Canadian Journal of Surgery 1997; 40: 209–212.

410. Gilbert AI, Graham MF, Voigt WJ. A bilayer patch device for inguinal hernia repair. Hernia 1999; 3: 161–166.

411. Gilbert AI, Graham MF, Voigt WJ. Personal communication, 2002.

412. Gilbert M, Clatworthy HW. Bilateral operations for inguinal hernia and hydrocele in infancy and childhood. American Journal of Surgery 1959; 97: 255–259.

413. Gill P, Kiami S. Pre-emptive analgesia with local anaesthetic for herniorrhaphy Anaesthesia 2001; 56; 414–417.

414. Gilliam A, O'Boyle CJ, Wai D, Perry EP. Ultrasonic diagnosis of strangulated obturator hernia. European Journal of Surgery 2000; 166: 420–421.

415. Gilmore OJA. Groin disruption in sportsmen. In: Kurzer M, Kark AE, Wantz GE, eds. Surgical Management of Abdominal Wall Hernias. London: Martin Dunnitz, 1999: 151–157.

416. Gilsdorf JR, Friedman RH, Shapiro P. Electromyographic evaluation of the inguinal region in patients with hernia of the groin. Surgery, Gynecology and Obstetrics 1988; 167: 466–468.

417. Glassow F. Inguinal hernia in the female. Surgery, Gynecology and Obstetrics 1963; 116: 701–704.

418. Glassow F. Is post-operative wound infection following simple inguinal herniorrhaphy a predisposing cause of recurrent hernia? Canadian Medical Association Journal 1964; 91: 870–871.

419. Glassow F. Femoral hernia: review of 1143 consecutive repairs. Annals of Surgery 1966; 163: 227–232.

420. Glassow F. Femoral hernia following inguinal herniorrhaphy. Canadian Journal of Surgery 1970; 13: 27–30.

421. Glassow F. Femoral hernia in men. American Journal of Surgery 1971; 121: 637–640.

422. Glassow F. The surgical repair of inguinal and femoral hernias. Canadian Medical Association Journal 1973; 108: 308–313.

423. Glassow F. Short stay surgery (Shouldice technique) for repair of inguinal hernia. Annals of the Royal College of Surgeons of England 1976; 58: 133–139.

424. Glassow F. Inguinal hernia repair using local anaesthesia. Annals of the Royal College of Surgeons of England 1984; 66: 382–387.

425. Glassow F. Ambulatory hernia repair (a discussion with M. Ravitch and G. Wantz). Contemporary Surgery 1984; 24: 107–130.

426. Goepel R. Über die Verschliessung von Bruchpforten durch Einleilung geflochtener fertiger Silberdrahtnetze. Verhandlungen der Deutschen Gesellschaft fur Pathologie 1900; 29: 4.

427. Goldstein H. A university experience using mesh in inguinal hernia repair. Hernia 2002; 5: 182–185.

428. Goligher JC, Irvin TT, Johnston D, De Dombal FT, Hill GL, Horrocks JC. A controlled clinical trial of three methods of closure of laparotomy wounds. British Journal of Surgery 1975; 62: 823–827.

429. Goligher JC. Surgery of the Anus, Rectum and Colon, 4th edn. London: Bailliere Tindall, 1980.

430. Gong Y, Shao C, Sun Q *et al.* Genetic study of indirect inguinal hernia. Journal of Medical Genetics 1994; 31: 187–192.

431. Gray HT. Lesions of the isolated appendix vermiformis in the hernial sac. British Medical Journal 1910; 2: 1142–1145.

432. Gray SW, Skandalakis JE, Soria RE, Rowe JS. Strangulated obturator hernia. Surgery 1974; 75: 20–27.

433. Green BT. Strangulated obturator hernia: still deadly. Southern Medical Journal 2001; 94: 81–83.

434. Green EW. Colostomies and their complications. Surgery, Gynecology and Obstetrics 1966; 122: 1230–1232.

435. Greenawalt KE, Butler TJ, Rowe EA, Finneral AC, Garlick DS, Burns JW. Evaluation of a Sepramesh biosurgical composite in a rabbit repair model. Journal of Surgical Research 2000; 94: 92–98.

436. Griffith CA. Inguinal hernia: an anatomical surgical correlation. Surgical Clinics of North America 1959; 39: 531–556.

437. Griffiths JC, Toomey WF. Large bowel obstruction due to a herniated carcinoma of sigmoid colon. British Journal of Surgery 1964; 51: 715–717.

438. Griffiths M, Water WE, Acheson ED. Variation in hospital stay after inguinal herniorrhaphy. British Medical Journal 1979; 1: 787–789.

439. Grosfield JL. Current Concepts in Inguinal Hernia in Infants and Children. World Journal of Surgery 1989; 13: 506–515.

440. Grosfield JL. Groin hernia in infants and children. In: Nyhus LM, Condon RE, eds. Hernia. Philadelphia: Lippincott, 1994.

441. Grosfield JL, Cooney DR. Inguinal hernia after ventriculo-peritoneal shunt for hydrocephalus. Journal of Pediatric Surgery 1974; 9: 311–315.

442. Gross RE. Inguinal hernia. In: Surgery of Infancy and Childhood. Philadelphia: Saunders, 1955: 107–120.

443. Grotzinger U. Ambulante Herniechirurgie. Therapeutische Umschau 1992; 49: 478–481.

444. Grove A, Jensen ML, Donna A. Mesotheliomas of the tunica vaginalis testis and hernial sacs. Virchows Archives of Pathology, Anatomy and Histopathology 1989; 415: 283–292.

445. Grover VK, Nur AMA, Usha R, Farag TI, Sabry MA. Indirect inguinal hernia among Bedouins. Journal of Medical Genetics 1996; 33: 887.

446. Gue S. Development of right inguinal hernia following appendicectomy. British Journal of Surgery 1972; 59: 352–353.

447. Gui D, Giangiuliani G, Veneziani A, Giorgi G, Sganga G. Inguinal hernia repair in patients with peritoneo-venous shunt: risk of an embolism. British Journal of Surgery 1986; 73: 122.

448. Guivarc'h M. Traitment chirugical des hernies anterior-laterales dites de Spiegel. Presse Medicale 1989; 18: 177.

449. Guivarc'h M, Fonteny R, Boche O, Roullet-Audy JC. Hernies ventrles antero-laterales dites de Spiegel. 16 cas et revue de la literature. Chirugie 1988; 114: 572.

450. Gullmo A. Herniography. The diagnosis of hernia in the groin and incompetence of the pouch of Douglas and pelvic floor. Acta Radiologica Scandinavica (Suppl) 1980; 361.

451. Gullmo A. Herniography. World Journal of Surgery 1989; 13: 560–568.

452. Gullmo A, Broome A, Smedberg S. Herniography. Surgical Clinics of North America 1984; 64: 229–246.

453. Gunnarsson U, Degerman M, Davidsson A, Heuman R. Is elective hernia repair worthwhile in old patients? European Journal of Surgery 1999; 165: 326–332.

454. Guttman FM, Bertrand R, Ducharme JC. Herniography and the pediatric contralateral inguinal hernia. Surgery, Gynecology and Obstetrics 1972; 135: 551–555.

455. Hackney RG. The sports hernia: a cause of chronic groin pain. British Journal of Sports Medicine 1993; 27: 58–62.

456. Hahn-Pedersen J, Lund L, Hansen-Hojhus J, Bojsen-Moller F. Evaluation of direct and indirect inguinal hernia by computed tomography. British Journal of Surgery 1994; 81: 569–572.

457. Haidenthaller J. Die Radicaloperationen der Hernien in der Klinik des Hofraths Professor Dr. Billroth, 1877–1889. Archiv für Klinische Chirurgie 1890; 40: 493–555.

458. Hair A, Duffy K, McLean J et al. Groin hernia repair in Scotland. British Journal of Surgery 2000; 87: 1722–1726.

459. Hair A, Paterson C, O'Dwyer PJ. Diagnosis of a femoral hernia in the elective setting. Journal of the Royal College of Surgeons of Edinburgh 2001; 46: 117–118.

460. Hair A, Paterson C, Wright D, Baxter JN, O'Dwyer PJ. What effect does the duration of an inguinal hernia have on patient symptoms? Journal of the American College of Surgeons 2001; 193: 125–129.

461. Halsted WS. The radical cure of hernia. Bulletin of the Johns Hopkins Hospital 1889; i: 12–13.

462. Halsted WS. The operative treatment of hernia. American Journal of Medical Science 1895; 110: 13–17.

463. Halsted WS. An additional note on the operation for inguinal hernia. In: Surgical Papers by William Stuart Halsted, Vol 1. Baltimore: Johns Hopkins Press, 1924: 306–308.

464. Halverson K, McVay CH. Inguinal and femoral hernioplasty: a 22 year study of the author's methods. Archives of Surgery 1970; 101: 127–135.

465. Hamer DB, Duthie HL. Pneumoperitoneum in the management of abdominal incisional hernia. British Journal of Surgery 1972; 59: 372–375.

466. Hamer-Hodges DW, Scott NB. Replacement of an abdominal wall defect using expanding PTFE sheet (Gortex). Journal of the Royal College of Surgeons of Edinburgh 1985; 30: 65–67.

467. Hamilton RW. Spontaneous rupture of an incisional hernia. British Journal of Surgery 1966; 53: 477–479.

468. Hamlin JA, Kahn AM. Herniography in symptomatic patients following inguinal hernia repair. Western Journal of Medicine 1995; 162: 28–31.

469. Hamlin JA, Kahn AM. Herniography: a review of 333 herniograms. American Surgeon 1998; 64: 965–969.

470. Handley WS. A method for the radical cure of inguinal hernia (darn and stay-lace method). Practitioner 1918; 100: 466–471.

471. Hanley JA, Hanna BKB. Obturator hernia: A report of three cases with strangulation occurring twice in two patients. Journal of the Irish Medical Association 1970; 63: 396–398.

472. Hannington-Kiff JG. Absent thigh adductor reflex in obturator hernia. Lancet 1980; i: 180.

473. Hardie RM. Day surgery assessment nurse. Journal of One-Day Surgery 1993; 2: 19–20.

474. Harding KG, Mudge M, Leinster SJ, Hughes LE. Late development of incisional hernia: an unrecognised problem. British Medical Journal 1983; 286: 519–520.

475. Hardy JC, Costin JR. Femoral hernias: a ten year review. Journal of the American Osteopathic Association 1969; 68: 696–704.

476. Harper RC, Cacia A, Sin C. Inguinal hernia: a common problem of premature infants weighing 1000 gm or less at birth. Pediatrics 1975; 56: 112.

477. Harrison CA, Morris S, Harvey JS. Effect of ilioinguinal and iliohypogastric nerve block and wound infiltration with 0.5% bupivacaine on postoperative pain after hernia repair. British Journal of Anaesthesia 1994; 72: 691–693.

478. Harrison LA, Keesling CA, Martin NL, Lee KR, Wetzel LH. Abdominal wall hernias: Review of herniography and correlation with cross-sectional imaging. Radiographics 1995; 15: 315–332.

479. Harshaw DH, Gardner B, Vives A, Sundaram KN. The effect of technical factors upon complications from abdomino-perineal resections. Surgery, Gynecology and Obstetrics 1974; 139: 756–760.

480. Harth M, Bourne RB. Osteitis pubis: an unusual complication of herniorrhaphy. Canadian Journal of Surgery 1981; 24: 407–409.

481. Hartley RC. Spontaneous rupture of incisional herniae. British Journal of Surgery 1962; 49: 617–618.

482. Harvald B. Genetic epidemiology of Greenland. Clinical Genetics 1989; 36: 364–367.

483. Harvey MH, Johnston MJS, Fossard DP. Inguinal herniotomy in children: a five year survey. British Journal of Surgery 1985; 72: 485–487.

484. Hass BE, Schrager RE. Small bowel obstruction due to Richter's hernia after laparoscopic procedures. Journal of Laparoendoscopic Surgery 1993; 3: 421–423.

485. Haydorm WH, Velanovich V. A five year U.S. Army experience with 36,250 abdominal hernia repairs. American Surgeon 1990; 56: 596.

486. Healy TEJ, Un EN. General anaesthesia for day stay surgery. In: Healy TEJ, ed. Clinical Anaesthesiology; Anaesthesia for Day Case Surgery. 1990: 667–677.

487. Heasman MA, Carstairs V. In-patient management: variations in some aspects of practice in Scotland. British Medical Journal 1971; 1: 495–498.

488. Heikkinen TJ, Haukipuro K, Hulkko A. A cost and outcome comparison between laparoscopic and Lichtenstein hernia operations in a day-case unit. Surgical Endoscopy 1998;12: 1199.

489. Heise CP, Sproat IA, Starling JR. Peritoneography (herniography) for detecting occult inguinal hernia in patients with inguiniodynia. Annals of Surgery 2002; 235: 140–144.

490. Heister L. A General System of Surgery in Three Parts (translated into English from the Latin). London: Innys, Davis, Clark, Manby and Whiston, 1743.

491. Helwig H. von. Über sogenannte Spontanrupturen von Hernien. Schweizerische Medizinische Wochenschrift 1958; 27: 662–666.

492. Heniford BT, Park A, Ramshaw BJ, Voeller G. Laparoscopic ventral and incisional hernia repair in 407 patients. Journal of the American College of Surgeons 2000; 190 (6): 645–650.

493. Heniford BT, Ramshaw BJ. Laparoscopic ventral hernia repair. Surgical Endoscopy 2000; 14: 419–423.

494. Henry AK. Operation for femoral hernia by a midline extraperitoneal approach: with a preliminary note on the use of this route for reducible inguinal hernia. Lancet 1936; i: 531–533.

495. Henry X, Bouras-Kara Terki N. Should prostheses be used in emergency hernia surgery? In: Bendavid R, Abrahamson J, Arregui M, Flament JB, Phillips E, eds. Abdominal Wall Hernias: Principles and Management. New York: Springer-Verlag, 2001: 557–559.

496. Herlock DJ, Smith S. Complications resulting from a patent processus vaginalis in two patients on continuous ambulatory peritoneal dialysis. British Journal of Surgery 1984; 71: 477.

497. Herman RE. Abdominal wound closure using a new polypropylene monofilament suture. Surgery, Gynecology and Obstetrics 1974; 138: 84–86.

498. Hernandez-Richter T, Schardey HM, Rau HG, Schildberg FW, Meyer G. The femoral hernia: an ideal approach for the transabdominal preperitoneal technique (TAPP). Surgical Endoscopy 2000; 14: 736–740.

499. Herrman NIB. Tensile strength and knot security of surgical suture materials. American Surgeon 1971; 37: 209–217.

500. Herszage L. Personal communication, 2002.

501. Hertzfeld G. Hernia in infancy. American Journal of Surgery 1938; 39: 422–428.

502. Hesselbach FK. Neueste Anatomisch-Pathologische Untersuchungen über den Ursprung und das Fortschreiten der Leisten- und Schenkelbrüche. Warzburg: Baumgartner, 1814.

503. Hesselink VJ, Luijendijk RW, de Wilt JHW, Heide R, Jeekel J. An evaluation of risk factors in incisional hernia recurrence. Surgical Gynecology and Obstetrics 1993; 176: 228–234.

504. Heydorn WH, Velanovich V. A five year U.S. Army experience with 36,250 abdominal hernia repairs. American Surgeon 1990; 56: 596–600.

505. Hilton J. Case of Obturator Hernia with symptoms of intestinal obstruction within the abdomen, to relieve which the abdomen was opened. Lancet 1848; 2: 103.

506. Hodgson NCF, Malthaner RA, Ostbyc T. The search for an ideal method of abdominal fascial closure: a meta-analysis. Annals of Surgery 2000; 231: 436–442

507. Hoffman HC, Traverso ALV. Preperitoneal prosthetic herniorrhaphy: one surgeon's successful technique. Archives of Surgery 1993; 128: 964–970.

508. Hoguet JB. Direct inguinal hernia. Annals of Surgery 1920; 72: 671–674.

509. Hoguet JP. Right inguinal hernia following appendectomy. Annals of Surgery 1911; 54: 673–676.

510. Holder LE, Schneider HJ. Spigelian hernias: anatomy and roentgenographic manifestation. Radiologic Diagnosis 1974; 112: 309–313.

511. Holzman MD, Purut CM, Reintgen K, Eubanks S, Pappas TN. Laparoscopic ventral and incisional hernioplasty. Surgical Endoscopy 1997; 11: 32–35.

512. Homans J. Three Hundred and Eighty-four Laparotomies for Various Diseases. Boston: Nathan Sawyer, 1887.

513. Horgan K, Hughes LE. Para-ileostomy hernia: failure of a local repair technique. British Journal of Surgery 1986; 73: 439–440.

514. Horn TW, Harris JA, Martindale R, Gadacz T. When a hernia is not a hernia: the evaluation of inguinal hernias in the cirrhotic patient. American Surgeon 2001; 67(11): 1093–1095.

515. Horner CH et al. Cited in Van Mameren H, Go PMNYH. Anatomy and variations of the internal inguinal region. In: Schumpelick V, Wantz GE, eds. Inguinal Hernia Repair. Basel: Karger, 1994.

516. Horton MC, Florence MG. Simplified preperitoneal Marlex hernia repair. American Journal of Surgery 1993; 165: 595–599.

517. House MG, Goldin SB, Chen H. Perforated Amyand's hernia. Southern Medical Journal 2001; 94: 496–498.

518. Howes EL. Effects of suture material on the tensile strength of wound repair. Annals of Surgery 1933; 98: 153–155.

519. Howes EL. The strength of wounds sutured with catgut and silk. Surgery, Gynecology and Obstetrics 1933; 57: 309.

520. Hughson W. The persistent or preformed sac in relation to oblique inguinal hernia. Surgery, Gynecology and Obstetrics 1925; 41: 610–614.

521. Hulten L, Kewenter J, Kock NG. Komplikationen der Ileostomie und Colostomie und ihre Behandlung. Chirurg 1976; 47: 20.

522. Hunt DM. Primary defect in copper transport underlies mottled mutant in mouse. Nature 1974; 249: 852–854.

523. Hunt TK, Goodson WH III. In: Way LW, ed. Current Surgical Diagnosis and Treatment, 9th edn. Norwalk: Appleton and Lange, 1991: 95–108.

524. Hunter J. Palmer's Edition of Hunter's works, published 1837, London, vol. iv, p. 1.

525. Hunter RR. Anatomical repair of midline incisional hernia. British Journal of Surgery 1971; 58: 888–891.

526. Hurst JW. Measuring the benefits and costs of medical care – the contribution of health status measurement. Health Trends 1984; 16: 16–19.

527. Ianora AA, Midiri M, Vinci R, Rotondo A, Angelelli G. Abdominal wall hernias: imaging with spiral CT. European Radiology 2000; 10: 914–919.

528. Iason AH. Hernia. Philadelphia: Blakiston, 1941.

529. Ijiri R, Kanamaru H, Yokoyama H, Shirakawa M, Hashimoto H, Yoshino G. Obturator hernia: The usefulness of computed tomography in diagnosis. Surgery 1996; 119: 137–140.

530. Iles JDH. Specialisation in elective herniorrhaphy. Lancet 1965; i: 751–755.

531. Iles JDH. Mortality from elective hernia repair. Journal of Abdominal Surgery 1969; May: 87–95.

532. Immordino PA. Femoral hernia in infancy and childhood. Journal of Pediatric Surgery 1972; 7: 40.

533. Ingall JRF. Femoral hernia in childhood. British Journal of Surgery 1964; 51: 438–440.

534. Ingimarsson O, Spak I. Inguinal and femoral hernias: long-term results in a community hospital. Acta Chirurgica Scandinavica 1983; 149: 291–297.

535. Ingoldby JH. Laparoscopic and conventional repair of groin disruption in sportsmen. British Journal of Surgery 1997; 84: 213–215.

536. Irvin TT, Koffman CG, Duthie HL. Layer closure of laparotomy wounds with absorbable and non-absorbable suture materials. British Journal of Surgery 1976; 63: 793–796.

537. Ismail W, Taylor SJC, Beddow E. Advice on driving after groin hernia surgery in the United Kingdom: questionnaire survey. British Medical Journal 2000; 321: 1056.

538. Israelsson L. Wound complications in the midline laparotomy incisions: the importance of suture technique. Thesis. The department of surgery, Lund University, Malmo, Sweden, 1995.

539. Israelsson LA, Jonsson T. Overweight and healing of midline incisions: the importance of suture technique. European Journal of Surgery 1997; 163: 175–186.

540. Israelsson LA. The surgeon as a risk factor for complications of midline incisions. European Journal of Surgery 1998; 164: 353–359.

541. Ivanov NT, Losanoff JE, Kjossev KT. Recurrent sciatic hernia treated by prosthetic mesh, reinforcement of the pelvic floor. British Journal of Surgery 1994; 81: 447.

542. Jackson DJ, Mocklen LH. Umbilical hernia: a retrospective study. California Medicine 1970; 113.

543. Jacoby HI, Brodie DA. Laparoscopic Herniorrhaphy. American Medical Association, 1996.

544. James PM Jr. The problem of hernia in infants and adolescents. Surgical Clinics of North America 1971; 51: 1361–1370.

545. James T. Umbilical hernia in Xhosa infants and children. Journal of the Royal Society of Medicine 1982; 75: 537–541.

546. Janik J, Shandling B. The vulnerability of the vas deferens (II): the case against routine bilateral inguinal exploration. Journal of Pediatric Surgery 1982; 17: 585–588.

547. Jarrett MED, personal communication.

548. Jenkins TPN. The burst abdominal wound: a mechanical approach. British Journal of Surgery 1976; 63: 873–876.

549. Jenkins TPN. Incisional hernia repair: a mechanical approach. British Journal of Surgery 1980; 67: 335–336.

550. Jenner RE. Strangulated obturator hernia. Annals of the Royal College of Surgeons of England 1975; 56: 266–269.

551. Johansson B, Hallerback B, Glise H, Anesten B, Smedberg S, Roman J. Laparoscopic mesh repair vs. open w/wh mesh graft for inguinal hernia (SCUR hernia repair study) – preliminary results. Surgical Endoscopy 1997; 11: 170.

552. Johansson B, Hallerback B, Glise H, Anesten B, Smedberg S, Roman J. Laparoscopic mesh versus open preperitoneal versus open conventional technique for inguinal hernia repair: a randomized multicenter trial (SCUR hernia repair study). Annals of Surgery 1999; 230: 225–231.

553. Jones DJ. Braided versus monofilament sutures in inguinal hernia. British Journal of Surgery 1986; 73: 414.

554. Jones KR, Burney RE, Peterson M, Christy R. Return to work after inguinal hernia repair. Surgery 2001; 129: 128–135.

555. Jones ME, Swerdlow AJ, Griffith M, Goldacre MJ. Risk of congenital inguinal hernia in siblings: a record linkage study. Paediatric and Perinatal Epidemiology 1998; 12: 288–296.

556. Jones PF, Towns FM. An abdominal extraperitoneal approach for the incarcerated inguinal hernia of infancy. British Journal of Surgery 1983; 70: 719–720.

557. Jones TCL. Partial enterocele: strangulated. Lancet 1904; i: 1280.

558. Judd ES. The prevention and treatment of ventral hernia. Surgery, Gynecology and Obstetrics 1912; 14: 175–182.

559. Julsrud ME. Osteitis pubis. Journal of the American Pediatric Medical Association 1986; 76: 562–565.

560. Junge K, Klinge U, Prescher A, Giboni P, Niewera M, Schumpelick V. Elasticity of the anterior abdominal wall and impact for reparation of incisional hernias using mesh implants. Hernia 2001; 5: 113–118.

561. Kapadia CR. Ligatures and suture materials. In: Dudley HAF, Poirees WJ, eds. Rob and Smith's Operative Surgery, vol. 1. London: Butterworths, 1983: 119–123.

562. Kaplan GW. Iatrogenic cryptorchism resulting from hernia repair. Surgery, Gynecology and Obstetrics 1976; 142: 671–672.

563. Kaplan SA, Snyder WH Jr, Little S. Inguinal hernia in females and the testicular feminization syndrome. American Journal of Diseases of Children 1969; 117: 243–251.

564. Kapris SA, Brough WA, Royston CMS, O'Boyle C, Sedman PC. Laparoscopic transabdominal preperitoneal (TAPP) hernia repair. Surgical Endoscopy 2001; 15: 972–975.

565. Kapur BML, Shah DK. Strangulated obturator presenting as subcutaneous emphysema of the thigh. Canadian Journal of Surgery 1969; 12: 233–235.

566. Karatassas A, Morris RG, Walsh D, Hung P, Slavotinek AH. Evaluation of the safety of inguinal hernia repair in the elderly using lignocaine infiltration anaesthesia. Australian and New Zealand Journal of Surgery 1993; 63: 266–269.

567. Kark AE, Kurzer M, Waters KJ. Tension-free mesh hernia repair: review of 1,098 cases using local anaesthesia in a day unit. Annals of the Royal College of Surgeons of England 1995; 77: 299–304.

568. Kasirajan K, Lopez J, Lopez R. Laparoscopic technique in the management of Spigelian hernia. Journal of Laparoscopy and Advanced Surgical Technique 1997; 7: 385.

569. Kasson MA, Munoz E, Laughlin A, Margolis IB, Wise L. Value of routine pathology in herniorraphy performed upon adults. Surgery, Gynecology and Obstetrics 1986; 163: 518–522.

570. Kastrissios H, Triggs EJ, Sinclair F, Moran P, Smithers M. Plasma concentrations of bupivacaine after wound infiltration of a 0.5% solution after inguinal herniorrhaphy; a preliminary study. European Journal of Clinical Pharmacology 1993; 44: 555–557.

571. Kathouda N, Mavor E, Friedlander MH et al. Use of fibrin sealant for prosthetic mesh fixation laparoscopic extraperitoneal inguinal hernia repair. Annals of Surgery 2001; 233(1): 18–25.

572. Kavey NB, Altshuler KZ. Sleep in herniorrhaphy patients. American Journal of Surgery 1979; 138: 682–687.

573. Kavic MS. Laparoscopic hernia repair. Surgical Endoscopy 1993; 7: 163–167.

574. Kavic MS. Laparoscopic hernia repair. Amsterdam: Harwood Academic Publishers, 1997: 33–40.

575. Kawji R, Feichter A, Fuchsjager N, Kux M. Postoperative pain and return to activity after five different types of inguinal herniorrhaphy. Hernia 1999; 3: 31–35.

576. Kehlet H. Balanced analgesia: a prerequisite for optimal recovery. British Journal of Surgery 1998; 85: 3–4.

577. Kehlet H, White PF. Optimizing anaesthesia for inguinal herniorrhaphy: general, regional, or local anaesthesia. Anaesthesia and Analgesia 2001; 93: 1367–1369.

578. Keith A. On the origin and nature of hernia. British Journal of Surgery 1924; 11: 455–475.

579. Kemler MA, Oostvogel HJM. Femoral hernia: is a conservative policy justified? European Journal of Surgery 1997; 163: 187–190.

580. Kemp DA, ed. Kemp and Kemp: The Quantum of Damages, revised edn, vol. 1. London: Sweet and Maxwell, 1975.

581. Kennedy CM, Matyas JA. Use of expanded polytetrafluoroethylene in the repair of the difficult hernia. American Journal of Surgery 1994; 168: 304–306.

582. Kennedy EM, Harms BA, Starling JB. Absence of maladaptive neuronal plasticity after genito-femoral-ilioinguinal neurectomy. Surgery 1994; 116: 665–671.

583. Kesek P, Ekberg O. Herniography in women under 40 years old with chronic groin pain. European Journal of Surgery 1999; 165: 573–578.

584. Keynes G. The modern treatment of hernia. British Medical Journal 1927; 173–179.

585. Khajanchee YS, Urbach DR, Swanstrom LL, Hansen PD. Outcomes of laparoscopic herniorrhaphy without fixation of mesh to the abdominal wall. Surgical Endoscoscopy 2001; 15: 1102–1107.

586. Khoury N. A randomized prospective controlled trial of laparoscopic extraperitoneal hernia repair and mesh-plug hernioplasty: a study of 315 cases. Journal of Laparoendoscopy and Advanced Surgical Technique 1998; 8: 367–372.

587. Kiely EM, Spitz L. Layered versus mass closure of abdominal wounds in infants and children. British Journal of Surgery 1985; 72: 739–740.

588. Kienzle HF, Staemmler S. Die Spighel-Hernie und ihre Behandlung. Fortschritte der Medizin 1978; 96: 876.

589. Kieswetter WB, Oh KS. Unilateral inguinal hernias in children. Archives of Surgery 1980; 115: 1443–1445.

590. Kieswetter WB, Parenzan L. When should inguinal hernia in the infant be treated bilaterally? Journal of the American Medical Association 1959; 171: 287–290.

591. King LR. Optimal treatment of children with undescended testicles. Journal of Urology 1984; 131: 734–735.

592. Kingsnorth AN, Britton BJ, Morris PJ. Recurrent inguinal hernia after local anaesthetic repair. British Journal of Surgery 1981; 68: 273–275.

593. Kingsnorth AN, Gray MR, Nott DM. Prospective, randomized trial comparing the Shouldice technique and plication darn for inguinal hernia. British Journal of Surgery 1992; 79: 1068–1070.

594. Kingsnorth AN, Hyland ME, Porter Sodergren S. Prospective double-blind randomized study comparing Perfix plug-and-patch with Lichtenstein patch in inguinal hernia repair: one-year quality-of-life results. Hernia 2000; 4: 255–258.

595. Kingsnorth AN, Porter C, Bennett DH. The benefits of a hernia service in a public hospital. Hernia 2000; 4: 1–5.

596. Kingsnorth AN, Porter CA, Cummings GC, Bennett DH. A randomized, double-blind study to compare the efficacy of levobupivacaine with bupivacaine in elective inguinal herniorrhaphy. European Journal of Surgery 2002; 168: 391–396.

597. Kingsnorth AN, Skandalakis PN, Colborn GL, Weidman TA, Skandalakis LJ, Skandalakis JE. Embryology, anatomy and surgical applications of the preperitoneal space. Surgical Clinics of North America 2000; 80: 1–24.

598. Kingsnorth AN, Wijesinha SS, Grixti CJ. Evaluation of dextran with local anaesthesia for short stay inguinal herniorrhaphy. Annals of the Royal College of Surgeons of England 1979; 61: 456–458.

599. Kirk RM. Which inguinal hernia repair? British Medical Journal 1983; 287: 4–5.

600. Kirk RM. The incidence of burst abdomen: comparison of layered opening and closing with straight through one layered closure. Proceedings of the Royal Society of Medicine 1973; 66: 1092.

601. Kirschner M. Die praktischen Ergebnisse der freien Fascien-Transplantation. Archiv für Klinische Chirurgie 1910; 92: 889–912.

602. Klinge U, Prescher A, Klosterhalfen B, Schumpelick V. Origin and pathophysiology of abdominal wall defects. Chirurgie 1997; 68: 293–303.

603. Klinge U, Zheng H, Si ZY, Bhardwaj R, Klosterhalfen B, Schumpelick V. Altered collagen synthesis in fascia transversalis of patients with inguinal hernia. Hernia 1999; 4: 181–187.

604. Klinkosch JT. Programma Quo Divisionem Herniarum, Novumque Herniae Ventralis Specium Proponit. Rotterdam: Beman, 1764.

605. Knapp RW, Mullen JT. Clinical evaluation of the use of local anaesthesia for the repair of inguinal hernia. American Surgeon 1976; 42: 908–910.

606. Knox G. The incidence of inguinal hernia in Newcastle children. Archives of Diseases in Childhood 1959; 34: 482–484.

607. Kocher T. Chirurgische operationslehre. Jena: Verlag von Gustav Fischer, 1907.

608. Kochler RH, Voeller G. Recurrences in laparoscopic incisional hernia repairs: a personal series and review of literature. Journal of the Society of Laparoendoscopic Surgeons 1999; 3: 293–304.

609. Kodner IJ. Colostomy and ileostomy. Ciba Clinical Symposia 1978; 30: 2–36.

610. Koehler RH. Diagnosing the occult contralateral inguinal hernia. Surgical Endoscopy 2002; 16: 512–520.

611. Koehler RH, Begos D, Berger D, Carey S, LeBlanc KA, Ramshaw B, Smoot R. Adhesion formation to intraperitoneally-placed mesh: reoperative clinical experience after laparoscopic ventral incisional hernia repair. (Submitted for publication).

612. Koehler RH, Voeller G. Recurrences in laparoscopic incisional hernia repairs: a personal series and review of the literature. Journal of the Society of Laparoendoscopic Surgeons 1999; 3: 293–304.

613. Komura JI, Yano H, Uchida M, Shima I. Pediatric spigelian hernia: reports of three cases. Surgery Today 1994; 24: 1081–1084.

614. Koontz AR. Preliminary report on the use of tantalum mesh in the repair of ventral hernias. Annals of Surgery 1948; 127: 1079–1085.

615. Koontz AR. Hernia. New York: Appleton-Century-Crofts, 1963.

616. Koontz AR. Atrophy of the testicle as a surgical risk. Surgery, Gynecology and Obstetrics 1965; 120: 511–513.

617. Kretschmer HL. Lumbar hernia of the kidney. Journal of Urology 1851; 65: 944–948.

618. Kreymer M. Inguinal hernien bei Centralafrikanern. Münchenener Medizinische Wochenschrift 1968; 110: 1750–1755.

619. Kronberg O, Kramhohft J, Backer O, Sprechler M. Late complications following operations for cancer of the rectum and anus. Diseases of the Colon and Rectum 1974; 17: 750.

620. Krug F, Herold A, Wenk H, Bruch HP. Nabenhernien nach laparoskopischen eingriffen. Der Chirurgie 1995; 66: 419–423.

621. Krukowski ZH, Matheson NA. Button-hole incisional hernia: a late complication of wound closure with continuous non-absorbable sutures (case report). British Journal of Surgery 1987; 74: 824–825.

622. Kugel RD. Minimally invasive, nonlaparoscopic, perperitoneal and sutureless inguinal herniorrhaphy. American Journal of Surgery 1999; 178: 298–302.

623. Kugel RD. The Kugel repair for groin hernias. In: Bendavid R, ed. Abdominal Wall Hernias. London: Springer-Verlag, 2001: 504–507.

624. Kugel RD. Ventral hernias: use of the Kugel patch. In: Bendavid R, Abrahamson J, Arregui M, Flament JB, and Phillips E, eds. Abdominal Wall Hernias, Principles and Management. New York: Springer-Verlag, 2001.

625. Kugel RD. Personal communication, 2001.

626. Kugel RD. Personal communication, 2002.

627. Kulah B, Kulacoghu IH, Oruc MT, Duzgun AP, Moran M, Ozmen MM, Coskum F. Presentation and outcome of incarcerated external hernias in adults. American Journal of Surgery 2001; 181: 101–104.

628. Kux M, Fuchsjager N, Schemper M. Shouldice is superior to Bassini inguinal herniorrhaphy. American Journal of Surgery 1994; 168: 15–18.

629. Kwong KH, Ong GB. Obturator hernia. British Journal of Surgery 1966; 53: 23–25.

630. Kyzer S, Alis M, Aloni Y, Charuzi I. Laparoscopic repair of postoperation ventral hernia. Surgical Endoscopy 1999; 13: 928–931.

631. Lancet Editorial. Country profile: United Kingdom. Lancet 1997; 350: 48–58.

632. Langenbuch. Quoted in Ponka (1980).

633. Laparoscopic and open hernia repair: randomized controlled trial of early results. World Journal of Surgery 1999; 23: 1004–1009.

634. LaRoque GP. The permanent cure of inguinal and femoral hernia. A modification of the standard operative procedures. Surgery, Gynecology and Obstetrics 1919; 29: 507–511.

635. Larson GM, Harrower HW. Plastic mesh repair of incisional hernia. American Journal of Surgery 1978; 135: 559–563.

636. Larson GM, Vandertoll DJ. Approaches to repair of ventral hernia and full thickness loss of the abdominal wall. Surgical Clinics of North America 1984; 64: 335–350.

637. Lassaletta L, Fonkalsrud EW, Tover JA, Dudgeon D, Asch MJ. The management of umbilical hernias in infancy and childhood. Journal of Pediatric Surgery 1975; 10: 405–409.

638. Lau H, Lee F. Determinant factors of pain after ambulatory inguinal herniorrhaphy: a multi-variate analysis. Hernia 2001; 5: 17–20.

639. Laugier S. Note sur une nouvelle espece de hernie de l'abdomen a travers le ligament de Gimbernat. Archives Generales de Medecine, Paris 1833; 2: 27–37.

640. Laurell CB, Ericksson S. The electrophoretic alpha-l-globulin pattern of serum alpha-l-antitrypsin deficiency. Scandinavian Journal of Clinical and Laboratory Investigation 1963; 15: 132–140.

641. Law NW, Trapnell JE. Does a truss benefit a patient with inguinal hernia? British Medical Journal 1992; 304: 1092.

642. Lawrenz K, Hollman AS, Carachi R, Cacciagnerra S. Ultrasound assessment of the contralateral groin in infants with unilateral inguinal hernia. Clinical Radiology 1994; 49: 546–548.

643. Lawrence K, Jenkinson C, McWhinnie D, Coulter A. Quality of life in patients undergoing inguinal hernia repair. Annals of the Royal College of Surgeons of England 1997; 79: 40–45.

644. Lawrence K, McWhinnie D, Goodwin A et al. Randomised controlled trial of laparoscopic versus open repair of inguinal hernia: early results. British Medical Journal 1995; 311: 981–985.

645. Lawrence K, McWhinnie D, Goodwin A et al. An economic evaluation of laparoscopic vs open inguinal hernia repair. Journal of Public Health Medicine 1996; 18: 41–48.

646. Lawrie P. A survey of the absorbability of commercial surgical catgut. British Journal of Surgery 1959; 46: 634–637.

647. Lawrie P, Angus G-E, Reese AJM. The absorption of surgical catgut. British Journal of Surgery 1959; 46: 638–642.

648. Leander P, Ekberg O, Sjoberg S, Kesek P. MR imaging following herniography in patients with unclear groin pain. European Radiology 2000; 10: 1691–1696.

649. Leaper DJ, Allan A, May RE, Corfield AP, Kennedy RH. Abdominal wound closure: a controlled trial of polyamide (nylon) and polydioxanone suture (PDS). Annals of the Royal College of Surgeons of England 1985; 67: 273–275.

650. Leaper DJ, Pollock AV, Evans M. Abdominal wound closure: a trial of nylon, polyglycolic acid and steel sutures. British Journal of Surgery 1977; 64: 603–606.

651. Leaper DJ. Laparotomy closure. British Journal of Hospital Medicine 1985; 33: 317–322.

652. Leber GE, Garb JL, Alexander AI, Reed WP. Long-term complications associated with prosthetic repair of incisional hernias. Archives of Surgery 1998; 133: 378–382.

653. LeBlanc KA. Two phase in vivo comparison study of adhesion formation of the Goretex soft tissue patch, Marlex mesh and Surgipro using a rabbit model. In: Arregui ME, Nagan RF, eds. Inguinal Hernia: Advances or Controversies? London: Radcliffe Medical Press, 1994: 515–517.

654. LeBlanc KA. Two-phase in vivo comparison studies of the tissue response to polypropylene, polyester, and expanded polytetrafluoroethylene grafts used in the repair of abdominal wall defects. In: Truetner KH, Schumpelick V, eds. Peritoneal Adhesions. London: Springer-Verlag, 1997: 352–362.

655. LeBlanc KA. Current considerations in laparoscopic incisional and ventral herniorraphy. Journal of the Society of Laparoendoscopic Surgeons 2000; 4: 131–139.

656. LeBlanc KA. Complications associated with the plug-and-patch method of inguinal herniorrhaphy. Hernia 2001; 5: 135–138.

657. LeBlanc KA. The critical technical aspects of laparoscopic repair of ventral and incisional hernias. American Surgeon 2001; 67(8): 809–812.

658. LeBlanc, KA. Personal experience, 2002.

659. LeBlanc KA. 'Tack' hernia – a new entity (submitted for publication).

660. LeBlanc KA. A new method to insert the Dualmesh prosthesis for laparoscopic ventral herniorrhaphy. JSLS 2002; 6(4): 349–352.

661. LeBlanc KA, Bellanger DE, Rhynes KV, Baker DS, Stout R. Tissue attachment strength of prosthetic meshes used in ventral and incisional hernia repair: a study in the New Zealand white rabbit adhesion model. Surgical Endoscopy 2002; 16(11): 1542–1546.

662. LeBlanc KA, Bellanger DE. Laparoscopic repair of paraostomy hernias: early results. Journal of the American College of Surgeons 2002; 194(2): 232–239.

663. LeBlanc KA, Booth WV, Bellanger DE, Whitaker JM. Laparoscopic incisional and ventral herniorrhaphy: our initial 100 patients. Hernia 2001; 5: 41–45.

664. LeBlanc KA, Booth WV, Spaw AT. Laparoscopic ventral herniorrhaphy using an intraperitoneal onlay patch of expanded polytetrafluoroethylene. In: Arregui ME, Nagan RF, eds. Inguinal Hernia: Advances or Controversies? Oxford: Radcliffe Medical Press, 1994: 501–510.

665. LeBlanc KA, Booth WV, Whitaker JA, Bellanger DE. Laparoscopic incisional and ventral herniorrhaphy: our initial 100 patients. American Journal of Surgery 2000; 180(3): 193–197.

666. LeBlanc KA, Booth WV, Whitaker JM, Baker D. In vivo study of meshes implanted over the inguinal ring and external iliac vessels in uncastrated pigs. Surgical Endoscopy 1998; 12: 247–251.

667. LeBlanc KA, Booth WV, Whitaker JM. Laparoscopic repair of ventral hernias using an intraperitoneal onlay patch: report of current results. Contemporary Surgery 1994; 45(4): 211–214.

668. LeBlanc KA, Booth WV. Avoiding complications with laparoscopic herniorrhaphy. Surgical Laparoscopy and Endoscopy 1993; 3(5): 420–424.

669. LeBlanc KA, Booth WV. Laparoscopic repair of incisional abdominal hernias using expanded polytetrafluoroethylene: preliminary findings. Surgical Laparoscopy and Endoscopy 1993; 3(1): 39–41.

670. LeBlanc KA, Spaw AT, Booth WV. Inguinal herniorrhaphy using intraperitoneal placement of an expanded polytetrafluoroethylene patch. In: Arregui ME, Nagan RF, eds. Inguinal Hernia: Advances of Controversies? Oxford: Radcliffe Medical Press, 1994: 437–439.

671. LeBlanc KA, Whitaker JM, Bellanger DE, Rhynes VK. Laparoscopic incisional and ventral hernia repair: lessons learned from 200 patients. Presented at the fifth annual American Hernia Society Meeting, Tuscon AZ, USA. Hernia (in press).

672. LeBlanc KE, LeBlanc KA. Groin pain in athletes. Hernia (in press).

673. Le Dran HF. The Operations in Surgery. London: Dodsley and Lay, 1781: 59–60.

674. Lee JR, Hancock SM, Martindale RG. Solitary fibrous tumours arising in abdominal wall hernia sacs. American Surgeon 2001; 67: 577–581.

675. Lee SL, Du Bois JJ. Laparoscopic diagnosis and repair of pediatric femoral hernia. Surgical Endoscopy 2000; 14: 1110–1113.

676. Leech P, Waddell G, Main RG. The incidence of right inguinal hernia following appendicectomy. British Journal of Surgery 1972; 59: 623.

677. Lees W. Carcinoma of colon in inguinal hernial sacs. British Journal of Surgery 1966; 53: 473–474.

678. Legorreta AP, Silber JH, Constantino GN et al. Increased cholecystectomy rate after the introduction of laparoscopic cholecystectomy. Journal of the American Medical Association 1993; 270: 1429–1432.

679. Lehnert B, Wadouh F. High coincidence of inguinal hernias and abdominal aortic aneurysms. Annals of Vascular Surgery 1992; 6: 134–137.

680. Leibl B, Schwarz J, Däubler P, Ulrich M, Bittner R. Standardisierte Laparoskopische Hernioplastik versus Shouldice-Reparation. Chirurgie 1995; 66: 895–898.

681. Lejars F. Neoplasmes herniares et peri-herniares. Gazette des Hopitaux Civils et Militaires 1889; 62: 801–811.

682. Lentz SM. Osteitis pubis: a review. Obstetrics and Gynecology Survey 1995; 50: 310–315.

683. Leonetti JP, Aranha GV, Wilkinson WA, Stanley M, Greenlee HB. Umbilical herniorrhaphy in cirrhotic patients. Archives of Surgery 1984; 119: 442–445.

684. Lerwick E. Studies of the efficacy and safety of polydioxanone monofilament absorbable suture. Surgery, Gynecology and Obstetrics 1983; 156: 51–55.

685. Leslie MD, Slater ND, Smallwood CI. Small bowel fistula from a Littre's hernia. British Journal of Surgery 1983; 70: 244.

686. Lestor R, Bourke JR. Strangulated femoral hernia containing appendices. Journal of the Royal College of Surgeons of Edinburgh 1979; 24: 102–103.

687. Levack JH. En masse reduction of strangulated hernia. British Journal of Surgery 1963; 50: 582–585.

688. Levene CL, Ockleford CD, Harber CL. Scurvy: a comparison between ultrastructural and biochemical changes observed in cultured fibroblasts and the collagen they synthesize. Virchows Archiv pt B, Cell Pathology 1977; 23: 325–338.

689. Lichtenstein IL. Hernia Repair Without Disability. St Louis: C.V. Mosby, 1970.

690. Lichtenstein IL. Hernia Repair Without Disability, 2nd edn. St Louis/Tokyo: Ishiyaku Euromerica, 1986.

691. Lichtenstein IL. Herniorrhaphy – a personal experience with 6321 cases. American Journal of Surgery 1987; 153: 553–559.

692. Lichtenstein IL, Shore JM. Simplified repair of femoral and recurrent inguinal hernias by a 'plug' technique. American Journal of Surgery 1974; 128: 439–444.

693. Lichtenstein IL, Shore JM. Exploding the myths of hernia repair. American Journal of Surgery 1976; 132: 307–315.

694. Lichtenstein IL, Shulman AG, Amid PK, Montilier MM. The tension-free hernioplasty. American Journal of Surgery 1989; 157: 188–193.

695. Lickley HLA, Trusler GH. Femoral hernia in children. Journal of Pediatric Surgery 1966; 1: 338.

696. Liem MS, Van Steensel CJ, Boelhouwer RU et al. The learning curve for totally extraperitoneal laparoscopic inguinal hernia repair. American Journal of Surgery 1996; 171: 281–285.

697. Liem MSL, Van der Graaf Y, Van Steensel CJ et al. Comparison of conventional anterior surgery and laparoscopic surgery for inguinal hernia repair. New England Journal of Medicine 1997; 336: 1541–1547.

698. Liem MSL, Van der Graaf Y, Zwart RC, Geurts I, van Vroonhaven TJMV. Risk factors for inguinal hernia in women: a case-controlled study. American Journal of Epidemiology 1997; 146: 721–726.

699. Lifschutz H, Juler GL. The inguinal darn. Archives of Surgery 1986; 121: 717–719.

700. Lister J. Note on the preparation of catgut for surgical purposes. British Medical Journal 1908; 1: 125–126.

701. Littré A. Observation sur une nouvelle espece de hernie. Histoire de l'Academie des Sciences (1700), Paris Mem., 300–310.

702. Lockwood CB. The radical cure of femoral and inguinal hernia. Lancet 1893; 2: 1297–1302.

703. Lockwood CB. The Radical Cure of Hernia, Hydrocele and Varicocele. Edinburgh and London: Young, 1898.

704. Loder R. A local anaesthetic solution with longer action. Lancet 1960; 2: 346–347.

705. Loftus IM, Rodgers PM, Ubhi SS, Watkin DFL. A negative herniogram does not exclude the presence of a hernia. Annals of the Royal College of Surgeons of England 1997; 79: 372–375.

706. Logan MT, Nottingham JM. Amyand's hernia: a case report of an incarcerated and perforated appendix within an inguinal hernia and review of the literature. American Surgeon 2001; 67: 628–629.

707. Loh A, Rajkumar JS, South LM. Anatomical repair of large incisional hernias. Annals of the Royal College of Surgeons of England 1992; 74: 100–105.

708. Londono-Schimmer EE, Leong APK, Phillips RKS. Life Table analysis of complications following colostomy. Diseases of the Colon and Rectum 1994; 37: 916–920.

709. Lorenz D, Stark E, Oestreich K, Richter A. Laparoscopic hernioplasty versus conventional hernioplasty (Shouldice): Results of a prospective randomized trial. World Journal of Surgery 2000; 24: 739–745.

710. Losanoff JE, Kjossev KT. Incarcerated spigelian hernia in morbidly obese patients: the role of intraoperative ultrasonography for hernia localization. Obesity Surgery 1997; 7: 211.

711. Lotheissen G. Zur Radikaloperation der Schenkel-hernien. Centralblatt für Chirurgie 1898; 21: 548–549.

712. Lubbers EJC, Devlin HB. The complications of a permanent ileostomy. Poster: 8th World Congress of Collegium Internationale Chirurgiae Digestivae, Amsterdam, 11–14 September, 1984.

713. Lucas-Championniere J. Chirurgie operatoire: Cure radicale des hernies; avec une etude statistique de deux cents soixante-quinze

operations et cinquante figures intercalees dans le texte. Paris: Rueff, 1892.

714. Luchs JS, Halpern D, Katz DS. Amyand's hernia: prospective CT diagnosis. Journal of Computer Assisted Tomography 2000; 24: 884–886.

715. Luijendijk RW, Hop WCJ, van den Tol P et al. A comparison of suture repair with mesh repair for incisional hernia. New England Journal of Medicine 2000; 343(6): 393–398.

716. Lung NG, Kit HK, Collins REC. Leiomyoma of the broad ligament in an obturator hernia presenting as a lump in the groin. Journal of the Royal Society of Medicine 1986; 79: 174–175.

717. Lynn HB, Johnson WW. Inguinal herniorrhaphy in children: a critical analysis of 1,000 cases. Archives of Surgery 1961; 83: 573.

718. Lytle WJ. Internal inguinal ring. British Journal of Surgery 1945; 32: 441–446.

719. Lytle WJ. Femoral hernia. Annals of the Royal College of Surgeons of England 1957; 21: 244–262.

720. Lytle WJ. The deep inguinal ring, development, function and repair. British Journal of Surgery 1970; 57: 531–536.

721. Maas SM, Vries Reilingh TS, van Goor H, de Jong D, Bleichrodt RP. Endoscopically assisted 'component separation technique' for the repair of complicated ventral hernias. Journal of the American College of Surgeons 2002; 194(3): 388–390.

722. Mabogunje OA, Grundy DJ, Lawrie JH. Orchidectomy in a rural African population. Transactions of the Royal Society of Tropical Medicine and Hygiene 1980; 74: 749–751.

723. MacArthur DC, Greive DC, Thompson JD, Greig JD, Nixon SJ. Herniography for groin pain of uncertain origin. British Journal of Surgery 1997; 84: 684–685.

724. MacEwen W. On the radical cure of oblique inguinal hernia by internal abdominal peritoneal pad and the restoration of the valved form of the inguinal canal. Annals of Surgery 1886; 4: 89–119.

725. MacFadyen BV, Arregui ME, Corbitt JD. Complications of laparoscopic herniorrhaphy. Surgical Endoscopy 1993; 7: 155–158.

726. Mack NK. The incidence of umbilical hernia in Africans. East African Medical Journal 1945; 22: 369.

727. MacKenzie JW. Daycase anaesthesia and anxiety: a study of anxiety profiles amongst patients attending a day bed unit. Anaesthesia 1989; 44: 437–440.

728. Maclennan A. The radical cure of inguinal hernia in children. British Journal of Surgery 1921–22; 9: 445–449.

729. MacLeod DAD, Gibbon WW. The sportsman's groin. British Journal of Surgery 1999; 86: 849–850.

730. Madden JL, Hakim S, Agorogiannis AB. The anatomy and repair of inguinal hernias. Surgical Clinics of North America 1971; 1269–1292.

731. Maddern GJ, Rudkin G, Bessell JR, Devitt P, Ponte L. A comparison of laparoscopic and open hernia repair as a day surgical procedure. Surgical Endoscopy 1994; 8: 1404–1408.

732. Magnus R. Late bowel obstruction due to kinking of the damaged loop following reduction of a strangulated hernia. British Journal of Surgery 1965; 52: 121–122.

733. Maguire J, Young D. Repair of epigastric incisional hernia. British Journal of Surgery 1976; 63: 125–127.

734. Maingot R. A further report on the 'keel' operation for large diffuse incisional hernias. The Medical Press 1958; 240: 989–993.

735. Maingot R. Abdominal Operations, 4th edn. New York: Appleton-Century-Crofts, 1961: 939.

736. Maingot R. Operations for sliding herniae and large herniae. British Journal of Clinical Practice 1961; 15: 993.

737. Mair GB. Preliminary report on the use of whole skin grafts as a substitute for fascial sutures in the treatment of herniae. British Journal of Surgery 1945; 32: 381–385.

738. Malycha P, Lovell G. Inguinal surgery in athletes with chronic groin pain: The 'sportsman's hernia'. Australian and New Zealand Journal of Surgery 1992; 62: 123–125.

739. Maniatis AG, Hunt CM. Therapy for spontaneous umbilical hernia rupture. American Journal of Gastroenterology 1995; 90: 310–312.

740. Manninen MJ, Lavonius M, Perhoniemi VJ. Results of incisional hernia repair. A retrospective study of 172 unselected hernioplasties. European Journal of Surgery 1991; 157: 29–31.

741. Marcy HO. A new use of carbolized catgut ligatures. Boston Medical Surgical Journal 1871; 85: 315–316.

742. Marcy HO. The cure of hernia. Journal of the American Medical Association 1887; 8: 589–592.

743. Marcy HO. Note on mortality after operation for large incarcerated hernia. Annals of Surgery 1900; 31: 65–74.

744. Margoles JS, Braun RA. Pre-peritoneal versus classical hernioplasty. American Journal of Surgery 1971; 121: 641–643.

745. Margotta R. An Illustrated History of Medicine. Lewis L, ed. English translation. Middlesex: Hamlyn, 1968.

746. Marks CG, Ritchie J. The complications of synchronous combined excision for adenocarcinoma of the rectum at St Mark's Hospital. British Journal of Surgery 1975; 62: 901–905.

747. Marsden AJ. Inguinal hernia: a three year review of one thousand cases. British Journal of Surgery 1958; 46: 234–243.

748. Marsden AJ. The results of inguinal hernia repairs: a problem of assessment. Lancet 1959; i: 461–462.

749. Marsden AJ. Inguinal hernia: a three year review of two thousand cases. British Journal of Surgery 1962; 49: 384–394.

750. Marshall FF, Leadbetter WF, Dretler SP. Ileal conduit parastomal hernias. Journal of Urology 1975; 113: 40–42.

751. Martin MC, Welch TP. Obturator hernia. British Journal of Surgery 1974; 61: 547–548.

752. Martin RE, Max CC. Primary inguinal hernia repair with prosthetic mesh. Hospimedica 1984; 1.

753. Martínez Insua C, Costa Pereira JM, Cardoso de Oliveira M. Obturator hernia: the plug technique. Hernia 2001; 5: 161–163.

754. Mason ML, Allen HS. The rate of healing of tendons: an experimental study of tensile strength. Annals of Surgery 1941; 113: 424.

755. Masso-Misse P, Hamadiko Y, Mbakop A, Yao GS, Malonga E. A rare complication of inguinal hernia. Evisceration by rupture of the scrotum secondary to blunt trauma of the abdomen. Journal de Chirugie 1994; 131: 212–213.

756. Matsuda T, Horii Y, Yoshida O. Unilateral obstruction of the vas deferens caused by childhood inguinal herniorrhaphy in male infertility patients. Fertility and Sterility 1992; 58: 609–613.

757. Matsumoto GM, Ise H, Inoue H, Ogawa H, Suzuki N, Matsuno S. Metastatic colon carcinoma found within an inguinal hernia sac: report of a case. Surgery Today 2000; 30: 74–77.

758. Mattson H. Use of rectus sheath and superior pubic ligament in direct and recurrent inguinal hernia. Surgery 1946; 19: 498–503.

759. Maydl C. Ueber retrograde Incarceration der Tuba und des Processus Vermiformis in Leisten und Schenkelhernien. Wiener Klinische Rundschau 1895; 9: 17–18 and 33–35.

760. Mayer AD, Ausobsky JR, Evans M, Pollock AV. Compression suture of the abdominal wall: a controlled trial in 302 major laparotomies. British Journal of Surgery 1981; 68: 632–634.

761. Mayo WJ. An operation for the radical cure of umbilical hernia. Annals of Surgery 1901; 31: 276–280.

762. Mayo WJ. Further experience with the vertical overlapping operation for the radical cure of umbilical hernia. Journal of the American Medical Association 1903; 41: 225–228.

763. McArdle G. Is inguinal hernia a defect in human evolution and would this insight improve concepts for methods of surgical repair. Clinical Anatomy 1997; 10: 47–55.

764. McArthur LL. Autoplastic suture in hernia and other diastases. Journal of the American Medical Association 1901; 37: 1162–1165.

765. McCarthy MP. Obturator hernia of the urinary bladder. Urology 1976; 7: 312–314.

766. McCarthy MC, Lemmon GW. Traumatic lumbar hernia: a seat belt injury. Journal of Trauma, Injury, Infection and Critical Care 1996; 40: 121–122.

767. McCleane G, Mackle E, Stirling I. The addition of triamcinalone acetonide to bupivacaine has no effect on the quality of analgesia produced by ilioinguinal nerve block. Anaesthesia 1994; 49: 819–820.

768. McDowell E. Quoted in Scharchner, A. Ephraim McDowell: Father of Ovariotomy and Father of Abdominal Surgery. Philadelphia: Lippincott, 1921.

769. McEntee GP, O'Carroll A, Mooney B, Egan TJ, Delaney PV. Timing of strangulation in adult hernias. British Journal of Surgery 1989; 76: 725–726.

770. McEvedy PG. Femoral hernia. Annals of the Royal College of Surgeons of England 1950; 7: 484–496.

771. McGavin L. The double filigree operation for the radical cure of inguinal hernia. British Medical Journal 1909; 2: 357–363.

772. McGregor D, Halverson K, McVay C. The unilateral pediatric inguinal hernia: should the contralateral side be explored? Journal of Pediatric Surgery 1980; 15: 313–317.

773. McKernan JB, Laws HL. Laparoscopic repair of inguinal hernias using a totally extraperitoneal prosthetic approach. Surgical Endoscopy 1993; 7: 26–28.

774. McLean AB. Spontaneous rupture of an umbilical hernia in an infant. British Journal of Surgery 1950; 37: 239.

775. McPherson K, Coulter A, Stratton I. Increasing use of private practice by patients in Oxford requiring common elective surgical operations. British Medical Journal 1985; 291: 797–799.

776. McVay CB. The anatomy of the relaxing incision in inguinal hernioplasty. Quarterly Bulletin of North West University Medical School 1962; 36: 245–252.

777. McVay CB. The normal and pathologic anatomy of the transversus abdominis muscle in inguinal and femoral hernia. Surgical Clinics of North America 1971; 51: 1251–1261.

778. McVay CB. The anatomic basis for inguinal and femoral hernioplasty. Surgery, Gynecology and Obstetrics 1974; 139: 931–945.

779. McVay CB, Anson BJ. Inguinal and femoral hernioplasty. Surgery, Gynecology and Obstetrics 1949; 88: 473–485.

780. McVay CB, Chapp JD. Inguinal and femoral hernioplasty. Annals of Surgery 1958; 148: 499–512.

781. Meckel JF. Ueber die Divertikel am Darmkanal. Archiv für die Physiologie 1809; 9: 421.

782. Medical Research Council Laparoscopic Groin Hernia Trial Group. Cost–utility analysis of open versus laparoscopic groin hernia repair: results from a multicentre randomized clinical trial. British Journal of Surgery 2001; 88: 653–661.

783. Meier DE, OlaOlorun DA, Omodele RA, Nkoi SK, Tarpley JL. Incidence of umbilical hernia in African children: redefinition of 'normal' and reevaluation of indications for repair. World Journal of Surgery 2001; 25: 645–648.

784. Melone JH, Schwartz MZ, Tyson KRT, Marr CC, Greenholz SK, Taub JE, Hough VJ. Outpatient inguinal herniorrhaphy in premature infants: is it safe? Journal of Pediatric Surgery 1992; 27: 203–208.

785. Menardi G, Saur H. Hodengangran als Komplikation der Inkarzeration der Säuglingshernie. Zeitschrift fur Kinderchirurgie 1975; 16: 421–425.

786. Metzger J, Lutz N, Laidlaw I. Guidelines for inguinal hernia repair in everday practice. Annals of the Royal College of Surgeons of England 2001; 83: 209–214.

787. Miki Y, Sumimura J, Hasegawa T et al. A new technique of laparoscopic obturator hernia repair: report of a case. Surgery Today 1998; 28: 652–656.

788. Mikkelsen WP, Berne CJ. Femoral hernioplasty: suprapubic extraperitoneal (Cheatle–Henry) approach. Surgery 1954; 35: 743–748.

789. Miklos JR, O'Reilly MJ, Saye WB. Sciatic hernia: a cause of chronic pelvic pain in women. Obstetrics and Gynecology 1998; 91(6): 998–1001.

790. Milamed DR, Hedley-White J. Contributions of the surgical sciences to a reduction of the mortality rate in the United States for the period 1968 to 1988. Annals of Surgery 1994; 219: 94–102.

791. Millat B, Fingerhut A, Gignoux M, Hay JM. The French Associations for Surgical Research. Factors associated with early discharge after inguinal hernia repair in 500 consecutive unselected patients. British Journal of Surgery 1993; 80: 1158–1160.

792. Miller AR, Van Heerden JA, Naessens JM, O'Brien PC. Simultaneous bilateral inguinal hernia repair: a case against conventional wisdom. Annals of Surgery 1991; 213: 272–276.

793. Milligan ETC. The inguinal route for radical cure of obturator hernia. British Medical Journal 1919; 2: 134–135.

794. Millikan KW, Cummings B, Doolas A. A prospective study of the mesh-plug hernioplasty. American Surgeon 2001; 67: 285–289.

795. Millikan KW, Deziel DJ. The management of hernia: considerations in cost-effectiveness. Surgical Clinics of North America 1996; 76: 105–116.

796. Miltenburg DM, Nuchern JG, Jaksic T et al. Meta-analysis of the risk of metachronous hernia in infants and children. American Journal of Surgery 1997; 174: 741–744.

797. Misra D. Inguinal hernias in premature babies: wait or operate. Acta Paediatrica 2001; 90: 370–371.

798. Misra D, Hewitt G, Potts SR et al. Inguinal herniotomy in young infants, with emphasis on premature neonates. Journal of Pediatric Surgery 1994; 29: 1496–1498.

799. Moiniche S, Mikkelsen S, Wetterslev J, Dahl JB. A qualitative systematic review of incisional local anaesthesia for postoperative pain relief after abdominal operations. British Journal of Anaesthesia 1998; 81: 377–383.

800. Montagu AMF. A case of familial inheritance of oblique inguinal hernia. Journal of Heredity 1942; 33: 355–356.

801. Montupet P, Esposito C. Laparoscopic treatment of congenital inguinal hernia in children. Journal of Pediatric Surgery 1999; 34(3): 420–423.

802. Moore CA. Hypertrophic fibrosis of the gut causing chronic obstruction: a sequel to a strangulated hernia. British Journal of Surgery 1913; 1: 361–365.

803. Moore CR, Oslund R. Experiments on sheep testis, cryptorchidism, vasectomy and scrotal insulation. American Journal of Physiology 1924; 67: 595–607.

804. Morales-Conde S. Personal communication, 2001.

805. Moreno IG. Chronic eventuation and large hernias. Surgery 1947; 22: 945–953.

806. Moreno-Egea A, Lirón R, Girela E, Aguayo JL. Laparoscopic repair of ventral and incisional hernias using a new composite mesh (Parietex). Surgery, Laparoscopy, Endoscopy and Percutaneous Technology 2001; 11(2): 103–106.

807. Morgan M, Beech R, Reynolds A, Swan AV, Devlin HB. Surgeons' view of day surgery: is there a consensus among providers. Journal of Public Health Medicine 1992; 14: 192–198.

808. Morgan M, Paul E, Devlin HB. Lengths of stay for three common surgical procedures: variations between districts. British Journal of Surgery 1987; 74: 884–889.

809. Morris D, Ward AWM, Handyside AJ. Early discharge after hernia repair. Lancet 1968; 1: 681–685.

810. Morris GE, Jarrett PEM. Recurrence rates following local anaesthetic day case inguinal hernia repair by junior surgeons in a DGH. Annals of the Royal College of Surgeons of England 1987; 69: 97–99.

811. Morris JM. The syndrome of testicular feminization in male pseudohermaphrodites. American Journal of Obstetrics and Gynecology 1953; 65: 1192–1211.

812. Morrison AS. Cryptorchidism, hernia and cancer of the testis. Journal of the National Cancer Institute 1976; 56: 731–733.

813. Morris-Stiff G, Coles G, Moore R, Jurewicz A, Lord R. Abdominal wall hernia in autosomal dominant polycystic kidney disease. British Journal of Surgery 1997; 84: 615–617.

814. Morton NS, Raine PAM. Paediatric Day Case Surgery. Oxford: Oxford University Press, 1995.

815. Moschowitz AV. Femoral hernia: a new operation for radical cure. New York Journal of Medicine 1907; 396–400.

816. Moschowitz AV. The rational treatment of sliding hernia. American Journal of Surgery 1966; 112: 52.

817. Moss CM, Levine R, Messenger N, Dardik I. Sliding colonic Maydl's hernia: report of a case. Diseases of the Colon and Rectum 1976; 19: 636–638.

818. Moure P, Martin R. Le role du ligament du foie dans les hernies epigastrique et ombilicales douloureuses. Bulletin et Memoires de la Societe Nationale de Chirurgie (19••); 59: 1011–1017.

819. Moynihan BGA. The ritual of a surgical operation. British Journal of Surgery 1920; 8: 27–35.

820. Mozingo DW, Walters MJ, Otchy DP, Rosenthal D. Properitoneal synthetic mesh repair of recurrent inguinal hernias. Surgery, Gynecology and Obstetrics 1992; 174: 33–35.

821. MRC Laparoscopic Groin Hernia Trial Group. Laparoscopic versus open repair of groin hernia: a randomised comparison. Lancet 1999; 354: 185–190.

822. Mudge M, Harding KG, Hughes LE. Incisional hernia. British Journal of Surgery 1986; 73: 82.

823. Mudge M, Hughes LE. Incisional hernia and post-thrombotic syndrome – an observed association. Annals of the Royal College of Surgeons of England 1984; 66: 351–352.

824. Mudge M, Hughes LE. Incisional hernia: a ten year prospective study of incidence and attitudes. British Journal of Surgery 1985; 72: 70–71.

825. Mufid MM, Abu-Yousef MM, Kakish ME et al. Spigelian hernia: diagnosis by high-resolution real-time ultrasonography. Journal of Ultrasound Medicine 1997; 16: 183.

826. Murdoch RWG. Testicular strangulation from incarcerated inguinal hernia in infants. Journal of the Royal College of Surgeons of Edinburgh 1979; 24: 97–101.

827. Muschaweck U. Umbilical hernia – How to do it! The Munich method. Presented at the combined meeting of the American and European Hernia Societies, Toronto, Canada, 2000.

828. Muschaweck U. Plug repair of inguinal hernia: indications, techniques, and results. In: Fitzgibbons and Greenburg, eds. Hernia. New York: Lippincott Williams and Wilkins, 2001: 163–172.

829. Musella M, Milone F, Chello M, Angelini P, Jovino R. Magnetic resonance imaging and abdominal wall hernias in aortic surgery. Journal of the American College of Surgeons 2001; 1993: 392–395.

830. Musgrove JE, McReady FJ. The Henry approach to femoral hernia. Surgery 1949; 26: 608–611.

831. Myers B, Rightor M, Donovan W. Inguinal hernia repair: an experimental model in the rat to evaluate technical factors. Archives of Surgery 1981; 116: 463–465.

832. Myers RN, Shearburn EW. The problem of recurrent inguinal hernia. Surgical Clinics of North America 1973; 53: 555–558.

833. Mynors JM. A large lumbar hernia. British Journal of Surgery 1955; 42: 554–555.

834. Nagahama T, Nakashima A, Ashikawa T et al. Obturator hernia diagnosed by herniography. In: Arregui ME, Nagan RF, eds. Inguinal Hernia: Advances or Controversies? Oxford: Radcliffe Medical Press, 1994: 333–341.

835. Narath A. Ueber eine Eigenartige Form von Hernia Cruralis (prevascularis) im Anschlusse an die unblutige Behandlung angeborener Hüftgelenksverrenkung. Archiv für Klinische Chirurgie 1899; 59: 396–424.

836. National Centre For Health Statistics. Health Interview responses compared with medical records. Health Statistics from the US. National Health Survey Series D. Washington DC: US Dept of Health, Education and Welfare, 1961.

837. National Confidential Enquiry into Perioperative Deaths. London, 1995.

838. National Institute for Clinical Excellence: Technology Appraisal Guidance No. 18. Guidance on the use of laparoscopic surgery for inguinal hernia. London, UK.

839. Naude GP, Ocon S, Bongard F. Femoral hernia: the dire consequences of a missed diagnosis. American Journal of Emergency Medicine 1997; 15: 680–682.

840. Naylor J. Combination of Spigelian and Richter's hernias: a case report. The American Surgeon 1978; 44: 750–752.

841. Nayak RN. Malignant mucocele of the appendix in a femoral hernia. Postgraduate Medical Journal 1974; 50: 24, 249.

842. Neuhauser D. Elective inguinal herniorrhaphy versus truss in the elderly. In: Bunker JP, Barnes BA, Mosteller F, eds. Costs, Risks and Benefits of Surgery. New York: Oxford University Press, 1977: 223–229.

843. Neutra RR. See Neuhauser (1977).

844. Nichol JH. The surgery of infancy. British Medical Journal 1909; 2: 753–754.

845. Nicholl JP, Beeby NR, Williams BT. Comparison of the activity of short stay independent hospitals in England and Wales, 1981 and 1986. British Medical Journal 1989; 298: 239–242.

846. Nicholls JC. Necessity into choice: an appraisal of inguinal herniorrhaphy under local anaesthesia. Annals of the Royal College of Surgeons of England 1977; 59: 124–127.

847. Nicholson S, Keane TE, Devlin HB. Femoral hernia: an avoidable sense of surgical mortality. British Journal of Surgery 1990; 77: 307–308.

848. Nielsen DF, Bulow S. The incidence of male hermaphroditism in girls with inguinal hernia. Surgery, Gynecology and Obstetrics 1976; 142: 875–876.

849. Nilsson E, Kald A, Anderberg B et al. Hernia surgery in a defined population: a prospective three year audit. European Journal of Surgery 1997; 163: 823–829.

850. Nilsson F, Anderberg B, Bragmark M et al. Hernia surgery in a defined population: improvements possible in outcome and cost-effectiveness. Ambulatory Surgery 1993; 1: 150–153.

851. Normington EY, Franklin DP, Brotman SI. Constriction of the femoral vein after McVay inguinal hernia repair. Surgery 1992; 111: 343–347.

852. Nussbaum A. Ein einfaches Hilfsmittel bei der Reposition der Säuglinge. München Medizinische Wochenschrift 1913; 60: 1434.

853. Nyhus L. Ubiquitous use of prosthetic mesh in inguinal hernia repair: the dilemma. Hernia 2000; 4: 184–186.

854. Nyhus LM, Condon RE, Harkins HN. Clinical experiences with pre-peritoneal hernial repair for all types of hernia of the groin. American Journal of Surgery 1960; 100: 234–244.

855. Nyhus LM, Donohue PE. Groin hernia repair: past, present and future. Problems in General Surgery 1995; 12: 7–11.

856. Nyhus LM, Harkins HN. Hernia. London: Pitman Medical/Philadelphia; Lippincott, 1965. Also ibid., 2nd edn., Condon RE, ed. Philadelphia: Lippincott, 1978.

857. Nyhus LM, Pollak R, Bombeck T, Donahue PE. The preperitoneal approach and prosthetic buttress repair for recurrent hernia: the evolution of a technique. Annals of Surgery 1988; 208: 733–737.

858. O'Donnell KA, Glick PL, Caty MG. Pediatric umbilical problems. Pediatric Clinics of North America 1998; 45: 791–799.

859. O'Donoghue PD. Strangulation of an ulcerated incisional hernia. British Journal of Surgery 1955; 43: 329–330.

860. O'Riordan DC, Kingsnorth AN. Audit of patient outcomes after herniorrhaphy. Surgical Clinics of North America 1998; 78: 1129–1139.

861. Oakley MJ, Smith JS, Anderson JR, Fenton-Lee, D. Randomized placebo-controlled trial of local anaesthetic infusion in day-case inguinal hernia repair. British Journal of Surgery 1998; 85: 797–799.

862. Obney N. Hydroceles of the testicle complicating inguinal hernias. Journal of the Canadian Medical Association 1956; 75: 733–736.

863. Obney N. An analysis of 192 consecutive cases of incisional hernia. Journal of the Canadian Medical Association 1957; 77: 463–469.

864. Ogilvie H. Hernia. London: Edward Arnold, 1959.

865. Ogundiran TO, Ayantunde AA, Akute OO. Spontaneous rupture of incisional hernia – a case report. West African Journal of Medicine 2001; 20: 176–178.

866. Okada T, Yoshida H, Iwai J, Matsunaga T, Ohtsuka Y, Kouchi K, Ohnuma N. Strangulated umbilical hernia in a child: report of a case. Surgery Today 2001; 31: 546–549.

867. Ollero Fresno JC, Alvarez M, Sanchez M. Femoral hernia in childhood: review of 38 cases. Pediatric Surgery International 1997; 12: 520–521.

868. Onukak EE, Grundy DJ, Lawrie JH. Hernia In Northern Nigeria. Journal of the Royal College of Surgeons of Edinburgh 1983; 28: 147–150.

869. Ordonez NG, Ro JV, Ayala AG. Lesions described as nodular mesothelial hyperplasia are primarily composed of histiocytes. American Journal of Surgical Pathology 1998; 22: 285–292.

870. Orr KB. Perforated appendix in an inguinal hernial sac: Amyand's hernia. Medical Journal of Australia 1993; 159: 762–763.

871. Ortiz H, Sara MJ, Armedariz M, de Miguel M, Marti J, Chocarro C. Does the frequency of para-colostomy hernias depend on the position of the colostomy in the abdominal wall? International Journal of Colorectal Disease 1994; 9: 65–67.

872. Oudesluys-Murphy AM, Teng HT, Boxma H. Spontaneous regression of clinical inguinal hernias in preterms female infants. Journal of Pediatric Surgery 2000; 35: 1220–1221.

873. Owings EP, Georgeson KE. A new technique for laparoscopic explorations to find contralateral patent processus vaginalis. Surgical Endoscopy 2000; 14: 114–116.

874. Page CM, Edwards H, Lloyd Williamson JCF, Parker GE, Badenoch AW, Wright AD, Heritage K. Discussion on hernia. Proceedings of the Royal Society of Medicine 1942; 36: 185–189.

875. Paillier JL, Baranger B, Darrieu H, Schill H, Neveux Y. Clinical analysis of expanded PTFE in the treatment of recurrent and complex groin hernias. Postgraduate Medical Journal 1992; 4: 168–170.

876. Pajotin P. Laparoscopic groin hernia repair using a curved prosthesis without fixation. Journal de Coelio-Chirurgie 1998; 28: 64–68.

877. Palmer BV. Incarcerated inguinal hernia in children. Annals of the Royal College of Surgeons of England 1978; 60: 121–124.

878. Palot JP, Avisse C, Cailliez-Tomasi JP, Greffler D, Flament JB. The mesh plug repair of groin hernias: a three year experience. Hernia 1998; 2: 31–34.

879. Palot JP, Flament JB, Avisse C et al. Utilisation des prothèses dans les conditions de la chirurgie d'urgence. Chirurgie 1996; 121: 48–50.

880. Palumbo LT, Sharp WS. Primary inguinal hernioplasty in the adult. Surgical Clinics of North America 1971; 51: 1293–1308.

881. Pananini AM, Lezoche E, Carle F et al. A randomized, controlled, clinical study of laparoscopic vs open tension-free inguinal hernia repair. Surgical Endoscopy 1998; 12: 979–986.

882. Panos RG, Beck DE, Maresh JF, Harford FJ. Preliminary results of a prospective randomized study of Cooper's ligament versus Shouldice herniorrhaphy technique. Surgery, Gynecology and Obstetrics 1992; 175: 315–319.

883. Pans A, Desaive C, Jacquet N. Use of a preperitoneal prosthesis for strangulated groin hernia. British Journal of Surgery 1997; 84: 310–312.

884. Pans A, Pierard GE, Albert A. Adult groin hernias: new insight into their biomechanical characteristics. European Journal of Clinical Investigation 1997; 27: 863–868.

885. Papagrigoriadis S, Browse DJ, Howard ER. Incarceration of umbilical hernia in children: a rare but important complication. Pediatric Surgery International 1998; 14: 231–232.

886. Park A, Birch DW, Lovrics P et al. Laparoscopic and open incisional hernia repair: a comparison study. Surgery 1998; 124: 816–822.

887. Park A, Gagner M, Pomp A. Laparoscopic repair of large incisional hernias. Surgical Laparoscopy and Endoscopy 1996; 6(2): 123–128.

888. Partrick DA, Bensard DD, Karrer FM et al. Is routine pathological evaluation of pediatric hernia sacs justified? Journal of Pediatric Surgery 1998; 33: 1090–1094.

889. Paterson-Brown S, Dudley HAF. Knotting in continuous mass closure of the abdomen. British Journal of Surgery 1986; 73: 676–680.

890. Payne JH, Grininger LM, Izawa MT, Podoll EF, Lindahl PJ, Balfour J. Laparoscopic or open inguinal herniorrhaphy? A randomised prospective trial. Archives of Surgery 1994; 129: 973–981.

891. Peacock EE. Here we are: behind again! American Journal of Surgery 1989; 157: 187.

892. Peacock EE, Madden JW. Studies on the biology and treatment of recurrent inguinal hernia: 11. Morphological changes. Annals of Surgery 1974; 179: 567–571.

893. Pearl RK, Prasad ML, Orsay CP, Abcarian H, Tan AB, Melzl MT. Early local complications from intestinal stomas. Archives of Surgery 1985; 120: 1145.

894. Pearl RK, Prasad ML, Orsay CP, Abcarian H, Tan AB. A survey of technical considerations in the construction of intestinal stomas. Annals of Surgery 1988; 51: 462–465.

895. Pearse HE. Strangulated hernia reduced en masse. Surgery, Gynecology and Obstetrics 1931; 53: 822–828.

896. Pedersen VM, Jensen BS, Hansen B. Skin closure in abdominal incisions: continuous nylon suture versus Steristrip tape suture. Acta Chirurgica Scandinavica 1981; 147: 619–622.

897. Peevy KJ, Speed FA, Hoff CJ. Epidemiology of inguinal hernia in pre-term neonates. Paediatrics 1986; 77: 246–247.

898. Pelissier EP, Blum D. The plug method in inguinal hernia: prospective evaluation of postoperative pain and disability. Hernia 1997; 1: 185–189.

899. Pelosa OA, Wilkinson LH. The chain stitch knot. Surgery, Gynecology and Obstetrics 1974; 139: 599–600.

900. Pemberton J, De J, Curry FS. The symptomatology of epigastric hernia: analysis of 296 cases. Minnesota Medicine 1936; 19: 109–112.

901. Percival WL. Ureter within a sliding inguinal hernia. Canadian Journal of Surgery 1983; 26: 283–286.

902. Pergament E, Himler A, Shah P. Testicular feminisation and inguinal hernia. Lancet 1973; 2: 740–741.

903. Perlstein J, DuBois JJ. The role of laparoscopy in the management of suspected recurrent pediatric hernias. Journal of Pediatric Surgery 2000; 35: 1205–1208.

904. Pescovitz MO. Umbilical hernia repair in patients with cirrhosis. No evidence for increased evidence of variceal bleeding. Annals of Surgery 1984; 199–325.

905. Petros JG, Rimm EB, Robillard RJ, Argy O. Factors influencing postoperative urinary retention in patients undergoing elective inguinal herniorrhaphy. American Journal of Surgery 1991; 161: 421–423.

906. Phelps S, Agrawal M. Morbidity after neonatal inguinal herniotomy. Journal of Pediatric Surgery 1997; 32: 445–447.

907. Philip PJ. Afferent limb internal strangulation in obstructed inguinal hernia. British Journal of Surgery 1967; 54: 96–99.

908. Phillips EH, Carroll BJ, Fallas MJ. Laparoscopic preperitoneal inguinal hernia repair without peritoneal incision: technique and early clinical results. Surgical Endoscopy 1993; 7: 159–162.

909. Phillips P, Pringle W, Evans C, Keighley M. Analysis of hospital based stomatherapy service. Annals of the Royal College of Surgeons of England 1985; 67: 37–40.

910. Picchio M, Lombardi A, Zolovkins A, Mihelsons M, La Torre G. Tension-free laparoscopic and open hernia repair: randomized controlled trial of early results. World Journal of Surgery 1999; 23: 1004–1009.

911. Pickford IR, Brennan SS, Evans M, Pollock AV. Two methods of skin closure in abdominal operations: a controlled clinical trial. British Journal of Surgery 1983; 70: 226–228.

912. Pollack HM, Popky GL, Blumberg ML. Hernias of the ureter: an anatomic roentgenographic study. Radiology 1975; 117: 275.

913. Ponka JL. Hernias of the Abdominal Wall. Philadelphia: WB Saunders, 1980.

914. Ponka JL. Spigelian hernias. In: Joseph K, Ponka MD, eds. Hernias of the Abdominal Wall. Philadelphia: WB Saunders, 1980: 478.

915. Ponka JL, Brush BE. Problems of femoral hernia. Archives of Surgery 1971; 102: 417–423.

916. Ponka JL, Brush BE. Experiences with the repair of groin hernia in 200 patients aged 70 or older. Journal of the American Geriatrics Society 1974; 22: 18–24.

917. Ponka JL, Sapala JA. Bupivacaine as a local anaesthetic for hernia repair. Henry Ford Hospital Medical Journal 1976; 24: 31.

918. Popp LW. Endoscopic patch repair of inguinal hernia in a female patient. Surgical Endoscopy 1990; 5: 10–12.

919. Popp LW. Improvement in endoscopic hernioplasty: transcutaneous aquadissection of the musculo fascial defect and preperitoneal endoscopic patch repair. Journal of Laparoendoscopic Surgery 1991; 1(2): 83–90.

920. Porcheron J, Payan B, Balique JG. Mesh repair of paracolostomal hernia by laparoscopy. Surgical Endoscopy 1998; 12: 1281.

921. Pories WJ. Personal communication, 1983.

922. Pott P. Treatise on Ruptures. London: Hitch and Hawes, 1757.

923. Powell J. All on our own: away from the district hospital. Journal of One-Day Surgery 1995; 2: 11.

924. Powers JH. Early ambulation: its influence on post-operative complications and return to work following hernioplasty in a rural population. Annals of the New York Academy of Sciences 1954; 524–535.

925. Prian GW, Sawyer RB, Sawyer KC. Repair of peristomal colostomy hernias. American Journal of Surgery 1975; 130: 694–696.

926. Primatesta P, Goldacre MJ. Inguinal hernia repair: incidence of elective and emergency surgery, readmission and mortality. International Journal of Epidemiology 1996; 25: 835–839.

927. Puri P, Guiney EJ, O'Donnell B. Inguinal hernia in infants: the fate of the testis following incarceration. Journal of Pediatric Surgery 1984; 19: 44–46.

928. Pye JK, Wijewardane PA, Crumplin MKH. Skin discolouration following inguinal hernia repair. British Journal of Surgery 1987; 74: 1171–1173.

929. Quagliarello J, Coppa G, Bigelow B. Isolated endometriosis in an inguinal hernia. American Journal of Obstetrics and Gynecology 1985; 152: 688–689.

930. Quill DS, Devlin HB, Plant JA, Denham KR, McNay RA, Morris D. Surgical operations rates: a twelve year experience in Stockton-on-Tees. Annals of the Royal College of Surgeons of England 1983; 65: 248–253.

931. Qvist G. Saddlebag hernia. British Journal of Surgery 1977; 64: 442–444.

932. Radcliffe G, Stringer MD. Reappraisal of femoral hernia in children. British Journal of Surgery 1997; 84: 58–60.

933. Rains AJH. Contribution to the principles of the surgery of inguinal hernia. British Journal of Surgery 1951; 39: 211.

934. Rajput A, Gauderer MWL, Hack M. Inguinal hernias in very low birth weight infants: incidence and timing of repair. Journal of Pediatric Surgery 1992; 27: 1322–1324.

935. Ralph-Edwards A, Maziak D, Deitel M, Thompson DA, Kucey DS, Bayley TA. Sudden rupture of an indirect inguinal hernial sac with extravasation in two patients on continous ambulatory peritoneal dialysis. Canadian Journal of Surgery 1994; 37: 70–72.

936. Ralphs DNL, Cannon SR, Bolton JB. Skin closure of inguinal herniorrhaphy wounds in short stay patients. British Journal of Surgery 1982; 69: 341–342.

937. Ramayya GR. Volvulus of an ileal conduit in an inguinal hernia. British Journal of Surgery 1984; 71: 637.

938. Ramirez OM, Ruas E, Dellon AL. 'Components separation' method for closure of abdominal wall defects: an anatomic and clinical study. Plastic and Reconstructive Surgery 1990; 86: 519–526.

939. Ramshaw BJ, Escartia P, Schwab J et al. Comparison of laparoscopic and open ventral herniorrhaphy. American Surgeon 1999; 65: 827–832.

940. Rath AM, Chevrel JP. The healing of laparotomies: review of the literature. Part 1. Hernia 1998; 2: 145–149.

941. Ravitch MM, Ventral hernia. Surgical Clinics of North America 1971; 51: 1341–1346.

942. Ray IA, Doddi N, Regula D, Williams JA, Melveger A. Polydioxanone (PDS) a novel monofilament synthetic absorbable suture. Surgery, Gynecology and Obstetrics 1981; 153: 497–507.

943. Read RC. Attenuation of the rectus sheath in inguinal herniation. American Journal of Surgery 1970; 120: 610–614.

944. Read RC. Marcy's priority in the development of inguinal herniorraphy. Surgery 1980; 88: 682–685.

945. Read RC. Can relaxing rectus sheath incision predispose to recurrent direct inguinal hernia? Archives of Surgery 1981; 116: 1493.

946. Read RC. The development of inguinal herniorrhaphy. Surgical Clinics of North America 1984; 64: 185–196.

947. Read RC. Cooper's Posterior lamina of transversalis fascia. Surgery, Gynecology and Obstetrics 1992; 174: 426–434.

948. Read RC. Metabolic factors contributing to herniation: a review. Hernia 1998; 2: 51–55.

949. Read RC, Schaefer RF. Lipoma of the spermatic cord, fatty herniorraphy, liposarcoma. Hernia 2000; 4: 149–154.

950. Read RC, White HJ. Inguinal herniation 1777–1977. American Journal of Surgery 1978; 136: 651–654.

951. Reardon PR, Preciado A, Scarborough T, Matthews B, Marti JL. Hernia at 5-mm laparoscopic port site presenting as early postoperative small bowel obstruction. Journal of Laparoscopy and Advanced Surgical Technique 1999; 9(6): 523–525.

952. Reid I, Devlin HB. Testicular atrophy as a consequence of inguinal hernia repair. British Journal of Surgery 1994; 81: 91–93.

953. Reinhard W. Surgical treatment of infantile hernia. Archiv für Klinische Chirurgie 1939; 195: 678–681.

954. Reinhoff WF Jr. The use of the rectus fascia for closure of the lower or critical angle of the wound in the repair of inguinal hernia. Surgery 1940; 8: 326–339.

955. Reynolds RD. Intestinal perforation from trauma to an inguinal hernia. Archives of Family Medicine 1995; 4: 972–974.

956. Richter A. Abhandlung von den Brüchen. Göttingen; I.C. Dietrich, 1785.

957. Rider MA, Baker DM, Locker A, Fawcett AN. Return to work after inguinal hernia repair. British Journal of Surgery 1993; 80: 745–746.

958. Ries E. Some radical changes in the after treatment of celiotomy cases. Journal of the American Medical Association 1899; 33: 454–459.

959. Rignault DP. Properitoneal prosthetic inguinal hernioplasty through a Pfannenstiel approach. Surgery, Gynecology and Obstetrics 1986; 163: 465–468.

960. Robbins AW, Rutkow IM. The mesh-plug herniaplasty. Surgical Clinics of North America 1993; 73: 501–511.

961. Robbins AW, Rutkow IM. Mesh plug repair and groin hernia surgery. Surgical Clinics of North America 1998; 78: 1007–1023.

962. Robertson GSM, Hayes IG, Burton PR. How long do patients convalesce after inguinal hernioplasty? Current principles and practice. Annals of the Royal College of Surgeons of England 1993; 75: 30–33.

963. Robin AP. Epigastric hernia. In: Nyhus LM, Condon RE, eds. Hernia, 4th edn. Philadelphia: Lippincott, 1995.

964. Rockwell E. Out-patient repair of inguinal hernia. American Journal of Surgery 1982; 143: 559–560.

965. Rodighiero D, Fusato G, Omodei Sale S et al. Surgical anatomy, diagnosis and treatment of Spigelian hernia. Giornale di Chirurgia 1996; 17: 485.

966. Rogers DA, Hattey RM, Howell CG. A prospective, randomized comparison of traditional and laparoscopic inguinal exploration in children. American Surgeon 1998; 64: 119–121.

967. Rogers FB, Camp PC. A strangulated Spigelian hernia mimicking diverticulitis. Hernia 2001; 5: 51–52.

968. Rosai J, Dehner LP. Nodular mesothelial hyperplasia in hernia sacs. A benign reactive condition simulating a neoplastic process. Cancer 1975; 35: 165–175.

969. Rosai J. Ackerman's Surgical Pathology, 6th edn, vol. 2. St Louis: Mosby, 1981.

970. Rose E, Santull TV. Sliding appendiceal inguinal hernia. Surgery, Gynecology and Obstetrics 1978; 146: 626–627.

971. Rosen M, Garcia-Ruiz A, Malm J, Mayes JT, Steiger E, Ponsky J. Laparoscopic hernia repair enhances early return of physical work capacity. Surgical Laparoscopy, Endoscopy and Percutaneous Techniques 2001; 11(1): 28–33.

972. Rosin J, Bonardi RA. Paracolostomy hernia repair with Marlex mesh: a new technique. Diseases of the Colon and Rectum 1977; 20(4): 299–302.

973. Roslyn JJ, Stable BE, Rangeneath C. Cancer in inguinal and femoral hernias. American Surgeon 1980; 46: 358–362.

974. Ross APJ. Incidence of inguinal hernia recurrence: effect of time off work after repair. Annals of the Royal College of Surgeons of England 1975; 57: 326–328.

975. Roth JS, Park AE, Witzke D, Mastrangelo MJ. Laparoscopic incisional/ventral herniorrhaphy: a five year experience. Hernia 1999; 4: 209–214.

976. Rowe MI, Copelson LW, Clatworthy HW. The patent processus vaginalis and the inguinal hernia. Journal of Pediatric Surgery 1969; 4: 102–107.

977. Rowe MI, O'Neill JA, Grosfeld JL et al. Disorders of the umbilicus. In: Essentials of Pediatric Surgery. St Louis: Mosby, 1995; 444–445.

978. Royal College of General Practitioners, OPCS. 1981–82. Morbidity Statistics from General Practice. Third National Study. London: HMSO, 1986.

979. Royal College of General Practitioners: Royal College of Surgeons of England. Clinical Guidelines for the Management of Groin Hernia in Adults. London: RCGP, 1997.

980. Royal College of Surgeons of England. Guidelines for Day Case Surgery, 1985.

981. Royal College of Surgeons of England. Guidelines for Day Case Surgery, 1992.

982. Royal College of Surgeons of England. Clinical Guidelines for the management of groin hernias in adults. London, 1993.

983. Rubin M, Schoetz DJ, Matthews JB. Parastomal hernia: is the stoma relocation superior to fascial repair? Archives of Surgery 1994; 129: 413–419.

984. Ruckley CV. Day care and short stay surgery for hernia. British Journal of Surgery 1978; 65: 1–4.

985. Ruckley CV, Cuthbertson C, Fenwick N, Prescott RJ, Garraway WM. Day care after operations for hernia or varicose veins: a controlled trial. British Journal of Surgery 1978; 65: 456–459.

986. Ruge, 1908. Cited in Rauber's Lehrbuch der Anatomie des Menschen, Kopsch FR. Abt 5; Nervensystem: 388, 1920.

987. Russell H. The saccular theory of hernia and the radical operation. Lancet 1906; 3: 1197–1203.

988. Russell IT, Devlin HB, Fell M, Glass NJ, Newell DJ. Day case surgery for hernias and haemorrhoids. Lancet 1977; 1: 844–847.

989. Rutkow I. A selective history of groin herniorrhaphy in the 20th century. Surgical Clinics North America 1993; 73: 395–411.

990. Rutkow I. Surgery, An Illustrated History. St Louis: Mosby, 1993.

991. Rutkow IM. The recurrence rate in hernia surgery: how important is it? Archives of Surgery 1995; 130: 575–577.

992. Rutkow IM, Robbins AW. Mesh plug technique for recurrent groin herniorrhaphy: a nine year experience or 407 patients. Surgery 1998; 124: 844–847.

993. Rutkow IM, Robbins AW. Demographic, classificatory, and socio-economic aspects of hernia repair in the United States. Surgical Clinics of North America 1993; 73: 413–426.

994. Rutkow IM, Robbins AW. Groin hernia. In: Cameron BC, ed. Current Surgical Therapy. London: Marcel Decker, 1995: 481–486.

995. Rutkow IM, Robbins AW. Hernia repair: the mesh plug hernia repair. In: Carter D, Russell RCG, Pitt HA, eds. Atlas of General Surgery, 3rd edn. London and New York: Chapman and Hall Medical, 1996: 59–67.

996. Rutkow IM, Robbins AW. Mesh plug repair: a follow-up report. Surgery 1995: 117: 597–598.

997. Rutkow IM, Robbins AW. Mesh plug repair and groin hernia surgery. Surgical Clinics of North America 1998; 78(6): 1007–1023.

998. Rutkow IM. Epidemiologic, economic, and sociologic aspects of hernia surgery in the United States in the 1990s. Surgical Clinics of North America 1998; 78: 941–951.

999. Rutkow IM, Robbins AW. Open mesh plug hernioplasty. Problems in General Surgery 1995; 12: 121–127.

1000. Rutledge RH. Cooper's ligament repair for adult groin hernias. Surgery 1980; 87: 601–610.

1001. Rutledge RH. Technique for all groin hernias in adults. Surgery 1988; 103: 1–10.

1002. Rutledge RH. Theodor Billroth: a century later. Surgery 1995; 118: 36–43.

1003. Rutten P, Ledecq M, Hoebeke Y, Roeland A, van den Oever R, Croes I. Hernie inguinal primaire: hernioplastie ambulatoire selon Lichtenstein: premiers resultats cliniques et implications economiques etude des 130 premiers cas operes. Acta Chirurgica Belgica 1992; 92: 168–171.

1004. Ryan EA. An analysis of 313 consecutive cases of indirect sliding inguinal hernias. Surgery, Gynecology and Obstetrics 1956; 102: 45–58.

1005. Ryan EA. Hernias related to pelvic fractures. Surgery Gynecology and Obstetrics 1971; 133: 440–446.

1006. Ryan WJ. Hernia of the vermiform appendix. Annals of Surgery 1937; 105: 135.

1007. Saha SP, Rao N, Stephenson SE Jr. Complications of colostomy. Diseases of the Colon and Rectum 1973; 16: 515–516.

1008. Salcedo-Wasicek CM, Thirlby RC. Postoperative course after inguinal herniorrhaphy: a case-controlled comparison of patients receiving worker's compensation vs patients with commercial insurance. Archives of Surgery 1995; 130: 29–32.

1009. Salerno GM, Fitzgibbons RJ, Filipi C. Laparoscopic inguinal hernia repair. In: Zucker KA, ed. Surgical Laparoscopy. St Louis: Quality Medical Publishing, 1991: 281–293.

1010. Salter RB. Innominate osteotomy in the treatment of dislocation and subluxation of the hip. Journal of Bone and Joint Surgery 1961; 43-B: 518–539.

1011. Sanchez-Montes I, Deysine M. Spigelian hernias. Archives of Surgery 1998; 133: 670–672.

1012. Sandblom P. The tensile strength of healing wounds. Acta Chirurgica Scandinavica 1944; suppl. 89–90: 1.

1013. Santora TA, Roslyn JJ. Incisional hernia. Surgical Clinics of North America 1993; 73: 557–570.

1014. Sarli L, Iusco DR, Sansebastiano G, Costi R. Simultaneous repair of bilateral inguinal hernias. Surgical Laparoscopy, Endoscopy and Percutaneous Techniques 2001; 11(4): 262–267.

1015. Savatguchi S, Matsunaga E, Honna T. A genetic study on indirect inguinal hernia. Japanese Journal of Human Genetics 1975; 20: 187–195.

1016. Scales JT. Discussion on metals and synthetic materials in relation to soft tissues: tissue reactions to synthetic materials. Proceedings of the Royal Society of Medicine 1953; 46: 647.

1017. Scarpa A. Sull'ernia, memorie anatomico-chirurgiche. Pavia Galleazzi, 1819.

1018. Schapp HM, Van De Pavoordt HDWM, Bast TJ. The preperitoneal approach in the repair of recurrent inguinal hernias. Surgery, Gynecology and Obstetrics 1992; 174: 460–464.

1019. Scheyer M, Arnold S, Zimmermann G. Minimally invasive operation techniques for inguinal hernia: spectrum of indications in Austria. Hernia 2001; 5: 73–79.

1020. Schier F. Laparoscopic surgery in inguinal hernias in children – initial experience. Journal of Pediatric Surgery 2000; 35: 1331–1335.

1021. Schier F, Danzer E, Bondartschuk M. Incidence of contralateral patent processus vaginalis in children with inguinal hernia. Journal of Pediatric Surgery 2001; 36: 1561–1563.

1022. Schilling JA. Advances in knowledge related to wounding, repair and healing: 1885–1984. Annals of Surgery 1985; 201: 268–277.

1023. Schmedt C-G, Däubler P, Leibl BJ, Kraft K, Bittner R. Simultaneous bilateral laparoscopic inguinal hernia repair. Surgical Endoscopy 2002; 16: 240–244.

1024. Schofield TL. Polyvinyl alcohol sponge: an inert plastic for use as a prosthesis in the repair of large hernias. British Journal of Surgery 1955; 42: 618–621.

1025. Schoots IG, van Dijkman D, Butzelaar RMJM, van Geldere D, Simons MP. Inguinal hernia repair in the Amsterdam region 1994–1996. Hernia 2001; 5: 3–40.

1026. Schultz L, Graber J, Pietraffita et al. Laser laparoscopic herniorraphy: a clinical trial. Preliminary results. Journal of Laparoendoscopic Surgery 1991; 1: 41–45.

1027. Schumpelick V, Ault G. The Aachen Classification of Inguinal Hernia. Problems in General Surgery 1995; 12: 57–58.

1028. Schumpelick V, Treutner KH, Arit G. Inguinal hernia repair in adults. Lancet 1994; 344: 375–379.

1029. Schurgers ML, Boelaert JRO, Daneels RF, Robbens EJ, Vandelanotte MM. Genital oedema in patients treated by continuous ambulatory peritoneal dialysis: an unusual presentation of inguinal hernia. British Medical Journal 1983; 388: 358–359.

1030. Scorer CG, Farrington GH. Congenital Deformities of the Testis and Epididymis. London: Butterworths, 1971.

1031. Scotte M, Majerus B, Sibert L, Teniere P. Incarceration vesicale dans une hernie de spiegel. Journal de Chirurgie (Paris) 1991; 128: 74–75.

1032. Scottish Health Service. Scottish in-patient statistics 1974. Edinburgh: Common Services Agency, Information Services Division, 1974.

1033. Schrenk P, Bettelheim P, Woisetschläger R, Reiger R, Wayand WU. Metabolic responses after laparoscopic or open hernia repair. Surgical Endoscopy 1996; 10: 628–632.

1034. Sculpher M, Drummond M, O'Brien B. Effectiveness, efficiency and NICE. British Medical Journal 2001; 322: 943–4.

1035. Sculpher M. Phase II Medical Laser Technology Assessment. HERG Research Report No 15, Brunel University, 1993.

1036. See WA, Cooper CS, Fisher RJ. Predictors of laparoscopic complications after formal training in laparoscopic surgery. Journal of the American Medical Association 1993; 270: 289–2692.

1037. Semmence A, Kynch J. Hernia repair and time off work in Oxford. Journal of the Royal College of General Practitioners 1980; 30: 90–96.

1038. Senapati, A. Spontaneous dehiscence of an incisional hernia. British Journal of Surgery 1982; 69: 313.

1039. Serpell JW, Jarrett PEM, Johnson CD. A prospective study of bilateral inguinal hernia repair. Annals of the Royal College of Surgeons of England 1990; 72: 299–303.

1040. Seymour DG, Garthwaite PH. Age deprivation and rates of inguinal hernia surgery in men. Age and Aging 1999; 28: 485–490.

1041. Shaw A, Santulli TV. Management of sliding hernias of the urinary bladder in infants. Surgery, Gynecology and Obstetrics 1967; 124: 1315–1316.

1042. Shearburn EW, Myers RN. Shouldice repair for inguinal hernia. Surgery 1969; 66: 450–459.

1043. Sheehan V. Spigelian hernia. Journal of the Irish Medical Association 1951; 29: 87–91.

1044. Shepherd JA. Acute appendicitis. A historical survey. Lancet 1954; ii: 299–302.

1045. Sherer DM, Dar P. Prenatal ultrasonographic diagnosis of congenital umbilical hernia and associated patent omphalomesenteric duct. Gynecologic and Obstetric Investigations 2001; 51: 61–68.

1046. Shouldice EE. Obesity and ventral hernia repair. Modern Medicine of Canada 1953; August: 89.

1047. Shouldice EE. The treatment of hernia. Ontario Medical Review 1953; 1–14.

1048. Shrock P. The processus vaginalis and gubernaculum. Their raison d'etre redefined. Surgical Clinics of North America 1971; 51: 1263–1268.

1049. Shulman A, Amid P. Which Lichtenstein method? Archives of Surgery 1994; 129: 561.

1050. Shulman AG, Amid PK, Lichtenstein IL. The 'plug' repair of 1402 recurrent inguinal hernias: 20-year experience. Archives of Surgery 1990; 125: 265–267.

1051. Shulman AG, Amid PK, Lichtenstein IL. The safety of mesh repair for primary inguinal hernias: results of 3019 operations from five diverse surgical sources. American Surgeon 1992; 58: 255–257.

1052. Shulman AG, Amid PK, Lichtenstein IL. Patch or plug for groin hernia – which? American Journal of Surgery 1994; 167: 331–336.

1053. Shulman AG, Amid PK, Lichtenstein IL. Returning to work after herniorrhaphy. British Medical Journal 1994; 309: 216–217.

1054. Silverman R. The use of AlloDerm in ventral hernia repair (rabbit model AlloDerm vs. Gore-Tex). (Submitted for publication).

1055. Simpson JG, Gunnlangsson GH, Dawson B, Lynn HB. Further experience with bilateral operations for inguinal hernia in infants and children. Annals of Surgery 1969; 169: 450.

1056. Simpson PI, Hughes DR, Long DH. Prolonged local analgesia for inguinal herniorrhaphy with bupivacaine and dextran. Annals of the Royal College of Surgeons of England 1982; 64: 243–246.

1057. Sinha SN, De Costa AE. Obturator hernia. Australian and New Zealand Surgery 1983; 53: 349–351.

1058. Sjodahl R, Anderberg B, Bolin T. Parastomal hernia in relation to the site of the abdominal wall stoma. British Journal of Surgery 1988; 75: 339–341.

1059. Skandalakis JE, Gray SW, Burns WB, Sangmalee U, Sorg JL. Internal and external supra-vesical hernia. American Surgeon 1976; 42: 142.

1060. Skandalakis LJ, Gadacz TR, Mansberger AR, Mitchell WE, Colborn GL, Skandalakis IE. Modern Hernia Repair. New York: Parthenon Publishing, 1996.

1061. Skandalakis PN, Skandalakis LJ, Gray SW, Skandalakis JE. Supra-vesical hernia. In: Nyhus LM, Condon RE, eds. Hernia, 4th edn. Philadelphia: Lippincott, 1995.

1062. Skidmore FD. Umbilical hernia in child swimmers. British Medical Journal 1979; 2: 494.

1063. Smedberg SGG. Herniography. In: Nyhus LM, Condon RE, eds. Hernia, 4th edn. Philadelphia: Lippincott, 1995.

1064. Smedberg S, Broome A, Elmer O, Gullmo A. Herniography in the diagnosis of obscure groin pain. Acta Chirurgica Scandinavica 1985; 151: 663–667.

1065. Smedberg SGG, Broome AEA, Gullmo A, Roos H. Herniography in athletes with groin pain. American Journal of Surgery 1985; 149: 378–382.

1066. Smith GD, Crosby DL, Lewis PA. Inguinal hernia and a single strenuous event. Annals of the Royal College of Surgeons of England 1996; 78: 367–368.

1067. Smith I. Irreducible inguinal herniae in children. British Journal of Surgery 1954; 42: 271–274.

1068. Smith MP, Sparkes RS. Familial inguinal hernia. Surgery 1965; 57: 807–812.

1069. Snyder WH. Paediatric Surgery, vol I. Chicago: Year Book, 1962: 573.

1070. Somell A, Ljungdahl L, Spangen L. Thigh neuralgia as a symptom of obturator hernia. Acta Chirurgica Scandinavica 1976; 142: 457–459.

1071. Song D, Greilich NB, White PF, Watcha MF, Tongier WK. Recovery profiles and costs of anesthesia for outpatient unilateral herniorrhaphy. Anesthesia and Analgesia 2000; 91: 876–881.

1072. Soper NJ, Brunt LM, Kerbl K. Laparoscopic general surgery. New England Journal of Medicine 1994; 330: 409–419.

1073. Spaeth JP, O'Hara IB, Kurth CD. Anesthesia for the micropremie. Semin Perinatol 1998; 22: 390–401.

1074. Spangen L. Spigelian hernia. Acta Chirurgica Scandinavica Suplementum 1976; 462: 1–47.

1075. Spangen L. Spigelian hernia. Surgical Clinics of North America 1984; 64: 351–366.

1076. Spangen L. Spigelian hernia. World Journal of Surgery 1989; 13: 573–580.

1077. Spangen L, Andersson R, Ohlsson L. Nonpalpable inguinal hernia in women. In: Nyhus LM, Condon RE, eds. Hernia, 3rd edn. Philadelphia: Lippincott, 1989.

1078. Sparkman RJ. Bilateral exploration of inguinal hernias in juvenile patients. Surgery 1962; 51: 393–402.

1079. Sparnon AL, Kiely EM, Spitz L. Incarcerated inguinal hernia in infants. British Medical Journal 1986; 293: 376–377.

1080. Spaw AT, Ennis BW, Spaw LP. Laparoscopic hernia repair: the anatomical basis. Journal of Laparoendoscopic Surgery 1991; 1: 269–277.

1081. Spiegel A. Opera Quae Extant Omnia. Amsterdam: John Bloew, 1645.

1082. Spittal MJ, Hunter SJ. A comparison of bupivacaine instillation and inguinal field block for control of pain after herniorrhaphy. Annals of the Royal College of Surgeons of England 1992; 74: 85–88.

1083. Stanton E, Mac D. Post-operative ventral hernia. New York Journal of Medicine 1916; 16: 511–515.

1084. Steele C. On operations for the radical cure of hernia. British Medical Journal 1874; 2: 584.

1085. Steigman CK, Sotelo-Avila C, Weber TR. The incidence of spermatic cord structures in inguinal hernia sacs from male children. American Journal of Surgical Pathology 1999; 23: 880–885.

1086. Steinke W, Zellweger R. Richter's hernia and Sir Frederick Treves: an original clinical experience, review, and historical overview. Annals of Surgery 2000; 232: 710–718.

1087. Stephens FC, Dudley HAF. An out-patient organisation for out-patient surgery. Lancet 1961; 1: 1042–1045.

1088. Stephenson BM, Phillips RKS. Para-stomal hernia: local resiting and mesh repair. British Journal of Surgery 1995; 82: 1395–1396.

1089. Sternhill B, Schwartz S. Effect of hypaque on mouse peritoneum. Radiology 1960; 75: 81–84.

1090. Steward DJ. Preterm infants are more prone to complications following minor surgery than are term infants. Anesthesiology 1982; 56(4): 304–306.

1091. Stirk DI. Strangulated inguino-femoral hernia with descent of the testis through the femoral canal. British Journal of Surgery 1955; 43: 331–332.

1092. Stirnemann H. Die Spigelische Hernie: Verpasst? Selten? Verlegenheitsdiagnose? Der Chirurg 1982; 53: 314.

1093. Stock FE. Faecal fistula and bilateral strangulated hernia in an infant. British Medical Journal 1951; 1: 171.

1094. Stoker DL, Spiegelhalter DJ, Singh R, Wellwood JM. Laparoscopic versus open inguinal hernia repair: Randomised prospective trial. Lancet 1994; 343: 1243–1245.

1095. Stoppa R. Reinforcement of the visceral sac by a preperitoneal bilateral mesh prosthesis in groin hernia repair. In: Bendavid R, ed. Abdominal Wall Hernias. London: Springer-Verlag, 2001; 428–436.

1096. Stoppa R, Wantz GE, Munegato G, Pluchinotta A. Hernia Healers: An Illustrated History. France: Arnette, 1998.

1097. Stoppa R, Wantz GE. Henri Fruchaud (1894–1960): a man of bravery, an anatomist, a surgeon. Hernia 1998; 2: 45–47.

1098. Stoppa R, Warlaumont CR, Verhaeghe PJ, Odimba BKFE, Henry X. Comment, pourquoi, quand utiliser les prostheses de tulle de Dacron pour traiter les hernies et les eventrations. Chirurgie 1982; 108: 570–575.

1099. Stoppa RE, Rives JL, Warlaumont CR, Palot JP, Verhaeghe PJ, Delattre JF. The use of Dacron in the repair of hernias of the groin. Surgical Clinics of North America 1984; 64: 269–285.

1100. Storling JR, Harms BA. The diagnosis and treatment of genito-femoral and ilio-inguinal neuralgia. World Journal of Surgery 1989; 13: 586–591.

1101. Stotter AT, Kapadia CR, Dudley HAF. Sutures in surgery. In: Russell RCG, ed. Recent Advances in Surgery. London: Churchill Livingstone, 1986.

1102. Strange SL. Spontaneous rupture of an umbilical hernia in an infant. Postgraduate Medical Journal 1956; 32: 39.

1103. Stromayr. Practica Copiosa – Lindau 1559. Cited by Rutkow IM. Surgery, An Illustrated History. Mosby: St Louis, 1993.

1104. Stuckej AL, Lutjko GD, Tivarovskij VI. Hernias of the spigeli line. Tsitologiia 1973; 15: 10–13.

1105. Sturdy DE. Incarcerated inguinal hernia in infancy with testicular gangrene. British Journal of Surgery 1960; 48: 210–211.

1106. Sugarbaker PH. Prosthetic mesh repair of large hernias at the site of colonic stomas. Surgical and Gynecological Obstetrics 1980; 150: 576–578.

1107. Sugarbaker PH. Peritoneal approach to prosthetic mesh repair of paraostomy hernias. Annals of Surgery 1985; 201(3): 344–346.

1108. Surana R, Puri P. Is contralateral exploration necessary in infants with unilateral inguinal hernia? Journal of Pediatric Surgery 1993; 28(8): 1027.

1109. Susmallian S, Gerwurtz G, Ezri T, Charuzi. Seroma after laparoscopic repair of hernia with ePTFE patch: is it really a complication? Hernia 2001; 5: 139–141.

1110. Syme G, Gibbon W. Groin pain in athletes. Lancet 1999; 353: 1444–1445.

1111. Szell K. Local anaesthesia and inginal hernia repair: a cautionary tale. Annals of the Royal College of Surgeons of England 1994; 76: 139–140.

1112. Tackett LD, Brewer CK, Luks FI et al. Incidence of contralateral inguinal hernia: a prospective analysis. Journal of Paediatric Surgery 1999; 34: 684–687.

1113. Tagart REB. The suturing of abdominal incisions. A comparison of monofilament nylon and catgut. British Journal of Surgery 1967; 54: 952–957.

1114. Tait L. A discussion on treatment of hernia by median abdominal section. British Medical Journal 1891; 2: 685–691.

1115. Tam PKH, Lister J. Femoral hernia in children. Archives of Surgery 1984; 119: 1161–1164.

1116. Tanner NC. A slide operation for inguinal and femoral hernia. British Journal of Surgery 1942; 29: 285–289.

1117. Tanyel FC, Dagdeviren A, Muftuoglu S, Gursoy MH, Yuruker S, Buyukpamukcu N. Inguinal hernia revisited through comparative evaluation of peritoneum, processus vaginalis and sacs obtained from children with hernia, hydrocele, and undescended testes. Journal of Paediatric Surgery 1999; 34: 552–555.

1118. Taube M, Porter RJ, Lord PH. A combination of subcuticular suture and sterile micropore tape compared with conventional interrupted sutures for skin closure. Annals of the Royal College of Surgeons of England 1983; 65: 164–166.

1119. Taylor EW, Dewar EP. Early return to work after repair of a unilateral inguinal hernia. British Journal of Surgery 1983; 70: 599–600.

1120. Tchupetlowsky S, Losanoff J, Kjossev K. Bilateral obturator hernia: a new technique and a new prosthetic material for repair-case report and review of the literature. Surgery 1995; 117: 109–112.

1121. Tepas JJ, Stafford PW. Timing of automatic contralateral groin exploration in male infants with unilateral hernias. American Journal of Surgery 1986; 52: 70–71.

1122. Thieme ET. Recurrent inguinal hernia. Archives of Surgery 1971; 103: 238–242.

1123. Thomas D. Strangulated femoral hernia. Medical Journal of Australia 1967; 1: 258–260.

1124. Thomas JM. Groin strain versus occult hernia: uncomfortable alternatives or incompatible rivals? Lancet 1995; 345: 1552–1553.

1125. Thomas WEG, Vowles KDL, Williamson RCN. Appendicitis in external herniae. Annals of the Royal College of Surgeons of England 1982; 64: 121–122.

1126. Thorndike A, Ferguson CF. Incarcerated inguinal hernia in infancy and childhood. American Journal of Surgery 1938; 39: 429–437.

1127. Tilson MD, Davis G. Deficiences of copper and a compound with iron exchange characteristics of pyridinoline in skin from patients with abdominal aortic aneurysms. Surgery 1983; 94: 134–141.

1128. Tingwald GR, Cooperman M. Inguinal and femoral hernia repair in geriatric patients. Surgery, Gynecology and Obstetrics 1982; 154: 704–706.

1129. Todd IP. Intestinal Stomas. London: Heinemann, 1978.

1130. Toms AP, Dixon AK, Murphy MP, Jamieson NV. Illustrated review of new imaging techniques in the diagnosis of abdominal wall hernias. British Journal of Surgery 1999; 86: 1243–1250.

1131. Ton JG. Tijdelijke prothesen bij het sluiten van geinfecteerde littekenbreuken. Nederlands Tijdschrift voor Geneeskunde 1967; 112: 972.

1132. Torzilli G, Carmana G, Lumachi V, Gnocchi P, Olivari N. The usefulness of ultrasonography in the diagnosis of the Spigelian hernia. International Surgery 1995; 80: 280.

1133. Torzilli G, Del Fabbro D, Felisi R, Leoni P, Gnocchi P, Lumachi V, Goglia P, Olivari N. Ultrasound-guided reduction of an incarcerated spigelian hernia. Ultrasound in Medicine and Biology 2001; 27(8): 1133–1135.

1134. Toy FK, Bailey RW, Carey S et al. Prospective, multicenter study of laparoscopic ventral hernioplasty. Surgical Endoscopy 1998; 12: 955–959.

1135. Toy FK, Smoot RT. Toy–Smoot laparoscopic hernioplasty. Surgical Laparoscopy and Endoscopy 1991; 1: 151–155.

1136. Toy FK, Smoot RT. Laparoscopic hernioplasty update. Surgical Laparoscopy and Endoscopy 1992; 2: 197–205.

1137. Trabucco EE. Sutureless inguinal mesh hernioplasty. Ospidale Italia Chirugia 2000; 6: 225–232.

1138. Trabucco EE, Trabucco AF. Flat plugs and mesh hernioplasty in the inguinal box: description of the surgical technique. Hernia 1998; 2: 133–138.

1139. Tran VK, Putz T, Rohde H. A randomized controlled trial for inguinal hernia repair to compare the Shouldice and the Bassini–Kirschner operation. International Surgery 1992; 77: 235–237.

1140. Treves F. Richter's hernia or partial enterocele. Medico-Chirurgical Transactions, London 1887; 52: 149–167.

1141. Trimbos JB. Factors relating to the volume of surgical knots. International Journal of Gynecology and Obstetrics 1989; 30: 355–359.

1142. Trotter C, Martin P, Youngson G, Johnston G. A comparison between ilioinguinal–iliohypogastric nerve block performed by anaesthetist or surgeon for postoperative analgesia following groin surgery in children. Paediatric Anaesthesia 1995; 5: 363–367.

1143. Truong SN, Pfingsten F, Dreuw B, Schumpelick V. Value of ultrasound in the diagnosis of undetermined findings in the abdominal wall and inguinal region. In: Schumpelick V, Wantz GE, eds. Inguinal Hernia. Basel: Karger, 1995; 29–41.

1144. Tsimoyiannis EC, Siakas P, Glantzounis G, Koulas S, Mavridou P, Gossios KI. Seroma in laparoscopic ventral hernioplasty. Surgical Laparoscopy, Endoscopy and Percutaneous Technique 2001; 11(5): 317–321.

1145. Tsimoyiannis EC, Tassis A, Glantzounis G, Jabarin M, Siakas P, Tzourou H. Laparoscopic intraperitoneal onlay mesh repair of incisional hernia. Surgical Laparoscopy and Endoscopy 1998; 8(5): 360–362.

1146. Tsutsui S, Kitamura M, Shirabe K, Yoshizawa S, Yoshida M. Radiographic diagnosis of obturator hernia. British Journal of Surgery 1994; 81: 1371–1372.

1147. Turnbull RB, Weakley FI. Atlas of Intestinal Stomas. St Louis: Mosby, 1967.

1148. Turnock RR. Preperitoneal approach to irreducible inguinal hernia in infants. British Journal of Surgery 1994; 81: 251.

1149. Ugahary F. The gridiron hernioplasty. In: Bendavid R, ed. Abdominal Wall Hernias. London: Springer-Verlag, 2001; 407–411.

1150. Ugahary F, Simmermacher R. Groin hernia repair via a grid-iron incision: an alternative technique for preperitoneal mesh insertion. Hernia 1998; 2: 123–125.

1151. Ugahary F. The gridiron hernioplasty. In: Bendavid R, ed. Abdominal Wall Hernias. London: Springer-Verlag, 2001; 408.

1152. Ulbak S, Ornsholt J. Para-inguinal hernia: an atypical spigelian variant. Acta Chirurgica Scandinavica 1983; 149: 335–336.

1153. Ulman I, Demircan M, Avanghu AA, Ergun O, Ozok G, Erdener A. Unilateral inguinal hernia in girls: is routine, contralateral exploration justified? Journal of Pediatric Surgery 1995; 30: 1684–1686.

1154. Underhill BML. Strangulated femoral hernia in an infant boy aged five weeks. British Journal of Surgery 1954; 42: 332–333.

1155. Usher FC. Further observations on the use of Marlex mesh. A new technique for the repair of inguinal hernias. American Surgeon 1959; 25: 792–795.

1156. Usher FC. Hernia repair with Marlex mesh. Archives of Surgery 1962; 84: 73–76.

1157. Usher FC. The repair of incisional and inguinal hernias. Surgery, Gynecology and Obstetrics 1970; 131: 525–530.

1158. Usher FC. New technique for repairing incisional hernias with Marlex mesh. American Journal of Surgery 1979; 138: 740–741.

1159. Valenti G, Capnano G, Testa A, Barletta N. Dynamic self regulating prosthesis (protesi autoregolantesi dinamica – PAD): a new technique in the treatment of inguinal hernias. Hernia 1999; 3: 5–9.

1160. van den Berg JC, de Valois JC, Go PMNYH, Rosenbusch G. Radiological anatomy of the groin region. European Radiology 2000; 10: 661–670.

1161. van den Berg JC, Strijk SP. Groin hernia: role of herniography. Radiology 1992; 184: 191–194.

1162. van der Hem JA, Hamming JF, Meeuwis JD, Oostvogel HJM. Totally extraperitoneal endoscopic repair of recurrent inguinal hernia. British Journal of Surgery 2001; 88: 884–886.

1163. Van Hee R, Goverde P, Hendrick L, Van der Schelling G, Totte E. Laparoscopic transperitoneal versus extraperitoneal inguinal hernia repair: a prospective clinical trial. Acta Chirurgica Belgica 1998; 98: 132–135.

1164. Van Meurs DPP. Strangulation of the ovary and fallopian tube in an obturator hernia. British Journal of Surgery 1945; 32: 539–540.

1165. Van Winkle W. The tensile strength of wounds and factors that influence it. Surgery, Gynecology and Obstetrics 1969; 129: 819–842.

1166. Van Winkle WJR, Hastings JC. Considerations in the choice of suture materials for various tissues. Surgery, Gynecology and Obstetrics 1972; 135: 113–126.

1167. Van Winkle W, Hastings JC, Barker E, Hines D, Nichols W. Effect of suture materials on healing wounds. Surgery, Gynecology and Obstetrics 1975; 140: 7–12.

1168. Vervest AM, Eeftinck Schattenkerk M, Rietberg M. Richter's femoral hernia: a clinical pitfall. Acta Chirurgica Belgica 1998; 98: 87–89.

1169. Vogt DM, Curet MJ, Pitcher DE, Martin DT, Zucker KA. Preliminary results of a prospective randomized trial of laparoscopic onlay versus conventional inguinal herniorrhaphy. American Journal of Surgery 1995; 169: 84–90.

1170. Vohr BR, Rosenfield AG, Oh W. Umbilical hernia in low birthweight infants (less than 1500 gm). Journal of Pediatrics 1977; 90: 807–808.

1171. Voitk A. Simple technique for laparoscopic paracolostomy hernia repair. Diseases of the Colon and Rectum 2000; 43: 1451–1453.

1172. Vowles KDJ. Intestinal complications of strangulated hernia. British Journal of Surgery 1959; 47: 189–192.

1173. Vrijland WW, Bonthuis F, Steyerberg EW, Marquet RL, Jeckel J, Bonjer HJ. Peritoneal adhesions to prosthetic materials. Surgical Endoscopy 2000; 14: 960–963.

1174. Waddington RT. Femoral hernia: a recent appraisal. British Journal of Surgery 1971; 58: 920–922.

1175. Wagh PV, Leverich AP, Sun CN, White JH, Read RC. Direct inguinal herniation in man: a disease of collagen. Journal of Surgical Research 1974; 17: 425–433.

1176. Wagman ID, Barnhart GR, Sugerman HJ. Recurrent midline hernial repair. Surgery, Gynecology and Obstetrics 1985; 161: 181–182.

1177. Wakeley CPG. Obturator hernia: its aetiology, incidence and treatment with two personal operative cases. British Journal of Surgery 1939; 26: 515–525.

1178. Wakeley CPG. Treatment of certain types of external herniae. Lancet 1940; 1: 822–826.

1179. Wakeley C, Childs P. Spigelian hernia: hernia through the linea semilunaris. Lancet 1951; 1: 1290–1291.

1180. Walters GAB. A retropubic operation for femoral herniae. British Journal of Surgery 1965; 52: 678–682.

1181. Walton JM, Bass JA. Spigelian hernia in infants: reports of two cases. Canadian Journal of Surgery 1995; 38: 95–96.

1182. Wantz GE. Suture tension in Shouldice's hernioplasty. Archives of Surgery 1981; 116: 1238–1239.

1183. Wantz GE. Testicular atrophy as a risk of inguinal hernioplasty. Surgery, Gynecology and Obstetrics 1982; 154: 570–571.

1184. Wantz GE. Complications of inguinal hernia repair. Surgical Clinics of North America 1984; 64: 287–298.

1185. Wantz GE. Giant prosthetic replacement of the visceral sac. Surgery, Gynecology and Obstetrics 1989; 169: 408–417.

1186. Wantz GE. The operation of Bassini as described by Attilio Catterina. Surgery, Gynecology and Obstetrics 1989; 168: 67–80.

1187. Wantz GE. Ambulatory hernia surgery. British Journal of Surgery 1989; 76: 1228–1229.

1188. Wantz GE. Atlas of Hernia Surgery. Raven Press, 1991.

1189. Wantz GE. Testicular atrophy and chronic residual neuralgia as risks of inguinal hernioplasty. Surgical Clinics of North America 1993; 73: 571–581.

1190. Wantz GE, Fischer E. Is high ligation of the indirect hernia sac essential in inguinal hernioplasty. Hernia 1998; 2: 131–132.

1191. Wara P, Sorensen K, Berg V. Proximal fecal diversion: review of ten years experience. Diseases of the Colon and Rectum 1981; 24: 114–119.

1192. Watkins KM. Appendix abscess in a femoral hernia sac. Postgraduate Medical Journal 1981; 57: 306–307.

1193. Watkins RM, Leach RD, Ellis H. Bilateral obturator herniae and associated femoral hernia. Postgraduate Medical Journal 1981; 57: 466.

1194. Watson LF. Hernia: Anatomy, Etiology, Symptoms, Diagnosis, Differential Diagnosis, Prognosis, and the Operative and Injection Treatment, 2nd edn. London: Harry Kimpton, 1938.

1195. Webster TR, Tracy TF. Groin hernias and hydroceles. In: Paediatric Surgery, 2nd edn. Ashcraft KW, Holder TM, eds. Philadelphia: WB Saunders, 1993: 562–570.

1196. Wechsler R, Kurtz AB, Needleman L. Pictorial essay: cross-sectional imaging of abdominal wall hernias. American Journal of Roentgenology 1989; 153: 517–521.

1197. Weimer BR. Congenital inheritance of inguinal hernia. Journal of Heredity 1949; 40: 219–220.

1198. Weiner ES, Touloukian RJ, Rodgers BM et al. Hernia survey of the section on surgery of the American Academy of Pediatrics. Journal of Pediatric Surgery 1996; 31(8): 1166–1169.

1199. Weiss U, Lernau OZ, Nissan S. Spigelian hernia. Annals of Surgery 1974; 180: 836–839.

1200. Wells CA. Hernia – incisional and umbilical. Annals of the Royal College of Surgeons of England 1956; 19: 316–318.

1201. Wellwood J, Sculpher MJ, Stoker D, Nicholls GJ, Geddes C, Whitehead A, Singh R, Spieghalter D. Randomized controlled trial of laparoscopic versus open mesh repair for hernia: outcome and cost. British Medical Journal 1998; 317: 103–110.

1202. Welsh DRJ. Sliding inguinal hernias. Journal of Abdominal Surgery 1964; 6.

1203. Welsh DRJ. The Shouldice inguinal repair. Problems in General Surgery 1995; 12: 93–100.

1204. Welty G, Klinge U, Klosterhalfen B, Kasperk R, Schumpelick V. Functional impairment and complaints following incisional hernia repair with different polypropylene meshes. Hernia 2001; 5: 12–147.

1205. West LS. Two pedigrees showing inherited predisposition to hernia. Journal of Heredity 1936; 27: 449–455.

1206. Wheatley RG, Samaan AK. Postoperative pain relief. British Journal of Surgery 1995; 82: 292–295.

1207. Wheeler MH. Femoral hernia: analysis of the results of surgical treatment. Proceedings of the Royal Society of Medicine 1975; 68: 177–178.

1208. Whipple AO. The use of silk in the repair of clean wounds. Annals of Surgery 1933; 98: 662–671.

1209. White HJ, Sun CN, Read RC. Inguinal hernia: a true collagen disease. Laboratory Investigations 1977; 36: 359.

1210. Wijesinha SS. Inguinal hernia – the local experience. Sri Lanka Journal of Surgery 1991; 7: 7–9.

1211. Williams BT, Nicholl JP, Thomas KJ, Knowlenden J. Differences in duration of stay for surgery in the N.H.S. and private hospitals in England and Wales. British Medical Journal 1985; 290: 978–980.

1212. Williams DI. Urology in childhood. In: Encyclopaedia of Urology. New York, 1974.

1213. Williams JG, Etherington R, Hayward MWJ, Hughes LE. Para-ileostomy hernia: a clinical and radiological study. British Journal of Surgery 77: 1355–1357.

1214. Williams M, Frankel S, Nanchalal K, Coast J, Donovan J. Hernia Repair: Epidemiologically Based Needs Assessment. Health Care Evaluation Unit, University of Bristol Print Services, 1992.

1215. Williams-Russo P, Sharrock NE, Nattis S, Szatrowski TP. Cognitive effects after epidural vs general anaesthesia in older patients: a randomized trial. Journal of the American Medical Association 1995; 274: 44–50.

1216. Willis B, Kim LT, Anthony T, Bergen PC, Nwariaku F, Turnage RH. A clinical pathway for inguinal hernia repair reduces hospital admissions. Journal of Surgical Research 2000; 88: 13–17.

1217. Winslet MC, Obeid ML, Kumar V. On-table pneumoperitoneum in the management of complicated incisional hernias. Annals of the Royal College of Surgeons of England 1993; 75: 186–188.

1218. Witherington R. Cryptorchism and approaches to its surgical management. Surgical Clinics of North America 1984; 64: 367–384.

1219. Wobbes T. Chrassords-Koops H, Oldhoff J. Relationship between testicular tumours, undescended testicles and inguinal hernias. Journal of Surgical Oncology 1980; 14: 45–51.

1220. Wolfler A. Zur Radikaloperation des freien Leistenbruches. In: Beitr. Chir. (Festschr. Gewidmet Theodor Billroth). Stuttgart: Hoffman, 1892: 552–603.

1221. Wood J. On rupture, inguinal, crural and umbilical. London: JW Davies, 1863.

1222. Woods GE. Some observations on umbilical hernias in infants. Archives of Disease in Childhood 1953; 28: 450–462.

1223. Wright D, Paterson C, Scott N, Hair A, Grant A, O'Dwyer PJ. Five-year follow up of patients undergoing laparoscopic or open groin hernia repair – a randomized controlled trial. Annals of Surgery 2002; 235: 333–337.

1224. Wulkan ML, Wiener ES, Van Balen N, Vescio P. Laparoscopy through the open ipsilateral sac to evaluate presence of contralateral hernia. Journal of Pediatric Surgery 1996; 31: 1174–1177.

1225. Wysocki A, Pozniczek M, Krzywon J, Bolt L. Use of polypropylene prostheses for strangulated inguinal and incisional hernias. Hernia 2001; 5: 105–106.

1226. Yavetz H, Harash B, Yogev L, Hamomnai ZT, Paz G. Fertility of men following inguinal hernia repair. Andrologia 1991; 23: 443–446.

1227. Yeates WK. Pain in the scrotum. British Journal of Hospital Medicine 1985; 133: 101–104.

1228. Yeh H-C, Lehr-Janus C, Cohen BA, Rabinowitz JG. Ultrasonography and CT scanning of abdominal and inguinal hernias. Journal of Clinical Ultrasound 1984; 12: 479.

1229. Yip AWC, Ah Chong AK, Lam KH. Obturator hernia: A continuing diagnostic challenge. Surgery 1993; 113: 266–269.

1230. Yokoyama T, Munakata Y, Ogiwara M, Kamijima T, Kitamura H, Kawasaki S. Preoperative diagnosis of strangulated obturator hernia using ultrasonography. American Journal of Surgery 1997; 174: 76–78.

1231. Yokoyama Y, Yamaguchi A *et al.* Thirty-six cases of obturator hernia: does computed tomography contribute to postoperative outcome? World Journal of Surgery 1999; 23: 214–217.

1232. Yordanov YS, Stoyanov SK. The incidence of hernia on the Island of Pemba. East African Medical Journal 1969; 46: 687–691.

1233. Young D. Repair of epigastric incisional hernia. British Journal of Surgery 1961; 48: 514–516.

1234. Yuen JS, Chow PK, Koong HN, Ho JM, Girija R. Unusual sites (thorax and umbilical hernial sacs) of endometrosis. Journal of the Royal College of Surgeons of Edinburgh 2001; 46: 313–315.

1235. Zaman K, Taylor JD, Fossard DP. Femoral hernia in children. Annals of the Royal College of Surgeons of England 1985; 67: 249–250.

1236. Zhang GQ, Sugiyama M, Hagi H, Urata T, Shimamori N, Atomi Y. Groin hernias in adults: value of color Doppler sonography in their classification. Journal of Clinical Ultrasound 2001; 29: 429–434.

1237. Zimmerman LM, Anson BJ, Morgan EH, McVay CB. Ventral hernia due to normal banding of the abdominal muscles. Surgery, Gynecology and Obstetrics 1944; 78: 535–540.

1238. Zimmerman LM, Anson BJ. Anatomy and Surgery of Hernia, 2nd edn. Baltimore: Williams and Wilkins, 1967: 216–227.

1239. Zimmerman LM, Laufman H. Sliding hernia. Surgery, Gynecology and Obstetrics 1942; 75: 76–78.

1240. Zinanovic S. The anatomical basis for the high frequency of inguinal and femoral hernia in Uganda. East African Medical Journal 1968; 45: 41–46.

1241. Zollinger RM. A unified classification for inguinal hernias. Hernia 1999; 4: 195–2000.

1242. Zuckerkandl M. Hernia inflammata in Folge Typhilitis des Wurmfortsatzes in einem Leistenbruche. Wiener Klinische Wochenschrift 1891; 4: 305.

Index